BIOMEDICAL
ULTRASONICS

MEDICAL PHYSICS SERIES

BIOMEDICAL ULTRASONICS

P. N. T. Wells

Department of Medical Physics,
Bristol General Hospital, Bristol, England

1977

Academic Press

London · New York · San Francisco

A Subsidiary of Harcourt Brace Jovanovich, Publishers

ACADEMIC PRESS INC. (LONDON) LTD
24–28 Oval Road
London NW1 7DX

U.S. Edition published by
ACADEMIC PRESS INC.
111 Fifth Avenue
New York, New York 10003

Library of Congress Catalog Number: 77–071842
ISBN: 0–12–742940–9

Printed in Great Britain by
Adlard & Son Ltd., Bartholomew Press, Dorking, Surrey

PREFACE

The importance of biomedical ultrasonics has increased greatly during the six years which I have spent working on this book. The impact which ultrasonic methods now have on health care exceeds all early expectation. As an academic pursuit, the study of biomedical ultrasonics has attracted many accomplished scientists. I have the privilege of being acquainted with many of the doctors, physicists, biologists and engineers whose work I have tried to describe. I hope that *Biomedical Ultrasonics* will contribute to the development of the subject by serving as the primary source of reference for everyone interested in the basic principles and applications of ultrasonic energy in medicine and biology.

February 1977   P. N. T. WELLS

ACKNOWLEDGEMENTS

Many people contributed, wittingly or unwittingly, to the preparation of *Biomedical Ultrasonics*. Amongst those to whom I am especially grateful are Jim Aller, Peter Atkinson, Tom Brown, Maurice Bullen, Geoffrey Dawes, Gilbert Devey, Ian Donald, Ken Evans, John Fleming, Douglas Follett, Özgen Feizi, Herbert Freundlich, Ed Guibarra, Angus Hall, Michael Halliwell, Kit Hill, David Hughes, Jack Angell James, Ciaran McCarthy, Ken McCarty, Steve Morris, Dick Mountford, Robin Poore, Alan Read, Jack Reid, Frank Ross, Bob Skidmore, Shelley Stuart, Annette Campbell White, Denis White and John Woodcock. Anne Davies, Lily Davies, Rosemary Cardwell and Josephine Reynolds skilfully typed the manuscript. It is a pleasure to acknowledge both the help and the courtesy of the staff of Academic Press, who have worked hard and patiently to publish this book.

CONTENTS

To my family and friends

1. WAVE FUNDAMENTALS*

1.1 SIMPLE HARMONIC MOTION

Consider the situation represented in Fig. 1.1. A particle of mass m is supported on a surface free from friction, and attached to a weightless spring of compliance ζ. If the particle is displaced from its equilibrium position, a restoring force F acts on the particle, given by, according to Hooke's law:

$$F = -u/\zeta \tag{1.1}$$

where u is the displacement amplitude. The restoring force acts on the particle in such a direction as to return it to its equilibrium position. The magnitude of this force is proportional to the amplitude of the displacement (i.e. the distance between the position of the particle and its equilibrium position). This *direct proportionality* is the feature of simple harmonic motion which distinguishes it from other, more complicated vibrations.

In simple harmonic motion there is always an equilibrium situation at which the oscillating system could remain at rest. Although the oscillations dealt with in this Section are of the mechanical type, analogous oscillations occur in electrical circuits (see Appendix 1).

Applying Newton's second law of motion to Eqn. 1.1:

$$-u/\zeta = ma = m\frac{d^2u}{dt^2} \tag{1.2}$$

where a is the acceleration of the particle at time t. Equation 1.2 may be rearranged thus:

$$\frac{d^2u}{dt^2} + \frac{1}{\zeta m}u = 0 \tag{1.3}$$

The dimensions of $1/\zeta\, m$ are $[T^{-2}]$. In a vibrating system, the particle completes one cycle of oscillation in a period τ, which has dimensions $[T]$; the frequency, f (i.e. the number of cycles in unit time) $= 1/\tau$. The dimen-

* Generally the results presented in this Chapter are derived from first principles. Where results are quoted without derivation or reference to other works, a published text on acoustics may be consulted. These texts include those of Blitz (1963), Gooberman (1968), Hueter and Bolt (1955) and Kinsler and Frey (1962).

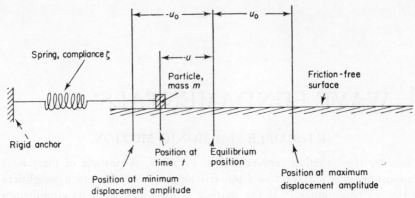

FIG. 1.1 Spring-particle system in simple harmonic motion.

sions of $1/\zeta m$ are therefore the same as those of f^2. Hence, Eqn. 1.3 may be rewritten:

$$\frac{d^2u}{dt^2} + (bf)^2 u = 0 \qquad (1.4)$$

where $(bf)^2 = 1/\zeta m$, b being a constant, and f being the frequency at which the particle oscillates. There are two possible solutions to Eqn. 1.4: these are:

$$u = A \cos bft = A \cos \omega t \qquad (1.5)$$

and

$$u = B \sin bft = B \sin \omega t \qquad (1.6)$$

These solutions satisfy Eqn. 1.4 because, from Eqn. 1.5;

$$\frac{d^2u}{dt^2} = -A\omega^2 \cos \omega t$$

and, from Eqn. 1.6;

$$\frac{d^2u}{dt^2} = -B\omega^2 \sin \omega t$$

where A and B are constants with the same dimensions as u, and $\omega = bf = 2\pi f$, where ω is defined as the angular frequency of the system.

The general solution to Eqn. 1.4 is given by superposition of the values of u in Eqns. 1.5 and 1.6:

$$u = A \cos \omega t + B \sin \omega t \qquad (1.7)$$

Equation 1.7 becomes, if A is rewritten as $u_0 \sin \phi$, and B, as $-u_0 \cos \phi$, where $u_0 = (A^2 + B^2)^{1/2}$, and ϕ is a constant:

$$u = u_0 \sin \phi \cos \omega t - u_0 \cos \phi \sin \omega t$$
$$= u_0 \sin (\omega t - \phi) \qquad (1.8)$$

Expressed in words, Eqn. 1.8 means that the displacement amplitude u of a particle in simple harmonic motion from its equilibrium position is equal, at any time t, to the product of its peak displacement amplitude u_0, and the sine of a time-varying angle $(\omega t - \phi)$ in which ω is the angular frequency $2\pi f$ of the oscillation of the particle, and ϕ is the phase angle; ϕ defines the position in the cycle of oscillation at $t = 0$.

Velocity is equal to rate of change of position. Hence the particle velocity may be found by differentiating Eqn. 1.8:

$$v = \frac{du}{dt} = u_0\omega \cos{(\omega t - \phi)} \qquad (1.9)$$

Similarly, particle acceleration may be found by differentiating Eqn. 1.9;

$$a = \frac{dv}{dt} = -u_0\omega^2 \sin{(\omega t - \phi)} \qquad (1.10)$$

The significance of the negative sign in Eqn. 1.10 is that the particle is decelerating as it moves away from its equilibrium position.

In this simple analysis, it has been assumed that the total energy stored in the oscillating system remains constant. (The effect of energy dissipation in such a system is discussed in Section 1.4.) The energy is stored entirely in the kinetic energy of the particle when the spring is not stressed (i.e. when $u = 0$); likewise, the energy is stored entirely in the potential energy of the spring when the displacement of the particle is maximum or minimum (i.e. when $v = 0$). At other times during the cycle, the energy is shared between the kinetic and potential stores. At any time t,

potential energy stored in spring

$$= \int_0^u u/\zeta \, du = u^2/2\zeta \qquad (1.11)$$

kinetic energy stored in mass

$$= mv^2/2 \qquad (1.12)$$

total energy stored in spring and mass

$$= u_0^2/2\zeta = m(u_0\omega)^2/2 = e \qquad (1.13)$$

1.2 THE WAVE EQUATION

A wave is a disturbance, the position of which in space changes with time.

1.2.a Transverse Waves

For example, consider a long thin string (which is really a chain of particles), fixed at one end. The other end is attached to a vibrator, so that it moves with simple harmonic motion along a line perpendicular to the undisturbed position of the string. The vibrations move along the string: in this way, energy is transmitted at a finite velocity. This type of vibration is called a *travelling wave*. The situation is illustrated in Fig. 1.2. Figure 1.2(a) represents the variation in displacement in space (where z is the distance) at any instant in time t. The *wavelength*, λ, is the z-distance between consecutive particles where the displacement amplitudes are identical. Figure 1.2(b) represents the variation in displacement in time at any particular position in space z. The *period*, τ, is the time which is required for the wave to move forward a distance λ. During the time τ, the wave completes one cycle of oscillation. The *frequency*, f, of the wave is equal to the number of cycles which pass through a given point in space in unit time. Thus:

$$f = 1/\tau \qquad (1.14)$$

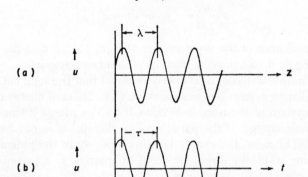

FIG. 1.2 Transverse waves on a string. (a) Distribution in space at time t; (b) distribution in time at position z.

The *velocity*, c, of the wave is equal to the distance travelled by the disturbance in unit time; thus:

$$c = f\lambda = \lambda/\tau \qquad (1.15)$$

The kind of wave which occurs on a string is called a *transverse wave*, because the particles oscillate in a direction normal to the direction in which the wave travels.

Next, consider the displacement of a very short section of the string, as illustrated in Fig. 1.3. The section is under constant tension ψ, and has a length δl given by

$$\delta l^2 = \delta z^2 + \delta u^2$$

hence

$$\delta l = \left\{ 1 + \left(\frac{\delta u}{\delta z} \right)^2 \right\}^{1/2} \delta z$$

and if $\delta u/\delta z$ is very small, $\delta l = \delta z$. The force acting in the u-direction on the element of string is equal to $\psi\{\sin(\theta + \delta\theta) - \sin\theta\}$; and, if θ is very small, $\sin\theta = \tan\theta = (\delta u/\delta z)_z$, where the subscript indicates the point at which the corresponding gradient is evaluated. Hence, the force is equal to

$$\psi\left\{\left(\frac{\partial u}{dz}\right)_{z+\delta z} - \left(\frac{\partial u}{dz}\right)_z\right\} \xrightarrow[\lim \delta z = 0]{} \psi\frac{\partial^2 u}{\partial z^2}\delta z$$

because the difference between the two terms in the bracket on the left-hand side of the expansion defines the differential coefficient of the gradient $\partial u/\partial z$ times the space interval δz.

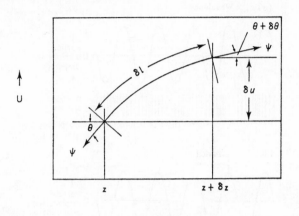

FIG. 1.3 An element of a string supporting a transverse wave.

If η is the mass per unit length of the string, then, according to Newton's second law of motion:

$$\psi\frac{\partial^2 u}{\partial z^2}\delta z = \eta\delta z\frac{\partial^2 u}{\partial t^2}$$

and hence

$$\frac{d^2 u}{\partial z^2} = \frac{1}{c^2}\frac{\partial^2 u}{\partial t^2} \tag{1.16}$$

where $c = (\psi/\eta)^{1/2}$, which has dimensions $[LT^{-1}]$ and is a velocity. Equation 1.16 is a *wave equation*. It relates the second differential of the participle displacement with respect to distance, to the acceleration of a simple harmonic oscillator. The significance of this is discussed in Section 1.3.

1.2.b Longitudinal Waves

Equation 1.16 was derived for transverse waves. Another *wave mode* occurs when the particles* in a medium supporting a wave oscillate backwards and forwards in the same direction as that in which the wave is travelling. This is called a *longitudinal wave*. The oscillation of the particles sets up periodic variations in pressure within the supporting medium and a pressure wave travels through the medium as neighbouring particles interact with each other, as illustrated in Fig. 1.4. Consider an unlimited liquid within which a plane is subjected to simple harmonic motion. (Non-viscous fluids cannot support shear stress, and so transverse waves cannot be generated.) The situation is illustrated in Fig. 1.5, which shows a small element of the liquid. In Fig. 1.5(a) the element is in equilibrium: it has

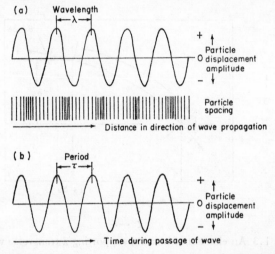

FIG. 1.4 Longitudinal waves in an extensive medium. (a) Particle displacement amplitude and particle spacing at time t: these are the distributions in space; (b) particle displacement amplitude at position z: this is the distribution in time.

length δz, cross-sectional area S, and density ρ. Figure 1.5(b) shows the element when subjected to longitudinal forces in simple harmonic motion: the out-of-balance of the forces on the opposite surfaces of the element is represented by a force δF on the right-hand surface. This force produces a displacement of $u + \delta u$ in the z-position of the right-hand surface. There is a gradient of force across the element; this is approximately linear because the element is small, and it is equal to $\partial F/\delta z$. Therefore,

$$\delta F = \frac{\partial F}{\partial z} \delta z \qquad (1.17)$$

*In this context, a *particle* is a volume element which is large enough to contain many millions of molecules, so that it is continuous with its surroundings; but it is so small that quantities variable within the medium (such as displacement amplitude) are constant within the particle.

According to Hooke's law,

$$F = KS \frac{\partial u}{\partial z} \qquad (1.18)$$

where K is the bulk modulus of the liquid; so that

$$\frac{\partial F}{\partial z} = KS \frac{\partial^2 u}{\partial z^2} \qquad (1.19)$$

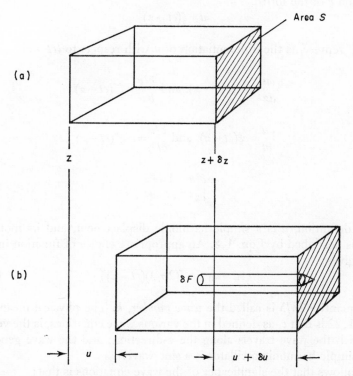

FIG. 1.5 An element of a medium. (a) In equilibrium; (b) in simple harmonic motion.

The mass of the element is $\rho S \delta z$ and its acceleration is given, to a close approximation, by $\partial^2 u / \partial t^2$. According to Newton's second law of motion, and substituting from Eqn. 1.19 in Eqn. 1.17,

$$KS \frac{\partial^2 u}{\partial z^2} \delta z = \rho S \delta z \frac{\partial^2 u}{\partial t^2}$$

and hence

$$\frac{\partial^2 u}{\partial z^2} = \frac{1}{c^2} \frac{\partial^2 u}{\partial t^2} \qquad (1.20)$$

where $c = (K/\rho)^{1/2}$. Equation 1.20 is the wave equation for longitudinal waves; it is identical in form to the Eqn. 1.16 which is the wave equation for transverse waves. Its significance is discussed in Section 1.3.

1.3 SOLUTION OF THE WAVE EQUATION

The wave equation, as expressed in Eqns. 1.16 and 1.20, is satisfied by a function ξ of the form

$$u = \xi(ct - z) \tag{1.21}$$

If ξ' represents the differentiation of u with respect to $(ct - z)$,

$$\frac{\partial u}{dz} = -\xi'(ct - z), \text{ and } \frac{\partial^2 u}{\partial z^2} = \xi''(ct - z)$$

also

$$\frac{\partial u}{\partial t} = c\xi(ct - z), \text{ and } \frac{\partial^2 u}{\delta t^2;} = c^2 \xi''(ct - z)$$

hence

$$\frac{\partial^2 u}{\partial z^2} = \frac{1}{c^2} \frac{\partial^2 u}{\partial t^2}$$

By definition, u is a simple harmonic displacement, and its motion at $z = 0$ is described by Eqn. 1.8. An appropriate choice of function in Eqn. 1.21 gives:

$$u = u_0 \sin \{(2\pi/\lambda)(ct - z)\} \tag{1.22}$$

The quantity $2\pi/\lambda$ is called the *wave number*, k. The physical meaning of Eqn. 1.22 is that c, as defined in the various wave equations, is the velocity at which the wave travels along the z-direction; and the wave generated by a simple harmonic oscillator is a sine wave.

It follows that the significance of the wave equations is that:

Eqn. 1.16: transverse waves travel along a string at a velocity

$$c = (\psi/\eta)^{1/2} \tag{1.23}$$

Eqn. 1.20: longitudinal waves travel in a medium at a velocity

$$c = (K/\rho)^{1/2} \tag{1.24}$$

Some typical values of longitudinal wave velocity in non-biological materials are given in Table 1.1. The variation with temperature of the velocity in water is shown in Fig. 1.6.

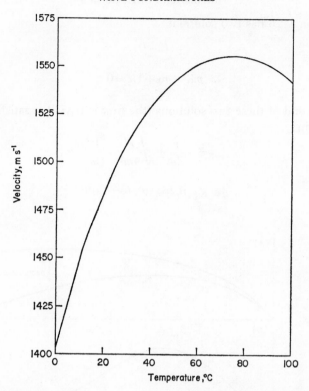

FIG. 1.6 Variation of propagation velocity with temperature in water. (Data of Grosso and Mader, 1972.)

1.4 DAMPED SIMPLE HARMONIC MOTION

In the lossless system discussed in Section 1.1, the peak displacement u_0 of the particle is constant. However, in practice such an ideal system cannot be realised, and energy is dissipated by processes such as friction, or imperfect elasticity. This results in an additional force, which is generally proportional to the velocity of the particle, so that Eqn. 1.3 must be modified thus:

$$\frac{d^2u}{dt^2}m + \frac{du}{dt}r + \frac{1}{\zeta}u = 0. \qquad (1.25)$$

where r is a constant with the dimensions of force per unit velocity.

Equation 1.25 can be solved by putting $u = Ke^{\alpha t}$; it follows that $du/dt = \alpha Ke^{\alpha t}$, and $d^2u/dt^2 = \alpha^2 Ke^{\alpha t}$. Hence:

$$Ke^{\alpha t}(m\alpha^2 + r\alpha + 1/\zeta) = 0 \qquad (1.26)$$

Equation 1.26 has two solutions:

$$K = 0$$

and

$$m\alpha^2 + r\alpha + 1/\zeta = 0$$

The second of these two solutions (the first is trivial) is satisfied by the relationship:

$$\alpha = -\frac{r}{2m} \pm \sqrt{\frac{r^2}{4m^2} - \frac{1}{\zeta m}}$$

and hence:

$$u = Ke^{-rt/2m}e^{\pm(r^2/4m^2 - 1/\zeta)^{\frac{1}{2}}t} \tag{1.27}$$

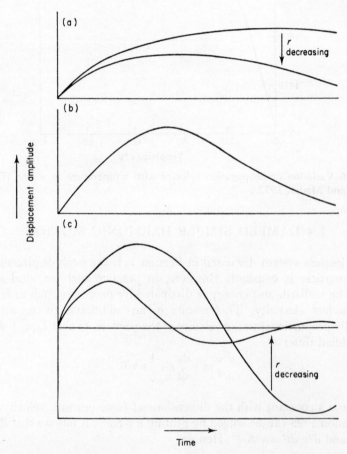

FIG. 1.7 Damped simple harmonic motion. (a) Heavy damping; (b) critical damping; (c) oscillatory damping.

The variation of u with t, described by Eqn. 1.27, can satisfy any one of three conditions illustrated in Fig. 1.7. The condition which applies in any particular situation is determined by the value of $(r^2/4m^2 - 1/\zeta m)$, which may be positive, zero, or negative.

(i) $(r^2/4m^2 > 1/\zeta m)$. The condition represents *heavy damping*; when such a system is disturbed from equilibrium by a sudden impulse. it returns slowly to equilibrium, without oscillation (i.e. the displacement never becomes negative).

(ii) $(r^2/4m^2 = 1/\zeta m)$. This condition represents *critical damping*; following a disturbance from equilibrium by the application of a sudden impulse, the system returns to equilibrium in the minimum time which is possible without oscillation.

(iii) $(r^2/4m^2 < 1/\zeta m)$. This condition represents *oscillatory damped simple harmonic motion*; following a disturbance from equilibrium by the application of a sudden impulse, the system oscillates, the displacement alternating between steadily decreasing positive and negative values. In this condition, $(r^2/4m^2 - 1/\zeta m)^{1/2}$ is imaginary, and the following relationship applies:

$$\left(\frac{r^2}{4m^2} - \frac{1}{\zeta m}\right)^{1/2} = (-1)^{1/2}\left(\frac{1}{\zeta m} - \frac{r^2}{4m^2}\right)^{1/2} = j\left(\frac{1}{\zeta m} - \frac{r^2}{4m^2}\right)^{1/2},$$

where $j = (-1)^{1/2}$. Substitution in Eqn. 1.27 gives:

$$u = Ke^{-rt/2m}e^{\pm j(1/\zeta m - r^2/4m^2)^{\frac{1}{2}}t} \qquad (1.28)$$

In Eqn. 1.28, the quantity $(1/\zeta m - r^2/4m^2)^{1/2}$ has the dimensions $[T^{-1}]$, and may be set equal to ω'. Thus

$$u = e^{-rt/2m}(K_1 e^{j\omega't} + K_2 e^{-j\omega't}) \qquad (1.29)$$

Now, $e^{jx} = j\cos x - \sin x$: by setting $K_1 = (U/2j)e^{j\phi}$, and $K_2 = -K_1$, where U and ϕ define the conditions at $t = 0$, Eqn. 1.29 becomes:

$$u = Ue^{-rt/2m}\sin(\omega't + \phi), \qquad (1.30)$$

so that $u = U\sin\phi$ when $t = 0$.

Equation 1.30 is of the same form as Eqn. 1.8, but modified by the term $(e^{-rt/2m})$, which determines the decay of u with time; u varies sinusoidally with time, but has an angular frequency ω' equal to $(1/\zeta m - r^2/4m^2)^{1/2}$.

In so far as the wave radiated into a medium by an oscillating source replicates the movement of the source, a wavetrain decaying in amplitude with time is radiated by an oscillator in damped simple harmonic motion.

1.5 RELATIONSHIPS OF THE WAVE PARAMETERS

The solution of the wave equation yields the following result:

$$u = u_0 \sin (\omega t - \phi) \qquad (1.31)$$

from Eqn. 1.22, putting $\omega = 2\pi f$, and $\phi = kz$, where $k = 2\pi/\lambda$. Equation 1.31 is identical to Eqn. 1.8. Hence, the wave radiated by a source in simple harmonic motion (or any other form of motion) replicates the movement of the source. The wave travels away from the source at a velocity given, for longitudinal waves, by

$$c = (K/\rho)^{1/2} \qquad (1.24)$$

The particle velocity v, and the particle acceleration a, may be derived using the procedures by which Eqns. 1.9 and 1.10 were obtained; thus:

$$v = u_0 \omega \cos (\omega t - \phi) \qquad (1.32)$$

and

$$a = -u_0 \omega^2 \sin (\omega t - \phi) \qquad (1.33)$$

Also, it has already been shown that

$$f = 1/\tau \qquad (1.14)$$

and

$$c = f\lambda = \lambda/\tau \qquad (1.15)$$

It now remains to derive the particle pressure p for longitudinal waves. During the course of the derivation of the wave equation, it is shown that

$$F = KS \frac{\partial u}{\partial z} \qquad (1.18)$$

The quantity $(-\partial u/\partial z)$ represents the mechanical strain applied to the medium, for cross-sectional area $S = 1$. If p is the particle pressure which causes this strain,

$$p = -K \frac{\partial u}{\partial z}$$

But, from Eqn. 1.24, $K = \rho c^2$; and hence

$$p = -\rho c^2 \frac{\partial u}{\partial z} \qquad (1.34)$$

Now,

$$u = u_0 \sin \{(2\pi/\lambda)(ct - z)\} \qquad (1.22)$$

so that

$$\frac{\partial u}{\partial z} = -u_0(2\pi/\lambda) \cos \{(2\pi/\lambda)(ct-z)\}$$

$$= -\frac{1}{c}.u_0\omega \cos (\omega t-\phi)$$

and, substituting from Eqn. 1.32,

$$\frac{\partial u}{\partial z} = -\frac{1}{c}.v$$

Substituting this value in Eqn. 1.34 gives

$$p = \rho c v \qquad (1.35)$$

Some typical values of wave parameters in water are given in Table 1.2.

1.6 CHARACTERISTIC IMPEDANCE

The relationship between pressure, velocity, and the quantity ρc, as described by Eqn. 1.35, is analogous to that which exists in electricity between voltage, current and impedance, as described by Ohm's law. For this reason, the quantity ρc is known as the characteristic impedance Z of the medium. Like electrical impedance, characteristic impedance may be a complex quantity. Thus:

$$Z = p/v = R + \mathcal{J}X \qquad (1.36)$$

where R and X are respectively the resistive and reactive components of Z. In the case of plane waves in a non-absorbent medium, $p/v = \rho c = Z$, and the medium behaves as a pure resistance. Some typical values for non-biological materials are given in Table 1.1.

1.7 INTENSITY

The total energy e of a particle oscillating with simple harmonic motion is equal to the sum of its potential and kinetic energies. In a lossless system, e does not vary with time; from Eqns. 1.9 and 1.13,

$$e = mv_0^2/2$$

The total mass of particles per unit volume is equal to the mean density ρ of the medium. The corresponding total energy E of all the particles in unit volume is the energy density. Hence

$$E = \rho v_0^2/2 \qquad (1.37)$$

TABLE 1.1

Properties of some non-biological materials

Material	Density, ρ [kg m^{-3}]	Velocity, c [m s^{-1}]	Characteristic impedance, Z [kg m^{-2} s^{-1}] ($\times 10^{-6}$)	Absorption coefficient, α [dB cm^{-1}] at 1 MHz	Approximate frequency dependence* of α
Air at STP	1·2	330	0·0004	12	f^2
Aluminium	2700	6400	17	0·018	f
Brass	8500	4490	38	0·020	f
Castor oil	950	1500	1·4	0·95	f^2
Mercury	13 600	1450	20	0·000 48	f^2
Polyethylene	920	2000	1·8	4·7	$f^{1.1}$
Polymethylmethacrylate	1190	2680	3·2	2·0	f
Water	1000	1480	1·5	0·0022	f^2

* For frequencies below about 10 MHz.
Data chiefly from Kaye and Laby (1968).

The energy travels through the medium with the wave velocity c. The energy which travels through unit area in unit time (which is the intensity I of the wave) is equal to the total energy contained in a column of unit area, and length equal to c.(unit time). Hence

$$I = cE \tag{1.38}$$

and

$$I = \rho c v_0^2 / 2 \tag{1.39}$$

In SI units, I has the dimensions [kg s^{-3}], which is equivalent to [watt per square metre], or [W m^{-2}]. This is an inconveniently large quantity in practice, and it is usual to express the intensity in units of [W cm^{-2}] or [mW cm^{-2}].

TABLE 1.2

Field parameters for plane waves in water: values for 1 W cm^{-2} at 1 MHz

Parameter	Value	Dependence
Heat equivalent	0·24 cal s^{-1} cm^{-2}	(intensity)
Peak particle acceleration, a_0	71 000 gravity	(intensity)$^{1/2}$, (frequency)
Peak particle displacement, u_0	0·018 μm	(intensity)$^{1/2}$, (frequency)$^{-1}$
Peak particle pressure, p_0	1·8 atmosphere	(intensity)$^{1/2}$
Peak particle velocity, v_0	12 cm s^{-1}	(intensity)$^{1/2}$
Radiation pressure,* F	0·069 g cm^{-2}	(intensity)
Velocity, c	1500 m s^{-1}	—
Wavelength, λ	1·5 mm	(frequency)$^{-1}$

* For complete absorption
Data from Wells (1969).

Some typical relationships between intensity and the other wave parameters are given in Table 1.2.

1.8 REFLEXION AND REFRACTION AT PLANE SURFACES

When a wave meets the interface between two different media, it may be partially reflected. The reflected wave returns in the negative direction through the incident medium, at the same velocity as that with which it approached the interface. The transmitted wave continues to move in the positive direction, but at the velocity corresponding to propagation in the medium beyond the interface. Just as in optics, the geometrical laws of reflexion apply, and the angles of incidence and reflexion are equal in the same plane for a longitudinal wave. However, if the ultrasonic wavelength is comparable with, or greater than, the dimensions of the reflecting object, the geometrical laws cease to apply. This situation is mentioned in Section

2.5; in the meanwhile, it is assumed that the wavelength is small compared with the dimensions of the interface, that the interface is plane and perpendicular to the propagation plane. In this case, any reflexion is said to be specular.

In Fig. 1.8, the suffixes i, r and t refer to the incident, reflected and transmitted waves. As in optics,

$$\theta_i = \theta_r \tag{1.40}$$

and, in order to maintain wavefront coherence (i.e. by the application of Snell's law),

$$(\sin \theta_i)/(\sin \theta_t) = c_1/c_2 \tag{1.41}$$

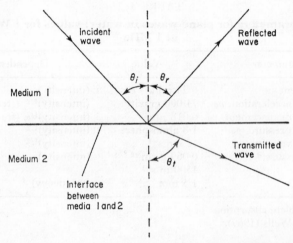

FIG. 1.8 The behaviour of a wave incident on the boundary between two media.

For any particular value of c_1/c_2, θ_t increases as θ_i is increased. If $c_2 > c_1$, θ_t reaches $\pi/2$ radians when $\theta_i < \pi/2$, and total reflexion occurs. When $\theta_t = \pi/2$, $\sin \theta_t = 1$, so that the critical angle for total reflexion is equal to $\sin^{-1}(c_1/c_2)$.

In a propagating wave, there are no sudden discontinuities in either particle velocity or particle pressure. Consequently, when a wave meets the interface between two media, both the particle velocity and the pressure are continuous across the interface. In physical terms, this ensures that the two media remain in contact. These conditions are satisfied when

$$v_i \cos \theta_i - v_r \cos \theta_r = v_t \cos \theta_t \tag{1.42}$$

and

$$p_i + p_r = p_t \tag{1.43}$$

The negative sign in Eqn. 1.42 arises because the direction of the reflected wave is reversed.

Now $p = \rho cv$ (Eqn. 1.35), so that Eqn. 1.42 becomes

$$(p_i/Z_1) \cos \theta_i - (p_r/Z_1) \cos \theta_i = (p_t/Z_2) \cos \theta_t \qquad (1.44)$$

The simultaneous solutions to Eqns. 1.43 and 1.44 are given by:

$$\frac{p_r}{p_i} = \frac{Z_2 \cos \theta_i - Z_1 \cos \theta_t}{Z_2 \cos \theta_i + Z_1 \cos \theta_t} \qquad (1.45)$$

and

$$\frac{p_t}{p_i} = \frac{2Z_2 \cos \theta_i}{Z_2 \cos \theta_i + Z_1 \cos \theta_t} \qquad (1.46)$$

The quantities (p_r/p_i) and (p_t/p_i) are respectively the pressure reflectivity and the pressure transmittivity of the interface.

At normal incidence, $\theta_i = \theta_t = 0$, and Eqns. 1.45 and 1.46 become:

$$p_r/p_i = (Z_2 - Z_1)/(Z_2 + Z_1) \qquad (1.47)$$

and

$$p_t/p_i = 2Z_2/(Z_2 + Z_1) \qquad (1.48)$$

If $Z_1 = Z_2$, $p_r/p_i = 0$ and there is no reflected wave.

If $Z_2 > Z_1$, the reflected pressure wave is in phase with the incident wave; but if $Z_2 < Z_1$, the reflected wave is π radians out of phase with the incident wave.

Now, from Eqn. 1.35,

$$p_0 = \rho c \, v_0$$

and substitution in Eqn. 1.39 gives:

$$I = p_0^2/(2\rho c)$$

so that, from Eqns. 1.45 and 1.46:

$$\frac{I_r}{I_i} = \left(\frac{Z_2 \cos \theta_i - Z_1 \cos \theta_t}{Z_2 \cos \theta_i + Z_1 \cos \theta_t} \right)^2 \qquad (1.49)$$

and

$$\frac{I_t}{I_i} = \frac{4Z_2 Z_1 \cos \theta_i \cos \theta_t}{(Z_2 \cos \theta_i + Z_1 \cos \theta_t)^2} \qquad (1.50)$$

The quantities (I_r/I_i) and (I_t/I_i) are respectively the intensity reflectivity and the intensity transmittivity of the interface. Some typical values of reflectivity for non-biological media (in decibels: see Appendix 2) are given in Table 1.3.

At normal incidence, $\theta_i = \theta_t = 0$ and Eqns. 1.49 and 1.50 become:

$$I_r/I_i = \{(Z_2 - Z_1)/(Z_2 + Z_1)\}^2 \tag{1.51}$$

and

$$I_t/I_i = 4Z_2 Z_1/(Z_2 + Z_1)^2 \tag{1.52}$$

TABLE 1.3

Reflectivities of some plane, non-biological boundaries, expressed in decibels below the level from a perfect reflector

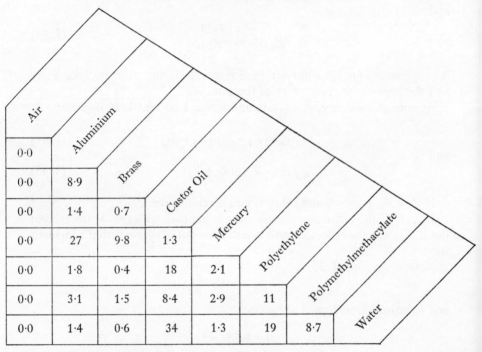

Air	Aluminium	Brass	Castor Oil	Mercury	Polyethylene	Polymethylmethacrylate	Water
0·0							
0·0	8·9						
0·0	1·4	0·7					
0·0	27	9·8	1·3				
0·0	1·8	0·4	18	2·1			
0·0	3·1	1·5	8·4	2·9	11		
0·0	1·4	0·6	34	1·3	19	8·7	

Based on data from Table 1.1.

If $Z_2 \gg Z_1$, or $Z_2 \ll Z_1$, $I_r/I_i = 1$, corresponding to total reflection at the interface.

1.9 WAVE MODE CONVERSION

Except in the case of normal incidence, the situations discussed in Section 1.8 apply only for longitudinal waves propagating in media which are unable to support other modes of wave. Fluids of negligible viscosity can support only longitudinal waves. In situations where wave modes can exist in addition to longitudinal waves, mode conversion may occur. The types of wave that are produced by a wave incident on an interface may be determined by resolving the stress and displacement components along the coordinates of the interface. Four separate boundary conditions exist in the general case. On both sides of the interface, the following quantities must each be equal: the normal displacements; the tangential displacements; the normal stresses; and the tangential stresses. The essential difference from the situation considered in Section 1.8 is that, in Eqn. 1.43, the pressure is considered to be acting only normally to the interface.

One important case of wave mode conversion may be mentioned. As explained in Section 1.8, total reflexion of a longitudinal wave occurs when $\theta_i \geqslant \sin^{-1}(c_1/c_2)$ if $c_2 > c_1$. Now in any medium the shear wave velocity is always less than that of the longitudinal wave. Therefore, even if $c_2 > c_1$ and $\theta_i > \sin^{-1}(c_1/c_2)$, it may still be possible for energy to be propagated in the second medium in the form of a shear wave. Increasing the value of θ_i so that it exceeds $\sin^{-1}(c_1/c_2)$ leads to an increase in the angle of transmission of the shear wave in the second medium until it travels along the interface as a surface wave.

Mathematical analysis of the conditions which arise with oblique incidence where mode conversion is possible is tedious. The analysis becomes difficult if the media are anisotropic, as in the case with many biological materials. Consequently, detailed analysis of idealized conditions is not particularly helpful in giving insight into biophysical problems.

1.10 STANDING WAVES

Standing waves are periodic waves having a fixed distribution in space, and result from the interference of travelling waves of the same frequency and mode. When the paths of two waves, travelling in different directions, cross each other, the particle displacements add together where they are in phase, and subtract one from the other where they are out of phase. The simplest case is that of a longitudinal wave normally incident on a perfect reflector. The reflected wave interferes with the incident wave so that the pressure in the resultant standing wave is zero at the nodes, and twice that in the travelling incident wave at the antinodes. There is no net flow of energy along the axis of the standing wave system, since all the energy of the incident wave is returned in the opposite direction by the reflected wave.

A travelling wave may be superimposed on a standing wave: for example, this occurs if the reflector returns only a fraction of the incident wave. The particle pressure at the nodes then has a finite value which is less than that of the incident travelling wave, and at the antinodes, it is less than twice that of the incident travelling wave. The situation may be quantitated in terms of the standing wave ratio, defined as the pressure amplitude at an antinode to that at the adjacent node. In a lossless medium, the relationship is:

$$SWR = (p_{oi} + p_{or})/(p_{oi} - p_{or}) \qquad (1.53)$$

The standing wave ratio cannot be less than unity. It is equal to unity when $p_{or} = 0$, which occurs when there is no reflexion at the interface. When $p_{oi} = p_{or}$, i.e. when there is perfect reflexion at the interface, $SWR = \infty$.

1.11 TRANSMISSION THROUGH LAYERS

If a wave is transmitted through three media separated by plane parallel surfaces, partial reflexion may occur at each interface. This leads to the establishment of standing waves in the first and second media. The standing wave in the second medium controls the reflexion into the first medium and the transmission into the third. The situation is very complicated at oblique incidence. At normal incidence, however, it can be shown (see, for example, Kinsler and Frey, 1962, pp. 136–9) that:

$$\frac{I_{t3}}{I_{i1}} = \frac{4Z_3Z_1}{(Z_3 + Z_1)^2 \cos^2 k_2 l_2 + (Z_2 + Z_3Z_1/Z_2)^2 \sin^2 k_2 l_2} \qquad (1.54)$$

where $k_2 = 2\pi/\lambda_2$, the wavelength constant of the second medium, and l_2 is the thickness of the second medium.

There are two situations which give solutions of Eqn. 1.54 which are of particular interest. Firstly, if $l_2 \ll \lambda_2/4$, or if $l_2 = n\lambda_2/2$ where n is an integer,

$$I_{t3}/I_{i1} = 4Z_1Z_3/(Z_1 + Z_3)^2 \qquad (1.55)$$

and transmission through the layer is independent of the properties of the layer material (but this simplication does not apply if $Z_2 \ll Z_1$ and $Z_2 \ll Z_3$, as is the case if Z_2 is a layer of gas trapped between liquids).

Secondly, if $l_2 = (2n - 1)\lambda_2/4$ where n is an integer, $I_{t3}/I_{i1} = 1$ when

$$Z_2 = (Z_1Z_3)^{1/2} \qquad (1.56)$$

Consequently it is possible to obtain complete transmission from one medium to another of different characteristic impedance, by the use of a layer of characteristic impedance equal to the geometric mean of the other two, and of thickness equal to an odd integral number of quarter wavelengths.

1.12 ABSORPTION

When a wave travels through a real medium, its intensity is reduced as a function of distance. In practice, several factors contribute to this attenuation. These factors include: deviation from a parallel beam, so that the energy per unit area is decreased (see Section 2.1); scattering by non-specular reflectors, so that a proportion of the energy no longer moves in the original direction of propagation (see Section 2.5); mode conversion resulting in the sharing of the energy between two or more waves travelling at different velocities and in different directions (see Section 1.9); and absorption, by which ultrasonic energy is converted to heat.

The amplitude of a plane wave propagating in the z-direction can be expressed in the form:

$$A_z = A_0 e^{-\mu_a z} \qquad (1.57)$$

where A_0 is the peak value at $z=0$ of a wave variable such as particle velocity, and A_z is the peak value at z of the same variable; μ_a is the amplitude attenuation coefficient, and has dimensions $[L^{-1}]$. In the literature, μ_a is often quoted in units of nepers per centimetre [Np cm^{-1}], so that:

$$\mu_a = -(1/z) \ln (A_0/A_z) \qquad (1.58)$$

In this book, attenuation is generally expressed in terms of an attenuation coefficient α, measured in units of decibels per centimetre [dB cm^{-1}], so that:*

$$\alpha = 20(\log_{10} e)\mu_a = 8.686\mu_a \qquad (1.59)$$

Some typical values of α in non-biological materials are given in Table 1.1.

Absorption is associated with the occurrence of a lag between the instantaneous pressure in the wave and the resultant change in the density of the propagating medium.

The classical mechanism (see, for example, Kinsler and Frey, 1962, pp. 221–5) of the absorption of ultrasound in fluids is due to the frictional forces which act to oppose the periodic motion of the particles in the medium. The situation arises because viscous fluids are able to transmit dynamic shearing forces, although they cannot, by definition, support static shear. Thus:

$$\mu_a = 2\eta\omega^2/3\rho c^3 \qquad (1.60)$$

where η is the viscosity of the fluid.

In addition to the classical theory of absorption due to viscosity, several other mechanisms may contribute to attenuation depending upon the properties of the propagating medium and the frequency of the wave. The

---

* Confusion sometimes arises as to whether a given attenuation coefficient refers to amplitude or to intensity. No difficulty should occur if the definition of α given here is used: for example, if $\alpha = 6$ dB cm^{-1}, inspection of a Table of Decibel Ratios (Appendix 2) shows that the amplitude of the wave is reduced almost exactly to one half by travelling through a distance of 10 mm, and the intensity, by travelling through 5 mm.

subject is discussed in detail in relation to absorption in biological materials in Chapter 4, so only a brief survey is given here.

(i) Relaxation processes

These are generally the most important contributors to ultrasonic absorption in biological materials. Energy in a system can exist in various forms, such as molecular vibrational energy, lattice vibrational energy, translational energy, and so on. When an ultrasonic wave passes through a medium, there is an increase in energy in one or more of these forms. All the different forms in which the energy can be stored are coupled in various ways. Consider, for example, a small element of volume in a medium supporting an ultrasonic wave. During the compressive part of the wave, a temperature rise occurs associated with an increase in the translational energy of the molecules in the element. If none of this energy flowed into another form, the increased translational energy would be returned to the vibrational energy of the wave during the decompressive part of the cycle, and no absorption would occur. However, it always happens that some of the excess translational energy flows into another form during the compression half-cycle. This process is not instantaneous, and so, during decompression, some of the energy returns out-of-phase with the travelling wave, and this results in absorption.

(ii) Relative motion

Relative motion produced by an altrasonic field between structured elements (such as biological cells) and their surrounding medium results in absorption of energy. In general, relative motion is due to radiation pressure (see Section 1.13) acting on in interface at which there is a change in characteristic impedance.

(iii) Bubble mechanisms

The presence of gas bubbles in the propagating medium may exert marked influences on biological materials (see Section 5.1.b), and may contribute to attenuation.

(iv) Hysteresis

In very viscous media and at frequencies greater than the viscous relaxation frequencies, there may be an excess absorption corresponding to a constant energy loss per cycle. This type of mechanism is known as hysteresis.

1.13 RADIATION PRESSURE

An ultrasonic wave exerts a static pressure on any interface or medium across which there is a decrease in ultrasonic intensity in the direction of wave propagation. This static pressure is quite distinct from the oscillating particle pressure of the wave. The theoretical aspect of the matter has received considerable attention, and its mechanism is still a subject of speculation. The physical processes which lead to the establishment of radiation pressure in an ultrasonic field are considerably more complex than is the situation with electromagnetic waves (see Appendix 1), although in both cases it happens that the force is proportional to the mean energy density of the wave motion. The difficulties arise because the mechanical wave equation is not linear in any real situation, and an ultrasonic beam of finite cross-section is subject to effects caused by the surrounding medium. Though many published papers have been devoted to the subject, and though various theoretical approaches have been used, some difficulties still stand in the way of a clear understanding of the physics of the problem.

The approach adopted here is not to reproduce one of the spurious arguments presented in many textbooks, but simply to present the result, which is supported both by experimental results and by some recent theoretical work. Thus, in the case of complete absorption of a finite beam of plane waves,

$$F = W/c \tag{1.61}$$

where F is the force due to radiation pressure, and W is the ultrasonic power.

The force F acts in the vector direction of the propagation of the wave. At normal incidence, the force on a perfect reflector is equal to twice the force which would act on a perfect absorber in the same situation; at oblique incidence, the direction of the resultant force may be resolved by taking into account the directions of the incident and the reflected waves. The situation may be clarified if it is appreciated that the transport of energy by a wave is associated with a flow of momentum across the plane normal to the ultrasonic beam. Thus, at a perfect absorber there is a single momentum change; but at a perfect reflector, there are two momentum changes because the reflected wave is returned unattenuated. For plane waves, the forces corresponding to oblique incidence and partial reflexion can be calculated from the corresponding momentum vectors; and similarly, the forces which cause streaming in an attenuating fluid can be calculated from the distance rates of momentum deposition.

Radiation pressure does not produce effects in lossless media in which plane waves of infinite extent are being propagated.

For an insight into the theoretical aspects of radiation pressure, reference may be made by Beyer (1950), Borgnis (1953) and Rooney and Nyborg (1972). Experimental comparisons of measurements made by calorimetric and radiation pressure methods have been made by Wells *et al.* (1963).

The independence of radiation pressure of the non-linearities of the medium has been demonstrated by Rooney (1973).

1.14 OTHER UNIDIRECTIONAL FORCES

In addition to the force due to radiation pressure, there are three other mechanisms which can cause unidirectional forces in an ultrasonic field. Although the magnitudes of these forces in biomedical situations are generally negligible, they deserve mention in a comprehensive review.

An obstacle suspended in a medium supporting an ultrasonic wave tends to move in sympathy with the particles of the medium, as a result of viscous coupling. Now the viscosity of the medium changes as a function of the wave amplitude, and so the force on the obstacle differs during the compression and rarefaction phases. The result is that a unidirectional force, called *Stokes' force*, acts on the obstacle in a direction normal to the wavefront.

Radiation pressure gives rise to a force which causes streaming along the axis of an ultrasonic wave travelling in an absorptive medium. If the medium thus set into motion has to pass between two obstacles, its velocity is increased. Consequently there is a decrease in the static pressure in the region where the velocity is increased, and this results in a unidirectional force which tends to move the particles in a direction parallel to the wavefront. This is called the *Bernoulli force*.

The linear wave equation is strictly applicable only in the case of a wave of infinitesimally small amplitude. If the wave amplitude is finite, the waveform becomes distorted by the generation and growth of harmonics. The result is that the wave develops a saw-tooth shape as it propagates; the shape returns to being sinusoidal as the amplitude is reduced with increasing range. An obstacle suspended in a medium supporting a wave distorted by this mechanism experiences momentum transfers at rates which differ during the fast leading edge, and during the trailing edge. This results in a unidirectional transfer of momentum. The corresponding force is called the *Oseen force*.

1.15 DOPPLER EFFECT

The apparent frequency of a constant frequency source is dependent on the motion of both the source and the receiver. If the effective path length is being reduced with time, the received frequency is greater than that of the source, and vice versa. The phenomenon is known as the *Doppler effect*. If all the velocities act along the same axis, the received frequency f_r is given by:

$$f_r = \left(\frac{c - v_r}{c - v_s}\right) f \qquad (1.62)$$

where v_r is velocity of the receiver, and v_s is the velocity of the source, both velocities being taken along the same direction as the propagation of the wave; and f is the frequency of the source.

Equation 1.62 can be rearranged to give the value of $f_D = (f_r - f)$, the Doppler shift frequency, thus:

$$f_D = \left(\frac{c - v_r}{c - v_s} - 1 \right) f \qquad (1.63)$$

1.16 NON-PLANAR WAVES

This Chapter is mainly concerned with the behaviour of plane, non-spreading waves. Such a wave can be represented in terms of a single space variable: the wavefront retains the same shape throughout space, and varies only in scale. In many practical situations, however, the shape of the wavefront is not uniform, and the plane wave relationships no longer apply.

The spherical wave is the simplest form of non-planar wave. Such a wave is generated by a source which is very much smaller than the wavelength of the ultrasound (see Section 2.1), and the wavefront (where the particle motion is in-phase) is in the form of a spherical surface. At large distances from the source, where the radius of the spherical surface is much larger than the wavelength, the wavefront may be considered to be plane over distances comparable with the wavelength.

The errors introduced by considering the waves due to practical sources to be planar depend upon the degree of deviation from wavefront uniformity over the plane of interest. If this deviation is negligible, the relationships derived in this Chapter for plane waves are applicable.

2. RADIATION

2.1. SPHERICAL WAVES

A vibrating source, which is very small in relation to the wavelength, radiates uniformly over a solid angle of 2π radians in the forward direction. Similarly a very small vibration detector is uniformly sensitive to disturbances arriving from any direction over a solid angle of 2π radians. *Huygen's principle* is that any wave phenomenon can be analysed by the addition of the contributions from some distribution of simple sources, or simple detectors, properly selected in phase and amplitude to represent the physical situation.

Spherical waves are non-planar: the energy which they carry is spread uniformly over a spherical surface. At any radius r from the source, the intensity I is related to the source power W by

$$I = W/4\pi r^2 \tag{2.1}$$

If $r \gg \lambda$, and $\lambda \gg a$, where a is the radius of the source, the wavefront (which is a surface over which the motion is everywhere in phase) may be considered to be plane over distances comparable with λ.

2.2 THE ULTRASONIC FIELD

The active surface of a transducer (see Chapter 3) of any shape and size may be considered to be represented by small areas, each of which acts as a simple transducer which radiates or receives energy in the manner appropriate for the application of Huygen's principle. The shape of the ultrasonic field corresponding to any particular transducer may be determined by geometrical calculation of the diffraction pattern which is set by the interference of the spherical wavelets radiated by all the Huygen's sources across the surface of the transducer. The same reasoning may be used to calculate the distribution of the sensitivity of a transducer acting as a receiver.

At any given point in space (r, θ) beyond the transducer, the ultrasonic field at any time is made up from all the separate contributions of each of the Huygen's sources. The situation for one of these simple sources is illustrated in Fig. 2.1. Where these contributions are in phase, they interfere to form amplitude maxima; but where they are in antiphase, destructive interference occurs and there are corresponding minima. The phase variations arise because of the differences in the path lengths between different points on the surface of the transducer and any single point in space. These distance differences generally have negligible attenuating effects.

In the following Sub-sections, consideration is given to some aspects of the radiation patterns of geometrically defined transducer shapes.

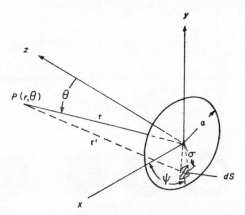

FIG. 2.1 Coordinate system showing the distribution of a Huygen's source dS, situated on a circular transducer radius a, to the ultrasonic field at a point (r, θ).

2.2.a Plane Disc Transducer

One of the most commonly used ultrasonic transducers is in the form of a disc, which is arranged to radiate or to receive energy at its plane surfaces. In the analysis of the corresponding ultrasonic field, it is assumed in the first instance that the surface of the disc may be considered to behave as piston vibrating with constant amplitude and phase, so that the hypothetical Huygen's wave sources are all identical, and distributed with uniform density.

The derivation of the field distribution involves the solution of the three-dimensional geometrical problem, as set out in several textbooks (see, for example, Kinsler and Frey, 1962, pp. 166–77). The beam is considered to be composed of two distinct regions, as shown in Fig. 2.2(a). The relationship which applies to the distribution along the central axis of the beam is

$$\frac{I_z}{I_0} = \sin^2 \frac{\pi}{\lambda} \{(a^2 + z^2)^{1/2} - z\} \tag{2.2}$$

where I_0 is the maximum intensity, I_z is the intensity at distance z from the piston, a is the radius of the piston, and λ is the wavelength in the

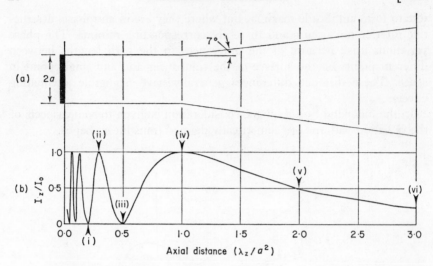

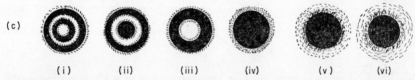

FIG. 2.2 The ultrasonic field of a plane disc transducer, $a/\lambda = 5.0$ (at 3 MHz in water this corresponds to $a = 2.5$ mm). (a) Conventional "textbook" representation of the field; (b) relative intensity distribution along the central axis of the beam; (c) ring diagrams showing the energy distributions of the beam sections at positions indicated in (b).

propagating medium. A typical graph of Eqn. 2.2 is shown in Fig. 2.2(b). Particular solutions of Eqn. 2.2 give the central axial positions respectively of the maxima as

$$z_{\max} = \frac{4a^2 - \lambda^2(2m+1)^2}{4\lambda(2m+1)} \quad (2.3)$$

and the minima as

$$z_{\min} = (a^2 - \lambda^2 n^2)/2n\lambda \quad (2.4)$$

where $m = 0, 1, 2$, etc., and $n = 1, 2, 3$, etc.

Moving along the central axis away from the source, the position of the last axial maximum occurs at a distance given by

$$z'_{\max} = (4a^2 - \lambda^2)/4\lambda \quad (2.5)$$

If $a^2 \gg \lambda^2$, this expression can be simplified to become

$$z'_{\max} = a^2/\lambda \quad (2.6)$$

The position z'_{max} of the last axial maximum is often taken to correspond to the beginning of the transition between the Frésnel zone (the near zone) and the Fraunhofer zone (the far zone): the matter is discussed later in this Sub-section.

The field in the far zone may be considered to be plane over distances comparable with λ (since $z \gg \lambda$ and $a \gg \lambda$). In the region where $z \gg z'_{max}$, the intensity follows the inverse square law, and $I_z \propto 1/z^2$. The relationship between the intensity and the angle θ defined in Fig. 2.2(a) contains a multiplying term, the directivity function D_s, given by

$$D_s = \frac{2\mathcal{J}_1(ka \sin \theta)}{ka \sin \theta} \qquad (2.7)$$

where $\mathcal{J}_1$ is Bessel's function of the first kind, and the wave number $k = 2\pi/\lambda$. (The wave number k plays the same role in space as ω does in time.)

Now $\mathcal{J}_1 (ka \sin \theta) = 0$ when $ka \sin \theta = 3\cdot83$, $7\cdot02$, $10\cdot17$, $13\cdot32$, etc. In physical terms, the energy is confined into lobes; the central lobe is reduced to zero at the angles $\pm \theta$ given by

$$\theta = \sin^{-1}(3\cdot83/ka) = \sin^{-1}(0\cdot61\lambda/a) \qquad (2.8)$$

If $ka < 3\cdot83$, D_s is not zero for any real value of θ, and only the main lobe occurs. In the long-wavelength limit, $ka \to 0$, and the source radiates Huygen's spherical waves.

The directivity function for the transducer the beam shape of which is represented in Fig. 2.2 is shown in Fig. 2.3. The energy in the side lobes is much lower than that in the main lobe. For example, the maximum

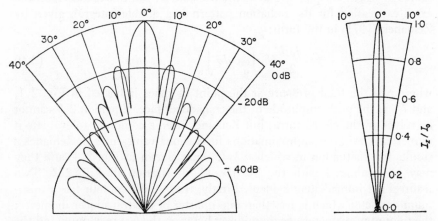

FIG. 2.3 Farfield beam pattern for a plane disc transducer, $a/\lambda = 5\cdot0$. (From data of Zemanek, 1971.)

intensity of the first side lobe (if it exists) is 18 dB below that of the main lobe.

Although the relationship given by Eqn. 2.7 can be extended without limitation into the far field, the reverse (i.e. unlimited extension in the direction towards the transducer) is certainly not valid. Consequently a boundary must exist which separates the far field from the near field. As already mentioned, most textbooks identify this boundary with the plane perpendicular to the central axis at z'_{max} as defined in Eqn. 2.6 (or, more generally, as in Eqn. 2.5). The first attempt thus to analyse the ultrasonic near field in a quantitative fashion seems to be that of Schoch (1941). He showed that the near field may be considered to be the convolution of two parts, one of which has the form of a plane wave, whilst the other depends on the shape of the edge of the radiator. This is a somewhat intractable approach. There is a relatively simple solution due to Dehn (1960), however, which gives a qualitative indication of the positions of the maxima. The maxima occur at positions at which the contributions of three rays, one perpendicular to the piston face, and one from each of its extreme edges, are most nearly in phase. Because of symmetry, the figure may be rotated about the beam axis to generate ring patterns representing the cross-section of the beam. Within the near field, the distribution of energy across the beam is not uniform, as indicated in Fig. 2.2(c). The number of maxima and minima across the beam diameter depends upon the values of z and a/λ. In general, the frequency of peaks increases with decreasing values of z, and with increasing values of a/λ. At successive axial maxima and minima, starting at z'_{max} and moving towards the source, there are one, two, three, etc., principal maxima across the beam. It is often stated that the ultrasonic beam is confined in the near field within a cylinder the radius of which is equal to that of the transducer. But this is incorrect: the exact expression for the radiation pattern is a double integral, given by Zemanek (1971) in the form:

$$p = \frac{j\rho ck}{2\pi} U_0 \int_0^a \sigma \, d\sigma \int_0^{2\pi} \frac{e^{j(\omega t - kr')}}{r'} \, d\psi \qquad (2.9)$$

where p is the total pressure at the point in space indicated in Fig. 2.1, and U_0 is the peak amplitude of the transducer face. Equation 2.9 cannot be solved in the closed form; but Zemanek used a computer to evaluate it numerically without approximations for various values of a/λ. Zemanek's results for a situation in which $a/\lambda = 5 \cdot 0$ are shown in Fig. 2.4, and they may be compared with the "textbook" illustration in Fig. 2.2. Two features are immediately evident. Firstly, the -3 dB contour has a minimum diameter which is less than one-quarter of the transducer diameter: the minimum diameter occurs midway between the last maximum and the last minimum of the axial distribution. Secondly, the contour behaves in a regular manner for a distance of up to $z = 0.75a^2/\lambda$ into the "conventional" near zone, and this is up to 25% closer to the transducer than the position of z'_{max}. This apparent separation defines a qualitative boundary between the region in which destructive interference does occur, and that in which it does not occur. The numerical choice of the boundary z-coordinate may be slightly modified by the choice of the value of the determining intensity contour.

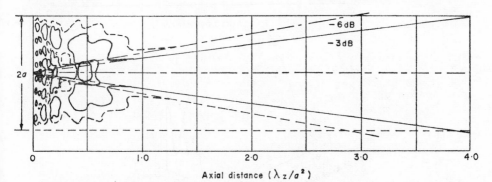

FIG. 2.4 Computed intensity contours in the plane of the central axis for a plane disc transducer, $a/\lambda = 5.0$. (Based on Zemanek, 1971.)

2.2.b Plane Rectangular Transducer

Although much less common than the disc transducer, a rectangular transducer is occasionally used. If l_1 and l_2 are the lengths of the sides of the rectangle, the far field directivity function is given by:

$$D_s = \frac{\sin\{(kl_1/2)\sin\theta\}}{(kl_1/2)\sin\theta} \cdot \frac{\sin\{(kl_2/2)\sin\phi\}}{(kl_2/2)\sin\phi} \qquad (2.10)$$

where θ is the angle normal to the source within the plane parallel to l_1, and ϕ is the corresponding angle within the plane parallel to l_2.

The near zone of a rectangular transducer is even less amenable to analysis than that of a circular transducer. The problem was first solved by Stenzel (1952), who reduced the analysis to an exact single integration of a tabulated function, which he performed by a graphical method. Another treatment of the rectangular transducer involves phase approximations (see, for example, Freedman, 1970). An approach to the problem of the near field analysis, however, which is equally applicable to both circular and rectangular transducers, has been described by Lockwood and Willette (1973a, b). They utilized an exact closed-form expression for the response of the pressure field to an impulse acceleration of the transducer, and obtained the transfer function of the system by evaluating the Fourier transform of the impulse response at the driving frequency. This requires

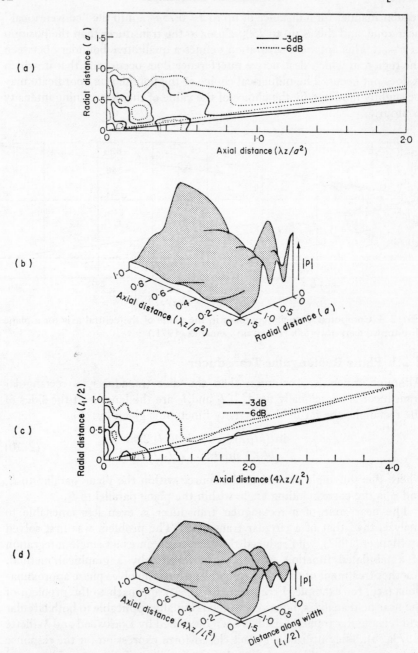

FIG. 2.5 Computed contours. (a) and (b) Data for a plane disc transducer $a/\lambda = 2\cdot5$; (c) and (d) data for a plane rectangular transducer, $l_1/\lambda = 2\cdot5$, $l_2/l_1 = 1\cdot5$. (Based on Lockwood and Willette, 1973.)

only a single numerical integration, whereas Zemanek's (1971) double integration requires more computational steps by a factor of a/λ. There is some slight and unexplained discrepancy between the far field contours calculated by the two methods. The results of Lockwood and Willette for both a circular and a rectangular transducer are illustrated in Fig. 2.5. The near field inhomogeneity of a rectangular transducer is less marked than that of a circular transducer of similar size. As a rough guide, the near field of a rectangular transducer extends for a distance somewhat beyond that of a circular transducer of diameter equal to the greater length of the rectangle. This is illustrated for a square and a circular transducer in Fig. 2.6.

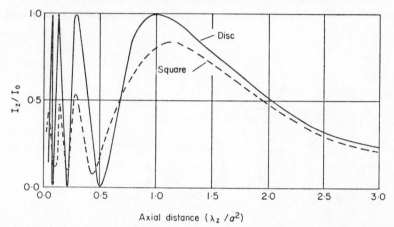

FIG. 2.6 Computed amplitude contours in the plane of the central axis of a plane disc transducer ($a/\lambda = 5\cdot0$) and a plane square transducer $1/2\lambda = 5\cdot0$). (Data of Stenzel, 1952.)

2.2.c Plane Disc Transducer: Transient Condition

The transient performance of the transducer is of central importance in ultrasonic diagnostic pulse–echo systems (see Chapter 6).

The steady state ultrasonic field of a plane disc transducer is discussed in Section 2.2(a); the directivity is determined by interference between the contributions from the entire surface of the transducer. When transient conditions apply, however, it is not sufficient to take account only of the phase of each elementary contribution of the transducer surface because the surface vibration is discontinuous in time. Consequently, all the contributions which combine together to form the field in the steady state may not be present at any particular point in space during a transient.

There are two popular approaches to the calculation of the ultrasonic field under transient conditions. Firstly, the computation can be based on time considerations and the knowledge of the form of the excitation of the transducer. At any point in the medium in which the wave is propagated, the field is zero until the arrival of the disturbance which originates from the surface of the transducer closest to the point under consideration. The field then changes continuously as contributions arrive from more distant points on the transducer. Filipczyński (1956) applied a geometrical analysis to the build-up of the far field resulting from the sudden commencement of constant-amplitude sinusoidal oscillation of the transducer. By summing the vector contributions of waves derived from elementary strips on the surface of the transducer, he showed that the initial directivity has the shape of an elongated cylinder, and that this alters continuously towards the steady state situation. This transition is very rapid, being substantially complete within about half a cycle. In practice, the instantaneous result of

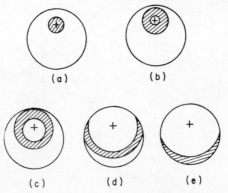

FIG. 2.7 Diagrams illustrating the regions (shaded) of the transducer which contribute to the ultrasonic field at some point lying on the perpendicular extended from the point + on the surface of the transducer, as time proceeds (a–e) during the pulse. (After Beaver, 1974.)

all the contributions depends on the changing amplitude of the emitted disturbance. The descriptions of the near field given by Kaspar'yants (1960), Christie (1962) and Kossoff (1963) did not take account of this factor, although it is included in the analyses of Oberhettinger (1961) and Farn and Huang (1968). The problem does not have a simple solution; as a rough guide, the transition to the steady state field distribution occupies between three and six half-cycles in the near field.

As the pulse develops in time, so the part of the surface which contributes to the field at any particular point in space moves radially outwards from the perpendicular extended from the transducer to the point. This is illustrated in Fig. 2.7. Beaver (1974) used this approach in his analysis of the transient ultrasonic field. A numerical-analysis algorithm equivalent to the equation describing the field in terms of the times of departure integrated over the entire surface of the transducer was computed for uniform excitation with pulsed carrier frequency. Calculations were made at sufficient points in time to define the shape of the field during the pulse. Figure 2.8 illustrates the beam profiles calculated for continuous wave excitation, and for two pulse shapes. Although these profiles are for a transducer of radius = 5λ, the field shapes of transducers of different

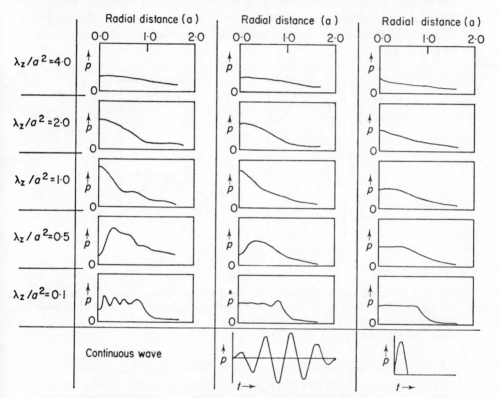

FIG. 2.8 Beam profiles for continuous-wave and two forms of pulsed ultrasonic fields, generated by a plane disc transducer ($a/\lambda = 5 \cdot 0$), at various distances from the transducer. (After Beaver, 1974.)

diameters are similar provided that their variation in departure time at the range under consideration does not exceed a quarter period.

Robinson *et al.* (1974) have discussed in more detail the physical processes involved during a transient ultrasonic field. They adopted a similar approach to that of Beaver (1974), but rely more on approximations in extrapolating from exact solutions of idealized conditions.

The second approach to the problem is to consider the time-averaged distribution of energy within the ultrasonic beam during the propagation of the pulse. This involves the concept of the frequency spectrum of the radiated energy, and can be solved as a single-aperture diffraction problem, utilizing a weighted superposition of the fields of single-frequency radiators at various frequencies within the band (Papadakis and Fowler, 1971). From the point of view of pulse–echo diagnostics, this method gives a result which corresponds to the square root of the effective beam distribution; but it may be somewhat misleading in discussions of biological effects, where the time-distribution of the field may be more relevant. The results of some calculations for various bandwidths of pulse excitation are given in Fig. 2.9.

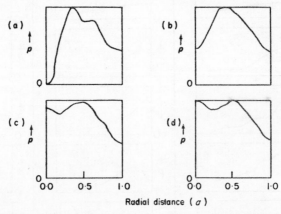

Radial distance (σ)

FIG. 2.9 Effective radial amplitudes in the plane corresponding to the last axial minimum ($z'_{min} = a^2/2\lambda$), for various bandwidths; the graphs show the maximum amplitude during the pulse. Bandwidths: (a) 0%; (b) 40%; (c) 80%; (d) 120%. (Based on Papadakis and Fowler, 1971.)

It is pointed out in the introduction to Section 2.2 that differences in propagation path length between a given point in space and the surface of the transducer generally introduce negligible modification of the ultrasonic field in an absorptive medium. Absorption merely reduces the field amplitude with increasing distance. Biological materials, however, have absorption coefficients which increase with frequency, and frequency-dispersive attenuation does modify the field of a pulsed beam in much the same way that the higher frequency components of the spectrum are increasingly reduced with distance (see Section 6.1(b)).

2.3 FOCUSING SYSTEMS

The directivity of an ultrasonic beam may be altered by focusing. The general principles are those which apply in elementary optics, but ray theory breaks down when the dimensions under consideration are not very much greater than the wavelength. The wavelength imposes the ultimate limitation on the dimensions of the focal region; the sharpness of the focus is determined by the ratio of the aperture of the radiator to the wavelength.

The methods commonly used to focus ultrasonic energy are described in the following Sub-sections.

2.3.a Curved Transducers

The theory of self-focusing radiators of curved section has been discussed by O'Neil (1949). In the case of a spherical concave radiator, vibrating with uniform normal velocity, and with radius a of the circular boundary large

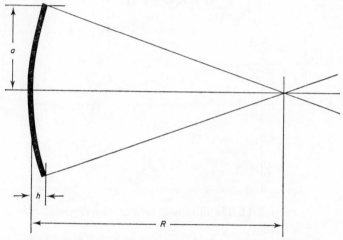

FIG. 2.10 The ultrasonic field of a self-focusing radiator.

in relation to both λ and the depth h (see Fig. 2.10) the ratio of the intensity at the centre of curvature to the intensity at the radiating surface is given by

$$I_r/I_0 = (kh)^2 \tag{2.11}$$

This ratio can be made large by suitable choice of dimensions, and the focusing is then very sharp.

The point of greatest intensity lies on the central axis. It is not at the centre of curvature, but it approaches this position from the radiator as kh becomes greater. The greatest intensity is not much greater than the intensity at the centre of curvature, however, except when kh is small. At the central part of the focal plane, the directivity function is identical to that of a plane disc transducer of radius a, as given in Eqn. 2.7.

2.3.b Lenses

The subject of ultrasonic lenses has been reviewed by Fry and Dunn (1962).

Lenses for ultrasonic applications are generally fabricated from solids, in which the velocity is greater than that in water. Therefore converging lenses are concave. The important dimensions of a spherical lens system are shown in Fig. 2.11. The focal length F is the distance from the point on the curved surface on the central axis to the midpoint of the region of convergence; R is the radius of curvature; a is the radius of the lens; and 2ψ is the aperture angle. Provided that $h < 0.1R$, and the angles of incidence and refraction are small enough for their sines to be not significantly different from their tangents,

$$F \simeq R/(1 - 1/n) \tag{2.12}$$

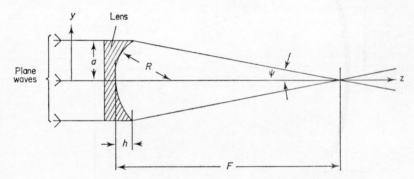

Fig. 2.11 The ultrasonic field of a lens system.

where the refractive index $n = c_1/c_2$, c_1 being the velocity in the lens, and c_2, that in the loading medium.

The rays leaving the spherical surface all converge at a distance F along the central axis. However, the rays originating from points of differing y-coordinate (or on annuli of differing y-coordinate generated by rotation about the plane perpendicular to the z-axis) are out of phase due to spherical aberration. (Elliptical lenses, on the other hand, do not suffer from this limitation, but they are more difficult to construct.) Consequently, the useful aperture of a spherical lens is restricted. If this limitation is chosen to correspond to the maximum aperture from which rays do not arrive at the focus with more than $\pi/2$ radians phase difference then

$$\lambda_2 \leqslant \frac{F^2 \tan^4\psi}{2Rn(n - 1 + n \tan^2 \psi)} \tag{2.13}$$

where λ_2 is the wavelength in the loading medium.

The lens should be made as thin as possible in order to minimize absorption losses. Transmission through a lens the characteristic impedance of which differs from the surrounding media is controlled by interference (see Section 1.11). Maximum transmission occurs in those regions where the lens thickness is an integral number of half wavelengths. Transmission is a minimum where the thickness is an odd integral number of quarter wavelengths. According to Tarnóczy (1965), the difference between interference maxima and minima is about 3 dB with a polymethylmethacrylate lens in water. The quarter-wave interference losses can be minimized by the use of a zone lens, in which the surface is stepped in half-wave increments. Experimental data for such a zone lens have been reported by Golis (1968) including results obtained with a plastic lens with an elliptical section.

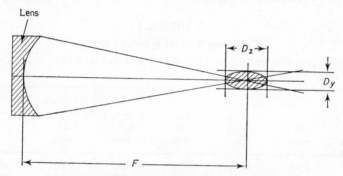

FIG. 2.12 The focal region of a focusing system.

The size and shape of the focal region depends upon the wavelength, in addition to the aperture and focal length of the lens. Consequently in practice a point focus cannot be achieved, and the situation illustrated in Fig. 2.12 exists. According to Fry and Dunn (1962), the focal volume is roughly ellipsoidal, the intensity being reduced by 3 dB from the maximum value in x–y plane where the diameter is given by

$$D_y = D_x \simeq k_t \lambda_2 F / 2a \qquad (2.14)$$

where k_t is a dimensionless factor the value of which is dependent upon ψ; if $\psi < 50°$, solutions to Eqn. 2.14 are correct to within 20% if k_t is taken to be equal to 1·0. Similarly, the length of the focal volume in the central z-axis is given by

$$D_s \simeq k_a D_y \qquad (2.15)$$

where k_a is a dimensionless factor; if $\psi < 50°$, an error of less than 15% in the value of k_a is introduced by taking it to be equal to $15(1 - 0·01\psi)$, ψ being expressed in degrees.

The intensity "gain" of a focusing system is defined as

$$G = I_F/I_0 \qquad (2.16)$$

where I_F is the intensity at the focus, and I_0 is the intensity at the entrance to the focusing system. If $\psi \leqslant 15°$

$$G = 0{\cdot}8 \, (2a/D_y)^2 \qquad (2.17)$$

Some typical values calculated from Eqns. 2.12–2.17 are given in Table 2.1. It is important to notice that these results do not take account of differences in the absorption coefficients of the lenses and the loading media. Generally the lens has the higher coefficient of absorption, and its increasing thickness towards its edge has the effect of reducing the radiated amplitude. This modifies the ultrasonic field (by reducing the side-lobe intensities: see Section 2.4), and reduces the gain of the system.

TABLE 2.1

Focusing lenses: typical values

Data for polystyrene lenses ($c_1 = 2350$ m s^{-1}) in water ($c_2 = 1500$ m s^{-1}), $n = 1{\cdot}57$; $F = 100$ mm, $R = 36{\cdot}3$ mm

				Values for ψ_{max}		
f MHz	λ_2 mm	ψ_{max} deg	a mm	$D_y = D_x$ mm	D_z mm	G
1	1·50	18·6	33·6	2·2	27·2	~750
3	0·50	14·0	24·8	1·0	13·0	2000
10	0·15	10·2	18·0	0·4	5·6	6500

The performance of a focusing system can be increased if a quarter-wave matching layer (see Section 1.11) is used to maximize the transmission between the transducer and the lens (Fry and Dunn, 1962).

The choice of the best material from which to construct a lens is determined by the optimum compromise between several conflicting factors. Ideally, the lens material should have an absorption coefficient of zero, a characteristic impedance equal to that of the loading medium, and the maximum value of refractive index. If water is the loading medium, there is no material at present available which satisfies all these conditions.

FIG. 2.13 Some typical focusing systems using mirrors. (a) A paraboloid, which focuses a parallel beam without aberration; (b) a system giving a forward focus (based on Fry and Dunn, 1962); (c) a system giving a forward focus, with a large effective aperture: the ellipsoid has two foci, the hyperboloid being placed to intercept the energy converging towards the minor focus (based on Olofsson, 1963).

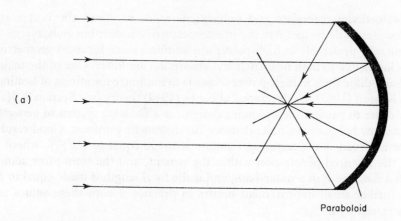

(a)

Paraboloid

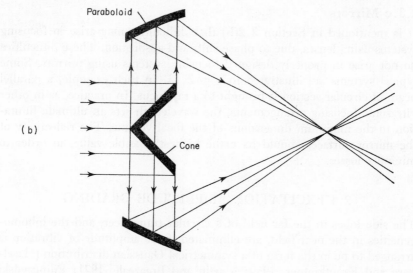

Paraboloid

(b)

Cone

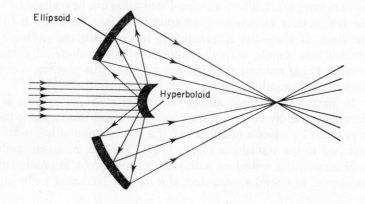

Ellipsoid

Hyperboloid

Polymethylmethacrylate and polystyrene seem to afford the best compromises. The former has the greater refractive index; but polystyrene is generally preferable in high-power applications, since for most geometries its losses due to both mismatch and absorption are lower. One of the major design difficulties in high-power lenses is to minimize the effects of heating.

Kossoff (1963) has developed O'Neil's (1949) theory (see Section 2.3(a)) in order to predict the optimum design for a focusing system to generate a narrow beam over a finite distance for diagnostic purposes. Good results are achieved if the transducer radius is made equal to $(\lambda P)^{1/2}$, where P is the required penetration within the patient, and the transducer stands off a distance P in a water-bath, and if the focal length is made equal to P. A further small improvement occurs in practice if both these values are increased by 20%.

2.3.c Mirrors

It is mentioned in Section 2.2(b) that difficulties may arise in focusing systems using lenses, due to phase shift and absorption. These difficulties do not arise in properly designed focusing systems using mirrors. Some typical systems are illustrated in Fig. 2.13. In each example, a parallel beam of circular section is brought to a ray focus. In practice, as in other ultrasonic focusing arrangements, the wavelength sets an ultimate limitation to the minimum dimensions of the focal volume. The reflectivity of the mirror surfaces should have the highest possible value, in order to minimize losses.

2.4 EXCITATION AMPLITUDE GRADING

The side lobes in the far field of a circular transducer, and the inhomogeneities in the near field, are eliminated if the amplitude of vibration is arranged to be in the form of a symmetrical Gaussian distribution (Haselberg and Krautkramer, 1959; Martin and Breazeale, 1971; Filipczyński and Etienne, 1973). The Gaussian distribution can be realized by arranging the rear surface electrode of the transducer (see Section 3.6.b) to be in the form of a rosette. Alternatively, the rear surface electrode may be divided into annuli, with the amplitude of the electrical drive to each annulus being reduced with increasing radius: in practice, a central disc with a single annulus may be satisfactory (Kossoff, 1971).

In narrow-band applications—and even with pulses of a few cycles duration—the divergence of the ultrasonic beam from a plane disc source is reduced by a factor of about two if a combination of half-wave plates is attached to the transducer (Lale, 1969). This improvement comes about because multiple reflexions within the plates remain in phase with normal incidence, but tend to interfere due to the increased path length with oblique incidence. Transducers with diameters of less than 15 wavelengths gain most from the phenomenon. Its principal disadvantage is that multiple reflexions, upon which the method depends, stretch the pulse.

2.5 SCATTER

In earlier Sections of this Chapter, certain wave phenomena are explained by consideration of the spatial and temporal distributions of the corresponding Huygen's wave sources. Firstly, in the case of an interface which is large in relation to the wavelength, the laws of reflexion and refraction may be derived by the application of the coincidence principle. Secondly, in the case of a vibrating source (or receiver), the beam distribution may be considered in terms of diffraction.

This Section is concerned with the converse situation in which an obstacle is placed in an infinite plane wave field. The total disturbance of the incident wave may be considered to be due to interference between the incident wave and a particular set of Huygen's wave sources distributed over the surface of the obstacle. The interfering radiation pattern of the obstacle is called the *scattered wave field*. This approach can be used to explain reflexion, diffraction and shadow formation by an obstacle.

Scattering of waves by an obstacle is a function of the *scattering cross-section S* of the obstacle. This is defined as the ratio of the total power scattered by the obstacle to the incident wave intensity. Three situations may be distinguished:

(i) Where the obstacle is very much larger than the wavelength, the radiation is reflected specularly and a shadow is formed. This situation differs only semantically from that in which the boundary of the field is determined by the size of the ultrasonic beam. The scattering cross-section $S = 1$ for a perfect reflector.

(ii) Where the obstacle is very much smaller than the wavelength, the radiation is scattered uniformly in all directions, and the incident wave is diffracted around the obstacle, suffering only minor perturbation. If the object is a spherical reflector,

$$S \propto k^4 a^6 \tag{2.18}$$

where a = radius of the sphere. This result follows the well-known relation in the Rayleigh scattering of light, where the intensity of the scattered wave is inversely proportional to the fourth power of the wavelength if $kr \ll 1$ since $k = 2\pi/\lambda$.

(iii) Where the obstacle has dimensions which are similar to the wavelength, the scattered radiation has a distribution which is both complex and critically dependent upon the dimensions and characteristic impedance of the obstacle. Scattering by cylinders and

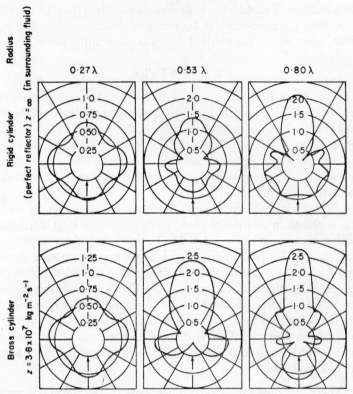

FIG. 2.14 Scattering polar diagrams for two types of cylinders in water. (From data of Faran, 1951.)

spheres has been reviewed by Faran (1951), on whose paper the data illustrated in Fig. 2.14 are based.

The situation often occurs in which an ultrasonic field is scattered by a uniformly random or pseudorandom distribution of relatively arbitrary discontinuities in characteristic impedance, which are individually small in size in relation to the wavelength. The subject has been reviewed by Twersky (1964), who has dealt with the bulk parameters of various scattering configurations. At megahertz frequencies, biological materials can generally be considered to correspond to this kind of model. In practice, experiments to test the theory are difficult to make, because the beam dimensions and attenuation introduce complications, as has been demonstrated with air bubbles in water by Mole *et al.* (1972). Sigelmann and Reid (1973) described a tone-burst method for the determination of scattering due to blood. The matter is discussed further in Chapter 5.

3. GENERATION AND DETECTION

3.1 TRANSDUCERS

A *transducer* is a device which can convert one form of energy into another. The ultrasonic transducers described in this Chapter are used to convert electrical energy into ultrasonic energy, and vice versa. Two types, magnetostrictive and piezoelectric, are discussed in this Section. Subsequent Sections deal with the generation and detection of ultrasonic energy. Other types of transducer are later described for the detection, visualization, and measurement of ultrasonic fields.

One of the factors which needs to be considered in choosing the type of transducer best suited to any particular application is the frequency. Ultrasonic waves have frequencies above the range of human hearing (i.e. above about 20 kHz).

3.1.a Magnetostrictive Transducers

Certain materials have the property that the application of a magnetic field causes a change in physical dimensions, and vice versa. This phenomenon is known as *magnetostriction*. It occurs in ferromagnetic materials and ferrites (which are synthetic ceramics). Magnetostriction was first described by J. P. Joule in 1847.

In the absence of an applied magnetic field, the magnetic domains of a magnetostrictive material are randomly orientated. The magnetism of such a material is caused by spin vectors of certain groups of electrons. These spins are more or less parallel within each domain. The shape of the domain is asymmetrical: the individual magnetic dipoles may be arranged either along the long axis, or the short axis, or some other axis of the domain, according to the particular material. The application of an external magnetic field tends to change the orientation of the spins by the rotation of the domains, and it is this rotation which causes the change which occurs in the dimensions of the material. This change may be either positive or negative, and for a given field strength it is in the same direction irrespective of the sign of the applied field.

The magnetic field is usually applied to the magnetostrictive material by means of a solenoid. The magnetic field H within a solenoid consisting of

n turns over a length l metres, carrying a current i amperes, is given by

$$H = in/l \qquad [\text{A m}^{-1}] \qquad (3.1)$$

The magnetic field H is related to the flux density B within the core as follows:

$$B = \mu\mu_0 H \qquad [\text{Wb m}^{-2}] \qquad (3.2)$$

where μ is the permeability of the core relative to μ_0, the permeability of free space. The value of μ_0 is constant (equal to $4\pi \times 10^{-7}$ J A^{-2} m^{-1}); but μ has a value which depends upon the ratio B/H for any particular material and degree of magnetization. The relationship between B and H may be represented by the shape of the magnetic hysteresis loop, as shown in Fig. 3.1.

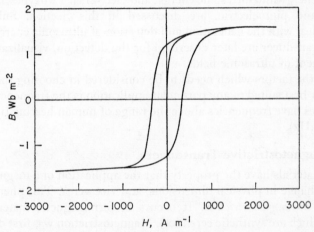

FIG. 3.1 Hysteresis loop for a typical magnetostrictive material (Permalloy 45).

The relationship between the mechanical strain and the applied magnetic field strength and flux density is illustrated, for three common magnetostrictive materials, in Fig. 3.2. (Values for representative points on these curves are given in Table 3.1.) The graphs indicate a square-law relationship of the form:

$$\delta l/l = \Delta = CB_0^2 \qquad (3.3)$$

where $\delta l/l$ is the mechanical strain (equal to Δ, the change in length per unit length) which results from the application of a static flux density B_0, and C is a factor which depends upon the material, and has units [m^{4}Wb^{-2}]. It should be noted that if an alternating magnetic field is applied—for example, by introducing the magnetostrictive material into the field of a solenoid carrying an alternating electric current—the magnetostrictor generally oscillates at twice the frequency of the magnetic field. (Some materials—for example, iron and cast cobalt—exhibit more complicated relationships between strain and applied field. In the case of iron, an increasing field produces first an increase and then a decrease in length; cast cobalt, on the other hand, first decreases in length, and then increases.) Although Eqn. 3.3 is non-linear, a linear relationship between Δ and B can be obtained if B, the alternating flux density, is both made very small and it is also superimposed on a larger, steady flux. By differentiating Eqn. 3.3 with respect to B, and setting $x = d\Delta$ and $B = dB_0$,

$$x = 2CB_0B \qquad (3.4)$$

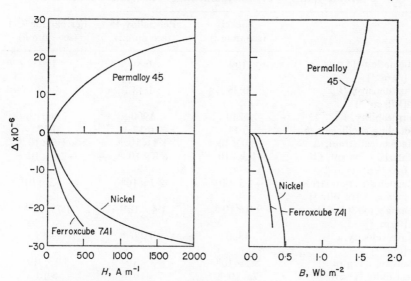

FIG. 3.2 Characteristics of some typical magnetostrictive materials. (Data from Hueter and Bolt, 1955; van der Burgt, 1957, 1958.)

Then, by defining the stress X thus:

$$X = \Lambda B \qquad (3.5)$$

where Λ is called the *magnetostriction stress factor*, with units [N Wb^{-1}], and by applying Hooke's law ($X = xY_0$, where Y_0 is Young's modulus), it follows that

$$\Lambda = 2CB_0Y_0 \qquad (3.6)$$

The ability of a magnetostrictive transducer to convert electrical to mechanical energy, and vice versa, is measured by its magnetomechanical coupling coefficient k_m, defined by

$$k_m^2 = \text{(stored mechanical energy)/(total stored energy)} \qquad (3.7)$$

The quantity k_m^2 is quite distinct from the efficiency of the transducer. If the transducer is lossless, its efficiency is unity: all the applied energy is stored, and none is converted to heat. The storage is either magnetic or elastic. The magnetomechanical coupling coefficient describes how the total energy is shared in storage: it is a measure of the magnetostrictive coupling. Only the energy which is stored elastically (i.e. mechanically) is available in the proper circumstances to appear as ultrasonic waves in a suitable load.

TABLE 3.1

Characteristics of some typical magnetostrictive materials

	Nickel (see note i)	Permalloy 45 (see note i)	Ferroxcube 7A1 (see note ii)
Magnetic field,* H [A m^{-1}]	160	600	190
Flux density, B [Wb m^{-2}]	0·25	1·43	0·23
Permeability, μ	1240	1900	960
Coupling coefficient, k_m	0·14	0·12	0·27
Mechanical strain, Δ	$-8\cdot0 \times 10^{-6}$	$1\cdot4 \times 10^{-5}$	$-1\cdot5 \times 10^{-5}$
Material constant, C [m^4 Wb^{-2}]	$-1\cdot3 \times 10^{-4}$	$6\cdot8 \times 10^{-6}$	$-2\cdot9 \times 10^{-4}$
Magnetostriction stress factor, Λ [N Wb^{-1}]	$-1\cdot3 \times 10^{7}$	$2\cdot7 \times 10^{6}$	$-2\cdot3 \times 10^{7}$
Young's modulus, Y_0 [N m^{-2}]	$2\cdot0 \times 10^{11}$	$1\cdot4 \times 10^{11}$	$1\cdot7 \times 10^{11}$
Wave velocity, c [m s^{-1}]	4850	4100	5440
Density, ρ [kg m^{-3}]	$8\cdot7 \times 10^{3}$	$8\cdot3 \times 10^{3}$	$5\cdot2 \times 10^{3}$
Resistivity [Ω m]	7×10^{-8}	7×10^{-7}	>10
Curie temperature [°C]	365	440	530

* Where relevant, other values correspond to this operating point.

(i) Data extracted chiefly from Hueter and Bolt (1955). *Permalloy* 45 is an alloy: 45% nickel, 55% iron.

(ii) Data from van der Burgt (1957, 1958). *Ferroxcube* is a ceramic ferrite developed by N. V. Philips' Gloeilampenfabricken, Eindhoven, Netherlands.

Note that the value of k_m is not constant; it depends upon the relationship between B and H corresponding to the instantaneous coordinates of the operating point on the hysteresis loop.

The magnetostrictive effect is temperature dependent. The coupling decreases with increasing temperature, disappearing altogether (i.e. $k_m = 0$) at temperatures above the *Curie* temperature.

In any particular application, the choice of the magnetostrictive material depends upon several factors, such as the operating frequency, the ultrasonic intensity, the environment, and economics. An important source of inefficiency in metallic transducers is due to eddy current losses. These are minimized by using a laminated construction. At a frequency of about 50 kHz, a laminated nickel transducer has an efficiency of about 40%, whereas a ferrite transducer is 80% efficient. The losses in metallic transducers become even less favourable at higher frequencies, and ferrites are the only satisfactory magnetostrictors. These materials have very high resistivity, and so they have relatively low eddy current losses. The maximum ultrasonic intensity is determined by the elastic limit and fatigue characteristic of the magnetostrictive material. In these respects, metals are generally superior to ceramics, which can be expected to operate safely only at intensities of less than about 20 W cm^{-2} in water. Metals tend to be more susceptible than ceramics to damage by the attack of the loading medium, for the latter are chemically inert and non-porous. Mass-produced ceramics are generally cheaper than metals.

3.1.b Piezoelectric Transducers

Certain materials have the property that the application of an electric field causes a change in physical dimensions, and vice versa. This phenomenon is known as the *piezoelectric effect*. It occurs in materials which are anisotropic, and which therefore lack centres of symmetry. The piezoelectric effect was first described by Pierre and Jacques Curie in 1880.

The electric charges bound within the crystal lattice of the material interact with the applied electric field, to produce a mechanical stress. In this way, piezoelectricity provides a coupling between electric and dielectric phenomena. Certain crystals which occur in nature are piezoelectric: quartz and tourmaline are the most common examples. Similar characteristics are found in many artificially grown crystals, such as those of ammonium dihydrogen phosphate, lithium sulphate, and lead niobate.

Another group of artificial materials, known as *ferroelectrics*, possess strong piezoelectric properties. In these materials, the individual charge domains are preferentially aligned along the polarization axis, in a manner analogous to the orientation of the magnetic domains in a ferromagnetic material in a magnetic field (see Section 3.1.a). The analogy leads to the term "ferroelectric". The phenomenon was discovered by Joseph Valasek in 1921.

There is a great variety of ferroelectric materials. Amongst the ceramic types, barium titanate was the first to be discovered. This has largely been replaced by lead zirconate titanate, which was originally developed by Jaffe *et al.* (1955). Several types of lead zirconate titanate are commercially available: although basically similar, during manufacture different chemicals are added and variations are made in thermal treatment in order to give the required properties. Mechanically, ceramic ferroelectrics are hard, light grey or brown materials, chemically inert and unaffected by humidity. Although somewhat brittle, they are extremely stiff and capable of exerting or sustaining large forces.

The electric field is usually applied to the piezoelectric material by means of two electrodes, one on each surface normal to the axis of polarization. (In ceramic ferroelectrics, the polarization process is carried out by first heating the material to a temperature in excess of the Curie temperature, and then allowing it to cool slowly with a strong electric field—typically 2 kV mm^{-1}—applied between the electrodes. As in magnetostriction, the Curie temperature is that above which the coupling coefficient is zero.)

The strain produced in a piezoelectric material by the application of unit electric field is called the piezoelectric coefficient d. Therefore the d coefficient is often called the *transmitting constant* of the material. Alternatively, the d coefficient may be defined by the converse relationship of the charge density output per unit applied stress under short-circuit conditions. It is measured in units $[\text{m V}^{-1}]$.

The piezoelectric coefficient g is defined as the electric field produced under open-circuit conditions per unit applied stress. The g coefficient is often called the *receiving constant* of the material, because receiving amplifiers fed from transducers are often voltage sensitive, rather than charge sensitive. It is measured in units $[\text{V m N}^{-1}]$.

The dielectric constant ϵ of a piezoelectric material depends upon the extent of mechanical freedom of the transducer. Two values are generally quoted. Firstly, the transducer is clamped so that it cannot move in response to an applied field: this value is designated as ϵ^S. Secondly, the transducer is allowed unrestricted movement: this value is designated as ϵ^T. These two values are related by the electromechanical coupling coefficient k_e, defined in the same way as the magnetomechanical coupling coefficient k_m (see Eqn. 3.7), as follows:

$$\epsilon^S/\epsilon^T = (1 - k_e^2) \tag{3.8}$$

Thus, the quantity k_e^2 is equal to the fractional decrease in the permittivity of the material due to the piezoelectric effect. Unlike magnetostrictive materials, k_e^2 has a constant value if the transducer is operated within its electrical and mechanical breakdown stress limits.

The piezoelectric coefficients d and g are related to the dielectric constant thus:

$$d/g = \epsilon^T \tag{3.9}$$

A stress applied to a solid in any direction can be resolved into six components, three of tensile stress and three of shear stress, each acting along one of three orthogonal axes. Piezoelectric coefficients are usually described in tensor notation, which enables the effect along any one axis to be expressed. A double subscript is used to describe each coefficient: the first subscript is in the electrical direction, and the second is in the mechanical direction. Subscripts 1, 2 and 3 apply to electric fields and tensile stresses and strains along the x, y and z axes respectively. Subscripts 4, 5 and 6 apply to shear stresses and strains, also along the x, y and z axes respectively. Thus d_{11} is the transmitting constant which relates voltage to tensile strain along the x-axis; d_{31} relates voltage along the z axis to tensile strain along the x-axis; and so on.

A thickness expanding quartz transducer is cut so that its thickness lies along the crystallographic x-axis. Such transducers are called "x-cut" plates; the corresponding piezoelectric transmitting and receiving constants are designated d_{11} and g_{11} respectively. However, it happens that the convention for piezoelectric ceramics corresponds to polarization and expansion along the z-axis for thickness expanding transducers, and the appropriate transmitting and receiving constants are d_{33} and g_{33}.

It can be seen from Eqn. 3.9 that, for a given value of g, the value of d is large if the dielectric constant is large, and vice versa. A large value of d is desirable for a transmitter, and a large value of g, for a receiver. A large value of dielectric constant is also desirable in a receiver operating at low megahertz frequencies, because this minimizes the relative shunting effect of the capacitance of the connecting cable and the input circuit of the receiving amplifier. For this reason, a large value of ϵ may in practice be a more desirable attribute of a receiver than a large value of g.

If a transducer is to operate both as a transmitter and as a receiver, it is desirable for both d and g to be large. It can be seen from Eqns. 3.8 and 3.9 that higher values of dg tend to be associated with higher values of k_e.

The more important mechanical and electrical coefficients of quartz, and of two typical lead zirconate titanates, are given in Table 3.2. The choice of the most suitable transducer material depends upon the particular application for which it is intended. The lead zirconate titanates listed in Table 3.2 have similar piezoelectric constants, but the mechanical Q-factor (see Section 3.3) of PZT-4 is substantially greater than that of PZT-5. Therefore PZT-4 is better suited for use in narrow-frequency-band systems, whereas PZT-5 may be chosen for short-pulse applications in which a broad-band frequency response is desirable. The lead zirconate titanates are superior to quartz in practically every respect at frequencies below about 15 MHz. For fundamental operation at higher frequencies (see Section 3.2), quartz may offer advantages because of its excellent mechanical properties and low electrical capacitance. Another material which may have significant advantages in certain situations is lithium sulphate. This has a g_{33} value which is seven times greater than that of PZT-5, but its ϵ value is 150 times lower. A disadvantage of lithium sulphate is that it is hygroscopic.

A great advantage of the piezoelectric ceramics is that they may be formed into any desired shape during manufacture, and polarized in any required direction. Although the most usual shape is a thickness-expanding disc, two other configurations are quite often used in ultrasonic applications. Firstly, spherical bowls are used, generally to produce focused ultrasonic fields. Secondly, cylinders with electrodes bonded on to their inner and outer curved surfaces are used as length expanders to drive various probes, and as omnidirectional receiving elements. In this con-

TABLE 3.2

Properties of some typical piezoelectric materials

	Quartz, x-cut (see note i)	PZT-4 (see note ii)	PZT-5A (see note ii)
Tensor subscript	11	33	33
Transmitting constant, d [m V^{-1}]	$2 \cdot 31 \times 10^{-12}$	289×10^{-12}	374×10^{-12}
Receiving constant, g [V m N^{-1}]	$5 \cdot 78 \times 10^{-2}$	$2 \cdot 61 \times 10^{-2}$	$2 \cdot 48 \times 10^{-2}$
Coupling coefficient, k_e	$0 \cdot 10$	$0 \cdot 70$	$0 \cdot 71$
Dielectric constant, ϵ^T [F m^{-1}]	$4 \cdot 00 \times 10^{-11}$	1150×10^{-11}	1500×10^{-11}
Wave velocity, c [m s^{-1}]	5740	4000	3780
Density, ρ [kg m^{-3}]	2650	7500	7750
Characteristic impedance, Z [kg m^{-2} s^{-1}]	$1 \cdot 52 \times 10^{7}$	$3 \cdot 00 \times 10^{7}$	$2 \cdot 93 \times 10^{7}$
Mechanical Q	> 25000	> 500	75
Curie temperature [°C]	573	328	365

(i) Data quoted by Cady (1946), Mason (1950), and from Bechman (1958).
(ii) Data extracted from Bulletin 66011/E, Vernitron Ltd., Southampton, UK. PZT is a registered trade name of Vernitron Ltd., Southampton, UK.

figuration, the transducer acts as a length expander because of the elastic coupling between radial and axial strains.

An interesting development, not new but only recently described in English, was the discovery of the piezoelectric effect in elongated and polarized films of polymers, particularly of polyvinylidene fluoride (Kawai, 1969). These polymers have the usual properties of flexible plastic films. Typical piezoelectric properties are: $k_e = 0 \cdot 1$; $Z = 4 \times 10^6$ kg m^{-2} s^{-1}; and $Q = 3$. These values may be compared with those listed in Table 3.2, for more conventional materials. In particular, the characteristic impedance of polyvinylidene fluoride is less than three times that of water, so that excellent matching is possible, and this combined with the low Q-factor implies that plastic transducers should be capable of operating with short pulses at quite high efficiencies.

3.2 RESONANCE

The application of a sinusoidal electrical driving signal to a transducer results in a corresponding variation in the thickness of the transducer. The movements of the faces of the transducer radiate energy into the media in contact with them, the quantity of energy radiated at each face being determined by the characteristic impedances at the boundary between the transducer and the medium, as described in Section 1.8. Therefore, some of the vibrational energy is reflected back into the transducer at each face, except in the unusual circumstance where the characteristic impedances are equal.

The energy reflected at each face of the transducer travels back across the transducer towards the opposite face. Meanwhile, if sinusoidal excitation is employed, the instantaneous value of the driving signal applied to the transducer is changing, so that when the energy reflected within the transducer arrives at the opposite face, a new stress situation exists due to the magneto- or electromechanical coupling. The total stress is equal to the sum of the instantaneous values of the stress due to mechanical coupling, and that due to the reflected wave. The phase relationship between these stresses depends upon the thickness and the propagation velocity in the transducer, and the frequency of the driving signal. If the thickness of the transducer is exactly half a wavelength, the stresses reinforce each other, and the transducer oscillates with maximum displacement amplitudes at its faces. This condition is known as *resonance*. The displacement amplitudes are minimum if the stresses oppose each other: this situation occurs where the transducer is of wavelength thickness.

The frequency which corresponds to half wavelength thickness is called the *fundamental* resonance frequency of the transducer. The transducer also resonates when driven at frequencies at which the thickness is equal to an odd integral number of half wavelengths. A transducer which is being driven at three times its fundamental frequency is three half wavelengths thick, and is said to be operating at its *third harmonic*, and so on. From similar reasoning, the transducer oscillates with minimum amplitude when it is driven at frequencies at which its thickness is equal to an integral number of wavelengths (i.e. an even integral number of half wavelengths).

Maximum efficiency for power generation is generally obtained by the use of a transducer of half wavelength thickness, arranged with a low impedance at the end further from the load. In practice, this backing medium is often air. Almost complete reflexion then occurs at the back face of the transducer, so that almost all the power is available for transmission into the load. The efficiency of the transmission into the load may be increased by an impedance matching layer of quarter wavelength thickness (see Section 1.11).

The mechanical constructions of some typical transducer assemblies for power generation are illustrated in Fig. 3.3. The thickness of a half wavelength transducer at a given frequency is directly proportional to the propagation velocity in the transducer. For example, a 25 kHz magneto-

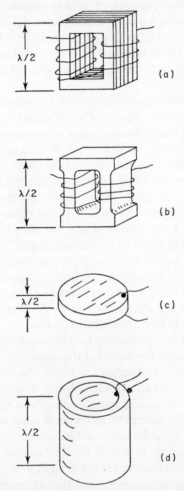

Fig. 3.3 Constructions of typical transducer types for ultrasonic power generation. (a) Window type magnetostrictive transducer, laminated metal construction; (b) window type magnetostrictive transducer, piezomagnetic ceramic construction; (c) disc type piezoelectric transducer; (d) length expanding cylinder type piezoelectric transducer.

strictive transducer constructed from nickel would have a thickness of 97 mm; and a 1 MHz piezoelectric transducer constructed from PZT-4 would have a thickness of 2·0 mm.

3.3 THE EQUIVALENT ELECTRICAL CIRCUIT

Any transducer may be represented by an equivalent electrical circuit. In order to derive such a circuit, it is necessary to consider all the factors which exist in the practical situation. A thorough treatment of the problem is

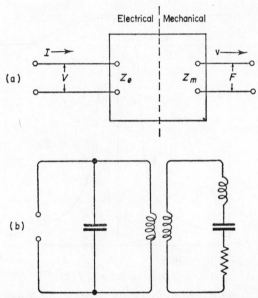

FIG. 3.4 Equivalent circuits of a transducer. (a) The four-terminal network; (b) the equivalent electrical circuit for a piezoelectric plate operating near resonance.

very complicated; but if radiation only takes place from one surface of the transducer, the situation may be represented by a four-terminal network with two electrical input terminals and two mechanical output terminals, as illustrated in Fig. 3.4(a). At the output terminals a mechanical force F applied over the transducer face of area A produces particle motion of velocity v. For plane waves their ratio is the *mechanical radiation resistance* Z_R given by:

$$Z_R = (\text{force})/(\text{particle velocity}) = pA/v = \rho cA \qquad (3.10)$$

by substitution from Eqn. 1.35. For most practical purposes, Z_R is a pure resistance. If the transducer is tuned to resonance, the mechanical radiation

3

resistance appears at the electrical terminals as a resistance R_e given by:

$$R_e = Z_R/4N^2 \qquad (3.11)$$

where N is the *amplitude transformation ratio*; the factor 4 arises from the doubling of velocity at the radiating face due to the low impedance at the opposite end.

The situation with a piezoelectric plate transducer may be represented by the equivalent circuit shown in Fig. 3.4(b). This is a simplification of the complete equivalent circuit, and is valid only at frequencies near resonance. For a rigorous treatment, see Gooberman (1968).

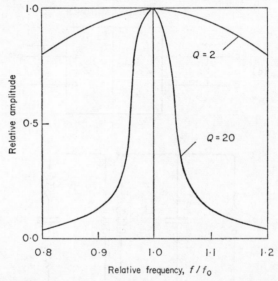

FIG. 3.5 The Q-factor related to frequency response, for two degrees of system damping.

The Q-factor of a transducer system describes its frequency response. Systems with a high Q have an output which is more critically dependent upon frequency than those with a low Q. The amplitude–frequency responses of two typical bandwidth-limited systems are illustrated in Fig. 3.5. The relationship is

$$Q = f_0/(f_2 - f_1) \qquad (3.12)$$

where f_0 is the resonance frequency (the frequency of maximum amplitude), and f_1 and f_2 are the frequencies below and above resonance at which the amplitude is reduced by $2^{1/2}$ (i.e. by approximately 3 dB).

A transducer system has two Q-factors, one mechanical and the other electrical. In the situation represented in Fig. 3.4, only the damping due to the load is considered: the losses due to the mounting of the transducer, and within the transducer, are neglected. In the case of many crystals, such as quartz, this may often be an adequate simplication; for magnetostrictive and piezoelectric ceramic transducers, however, these losses are seldom negligible (see Section 3.1).

3.4 IMPEDANCE MATCHING

The load presented by a transducer system may be represented by an electrical equivalent circuit, as discussed in Section 3.3. Losses occur if this load is not matched by the electrical impedance of the driving generator (or the receiver amplifier). Similarly, losses occur if the characteristic impedance of the mechanical load is not matched by that of the radiating surface of the transducer system. These two problems are dealt with separately in the following Sub-sections.

3.4.a Electrical Impedance Matching

Maximum efficiency is obtained when the electrical impedance of the generator (or the receiver) is matched to that of the transducer. This can be achieved by ensuring that the capacitance and inductance of the transducer (see Fig. 3.4(b)) form part of the tuned circuit of the associated electrical systems. In general,

$$f_0 = 1/\{2\pi(LC)^{1/2}\} \tag{3.13}$$

where L and C are the total parallel equivalent values of inductance and capacitance respectively.

3.4.b Mechanical Impedance Matching

The effects of matching the characteristic impedances of the backing and loading media to that of the transducer have been investigated amongst others by McSkimmin (1955) and Kossoff (1966). The frequency bandwidth of a transducer can be increased by the use of an impedance matching layer of appropriate thickness and characteristic impedance, included between the radiating surface of the transducer and the load. Such a layer acts as a mechanical transformer which reflects an increased load into the transducer (see Section 1.11). This would have no advantage in the case of an ideal transducer system with zero losses, because the input power could only be dissipated in the load. In a practical system, however, the losses due to absorption in a mechanical impedance matching layer may be less than those which occur in the transducer in the absence of matching, and the result may be an increase in efficiency. The matching layer is generally chosen to be of quarter wavelength thickness, and of characteristic impedance equal to the geometric mean of those of the transducer and of the loading medium. Such an arrangement is frequency selective, and this may further reduce the improvement of which it is potentially capable. The matter is discussed further in Section 3.6.b.v.

Mechanical impedance matching layers are seldom used with magneto-strictive transducers. Various materials have been used to match ferro-electric transducers to water-equivalent loads, including epoxy resin, both alone and supporting aluminium powder. For example, a characteristic impedance of 6.71×10^6 kg m^{-2} s^{-1} is required for the matching layer between PZT-4 and water, and this can be obtained by making a mixture of about 1·8 parts by weight of aluminium powder with 1 part of epoxy resin.

3.5 VELOCITY TRANSFORMERS

A velocity transformer is a mechanical device designed to match the impedance of the transducer to that of the load. This is achieved by funnelling the vibrations through a tapered structure. If the cross-sectional diameter of the taper is always less than half a wavelength, the particle velocity increases in inverse proportion to the taper diameter provided that no losses occur. Thus

$$v_i/v_0 = d_0/d_i \qquad (3.14)$$

where d is the diameter of the taper, and the suffixes i and o refer to the input and output planes respectively. Similarly,

$$I_i/I_0 = (d_0/d_i)^2 \qquad (3.15)$$

It may be seen from Eqns. 3.14 and 3.15 that the velocity transformer may be used to obtain very high ultrasonic particle velocities and intensities. For example, if $d_i = 50$ mm and $d_0 = 1$ mm, and $d_i < \lambda/2$, $v_0 = 50v_i$ and $I_0 = 2500 I_i$.

The length of a velocity transformer determines its operating frequency. This is because the material of which the transformer is constructed generally differs in characteristic impedance from that of the transducer and the load. Maximum efficiency occurs when the length is equal to an odd integral number of half-wavelengths, as this corresponds to the resonance frequency (see Section 3.2). The interface between the base of the taper and the transducer is located at a pressure node, whilst the tip of the taper vibrates with maximum amplitude.

The constructions of some typical velocity transformers are illustrated in Fig. 3.6. The exponential taper represented in Fig. 3.6(a) is generally the most satisfactory from the point of view of performance: the material is subjected to the minimum of stress for a given transformation ratio. In this case,

$$d_z^2 = d_i^2 e^{-sz} \qquad (3.16)$$

where s is the flare constant and z is the distance from the input end of the taper to the diameter d_z. It has been shown by Neppiras (1953) that the taper increases the propagation velocity to a value c' given by

$$c' = c_b/(1 - s^2 c^2/4\omega^2)^{1/2} \tag{3.17}$$

where c_b is the longitudinal bar velocity. This must be taken into account

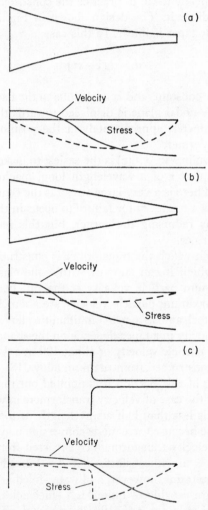

FIG. 3.6 Constructions of typical velocity transformers, showing stress and velocity distributions. (a) Exponential taper; (b) conical taper; (c) stepped taper.

in calculating the length of the transformer. Furthermore, the particle velocity is zero when

$$\tan (\omega z/c') = 2\omega/sc' \qquad (3.18)$$

The value of z given by Eqn. 3.18 corresponds to the position of the nodal plane. Velocity transformers are often mounted by means of a flange attached at the nodal plane. For most practical purposes it is adequate to take the position of the nodal plane to pass through the centre of gravity of the transformer.

Although theoretically ideal, in practice the construction of an exponential taper may be difficult. The design shown in Fig. 3.6(b) is relatively easy to make, as the taper is linear. In this case

$$d_z = d_i(1 - sz) \qquad (3.19)$$

where s is the taper constant, and is analogous to the flare constant in Eqn. 3.16. Similarly, the nodal plane is displaced towards the end of the taper with the larger diameter, approximately at the position of the centre of gravity of the transformer.

The system shown in Fig. 3.6(c) is the easiest to make. It consists of two cylinders, each a quarter of a wavelength long, machined from a single block of material. There is a very large stress at the centre of such a transformer, and there is a tendency for failure to occur in this plane. This risk may be reduced by radiusing the corner, but this reduces the effective ratio of the transformer.

The material from which the transformer is constructed determines the maximum stress which it can support within the elastic limit, and this controls the maximum particle velocity at the tip. In an untapered rod, typical values of maximum particle velocity are about 5·5 m s^{-1} in brass, 13.2 m s^{-1} in tool steel, and 32.6 m s^{-1} in titanium alloy 318. The maximum value of particle velocity in a taper depends on the shape of the taper: with optimum design, a particle velocity of about 100 m s^{-1} can be achieved at the tip of a taper constructed from titanium alloy 318.

At the beginning of this Section it is pointed out that the relationships given apply only in the case of velocity transformers in which largest cross-sectional diameter is less than half a wavelength. If $d_i > \lambda/2$, the situation is difficult to analyse because wave mode conversion may occur (see Section 1.9). In general, velocity transformers constructed from materials able to support shear waves are unsatisfactory if $d_i > \lambda/2$. Fluids are unable to support static shear strains, however, and water-filled velocity transformers in which $d_i > \lambda/2$ are capable of quite high efficiencies. For example, the velocity transformer of James et al. (1963) in which $d_i = 5$ mm and $d_0 = 2$ mm has an efficiency of about 80% at 3 MHz, which corresponds to $d_i/20 = \lambda/2$.

3.6 ULTRASONIC GENERATORS AND DETECTORS

This Section is concerned with the two kinds of transducer which are most commonly used to generate and detect ultrasonic waves.

3.6.a Magnetostrictive Generators

Examples of the two typical types of magnetostrictive generator are illustrated in Fig. 3.7. Both use magnetostrictive elements with winding windows. Velocity transformers (see Section 3.5) increase the amplitudes of the vibration at the outputs. The nodal supports are mounted through

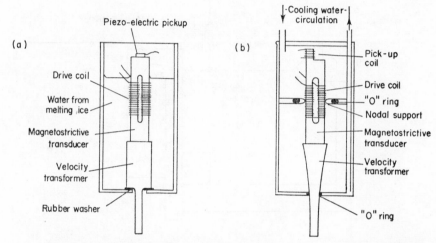

FIG. 3.7 Typical magnetostrictive generators. (a) An arrangement designed to irradiate small volumes of liquid: a piezoelectric transducer is used for positive feedback to the electrical oscillator (after Hughes and Cunningham, 1963); (b) an instrument which has a very high output amplitude at a small tip: a magnetically coupled pickup coil is used for feedback.

rubber, to minimize transmission losses. In higher-power systems it is necessary to cool the transducer by a heat exchanger; but this may not be required with lower powers.

The Q-factor of this type of generator is rather high, particularly when designed to operate at high power, and the resonance frequency is affected by the conditions of its mechanical loading. Therefore it may not be satisfactory to drive the generator from a fixed frequency source, since the frequency would be optimum only for a particular loading condition. The problem may be overcome by means of a vibration pick-up transducer arranged to optimize by positive feedback the frequency of an oscillatory loop. A typical circuit arrangement is illustrated in Fig. 3.8. The pickup transducer gives a voltage proportional to the motion of the magneto-strictor: this is fed back to the input of the power amplifier. The output power is determined by the characteristics of the amplifier.

An alternative method of automatic frequency control which does not require a pickup transducer has been described by, for example, Neppiras (1971). An electrical circuit is connected to the drive coil of the transducer which is the complex conjugate of the transducer electrical characteristics. The output from this circuit is proportional to the motion of the transducer.

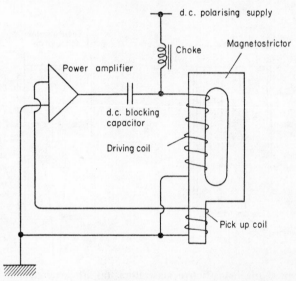

FIG. 3.8 Electrical driving arrangements for a magnetostrictive generator with mechanical pickup transducer. A magnetic pickup is illustrated, but the technique is equally applicable to a piezoelectric pickup.

The method has the advantages that no pick up transducer is required, there are no additional electrical connexions, and it is cheaper.

3.6.b Piezoelectric Generators and Detectors

Piezoelectric generators have a significant advantage in efficiency at frequencies in excess of about 500 kHz, in comparison with magneto-strictive types. Quite apart from this, the dimensions of a transducer operating at its fundamental resonance frequency decrease with increasing frequency, and it becomes increasingly difficult to construct a magneto-strictive system. Another advantage of the piezoelectric transducer is that it is possible to fabricate and to polarize non-planar shapes, such as are required for self-focusing (see Section 3.1.b).

(*i*) *Generators incorporating direct-radiating plane transducers*

At frequencies above about 500 kHz, the simplest source of ultrasonic energy is generally an electrically driven plane piezoelectric disc radiating directly into the load. The beam shape of such a source is discussed in Section 2.2.a. Three typical arrangements are illustrated in Fig. 3.9. The assembly of these units depends upon epoxy resin adhesive (such as Araldite*), which forms excellent bonds between metals and ceramics, and some plastics. Lead zirconate titanate (see Section 3.1.b) is often more satisfactory than quartz at frequencies below about 15 MHz: it has a low electrical impedance (requiring a relatively low driving voltage), a moderate Q-factor, and it is cheap.

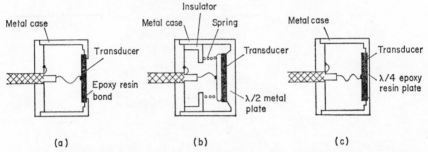

FIG. 3.9 Typical generators incorporating direct-radiating plane disc transducers. (a) No matching: the transducer radiates into the load through the front electrode only; (b) half-wave transmission layer, generally of metal; (c) quarter-wave transmission layer.

Air provides a low impedance backing, so that almost all of the energy is available for transmission into the load. Figure 3.9(a) shows the simplest system, in which only the front electrode lies between the transducer and the load. This has the advantage that there is very little to go wrong, but the assembly is rather fragile. This type of generator has been constructed by, amongst many others, Connolly (1968) and Wells (1968). An instrument with a transducer of only 1·5 mm diameter has been described by Kossoff *et al.* (1967).

A more robust arrangement is shown in Fig. 3.9(b): the transducer is protected from the load by a plate (usually of metal) of $\lambda/2$ thickness. The principal difficulty here is to ensure a continuous bond between the transducer and the plate, since any contained air greatly reduces the transmission into the load. In practice, the characteristic impedance of the

---

*Araldite is a trade name of CIBA-Geigy (UK) Ltd., Duxford, Cambridge, UK. For a typical epoxy resin, $c = 2800$ m s^{-1}, $\rho = 1200$ kg m^{-3}, and $\alpha = 2$ dB cm^{-1} at 1 MHz.

transducer is very different from that of the load, but this does not give rise to problems in continuous wave applications, since the systems operate at resonance and have high Q-factors. For moderately short-pulse work, however, the arrangement shown in Fig. 3.9(c) has the advantage that the characteristic impedance of the transducer is matched to that of the load by means of a quarter-wave layer (see Section 1.11). The disadvantages of this system are that it is necessary that the bonding should be perfect, and that the matching layer is often plastic-based, and so has a high absorption coefficient which limits the power which it can handle.

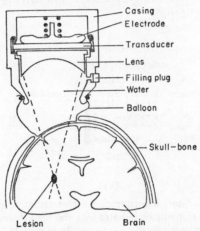

Fig. 3.10 A single-beam 2·7 MHz focused generator. In this example, the transducer is a 0·9 MHz quartz disc of 80 mm overall diameter, operating at the third harmonic frequency. (Based on Lele, 1962.)

(ii) Generators incorporating lenses

In much of the original work on ultrasonic neurosurgery (see Section 10.2), beams of ultrasound focused by lenses were used (see, for example, Fry 1958). A typical arrangement is shown in Fig. 3.10. The considerations which determine the lens design are discussed in Section 2.3.b. The coupling layer between the transducer and the lens is either castor oil or silicone oil. The lens is held so that it can expand sideways relative to the housing: this eliminates variations in the ultrasonic field due to flexure of the lens resulting from unequal coefficients of thermal expansion.

The maximum intensity which can be launched at the transducer surface of such a system is in the order of 10 W cm^{-2}. For a given size of transducer and irradiation configuration, this limits the intensity at the focus. In practice, the size of the transducer is limited by economics, and by the losses at the edge of the lens. If a greater focal intensity is required, several generators may be arranged so that their foci coincide both in position and in phase.

(iii) Generators incorporating velocity transformers

The arrangement illustrated in Fig. 3.11(a) is used to generate ultrasonics at a small tip at frequencies in the 0·1–1 MHz range. It is often called a *Mason horn*, after W. P. Mason, one of the pioneers of ultrasonic science. The transducer is a length-expanding cylinder of lead zirconate titanate, with silver electrodes bonded to the inside and outside curved surfaces.

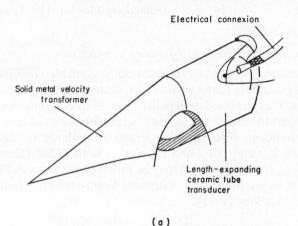

Electrical connexion

Solid metal velocity transformer

Length-expanding ceramic tube transducer

(a)

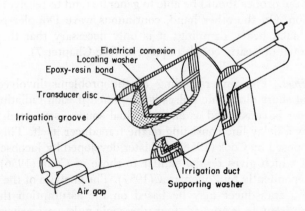

Electrical connexion
Locating washer
Epoxy-resin bond
Transducer disc
Irrigation groove
Irrigation duct
Supporting washer
Air gap

(b)

FIG. 3.11 Typical piezoelectric generators employing velocity transformers. (a) Solid cone; (b) water-filled cone (after James *et al.*, 1963).

The velocity transformer is bonded with epoxy resin to one end of the transducer, which is of length equal to $\lambda/2$. The considerations which determine the design of the solid metal velocity transformer are discussed in Section 3.5. It is mentioned in that Section that difficulties arise in solid velocity transformers if the dimensions are greater than about half a wavelength, and a solution to this problem is to use a liquid-filled velocity transformer. Such an arrangement is illustrated in Fig. 3.11(b). A refinement of this design is the air-filled cavity within the wall of the cone, which prevents the leakage of ultrasound. Water-filled velocity transformers of even larger sizes have been constructed by Gordon (1963) and Sjöberg et al. (1963).

(iv) Generators incorporating self-focusing transducers

Curved piezoelectric transducers are readily available commercially, and two typical generators based on them are illustrated in Fig. 3.12. In many applications, they are used to irradiate tissues in circumstances in which it is convenient to enclose the focused beam within a solid cone containing water (or physiological saline). The arrangement shown in Fig. 3.12(a) is the simplest, in that no cooling circulation is provided (Kossoff, 1964). Where cooling is necessary, this may be provided as shown in Fig. 3.12(b). A somewhat larger transducer, without a beam-enclosing cone, has been described by Coakley (1971).

(v) Generators designed for medical diagnostic applications

Most medical ultrasonic diagnostic probes fall into one of two categories. The first group is for pulse–echo applications (see Chapter 6): the requirement is that the probes should be able to generate (and to receive) pulses of short duration. On the other hand, continuous wave Doppler probes do not require such heavy damping; it is only necessary that they should operate at equal or nearly equal frequencies (see Chapter 7).

Basic principles. The understanding of the problems involved in the generation of short ultrasonic pulses is simplified if each radiating face of the transducer is considered as an individual source, separated from the other face by a delay line consisting of the transducer itself. This concept was first proposed by Cook (1956), and later developed by Jacobsen (1960). A treatment which gives results similar to those of Cook (1956) was developed independently by Ponomarev (1957). The analysis of the transient response of a transducer may be based on the assumption that, if an electrical step impulse is applied, four ultrasonic pulses are generated, two at each face. Of each of these two pairs of stress waves, one travels into the transducer, and the other travels into the loading or backing medium. The relative magnitudes of these pulses are determined by the characteristic

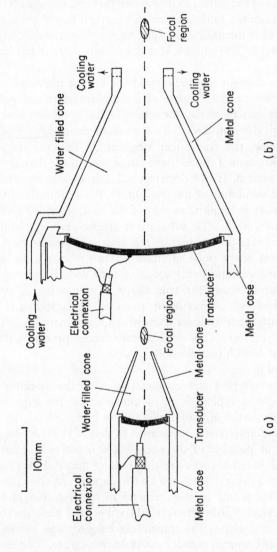

FIG. 3.12 Typical generators using self-focusing transducers. (a) Simple uncooled arrangement for operation at 3 MHz (after Kossoff, 1964); (b) 2 MHz system with water cooling.

impedances Z_t, Z_b and Z_l of the transducer, the backing and the load respectively. The two pulses within the transducer travel backwards and forwards, and are reflected and transmitted at the transducer faces. The stress wave in either the loading or the backing medium may be computed from the progress of the pulses as they move through the system. This kind of analysis is not limited to the case of an electrical step impulse, but it can be extended to other forms of excitation, such as the transient impulse and the gated sine wave. The process is described in more detail later in this Sub-section.

One of the commonest methods by which a short ultrasonic pulse may be generated is by the application of a transient electrical pulse to the transducer. This can be done, for example, by suddenly discharging a capacitor through the transducer. As a result of the sudden application of the electrical pulse, the transducer rings at its fundamental resonance frequency: the duration of the radiated stress wave pulse depends upon the Q-factor of the system. If the electrical pulse is short compared with the natural period of oscillation of the transducer, the amplitude of the second radiated stress wave is larger than that of the first, provided that the Q of the system permits this. The subsequent stress wave amplitudes decay exponentially at a rate determined by the system Q (see Section 3.3).

The observation of the pulse of stress waves presents some difficulties. A receiving transducer and oscilloscope of very wide frequency band are required in order to study the true shape of the pulse. A much more convenient method, which has many practical applications, is to reflect the pulse back into the transducer from which it originated, and to use this transducer as a receiver. This double transducing process has a double restriction on bandwidth (see Section 3.7.m).

It is mentioned in Section 3.4 that the mechanical Q of a transducer can be controlled by altering the characteristics of the backing medium. Figure 3.13 shows a typical form of construction for a probe for the generation and detection of short pulses. The backing material is chosen to have a similar characteristic impedance to that of the transducer, and to absorb as much as possible of the energy which enters it. Energy which enters, but which is not absorbed in the backing material may be reflected into the load after a delay determined by the dimensions and characteristics of the probe. This is one of the factors which determines the dynamic range of the device. Washington (1961) concluded that the best compromise for the material of the transducer backing was obtained with a 2 to 1 (by weight) tungsten powder in Araldite mixture. The compromise is between pulse duration and sensitivity: the shorter the pulse, the lower the sensitivity. This is because a large fraction of the total ultrasonic energy is absorbed by the backing in a device which generates a short pulse in the load. Lutsch (1962) investigated the properties of solid mixtures of tungsten and rubber powders in epoxy resins, from the point of view of providing the best backing material for pulse transducers. He recommended that the ratio of resin to tungsten powder should be chosen to satisfy the impedance specification, which determines the pulse length, and that rubber powder should be added to increase the attenuation. Rubber powder has similar characteristic impedance to that of epoxy resin, but, for example, the addition of 5% by volume of rubber powder to a 10% by volume mixture of tungsten powder in epoxy increases the attenuation from 5·6 to 8·0 dB cm^{-1} at 1 MHz. At this frequency, unloaded Araldite has an absorption coefficient of about 2·0 dB cm^{-1}.

The acoustic insulator shown in Fig. 3.13 between the case of the probe and the transducer and backing block assembly minimizes the coupling of ultrasonic energy into the case. This would be undesirable because the

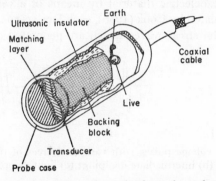

FIG. 3.13 Typical ultrasonic diagnostic probe for pulse–echo applications: mechanical damping is provided by the backing block of highly attenuating material (e.g. fine particles of tungsten suspended in epoxy resin).

case is often made of a low-loss material, such as a metal, and is likely to ring for some time in response to an ultrasonic transient. Ringing of the case would reduce the dynamic range of the device. Corprene (Higgs and Erikson, 1969), Nebar, cork, rubber, and plastics such as nylon and PTFE, are suitable acoustic insulators.

The radiating face of the transducer may be protected by a thin film of material, such as epoxy resin. The thickness of this film to some extent controls the performance of the device: this is discussed later in this Sub-section.

Figure 3.14 shows oscillograms of pulses, generated by the application of a fast electrical transient (about 0·05 μs rise time) to 2 MHz transducers with various backing materials. The degree of damping provided in the transducer used to obtain Fig. 3.14(a) was heavy, that in Fig. 3.14(c) light, and that in Fig. 3.14(b) an intermediate value. These oscillograms do not represent the real shapes of the corresponding ultrasonic stress waves, but they are the result of the double transducing process which has been previously described. Therefore, although the stress amplitudes of the third and subsequent half-cycles of the ultrasonic wave must be less than that of the second half-cycle (because of the form of excitation), nevertheless the observed pulse continues to build up for about six half-cycles in the case of the lightly damped transducer. This is because of the restricted bandwidth of the transducer when acting as a receiver. This theory is supported by the experimental results of Cook (1956), who demonstrated that the propagated stress wave from a transducer excited by a fast transient pulse consists of a series of stress transients with short rise times, alternating in polarity and separated by time intervals equal to one half the fundamental period of the transducer.

Single stress waves of very short duration may be generated by exciting a thick slab of piezoelectric material by means of a very short electrical transient. As postulated by Cook (1956), each face acts as a separate source. The duration of the stress waves which are generated depends upon the

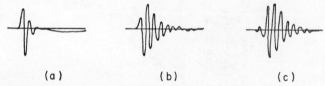

(a)   (b)   (c)

FIG. 3.14 Received voltage pulses with various degrees of transducer damping. (a) Heavy damping; (b) intermediate damping; (c) light damping.

duration of the electrical transient and the electrical loading of the system. For each excitation, an exponentially decaying train of stress waves is radiated into the load. The waves are separated by time intervals determined by the transit time (which may be made to be quite long) of a stress wave within the piezoelectric block. Details of some of the techniques involved have been given, for example, by Carome *et al.* (1964) and by Petersen and Rosen (1967). (It has been shown by Stuetzer (1967) that, in a short-circuited voltage-step excited plate, stress and current responses consist initially of alternating exponential pulses. These, in an unexpected manner, decay to a sine wave accompanied by a sequence of sharp spikes. Moreover, the spike and sinusoidal waveforms are characterized by different periods.)

It is possible to detect very fast stress waves in a similar manner, but confusion may arise if observation is attempted of several waves arriving spaced in time. If the wavetrain is sufficiently long, the later pulses are indistinguishable from secondary signals due to the earlier pulses travelling within the detector. In addition, the detector voltage is not a replica of the incident stress wave, but it is proportional to its time integral (Redwood,

1963; Carome *et al.*, 1964). This is because the voltage across the detector is proportional to the space integral of the strain within it, and the space profile of the strain is of the same form as the time profile of the incident stress wave. Thus, a voltage replica of the stress wave may be obtained by differentiation of the voltage output from the detector.

Detailed analysis. The mathematical analysis of the waveform of the stress wave generated by the application to the transducer of a given electrical voltage waveform is rather complicated. An extension of similar considerations applies to the case of a receiving transducer. The most thorough investigation seems to be due to Redwood (1961, 1963, 1964). For many practical applications, a graphical analysis described by Redwood (1963) will provide a sufficiently accurate result.

Redwood (1963) studied the specific case of a 10 mm diameter transducer of characteristic impedance 30×10^6 kg m^{-2} s^{-1} (barium titanate), radiating into a perfectly absorbent backing medium and a loading medium (water) of characteristic impedances 19×10^6 and $1\cdot5 \times 10^6$ kg m^{-2} s^{-1} respectively. The time of travel between the faces of the transducer was $0\cdot2$ μs corresponding to a fundamental resonance frequency of $2\cdot5$ MHz. Figure 3.15 shows the waveforms constructed by graphical analysis for this particular case. The exciting voltage waveform (Fig. 3.15(a)) was observed by means of a wide-band oscilloscope. Figure 3.15(b), which represents the radiated stress wave, was constructed from the voltage waveform, taking into account the external radiation from the front face of the transducer, the internal radiation from the back face, and the reflexion from the back face of the internal wave generated at the front face. Thus, the analysis is similar to that of Cook (1956), described earlier in this Sub-section. The fourth and subsequent terms were not included in the graphical construction, because they are small in amplitude and their estimation is subject to cumulative error.

Figure 3.15(b) was derived on the assumption that the voltage waveform is reproduced exactly as a stress waveform. However, the capacitive elements in the equivalent circuit of the transducer cannot be neglected in a rigorous analysis. Redwood (1963) calculated the effect of the transducer time constant on the radiated pulse. Figure 3.15(c) shows the modified waveform. The overall effect on shape is quite small, and the time positions of the wave peaks and zeros are negligibly affected. Thus, for most practical purposes, the effect of this time constant may be neglected. In this connexion, see also Stuetzer (1967).

If the stress wave shown in Fig. 3.15(c) is reflected back into the transducer, the output voltage depends upon the electrical load. With an open circuit transducer, the output voltage is proportional to the difference in the displacements of the surfaces, and the resultant voltage waveform is shown in Fig. 3.15(d). However, if the transducer is electrically loaded, the voltage waveform is modified by the introduction of a time constant in the equivalent circuit. Figure 3.15(e) shows the voltage waveform generated by the transducer in response to the stress wave shown in Fig. 3.15(c) with the transducer terminated by 37 Ω (two 75 Ω resistive loads in parallel) and an additional shunt capacitance of 800 pF.

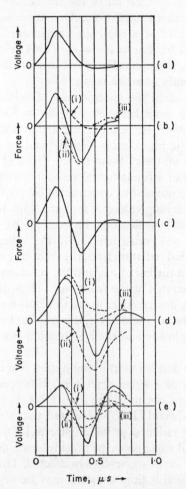

FIG. 3.15 Diagrams illustrating the pulse response of a 2·5 MHz transducer. (a) Exciting voltage waveform; (b) propagated stress wave; (c) propagated stress wave, modified by transducer time constant; (d) integration by open circuit detector; (e) effect of time constant in detection. (i), (ii) and (iii) correspond respectively to the contributions from the front face, the back face, and the front face by reflexion from the back face. (Adapted from Redwood, 1963.)

Redwood (1963) was able to verify the results of this analysis by experiment. For some measurements, a long block of piezoelectric ceramic was used as a non-resonant detector, and for others, the same transducer was used both to generate and to receive the pulses.

In principle, this method of analysis may be extended to other forms of electrical excitation and to the detection of other forms of stress wave. However, for conditions resulting from more complex excitations than the approximately half-sinusoid considered by Redwood (1963), graphical analysis becomes rather difficult.

Pulse frequency spectrum. The frequency associated with a continuous wave train of constant frequency has a single value: all the energy occurs at this single frequency. However, in a wavetrain which is discontinuous, the energy distribution is not monotonic, but it is spread over a frequency spectrum.

The analysis of the amplitude distribution of a wavetrain into its frequency spectrum is based on Fourier's theorem. In its simplest form, this states that any periodic variation which fulfils certain conditions regarding continuity may be considered as the sum of a number of sinusoids whose periods exhibit a simple relationship. In addition, the equivalent series of sinusoids is unique for any given periodic variation.

In the case of a pulse, graphical integration may be used to evaluate the amplitudes of the sine and cosine series for various values of frequency, as follows:

$$A_s(\omega) = \int_0^\infty F(t) \sin \omega t \, dt, \qquad (3.20)$$

and

$$A_c(\omega) = \int_0^\infty F(t) \cos \omega t \, dt, \qquad (3.21)$$

where $A_s(\omega)$ = amplitude of the sine term corresponding to f,

ω $= 2\pi f$, where f is the frequency,

$A_c(\omega)$ = amplitude of the cosine term corresponding to f, and

$F(t)$ = instantaneous value of the pulse amplitude corresponding to f.

The overall amplitude of the spectrum $A(\omega)$ at any particular frequency $\omega/2\pi$ may be calculated from the corresponding values of $A_s(\omega)$ and $A_c(\omega)$, as follows

$$A(\omega) = \{(A_s(\omega))^2 + (A_c(\omega))^2\}^{1/2} \qquad (3.22)$$

Redwood (1963) calculated the frequency spectrum of the pulse shown in Fig. 3.15(c). The corresponding amplitude distribution, for a repetition rate of 1000 s^{-1} is shown in Fig. 3.16. The frequency of maximum amplitude of the spectrum (1·9 MHz) is markedly shifted from the fundamental resonance frequency of the transducer (2·5 MHz). The pulse has a half-amplitude bandwidth of 2·5 MHz, and a half-power bandwidth of 1·8 MHz.

The frequency spectrum is of considerable importance in diagnostic systems employing pulsed ultrasonics. Pellam and Galt (1946) pointed out that the frequency spectrum is modified by transmission through a medium in which the absorption coefficient depends upon the frequency. If, as is usual, the absorption increases with increasing frequency, then the high frequency components of a pulse are attenuated more than those of low frequency, and there is a shift downwards of the centre frequency of the spectrum. Kolsky (1956) discussed this effect in some detail, and Redwood (1963) calculated, using the technique of Fourier synthesis, how a frequency

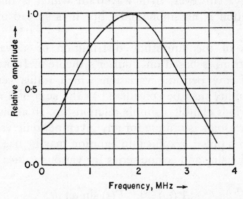

FIG. 3.16 Frequency amplitude spectrum of the pulse shown in Fig. 3.15(c). (Adapted from Redwood, 1963.)

dependent absorption alters the pulse shape. He concluded that large errors are possible in the measurement of absorption if the pulse has a broad spectrum, since its amplitude is maintained by the low frequency components. Accurate absorption measurements can only be achieved by the use of a narrow frequency spectrum, which in turn requires the use of a relatively large number of cycles. The corollary of this phenomenon, that the effective absorption coefficient in a medium depends upon the characteristics of the ultrasonic pulse, has important implications in diagnosis: see Chapter 6. Errors in velocity measurements are also possible, because of shifts in the time positions of the wave amplitude zeros due to pulse stretching, but these errors are not usually large, nor is their effect magnified by dispersion. The matter is discussed in Chapter 4.

The effect of absorption on the frequency spectrum is illustrated in Fig. 3.17. In this figure, curve (i) represents the same spectrum as that shown in Fig. 3.16, but redrawn with the amplitude expressed in decibels.

The maximum amplitude occurs at 1·9 MHz, and is chosen to correspond to 0 dB in Fig. 3.17. This spectrum is that for zero dispersive absorption. Curves (ii)–(v) show how the spectrum is shifted to lower frequencies, and the amplitude is decreased, for a pulse travelling through increasingly dispersive absorbers. For example, if the propagating medium has an absorption coefficient of 1 dB cm^{-1} MHz^{-1}, which is quite typical for a biological soft tissue (see Chapter 4), then an absorption rate of 5 dB MHz^{-1} is equivalent to a path length of 50 mm in the medium, and so on. Thus, these curves also illustrate the effect on the frequency spectrum which occurs as the pulse travels various distances in a dispersive absorber.

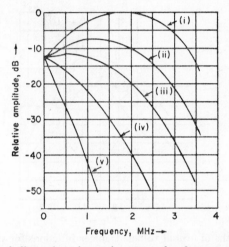

Fig. 3.17 Effect of dispersive absorption on pulse frequency spectrum. (i) No absorption (Fig. 3.16 redrawn with decibel scale); (ii) absorption 5 dB MHz^{-1}; (iii) absorption 10 dB MHz^{-1}; (iv) absorption 20 dB MHz^{-1}; (v) absorption 40 dB MHz^{-1}.

Mechanical impedance matching. As mentioned in Section 3.4.b, in relation to the continuous wave situation, the effects of matching the characteristic impedance of the transducer to the backing and loading media have been quite thoroughly investigated, particularly by Kossoff (1966). He used a rather sophisticated piezoelectric ceramic, PZT-7A, as the transducer, but his results are equally applicable to other transducer materials. His analysis is to some extent based on the earlier work of McSkimmin (1955), who showed that the bandwidth of a transducer can be increased by the use of a matching layer of suitable thickness and characteristic impedance, included between the tranducer and the load. Such a layer acts as a mechanical transformer which reflects an increased load into the transducer (see Section 1.11). Thus, the power is more efficiently absorbed by the load, and the system has a reduced loss. The matching layer is frequency selective, and optimization is based on a compromise between the efficiency of the system and bandwidth limitation due to the frequency selective components.

Various combinations of backing and matching are possible. Kossoff (1966) considered a 2 MHz transducer of 25 mm diameter, working into a water load, and presented his data mainly in the form of separate graphs of transmitting and receiving transducer voltage transfer functions, plotted against the fractional deviation from the open-circuit resonance frequency.

Walker and Lumb (1964) have described how the loop gain of a transducer system consisting of a transmitter and a receiver may be estimated.

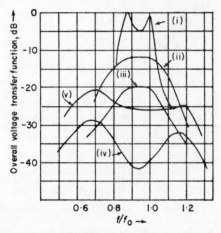

FIG. 3.18 Bandwidths of overall voltage transfer functions for various transducer systems (f/f_0 = fractional frequency deviation). (i) Air backed: unmatched to load; (ii) air backed: matched to load; (iii) tungsten powder in Araldite backed: unmatched to load; (iv) matched to tungsten powder in Araldite backing: unmatched to load; (v) matched to tungsten powder in Araldite backing: matched to load. (Adapted from Kossoff, 1966.)

The reflexion conditions in the definitions of loop gain and voltage transfer function as calculated by Kossoff (1966) are different, but the principles are the same. A simple calculation of loop gain or voltage transfer function, however, requires a simple transmitter voltage waveform which has the same shape as the propagated stress wave. This condition is not satisfied in the case of a shock excited transducer, and the calculation becomes much more difficult. Shock excited systems are most easily investigated by direct measurement, using some kind of standard reflecting surface.

Some of Kossoff's (1966) results have been recalculated for Fig. 3.18 to give the overall voltage transfer function, and so correspond to the output voltages obtained after perfect reflexion with zero loss of the ultrasonic wave generated by a given input voltage. The frequency response of the airbacked transducer has the narrowest bandwidth. The transducer with an unmatched tungsten powder in Araldite backing has a similar bandwidth to that of the unbacked transducer matched to the load, but it has an overall voltage transfer function corresponding to some 8 dB lower sensitivity. If poor sensitivity and some degree of ripple can be tolerated in the pass band, a transducer matched to both the load and backing has the widest bandwidth. A transducer which is matched to the backing but unmatched to the load has a similar bandwidth, but greater ripple and even lower sensitivity.

The tungsten powder in Araldite backing material used by Kossoff (1966) was made by adding 100–200 g of tungsten powder to 40 ml of Araldite (100 parts casting resin D and 50 parts polyamid 75), and centrifuging the mixture. The characteristic impedance varied from 6×10^6 to 16×10^6 kg m^{-2} s^{-1}. Kossoff (1966) quotes the value of the characteristic impedance of PZT-7A as 37.5×10^6 kg m^{-2} s^{-1}. Matching of the load (water, $Z = 1.48 \times 10^6$ kg m^{-2} s^{-1}) or the backing was accomplished by means of a quarter-wave layer of Araldite containing aluminium. This was prepared by mixing 1.5 parts by weight of aluminium powder with 1 part of Araldite (100 parts casting resin D and 10 parts of hardener 351), which gave an impedance of 5.5×10^6 kg m^{-2} s^{-1}.

Kossoff's (1966) analysis is based on a steady state situation. This is because the action of a matching layer depends upon the existence of an equilibrium standing wave system. The time required for the establishment of steady state conditions depends upon a number of factors, and in particular, upon the losses of the system: the greater the losses, the more rapidly does the transient situation approach that of the steady state. Therefore, although the steady state bandwidth can be improved by the techniques developed by Kossoff (1966), these improvements become less significant as the duration of the ultrasonic pulse is decreased. Kasai et al. (1973) have discussed this matter, and have developed a method of analysis which allows the optimum value of the characteristic impedance to be determined. It is not equal to the geometric mean of the characteristic impedances on each side of the layer, as predicted by continuous wave theory: the value depends on the dynamic range for which the system is optimized.

Theoretical prediction of the bandwidth of a transducer is apt to be rather inaccurate, on account of the difficulties involved in estimating the magnitudes of the various factors which control the frequency response. Therefore, it is generally better to measure the frequency response of a particular transducer by an experimental method. Gericke (1966) has described an automatic system in which the transducer is excited by gated pulses from a constant-amplitude oscillator, the frequency of which is swept through the range 0.3–12 MHz. A voltage proportional to the instantaneous value of the frequency is fed to the x-deflexion plates of a cathode ray oscilloscope. The transducer is arranged to transmit the pulses into a block of low-loss material, such as aluminium, and to receive the echoes from a reflecting surface. The thickness of the block is made large enough to give a delay which avoids ambiguity between the exciting pulses and the received echoes. The output from the transducer is fed to a wide-band amplifier, the output of which is connected to the y-deflexion plates of the oscilloscope. A bright-up pulse is applied to the z-modulation input of the oscilloscope for the duration of each received pulse. Thus, a display appears on the oscilloscope in which the x-deflexion is proportional to the frequency, and the y-deflexion, to the overall voltage transfer function.

It is important to understand the distinction between the frequency spectrum of an ultrasonic pulse, and the frequency response of a transducer. The frequency response describes the continuous-wave bandwidth of the transducer system, whereas the frequency spectrum depends not only upon the frequency response of the transducer, but also upon the form of the electrical excitation and the properties of the propagating medium.

The satisfactory generation and detection of very short pulses of ultra-sound by a resonant transducer can only be achieved by the use of a non-reflective backing medium. The best backing material currently available seems to be epoxy resin loaded to a high density with tungsten powder, but even if a mixture with the highest practical characteristic impedance of 16×10^6 kg m^{-2} s^{-1} is used, the reflexion at the transducer (lead zirconate titanate) to backing interface is only about 20 dB below that from an air backing. The internal reflexion at a water-loaded face is only about 0·5 dB down, and so the voltage transfer function is small with very short pulses. The Q-factor corresponding to the overall frequency response of the transducer has a value of about 2·5 with most heavily damped probes. It is hard to imagine how the situation could be improved unless transducer materials of much lower characteristic impedance than that of the ferro-electric ceramics were to be used. This appears to be a real possibility with the development of piezoelectric plastics (see Section 3.1.b).

Dynamic range. The dynamic range of a pulse transducer may be defined as the ratio of the amplitude of the main pulse to the amplitude of the ripple following this pulse, measured with the transducer receiving the echo from a flat reflector normal to the axis the ultrasonic beam. As explained in Chapter 6, a large dynamic range is desirable in certain diagnostic applications.

The dynamic range is controlled by a number of factors. The principal limitation arises in the mounting of the transducer. If energy is coupled into the probe casing (which is often constructed from metal), the casing may ring for some time after the main pulse has been generated. This ringing may be coupled back into the transducer, causing a reduction in dynamic range. The effect may be minimized by the presence of an acoustic insulator between the transducer and the case, as shown in Fig. 3.13. Any tendency of the casing to ring may be reduced by breaking up its profile, and by including bands of a damping material such as a plastic.

Another factor which limits the dynamic range is the coupling of energy into resonant radial modes within the transducer. Kossoff *et al.* (1965) have shown that this effect may be reduced by making the transducer radially asymmetrical. The method they used was to attach a small cube of rubber to the rear surface near the edge of the transducer, within the backing block. The portion of the transducer covered by the rubber was

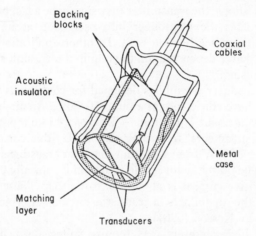

FIG. 3.19 Typical ultrasonic diagnostic probe for continuous wave Doppler applications: one transducer acts as the transmitter, the other as the receiver; in this situation, damping is not an important requirement.

not excited, thus destroying the radial symmetry. The addition of the rubber increased the dynamic range of a typical probe by 6 dB.

Arrays. Arrays of transducers have been used to steer the ultrasonic beam, and to focus it. Such specialized systems are discussed in Section 6.10.c.

Doppler probes. The construction of a typical Doppler probe is shown in Fig. 3.19. As explained by Wells (1974), the use of separate transducers for transmitting and receiving allows a proper choice to be made of their characteristics to achieve the maximum sensitivity. The constructions of Doppler probes designed for various clinical applications are discussed at the appropriate places in Chapter 7.

(vi) Generators producing transverse oscillations

A thin fibre (such as narrow glass capillary tube) can be set into transverse vibration (see Section 1.2.a) if it is attached at one end to a length-expanding cylindrical piezoelectric transducer, so that the axis of the fibre is at right angles to the axis of the transducer (Williams and Nyborg, 1970). The technique is referred to in Sections 9.7 and 9.11.h.

(vii) Electrical drivers for piezoelectric transducers

Unlike many applications of magnetostrictive transducers (see Section 3.6.a), it is generally unnecessary to use automatic frequency control in systems using piezoelectric transducers. A fixed frequency oscillator, with or without a power amplifier, is generally satisfactory. For pulse–echo diagnostic applications, the transmitter may simply be a fast pulse generator which shock–excites the transducer into oscillation at its fundamental resonance frequency (see Section 6.3). In other applications, the design of the electrical driver depends upon the required ultrasonic power and the conditions of pulsing.

Ultrasonic transducer assemblies designed for continuous wave or long-pulse operation have efficiencies of around 50–70%. An air-backed PZT-4 transducer delivers about 1 μW mm^{-2}(V $pk–pk$)$^{-2}$ into a water load when operating at a fundamental frequency of 3 MHz: this corresponds to an ultrasonic power of 1 W from a 10 mm diameter transducer when driven at 40 V r.m.s. The power factor in this situation is typically 0·5, so that the corresponding drive current is about 100 mA r.m.s. These requirements are well within the capabilities of transistor circuits. A typical system has been described by Kossoff (1964).

Substantially higher powers may require voltages which cannot conveniently be obtained with transistors. This is almost always the case with quartz transducers, which have much higher electrical impedances than the corresponding ceramic transducers. It also applies to ceramic transducers operating at the lower frequencies, and at high powers at the higher frequencies. The design of electrical driving systems gives much scope for ingenuity, and a typical versatile arrangement has been described by Connolly (1968).

3.7 METHODS OF DETECTING AND MEASURING ULTRASONIC WAVES

In this Section, most of the ultrasonic detectors, visualization and measuring systems relevant to biomedical work are described.

3.7.a Hydrophones

Hydrophones are detectors based on transducers which respond directly to the ultrasonic field. The output of a hydrophone is an electrical signal which follows the instantaneous value of the ultrasonic field at the ultrasonic frequency. Generally hydrophones are used to measure the intensities at points within ultrasonic fields: for this purpose, it is desirable that the detecting element should be small in relation to the wavelength, so that the hydrophone should have a negligible effect upon the field, and its response should be non-directional.

Hydrophones may be calibrated by either of two methods. Generally the simplest method is to measure the amplitude of the hydrophone output when it is situated in an ultrasonic field of known intensity (measured, for example, by a thermocouple probe: see Section 3.7.g).

The second method is based on the reciprocity theorem; it is seldom used, mainly because it involves assumptions concerning the directivity of the hydrophone. Self-reciprocity calibration may have advantages when plane waves are involved (Simmons and Urick, 1949; and see Section 3.7.m).

(i) Magnetostrictive hydrophones

Hydrophones based on magnetostrictive transducers are useful for measurements in ultrasonic fields at frequencies of up to about 500 kHz. As shown in Fig. 3.20(a), the instrument may simply be a rod of magnetostrictive material such as nickel, with a diameter of about 1% of the wavelength (for nickel, $c = 4800$ m s^{-1}), and with a length equal to an integral number of half wavelengths (Koppelmann, 1952). The polarizing magnetic field may be applied by a solenoid near the middle of the rod, and the ultrasonic signal may be picked up by a second solenoid at the end of the rod. The sensitivity of the hydrophone may be restricted to the tip at the opposite end by encasing the rod in a plastic sleeve. The frequency response of the hydrophone (which in this case is a resonant system) may be broadened by damping the vibration of the rod with an absorbent material such as rubber at the electrical pickup end.

(ii) Piezoelectric hydrophones

Hydrophones using piezoelectric transducers are capable of operating at much higher frequencies than those based on magnetostrictive transducers. There are two main types of piezoelectric hydrophone.

In the first type, the ultrasound is conducted from the field under investigation to the transducer by means of a waveguide, such as a slim metal rod, as shown in Fig. 3.20(b). This resembles the magnetostrictive hydrophone described in the preceding Sub-section, and has similar disadvantages: the diameter of the waveguide needs to be about 1% of the wavelength, and its length is resonant at the ultrasonic frequency. Instruments based on this principle have been described by Koppelmann (1952) and Saneyoshi *et al.* (1966).

In the second type of piezoelectric hydrophone, the transducer itself is introduced into the ultrasonic field at the end of a probe. Several typical constructions are illustrated in Fig. 3.21. Provided that the dimensions of the sensitive element are less than about $\lambda/10$ (i.e. $ka < \sim 0.5$), the directivity of the sensitivity is sufficiently uniform for most practical purposes. Where $ka > \sim 0.5$, the hydrophone is rather directional, and special pre-

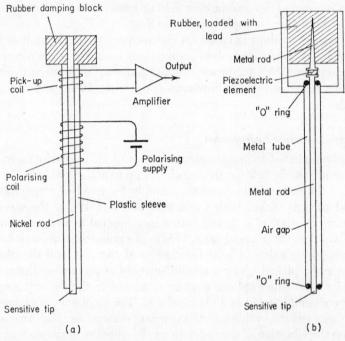

FIG. 3.20 Hydrophones using waveguide probes. (a) Magnetostrictive (after Koppelmann, 1952); (b) piezoelectric (after Saneyoshi *et al.*, 1966).

cautions may be necessary to avoid the introduction of errors into measurements of ultrasonic field distribution. In addition to errors due to nonuniform directivity functions, this type of hydrophone, in common with those using waveguides, has a response which is frequency-dependent. Where this may cause problems (i.e. when the hydrophone is being used to measure ultrasonic fields of wide frequency spectra, such as occur with short pulses), there are two techniques which can reduce the difficulty. Firstly, heavy damping may be employed to lower the Q of the system (see Section 3.3), and so increase its bandwidth. Secondly, the transducer dimensions may be chosen so that it operates at frequencies far removed

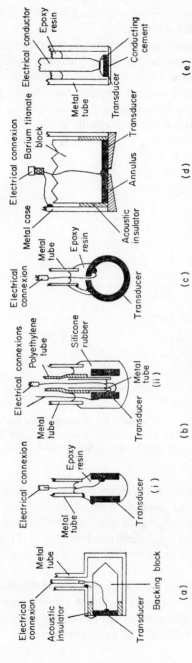

FIG. 3.21 Piezoelectric hydrophones, with the elements mounted at the sensitive ends of the probes. (a) Transducer diameter 1–5 mm, resonance frequency > 15 MHz: suitable for measurements in pulsed fields at frequencies below about 5 MHz (after Brendel, 1972); (b) transducers in the form of cylinders, 1·6 mm outside diameter, 1·6 mm length: two methods of construction, (i) after Ackerman and Holak, 1954; (ii) after Hill, 1970: suitable for measurements in slowly changing fields at frequencies below about 5 MHz (the directivity of a typical probe of this type is shown in Fig. 3.22); (c) spherical transducer, 0·2 mm outside diameter: suitable for measurements in slowly changing fields at frequencies below about 10 MHz (after Romanenko, 1957); (d) masked transducer: the central aperture has a diameter of about 3 mm: suitable for measurements in short pulse fields at frequencies below about 5 MHz (after Christie, 1962); (e) transducer mounted at the tip of a 21 gauge hypodermic needle: the transducer is 0·46 mm diameter, 10 MHz thickness resonance frequency (after Colbert et al., 1972).

from that of its natural resonance (see Section 3.2). In this latter case, it is usual for the hydrophone to have a higher resonance frequency, because this corresponds to smaller physical dimensions.

It is occasionally adequate to use an ordinary ceramic capacitor polarized with a high voltage as a piezoelectric hydrophone (Schmitt, 1961). Such capacitors are inexpensive, and quite small sizes can be obtained.

In practice, it is often difficult to construct a hydrophone which is small enough for $ka < \sim 0.5$ at megahertz frequencies. For example, at 1 MHz in water this requires that $a < \sim 0.1$ mm. As a result, it is seldom correct to assume that the directivity is uniform, even when the transducer is a

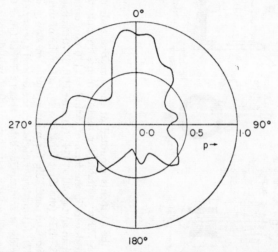

FIG. 3.22 Directivity of pressure amplitude sensitivity of cylindrical hydrophone (such as that illustrated in Fig. 3.15(b)) in the radial plane. Cylinder length = 1.6 mm, outside diameter = 1.5 mm; ultrasonic frequency = ~ 2.6 MHz, pulsed. (After Bom, 1972.)

cylinder which should in principle have a uniform sensitivity to ultrasound approaching from any direction in a plane parallel to the axis of the cylinder and passing through the centre of the cylinder (as should be realizable with hydrophones of the type illustrated in Fig. 3.21(b)). For example, Fig. 3.22 shows the directivity in this plane for a typical probe of this type.

To some extent, Okujima (1974) has solved the problem of the conflicting requirements of sensitivity and directivity by means of a probe curved with differing radii in two dimensions. The instrument has a frequency response which extends within 3 dB up to 4 MHz, and a directivity within 10 dB of ± 1.0°.

A hydrophone which differs from the two main types just described is illustrated in Fig. 3.23. The use of a focusing transducer allows the instrument to detect disturbances occurring at the focus, and the problem of directional non-uniformity is greatly reduced. A second advantage is that this type of hydrophone does not interfere with the ultrasonic field.

(iii) Beam plotting

A convenient hydrophone for plotting pulsed ultrasonic fields may be constructed by baffling a large transducer to a small aperture. The transducer may either have a wideband frequency response (Aveyard, 1962; Hodgkinson, 1966), or it may have its resonance frequency far removed from the centre frequency of the pulse under investigation (Christie, 1962).

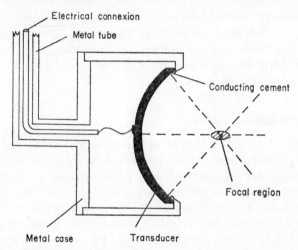

FIG. 3.23 Focused hydrophone. In this example, the transducer has diameter and radius of curvature both equal to 48 mm. It is most sensitive to disturbances at the focus. (Based on Coakley, 1971.)

Several systems for beam plotting using this kind of detector have been described in the literature. For example, Christie (1962) constructed a water tank in which the detector could be moved by a manually operated system to any point in the ultrasonic field. Measurements were made from an oscilloscope on which the detected pulse was displayed: the timebase of the oscilloscope was triggered by a pulse appropriately delayed in time from the instant of excitation of the source transducer. In this way, it was possible to deduce the field distribution at various stages during the propagation of the pulse (see Section 2.2.c).

Aveyard (1962) constructed an automatic beam plotting system, with a recorder* in which moist chemically treated paper is passed between two

---

* "Mufax" recorder: Muirhead Ltd., Morden, Surrey, UK.

electrodes. The application of a potential difference to these electrodes produces a proportional darkening of the paper. The system was arranged to reconstruct the intensity distribution of the ultrasonic beam by darkening the two-dimensional image according to the ultrasonic intensity. Hodgkinson (1966) devised a technique by which the write-out of Aveyard's (1962) system was quantized into six discrete grey levels. The quantizing circuiting was designed to accept a continuously variable signal, and to separate this into bands of 6 dB intensity range for presentation on the recorder. The lines of transition between adjacent areas of different grey level corresponded to lines of constant intensity separated by 6 dB. For this reason, the recordings were called "*isosonographs*".

In systems in which a hydrophone is used to plot the ultrasonic field, the amplitudes represented on the recording are generally peak amplitudes. Since the peak amplitude is normally that of at least the second, and frequently the third or some subsequent half-cycle, the beam pattern corresponds fairly closely with with that predicted by continuous wave theory (see Section 2.2).

3.7.b Electrokinetic Probes

An ultrasonic detector of simple construction and small size has been described by Dietrick *et al.* (1953). It is based on the so-called *electrokinetic effect*: if a wire covered with a fibre or porous coating is submerged in a dilute electrolytic solution and irradiated with ultrasonic waves, an alternating potential of the same frequency is produced on the wire relative to the bulk of the surrounding solution. This type of probe seems to have been neglected in recent years; but it might be useful in measuring ultrasonic intensities within living tissues.

3.7.c Electromagnetic Transducers

The absolute intensity of an ultrasonic wave may be determined by measuring the voltage induced in a conductor which is moved through a magnetic field as a result of the ultrasonic disturbance. Filipczyński (1967) has described such an instrument, consisting of a rectangular block of polymethylmethacrylate on which a conductor, in the form of 10 turns of aluminium, 2 μm thick, is evaporated. The block is arranged so that one of the flat surfaces on which the conductor is deposited is situated between the poles of a powerful magnet. If this surface is set into motion by the passage of an ultrasonic wave, a voltage is induced in the conductor which is proportional to the velocity of the surface. Problems with standing waves generally restrict the method to the measurement of the intensities of short pulses.

3.7.d Electrostatic Transducers

(i) *Capacitance transducers*

The absolute intensity of an ultrasonic wave may be determined by means of a parallel plate capacitor. One plate is kept stationary, and the other is displaced by the reflexion of the wave at its surface. A typical arrangement is illustrated in Fig. 3.24. The method is more suited to the measurement of the intensity of a short-duration pulse than continuous waves, because standing waves are set up with the latter.

If C_0 is the capacitance of the air gap, and C' is the parallel stray capacitance,

$$\delta = d_0 \frac{e}{E} \frac{C_0 + C'}{C_0} \tag{3.23}$$

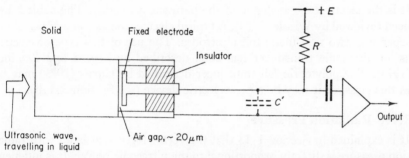

Fig. 3.24 Capacitance transducer and associated electronics for the measurement of ultrasonic intensity. A fraction of the ultrasonic wave travelling in the liquid enters the solid electrode, and is reflected at the interface with the air gap. This causes variations in the spacing between the electrodes, and the resultant capacitance changes lead to a variation in voltage across the resistor R. The capacitor C blocks the d.c. voltage, so that only the a.c. signals are fed to the amplifier.

where δ is the displacement of the moving electrode in response to the ultrasonic disturbance, and e is the corresponding change in voltage across the detector; and d_0 is the static width of the air gap, and E is the polarizing voltage. The shunting effect of the polarization supply resistor R is negligible if $\omega R(C_0 + C') \gg 1$. The wave is totally reflected at the interface with the air gap, and so the displacement amplitude δ is twice the displacement u_2 of the wave propagating in the moving electrode. Now if Z_1 and Z_2 are respectively the characteristic impedances of the liquid and the moving electrode, from Eqn. 1.48,

$$u_1 = u_2 \frac{Z_1 + Z_2}{2Z_2} \tag{3.24}$$

and the instantaneous intensity i_1 in the liquid is given by

$$i_1 = \frac{Z_1 (du_1/dt)^2}{2} \qquad (3.25)$$

The maximum pulse duration with this method is limited by the thickness of the moving electrode.

Transducers of this type have been described by Kolsky (1956), Filipczyński (1966) and Gauster and Breazeale (1966). An alternative arrangement using a fixed electrode of small size has been developed by Filipczyński and Lypacewicz (1972) for measuring displacement profiles of transducer surfaces.

(ii) Electrets

An electret is a piece of material which is permanently electrically polarized. It is the electrostatic analogue of the permanent magnet. The subject has been reviewed by Wintle (1973). A typical electret consists of a Mylar sheet separating two thin metal foil electrodes. The use of this type of electret as an ultrasonic transducer has been described by Legros and Lewiner (1973). The polymeric foil transducer described by Curtis (1974) may be in this class, or it may be a piezoelectric device (see Section 3.1.b).

3.7.e Radiation Pressure

It is explained in Section 1.13 that the vector force associated with radiation pressure is directly proportional to the ultrasonic power. It is independent of the ultrasonic frequency.

(i) Radiation pressure balances

Several instruments have been described in which ultrasonic power is measured by the determination of the force associated with its radiation pressure. Three typical examples are illustrated in Fig. 3.25. In the simple arrangement, shown in Fig. 3.25(a), a balance has a reflector arranged to intercept a vertical ultrasonic beam travelling in water, and to reflect the beam horizontally into an absorber. The reflector may consist of two thin sheets of metal, sealed together at their edges but elsewhere separated by a sheet of dry paper. The beam is brought into balance by a movable rider, adjusted so that the turning moment of the rider about the fulcrum is equal and opposite to the turning moment of the radiation force. The radiation force is, subject to certain errors, equal to that corresponding to perfect absorption at the inclined reflector, since in principle the momentum of the reflected beam produces a force acting through the fulcrum. Substitution in Eqn. 1.61 shows that an ultrasonic beam with a power of 1 W travelling in water at 20°C produces a force of 6.7×10^{-4} N when it is

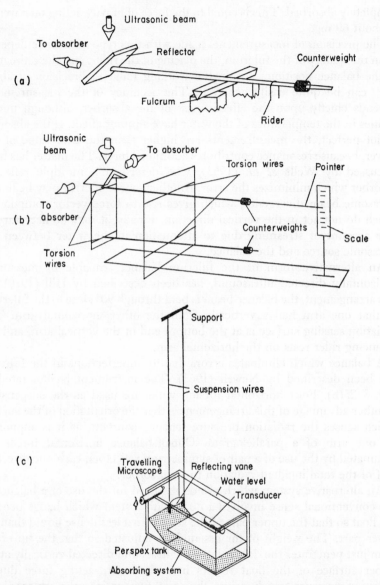

FIG. 3.25 Typical radiation pressure balances. (a) Simple beam balance (after Wells *et al.*, 1963); (b) Roberval balance with torsion wire suspension (after Newell, 1963); (c) suspension radiometer (after Wells *et al.*, 1964). Types (a) and (b) are suitable for measuring powers in the range 0·1–10 W, and (c) for powers between 0·002 and 0·1 W.

completely absorbed. This is equal to the force of gravity acting on a weight of about 69 mg.

The precision of measurements made with this type of balance depends upon the quality of the fulcrum, the placing of the rider, and the estimation of the balance position. Within the working range, a precision of about 15% can be quite easily achieved. The accuracy of the measurements depends chiefly upon the effectiveness of the absorber, although uncertainties in the temperature of the water have a minor effect. If the absorber is not perfect, the measurements are higher than the true value of the power, because resonance contributes additional force. The matter has been discussed by Wells *et al.* (1963), who described a multiple reflexion absorber which minimizes the error. Another source of error may be due to ultrasonic beam divergence, which gives rise to force vector components which do not act in the vertical direction. Finally, it may be necessary to take account of streaming due to attenuation in the water between the ultrasonic source and the balance.

An alternative form of the fulcrum balance, capable of measuring horizontally directed ultrasound, has been described by Hill (1970). In this arrangement, the balance beam is bent through 90° close to the fulcrum, so that one arm hangs vertically from the other, horizontal arm. The radiation sensing surface is at the bottom end of the vertical arm, and the balancing rider rests on the horizontal arm.

A balance which eliminates errors due to imperfections in the fulcrum has been described by Newell (1963). The instrument is illustrated in Fig. 3.25(b). Four horizontal torsion wires are used as the suspension. Another advantage of this arrangement is that the orientation of the surface which senses the radiation pressure remains constant, as it is supported on one arm of a parallelogram. Out-of-balance horizontal forces are eliminated by the use of a pair of symmetrical reflectors, each one directing half of the total incident radiation to an absorber.

An alternative system which avoids the need for the use of a balance in the conventional sense involves a float, with a stem which hangs beneath the float so that the upper part of the stem is in a less dense liquid than the lower part. The weight of the assembly is adjusted so that the tip of the stem just penetrates the denser liquid. Ultrasound directed vertically at the upper surface of the float results in a downward-acting force due to radiation pressure which drives the stem further into the denser liquid until balance is restored. If the upper surface of the float is in the form of a cone with its apex downwards, the device is self-centring around the ultrasonic beam. Such an arrangement has been described by Kossoff (1962).

More sensitive detectors are necessary in order to measure very low ultrasonic powers such as those used in most diagnostic systems. Three types of radiation pressure instrument capable of measuring powers of a few milliwatts have been described in the literature. One of these, due to Wells *et al.* (1964), is illustrated in Fig. 3.25(c). The radiometer consists of an air-filled aluminium box, 55 mm in diameter and 2 mm thick, suspended from two fine wires each about 1 m long. The vane itself is buoyant in water, but it is arranged to sink at an angle of 45° to the horizontal by means of two aluminium bars, attached to the vane at each end of its horizontal diameter. With all instruments of this type, errors may arise due to the temperature dependence of the effective weight of the radiation-sensing components. Measurements are made by observation of the distance of deflexion of the vane when it is struck by the horizontally directed ultrasonic beam. A travelling microscope is used. The vane behaves as if it were a perfect absorber, because the reflected ultrasound acts vertically and so produces no horizontal force component. At powers of around 2 mW, the accuracy is about 5%.

The second type of sensitive radiation pressure detector is based on a modified analytical balance, arranged to measure the very small force corresponding to absorption of the ultrasonic beam. Such instruments have been described by Kossoff (1965) and Hill (1970). At powers of around 2 mW the accuracy is about 7%.

Wemlén (1968) has constructed a balance in which a restoring force is applied through an electrical servo so that the instrument operates with negligible deflexion. At powers of around 10 mW, the accuracy is better than 5%. A somewhat similar instrument has been described by Rooney (1973).

(ii) Pressure on spheres

The theory of King (1934) for the force due to radiation pressure which is exerted by a plane progressive wave on a sphere has been used by Fox (1940) to compute data from which it is possible to estimate the intensity at any point in an ultrasonic field in a fluid, by measurement of the deflexion of a suspended sphere. The method is more suited to the measurement of intensity than total power, although the latter can be obtained by integration.

A small metal sphere is suspended from two filaments in the horizontally directed ultrasonic field, so that it is located at the point in space at which the intensity is to be measured. For small deflexions, and working in SI units, the intensity I is given by

$$I = \frac{Mg\Delta c}{\pi la^2 Y} \tag{3.26}$$

where M = effective weight of the sphere in water,

g = acceleration due to gravity,

Δ = horizontal displacement of the sphere,

l = length of supporting filament,

a = radius of sphere, and

Y = a numerical function the value of which depends on the material and dimensions of the sphere.

Values of Y which may be expected to give errors of not more than 10% may be read off from Fig. 3.26. If units of [W, cm, s, g] are used, the right-hand side of Eqn. 3.26 should be multiplied by a factor of 10^{-7}.

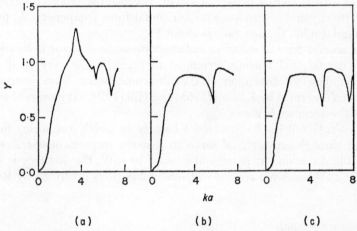

(a)   (b)   (c)

FIG. 3.26 Values of the parameter Y (see Eqn. 3.26) as functions of sphere diameters, for various materials in water: (a) brass; (b) steel; (c) stainless steel. (Data of Hasegawa and Yosioka, 1969.)

(iii) Streaming

When ultrasound travels through a liquid, a fraction of the energy carried by the wave is absorbed. The resultant radiation pressure causes the liquid to stream. An instrument for the measurement of ultrasonic power based on this effect has been described by Sjöberg *et al.* (1963): its construction is illustrated in Fig. 3.27. It consists of a glass tube formed into a "b" shape. The "b" is open at the top, the loop re-entering the upper part of the tube about 50 mm below the top. The short side of the loop of the "b" is slightly conical, about 3 mm in diameter at the bottom and opening upwards. This tube contains a spherical plastic bead of about 4 mm diameter. When an ultrasonic beam is introduced into the water-filled system through the open end at the top, the water is set into circulation under the influence of the radiation pressure. In the conical section, the velocity of streaming is greatest at the bottom, and least at the top. Consequently the bead rises up the conical section until the upward force due to the motion of the liquid is equal to the downward force due to gravity. A scale can be attached to the cone relating the position of the bead to the ultrasonic power.

(iv) Pohlman cell

The Pohlman cell is an ultrasonic detector consisting of fine metal flakes suspended in a transparent liquid between two membranes (Pohlman,

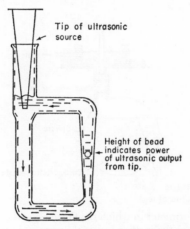

Tip of ultrasonic source

Height of bead indicates power of ultrasonic output from tip.

FIG. 3.27 Instrument for the measurement of ultrasonic power, based on the acoustic streaming phenomenon. The height of the bead indicates the power of the ultrasonic beam. (After Sjöberg *et al.*, 1963.)

1948). In a typical cell, the flakes have a diameter of 20 μm and a thickness of 1·5 μm, and are suspended in toluene in a cell with a diameter of 100 mm, the windows of which are polyethylene sheets of 50 μm thickness. In the absence of an irradiating ultrasonic field, the flakes are randomly orientated, and the cell has a uniformly grey appearance. The radiation pressure associated with an ultrasonic field, however, tends to align the orientation of the flakes so that a pattern appears in the cell which corresponds to the ultrasonic intensity distribution. The minimum intensity required to produce a change in brightness of about 50% of the background brightness is about 0·1 mW cm^{-2}, and the dynamic range of the cell is about 20 dB. Typically the image appears within 1–5 s after the exposure to the ultrasound has begun.

(v) *Liquid surface levitation*

Liquid surface levitation was one of the earliest methods to be devised for the real-time visualization of ultrasonic images. The historical background has been reviewed by Rozenberg (1955). A flat liquid–air horizontal surface is irradiated with the vertically directed ultrasonic field which it is desired to visualize. At each element of the surface, equilibrium exists when the force due to radiation pressure is equal to the restoring forces of gravity and surface tension. The deformed liquid surface serves as an optical phase-object, and a visible representation of the ultrasonic image may be produced by reflexion or refraction of light.

Green (1971) has reviewed the projected uses of this method in ultrasonic diagnostics. Apart from being inconvenient, the principal limitation

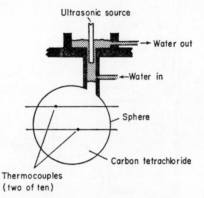

FIG. 3.28 A simple calorimeter in which the flow of cooling water eliminates errors due to heat resulting from the inefficiency of the ultrasonic source. The ten thermocouples within the calorimeter are connected in series with a further 10 thermocouples maintained at constant temperature. (After Wells *et al.*, 1963.)

is that of low sensitivity: around 10 mW cm^{-2} is necessary for a resolution with a spatial frequency of 1 cycle mm^{-1}.

3.7.f Calorimeters

When ultrasound is completely absorbed, all the energy carried in the wave is converted into heat. The calorimetric method is based on the measurement of this heat energy.

In practice, the principal difficulty is to separate the heat due to the inefficiency of the source from that due to the absorption of the ultrasound. The matter has been discussed by Wells *et al.* (1963), who designed the calorimeter illustrated in Fig. 3.28. The instrument consists of a hollow sphere of about 40 mm diameter, with thin plastic walls. The sphere contains 10 copper/constantan thermocouples each of about 10 μm diameter, and it is supported in air by means of a small tube. Ultrasonic radiation which enters the tube suffers multiple reflexions and absorption in the sphere. The sphere is filled with carbon tetrachloride (density 1·6 g cm^{-3}, absorption coefficient 0·05 dB cm^{-1} at 1 MHz), and the entry tube is fitted with two additional tubes for the upward circulation of cooling water past the source. Water is immiscible with carbon tetrachloride. There is little reflexion at the interface between the water and the carbon tetrachloride, since the difference in the characteristic impedances is only about 1%.

The importance of ensuring that the calorimeter responds only to heat generated by the absorption of ultrasound does not seem to have been widely realized. The precaution has been overlooked in many instruments of otherwise advanced design. Calorimeters capable of high accuracy have been described by Mikhailov and Shutilov (1957) and by Zieniuk (1965).

3.7.g Thermocouple Probes

The thermocouple probe was devised by Fry and Fry (1954a). In contrast to other detectors, it yields directly values of the particle velocity amplitude and pressure amplitude in ultrasonic fields of any configuration. In a travelling plane wave field, it measures the intensity. The instrument can be made with an extremely small measurement volume, it is insensitive to stray radio-frequency fields, and it has a low electrical impedance. Its disadvantages are that it has a relatively large overall size, it requires an intensity of at least about 1 W cm^{-2} to give a satisfactory output, and it does not respond to rapid changes in the ultrasonic field.

The constructions of two typical instruments are illustrated in Fig. 3.29. They differ only in size and in the characteristics of the absorbing media. In both, a thermocouple junction is embedded in an absorbing medium, chosen to have a characteristic impedance closely matching that of the liquid supporting the ultrasonic field under investigation, and possessing a relatively high value of absorption coefficient. The diameter of the wires in the neighbourhood of the thermojunction is made as small as possible— typically $\lambda/100$. The minimum diameter of the device with the liquid absorber is around 50 mm, but that with the solid absorber can be much smaller.

The source of ultrasound is excited to produce a single square-wave pulse of duration about 1 s. The corresponding change in thermoelectric voltage is recorded: a typical result is shown in Fig. 3.30. The initial, rapid increase in temperature is due to the conversion of ultrasonic energy into heat by viscous forces acting between the wire and the embedding medium. This is followed by a steady increase in temperature, which is approximately linear with time, caused by the absorption of ultrasound in the embedding medium. From this time rate of change of temperature it

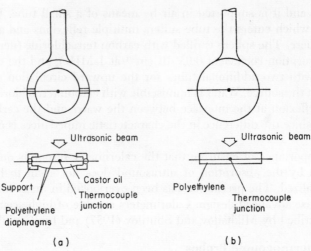

FIG. 3.29 Thermocouple probe constructions. (a) Liquid-filled type (castor oil absorber) (after Fry and Fry, 1954a); (b) solid type (polyethylene absorber) (after Yoskioka and Oka, 1965).

is possible to calculate either the absolute value of ultrasonic intensity if the absorption coefficient of the embedding medium is known, or vice versa. The subsequent exponential decrease in temperature is due to cooling when the ultrasound is switched off. It has been shown both theoretically (Fry and Fry, 1954a) and experimentally (Fry and Fry, 1954b) that the intensity I at the thermojunction is given by

$$I = \frac{H}{\mu_i} \left(\frac{dT}{dt} \right) \tag{3.27}$$

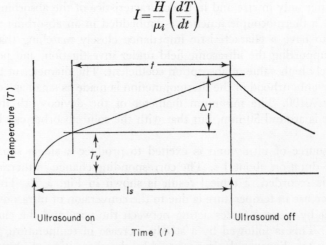

FIG. 3.30 Typical time course of temperature recording obtained with a thermocouple probe in response to a square pulse of ultrasound.

where H is the heat capacity per unit volume of the embedding medium, μ_i is the intensity absorption coefficient per unit path length ($\mu_i = 2\mu_a = 0{\cdot}230\alpha$: see Section 1.12), and dT/dt is the rate of change of temperature (from Fig. 3.29, $dT/dt = \Delta T/t$).

If the embedding medium is a liquid the response of a thermocouple probe is influenced at high intensities by streaming (see Section 1.13) in the boundary region around the wire. With castor oil, this effect causes the failure of Eqn. 3.27 at intensities in excess of about 350 W cm^{-2} (Hueter, 1957). Another disadvantage of a liquid embedding medium is that the mechanical arrangements required to seal the cell make the construction of a small probe rather difficult. The solid embedding medium (polyethylene) used in the probes constructed by Yoskioka and Oka (1965)

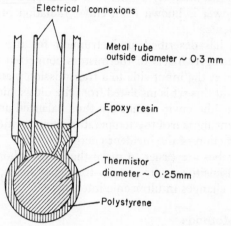

Electrical connexions

Metal tube
outside diameter ~ 0·3 mm

Epoxy resin

Thermistor
diameter ~ 0·25mm

Polystyrene

FIG. 3.31 Construction of a thermistor probe.

allows quite small sizes to be realized, and such probes might possibly be used for the measurement of intensity in living tissue.

3.7.h Thermistor Probes

A thermistor is an element of semiconductor material which has a large temperature coefficient of resistance. Thermistors can be obtained commercially with diameters as small as 250 μm, connected to wires of 30 μm diameter. Although a thermistor placed by itself in an ultrasonic field supported in a non-absorbent medium experiences no change in temperature, it can be made sensitive to the field if it is coated with a thin layer of absorbent material.

The construction of a probe based on this effect is illustrated in Fig. 3.31. The thermistor is mounted at the end of a stainless steel tube, to which it is attached by epoxy resin. The absorbent layer around the thermistor is deposited by dipping in model-maker's polystyrene cement, which dries to form a thin and resilient coating.

The thermistor is connected in one arm of a Wheatstone bridge. Typically the other resistors in the bridge may be of 1 kΩ each. The indicator may be a moving coil meter of 50 μA full-scale deflexion sensitivity, and the bridge may be supplied with about 1·5 V. The increase which occurs in the equilibrium temperature of the probe tip (or the out-of-balance current, to which the temperature change is proportional) when the ultrasound is switched on is proportional to the intensity, at low values of intensity.

The thermistor probe needs to be calibrated against some other measuring device, such as a thermocouple probe. Alternatively it may be calibrated by integration of the intensity profile of a beam plotted with the probe, when the total power is known from either radiation pressure or calorimetric measurements.

Szilard (1974) has described an instrument for the measurement of ultrasonic flux, using two sets of thermistors connected in a Wheatstone bridge. One set is at the input side to a transmission plate; the other is at the output side, but this set is insulated from the ultrasonic field. Temperature effects due to the environment are thus balanced and so eliminated, and the instrument measures the temperature increase due to the absorption of a small fraction of the incident energy.

Thermistor probes are easier to make than hydrophones of equivalent size. They are insensitive to stray radio-frequency fields, but they do not respond to rapid changes in ultrasonic intensity.

3.7.i Optical Methods

(i) Diffraction

The propagation of an ultrasonic wave is associated with changes in the density of the supporting medium. In a transparent medium, these variations in density lead to variations in refractive index. For a given frequency of light,

$$(n^2+2)(n^2-1)=A\rho \tag{3.28}$$

where n is the refractive index, and A is a constant which depends on the properties of the medium. Hence, for a variation in density,

$$dn/n=(d\rho/\rho)\{(n^2+2)(n^2-1)/6n^2\} \tag{3.29}$$

so that the relative change in refractive index is of the same order as the relative changes in density.

The dependence of the refractive index of a transparent medium upon the intensity of an ultrasonic field travelling through it forms the basis of the *schlieren* method for the visualization of ultrasonic disturbances. The method depends upon the deflexion of a ray of light from its undisturbed path when it passes through a medium in which there is a component of refractive index gradient normal to the ray.

Several schlieren systems have been described in the literature for the visualization of ultrasonic waves. They share the same basic principles: three typical arrangements are illustrated in Fig. 3.32. A beam of light passes through a transparent medium, usually water, in which is established the ultrasonic field to be investigated. The light is then focused on to an obstruction, so that none reaches the camera (or the observer) when the field is zero; alternatively, the focus falls in an aperture, so that all the light reaches the camera when there is no field. When ultrasound changes the refractive index of the medium, the light which passes through the disturbed areas no longer necessarily passes through the original focus, but may be deviated to change the proportion of light which reaches the camera. In more precise terms, when there is no ultrasonic disturbance, all the light is undiffracted and falls in the zero order. In a system where the zero order is occult, the light transmission is approximately proportional to the parallel plane wave ultrasonic amplitude within the range 10–80% transmission for white light (Willard, 1947). At greater ultrasonic intensities, the linear relationship fails and light reappears in the zero order.

The schlieren system illustrated in Fig. 3.32(a) uses lenses to shape the light beam. These lenses need to be free from spherical and other aberrations, and of at least the same diameter as the part of the ultrasonic field to be investigated. It is very difficult to obtain well-corrected lenses of adequate diameter. Therefore it is often better to use concave mirrors instead of lenses, as these can be made of relatively large size quite cheaply. Mirrors are free from chromatic aberration (but this is not important with monochromatic light such as that from a laser), and they can be made paraboloid in section, which eliminates spherical aberration.

The choice of occultation arrangement may be important. A spot of indian ink on a glass slide is suitable if symmetrical observation is required. It frequently happens, however, that a large proportion of the field acts along a main axis, and in this case satisfactory results can often be obtained using a knife-edge normal to the direction of the ultrasonic disturbance: for example, the system illustrated in Fig. 3.32(c) is sensitive to ultrasonic waves travelling in the plane of the diagram, as represented by the arrow.

The schlieren image may be photographed, thrown upon a suitable screen, or observed directly.

At low and medium ultrasonic intensities, the interpretation of the schlieren image is easy: the brighter that the image appears, the more intense is the corresponding part of the ultrasonic field. Unfortunately, quantitative analysis is much more difficult. The intensity of the deviated light depends not only upon the intensity of the ultrasonic disturbance, but also upon its physical extension. The analysis would be quite simple if each ray of light remained in a region of constant refractive index gradient during its passage through the ultrasonic disturbance. Since each ray is

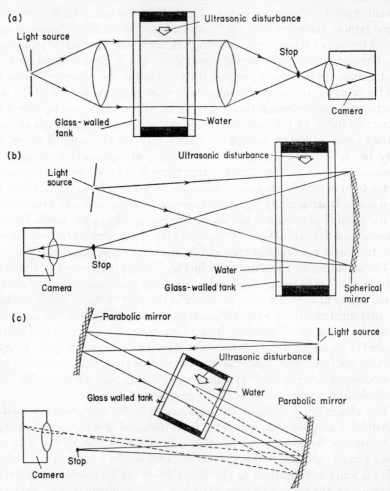

FIG. 3.32 Typical schlieren systems for ultrasonic field visualization in transparent media. (a) Lens system (after Harding and Baker, 1968); (b) and (c) systems with concave mirrors (after Sjöberg *et al.*, 1963, and James *et al.*, 1961, respectively). In the reflexion systems, it is important to ensure that the angles formed between the incident and reflected light beams along the optical axes are equal and as small as possible, in order to avoid coma and to minimize astigmatism. James *et al.* (1961) used cylindrical lenses close to the light source and the occultation plane, in order to correct for the astigmatism due to using the mirrors off their axes.

continuously refracted, however, this condition may not be satisfied even in a two-dimensional system if the disturbance contains large refractive index gradients (as it inevitably does at high ultrasonic intensities). The problem is further complicated in a three-dimensional system by the variation in refractive index across the disturbance.

Ordinary schlieren systems are incapable of visualizing very low intensity ultrasonic fields because the variation in image brightness is too small to be detectable. This applies not only to continuous wave fields, but also to pulsed beams in which the average intensity is low. Nevertheless, the ultrasonic energy in a single pulse may be quite substantial, and so it may be possible to visualize a pulsed field, which has a low average intensity, by synchronous pulsing of the light source. The time average light intensity diffracted by a pulse is equal to that for a continuous wave, reduced by the

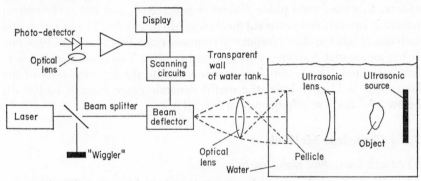

FIG. 3.33 Interference visualization system. (After Mezrich *et al.*, 1975.)

pulse duty-factor. Several such systems have been constructed: see, for example, Aldridge (1967).

In summary, schlieren techniques for the visualization of an ultrasonic field are generally useful only in so far as they give qualitative impressions of the extent of the field and variations of intensity within the field. Quantitative analysis of the schlieren image is extremely difficult, and is really only manageable when the ultrasonic field shape is very simple. An example of such an analysis has been given by Erikson (1972).

(ii) Interferometry

Optical interferometry can be used to study quite small displacements. Deferrari *et al.* (1967) used a laser interferometer to study the displacement of low-frequency transducers. The method has since been extended to higher frequencies, and holography is now also used.

Mezrich *et al.* (1975) have developed an ingenious visualization system based on interferometry, as illustrated in Fig. 3.33. The pellicle is a flexible, optically reflective membrane, with a thickness of about 6 μm and a diameter of up to 150 mm. The characteristic impedance of the pellicle is similar to that of the water in which it is suspended, and it therefore vibrates at the ultrasonic frequency according to the distribution of ultrasonic amplitude over its surface. These vibrations are detected by optical interference between a reference beam and a beam reflected by the pellicle. A two-dimensional image of the ultrasonic field is obtained by scanning the pellicle synchronously with a television-type raster display of the output from the photo-detector of the interferometer. This scanning is achieved with a mirror–galvanometer arrangement. A refinement of the system is the incorporation of the "wiggler". This is a vibrating mirror from which the reference beam is reflected. The amplitude and frequency of vibration of the wiggler are chosen so that the reference beam moves through at least 90° phase change whilst each element of the pellicle is being scanned. This ensures that maximum phase difference is detected, and makes the system relatively insensitive to external mechanical disturbances. The experimental instrument has a uniform frequency response extending to at least 10 MHz. It has an angular response which is flat to $\pm$ 40°. The resolution is wavelength-limited. The sensitivity is proportional to the light intensity of the laser; with a 15 mW laser, the useful dynamic range extends to 100 dB below 1 W cm^{-2} at a frequency of 1·5 MHz.

3.7.j Chemical Methods

(i) Starch iodine blue stain reaction

The chemical reaction whereby starch is stained blue by iodine liberated from potassium iodide is accelerated in the presence of ultrasonic radiation. This effect forms the basis of the method described by Kossoff (1962) for the visualization of ultrasonic field distributions. A suspension of starch in polyvinylacetate with small quantities of butyl plithate as plasticizer and gelatine as strengthener is spread thinly over a thin polyethylene sheet resting on a flat surface. The suspension dries to form a layer of about 70 μm thickness. Film prepared in this way can withstand water at temperatures of up to about 40°C.

In order to visualize the cross-section of an ultrasonic field, a piece of film is suspended in the plane of interest in a weak solution of potassium iodide and iodine in water. At ultrasonic intensities of between 0·1–10 W cm^{-2}, the film darkens in 5–10 s. The pattern on the film tends to fade after about 30 min, and so it has to be photographed to make a permanent record. The density of the darkening is directly proportional to the corresponding ultrasonic intensity–exposure time product. When calibrated against an absolute method of measurement, such as a thermocouple probe, accuracies of about $+15\%$ can be achieved.

(ii) Cholesteric liquid crystals

Cholesteric liquid crystals exhibit reversible irridescent colour effects at various temperatures. They have been used by Cook and Wercham (1971) to visualize the thermal pattern induced by an ultrasonic field in a polyethylene sheet floating on the surface of water. At megahertz frequencies, an intensity of around 0·25 W cm^{-2} produces a useful colour pattern within about 3–5 s, but the pattern is destroyed by lateral heat flow after about 10 s.

(iii) Structural changes in polymethylmethacrylate

Ultrasonic irradiation causes alterations within the plastic which are easily visualized with polarized light. It has been shown by Lele (1962) that there is a consistent and reproducible relationship between the size of the altered part of the plastic, and the ultrasonic "dosage". The method is particularly convenient for the demonstration of the production of trackless damage by a focused ultrasonic beam.

(iv) Lecithin solution breakdown

Ultrasonic irradiation breaks down the large particles of sols such as those of lecithin. The breakdown results in an increase in light transmission through the sol. It has been shown by Chapman and Christie (1972) that the increase in light transmission is directly proportional to the ultrasonic intensity in the range 0–16 W cm^{-2}, for conditions of constant irradiation time (30 s), at a frequency of 20 kHz.

(v) Reduction of ammonium nitrate

Trier *et al.* (1973) described how they irradiated a 10 ml solution of NH_4NO_3 (pH $= 3·9$) with ultrasound at pulse–echo intensities, and found that the formation of nitrite ions was proportional to the irradiated time (at fixed intensity) in the range 1–4 h. There seems to be no satisfactory explanation for this observation.

(vi) Enzyme systems

Unpublished data of I. V. Berezin indicate that it may be possible to devise an enzyme-based film possessing acoustochemical gain. (Indeed, it may be that the sound receptors in the ear operate as chemical amplifiers in which enzymes turn over substrate.) Enzyme-based film detectors for ultrasound would be analogous with photographic emulsions for light detection.

(vii) Other chemical systems

Various other chemical systems may be used for visualizing ultrasonic fields. They are based on temperature-sensitive chromotrophic compounds, dyes, and phosphors. They generally have low sensitivities (see Ernst and Hoffman, 1952).

3.7.k Ultrasonic Image Converters

Ultrasonic-to-electronic image conversion was first proposed in the 1930s by S. Y. Sokolov. The most common form of converter—and that discussed in this Section—is based on the property of a piezoelectric plate which allows it to resonate point by point in sympathy with an incident ultrasonic distribution, with negligible lateral spread in the thickness mode. The method has been developed in Russia (Semennikov, 1958), in Germany (Freitag *et al.*, 1960), in the UK (Smyth *et al.*, 1963), and in the USA (Jacobs *et al.*, 1963).

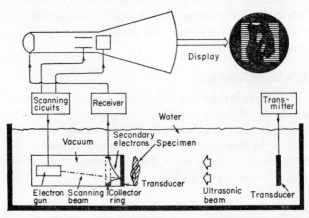

FIG. 3.34 Basic principles of ultrasonic image conversion. This system uses continuous wave ultrasound, and high energy electron scanning.

The basic principles of a typical system are illustrated in Fig. 3.34. The ultrasonic transmitting transducer irradiates the specimen with a continuous wave field, producing a "shadow" image on the transducer of the image converter (see Section 8.1.a). The acoustic image is thus converted to an electrical charge pattern on the inside surface of the transducer. The electron beam in the evacuated tube scans the charge pattern in a raster. If the scanning beam is of high energy (around 1000 V), the instantaneous current of secondary emission electrons which flows into the collector is proportional to the charge on each element of the transducer. In the design of Jacobs (1965), the performance is improved by the use of an electron multiplier which is integral with the converter. The secondary electrons from the transducer are collected by the multiplier, the output of which is fed into the video amplifier.

The converter of Smyth *et al.* (1963) uses a low energy scanning beam (around 200 V), which cannot generate secondary electrons. A sequential process is necessary in normal operation. The transducer is first scanned once with the electron beam, with no incident ultrasound. This depresses the potential of the inside surface of the transducer to that of the electron gun. The ultrasound is switched on during the next scanning frame, and more electrons can arrive at the transducer only during positive half-cycles at those points which are in vibration: the charging current is proportional to the corresponding ultrasonic amplitude. The transducer is prepared for the next sequence by allowing positive ions to be drawn to it until it is again at cathode potential.

The sensitivity of a practical ultrasonic image converter is around 10–100 nW cm^{-2} (Freitag *et al.*, 1960; Smyth *et al.*, 1963). The maximum sensitivity occurs when the transducer is $\lambda/2$ in thickness. In principle, the resolution may be improved by using a thinner transducer operating at a higher frequency, but in practice, the transducer cannot be made both large in diameter and thin in section, because it forms one of the walls of a vacuum enclosure. Consequently, most converters operate at frequencies below about 5 MHz, and have transducer diameters of less than 50 mm. Jacobs (1974) has developed discrete transducers assembled to form a large aperture, matched to the loading by plastic elements, and these have largely overcome these limitations of earlier designs. Possibly even better is the system developed by Brown *et al.* (1975), in which the transducers are mounted on the inside of a faceplate in the form of a mosaic.

Unfortunately, continuous wave operation of ultrasonic image converters is associated with image degradation due to multiple reflexions in the visualized volume. It is possible to use a pulsed system in which a separate pulse is used for each position of the scanning beam. This arrangement would require 2 s for 2000 resolution elements to be scanned at a rate of 1000 s^{-1}, which is probably about the maximum which could be achieved in practice. As one of the attractive features of the image converter is its potentially high speed, so slow a rate is unsatisfactory; and in any event, a similar performance could probably be obtained by mechanical scanning.

In order to maintain fast display rates with pulsed ultrasound, it is necessary to arrange for the entire image to be stored on some kind of sensitized plate, so that this plate can be scanned repetitively without the limitation that it would otherwise only be possible to extract information during irradiation. The stored pattern is erased after it has been scanned, just before the arrival of the next pulse. Two storage systems have been described by Goldman (1962), both of which could operate with 10 μs pulses of 1 MHz ultrasound. In the converter illustrated in Fig. 3.35(a), the flood gun is turned on at the instant that the leading edge of the pulse arrives at the transducer. If the outer surface of the transducer is at earth potential, the potential of the inner surface begins to alternate with respect to earth at the ultrasonic frequency. Each point on this surface exhibits a self-rectifying action and so stores an electron charge proportional to the corresponding ultrasonic amplitude. The flood gun is turned off at the end of the ultrasonic pulse, leaving a negative charge pattern on the inside of the transducer. This charge pattern is then scanned in a raster in the same way that a high energy continuous wave converter is scanned, the secondary electrons being collected by the mesh. When the scanning process has been completed, the charge pattern is erased by turning on the flood gun so that the inside surface of the transducer goes positive until it reaches earth potential. The converter is then ready to store the image of the next pulse.

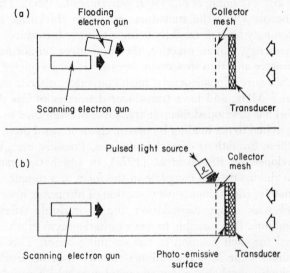

FIG. 3.35 Two types of pulsed ultrasonic image converters. (a) Secondary emission storage type; (b) photo-emission storage type.

The converter illustrated in Fig. 3.35(b) is both easier to manufacture and electronically simpler to operate than the secondary emission storage type. Goldman's (1962) design uses magnetic deflexion and focusing. The inside surface of the transducer is coated with a photoemissive layer of high lateral resistivity. The light source is turned on during the time that the ultrasonic pulse is arriving: this causes electrons to be emitted in proportion to the maximum negative voltage developed at each point on the transducer. Therefore a stored charge pattern is formed which is positive with respect to earth. Scanning at high energy not only provides the video signal, but also neutralizes the charge pattern so that no erasing process is necessary before the arrival of the next pulse.

3.7.1 Pulse Echo Methods

A method which is quite widely used for plotting the effective distribution of a pulsed ultrasonic beam is to measure the echo amplitudes from a small target situated in turn at many points in the field propagated in water, or some other liquid. The technique has been described by, for example, Panian and van Valkenburg (1961), Gordon (1964), and Wells (1966a, b). The essentials of the pulse–echo method are explained in Section 6.1.a. For echo amplitude measurement, it is usually best to employ a null method, using a calibrated attenuator in the connexion between the transducer and the receiver amplifier. The amplitude on the display is kept constant as the target is moved in the field, by making appropriate alterations in the attenuation. Relative echo amplitudes can then be expressed directly in decibels, read from the settings of the attenuator. Because the displayed amplitude is kept constant, any non-linearities in the receiver amplifier introduce only second-order errors due to alterations in the shape of the echo signal waveform. Alternatively, the attenuator may be inserted in the connexion to the transducer so that both the transmitted and received pulses are equally attenuated. In this arrangement, the relative echo amplitudes are equal to twice the difference in the corresponding attenuator settings, provided that the pulse shape is not intensity-dependent within the range investigated.

Lypacewicz and Hill (1974) have discussed the relative merits of various targets in this application. Not surprisingly, a small ball-bearing is generally an excellent choice. Such a target is self-aligning, because it is spherical in shape and so non-directional, presenting a similar surface to the beam independent of its position. The target may be attached to a wire soldered to its rear surface, which can be mounted on a coordinate measuring system. If this wire is made sufficiently long behind the target, no confusion arises between the echo from the target and those from the support. Usually the sphere should be chosen to be as small as is consistent with an adequate echo amplitude and a rigid mounting, and at low megahertz frequencies a diameter of about 3 mm is satisfactory. For sensitivity intercomparison, however, Gordon (1964) suggested the use of a steel sphere of 10 mm diameter, which could be considered to have an *"echo coefficient"* of zero decibels.

A great merit of the technique is that it produces a representation of the beam which is actually used in the pulse–echo application. The amplitude which is measured corresponds to the largest half-cycle in the received pulse, if full wave demodulation is employed. The displayed signal is generated by the system transmitter, ᵗransduced twice, and processed by the receiver which is used for diagnostic applications. Therefore, in many respects this technique for beam plotting is to be commended. Double transduction not only changes the bandwidth of the system, but also modifies the effective directivity of the beam.

An example of an ultrasonic beam plotted by this technique is shown in Fig. 3.36. In Fig. 3.36(a) the data are plotted as lines of equal echo amplitude (iso-echo amplitude curves), whereas in Fig. 3.36(b), the same data are shown in the form of echo amplitude distributions across the beam diameter at various distances from the transducer. It is not possible to measure the distribution very close to the transducer, partly because the

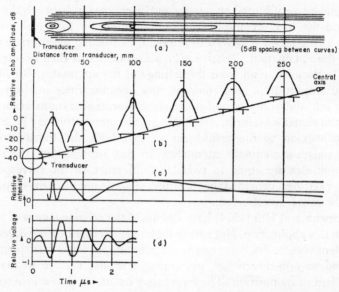

FIG. 3.36 Methods of plotting the ultrasonic field. These examples are for a 1·7 MHz (zero-crossing frequency) transducer of 20 mm diameter. (a) Iso-echo amplitude curves; (b) diametrical distributions; (c) theoretical axial intensity distribution for continuous waves; (d) echo from an extensive flat target normal to the beam. Diagrams (a) and (b) were plotted experimentally using a 3·2 mm diameter steel ball as the target in water.

pattern is rather complicated, and partly because of the paralysis of the receiver which results from the application of the transmitting pulse continues for a time which corresponds to 10–20 mm in front of the transducer.

3.7.m Reciprocity

Nowadays, the calibration of electroacoustic transducers—such as microphones and loudspeakers—by the free field reciprocity method is standard practice. The usual technique (MacLean, 1940) requires, besides the instrument to be calibrated, two additional transducers, one of which is a reversible transducer which satisfies specified reciprocity conditions. It is an attractive method because it enables acoustic quantities to be determined from electrical and length measurements. If, in a free field, an excess pressure p' produces a particle velocity v', and similarly p'' produces v'', the reciprocity theorem states that

$$p'v'' = p''v' \qquad (3.30)$$

The theorem is applicable to an electroacoustical system in its entirety, by analogies between pressure and voltage, and velocity and current.

The electroacoustic transducers used in ultrasonics are generally reversible, and Carstensen (1947) took advantage of this to develop the self-reciprocity method of calibration, which depends on reflecting the transmitted wave so that it is detected by the transducer from which it originated. No knowledge of the internal structure of the transducer is required. The receiving response M of the transducer is related to its transmitting response S by a parameter J_s which is essentially the volume current of a point source to its pressure produced at a distance d, as follows:

$$M/S = J_s = 2d\lambda/\rho c \qquad (3.31)$$

The use of this relationship requires that measurements should be made in the far field. It has been shown by Simmons and Urick (1949), however, that a similar relationship applies to plane waves in the near field, where

$$M/S = J_p = 2A/\rho c \qquad (3.32)$$

in which J_p is the plane wave reciprocity parameter, and A is the area of the transducer.

The application of this principle to the calibration of ultrasonic pulse–echo transudcers is fraught with difficulty. Some of the problems have been discussed by Reid (1974).

4. VELOCITY, ABSORPTION AND ATTENUATION IN BIOLOGICAL MATERIALS

4.1 PROPAGATION VELOCITY

In Chapter 1, the velocity of a wave is considered to have a single value. This is always true at any single value of frequency, although strictly there is no such thing in nature as a sinusoidal disturbance, because such a disturbance would be infinite in both space and time. Nevertheless, the concept is a useful one, and in practice sinusoidal wave motion may be assumed at the centre of a wave train of more than a few cycles in length. In certain circumstances, however, a number of waves of differing frequencies may be superimposed to form a *group*, and such a group *disperses* with time if the wave velocity is frequency-dependent. A group of waves exists in a pulse of short duration.

The extent to which velocity dispersion is important depends upon the absorption characteristics of the propagating medium. As pointed out in Section 1.12, absorption occurs when there is a lag between pressure and density in a wave. If a relaxation process is involved, it must be accompanied by a velocity dispersion near the relaxation frequency. This phenomenon is discussed in Section 4.5.b. In practice, the magnitude of the dispersion is very small (in the order of 0·7% of the velocity in soft tissues over a frequency range 1–10 MHz), so that the measurement is difficult and the effect is generally negligible.

Instruments designed for the measurement of velocity in non-biological materials may not be suitable for use with biological materials. This is because such materials are available only in shapes and sizes over which there is little, if any, control. The samples may be neither fluid nor rigid. Variability between different samples of similar tissues may be considerable. Many tissues are microscopically inhomogeneous. They are chemically unstable and very sensitive to environmental conditions so that measurements must be made with the minimum of disturbance to the material if reliable and reproducible results are to be obtained. Although the shape of a sample may be distorted to give a suitable geometrical configuration, as a general guide such compression should not exceed 20% of the sample thickness. Distortion beyond this may result in a significant expression of water, and it may produce irreversible changes in the tissues. Unfortunately, large homogeneous samples of tissue are unusual, particularly in small animals, although large samples are necessary for accurate measurements. Results are seldom satisfactory unless the sample is at least 5 wavelengths thick and 20 wavelengths in diameter, although velocity measurement may be possible with a sample of smaller diameter. Another factor of major importance is the temperature of the sample, since both velocity and absorption are generally temperature-dependent.

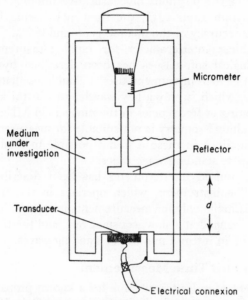

FIG. 4.1 A typical arrangement of a continuous-wave interferometer.

The experimental difficulties associated with measurements of solid tissues are much greater than those experienced with solutions and suspensions, which behave as structurally homogeneous liquids. It is relatively easy, however, to make measurements of fat, which may be substantially distorted in shape without significant alteration in structure.

4.2 METHODS OF VELOCITY MEASUREMENT

4.2.a Interferometry

The continuous-wave interferometer is suitable for the measurement of velocity in liquid and quasi-liquid materials such as blood and some other soft tissues (Andreae and Edmonds, 1961). A typical arrangement is illustrated in Fig. 4.1. The transducer generates plane longitudinal waves, and a standing wave system becomes established between the transducer and the reflector within the medium under investigation. The accuracy of the method depends on the parallelism of the opposite ends of the interferometer, and a high degree of mechanical precision is necessary. The standing wave system reacts through the transducer on to the electrical driving system, so that when the path length d is an integral number of half wavelengths, the detecting system indicates a corresponding minimum in the driving voltage. The distance d is normally made equal to around 100 half wavelengths, and an average is taken of several measurements made with the micrometer of the positions of consecutive minima. The velocity is then calculated from Eqn. 1.15, the frequency having been measured electrically. The accuracy of the method is around 0·5%.

A two-transducer interferometer for rapid measurement of sound velocity in biological soft tissues has been described by Goldman and Richards (1954). Their instrument uses a double-oscillator phase comparison detector, which is only a few wavelengths in thickness. It is also capable of operating at frequencies in the range 1–36 MHz.

Thick-sample interferometry is not suitable for measurements in highly absorbent media, since in these it is not possible to establish stationary fields with adequate standing wave ratios.

An automatic pulsed interferometer has been described by Kessler et al. (1971). The instrument, which operates in the frequency range 1–200 MHz, is suitable only for measurements in liquids. The path length is continuously changed at a slow, constant rate, and the time is measured for the passage of an integral number of standing waves.

4.2.b Pulse Transit Time Measurement

The measurement of pulse transit time for a known propagation distance gives a direct measurement of velocity (Pellam and Galt, 1946). There are two distinct methods. In the first, the pulse is transmitted by one transducer and detected by another, the axes of the two ultrasonic beam patterns being coincident. In the second method, which is based on the A-scope commonly used in medical diagnosis (Chapter 6), one transducer acts both as transmitter and receiver, with a reflector positioned normal to the ultrasonic beam axis. The transit time may be measured in either of two ways, as illustrated in Fig. 4.2. The measurement system shown in Fig. 4.2(a) uses a calibrated timebase, and a commercial oscilloscope may give an accuracy of around 3%. The comparison method shown in Fig. 4.2(b) uses the oscilloscope as a null detector, and depends for its accuracy upon the measurements of d, d' and c', and its accuracy may be around 0·5%. A variant of this latter method has been described by Kossoff et al. (1973). The distance between the transducer and the reflector is adjusted to accommodate the available length of specimen, and the echo displayed on the A-scope is photographed with an expanded timebase, by the use of an appropriate time-delay. The transducer and reflector are then placed, undisturbed in relative position, in a medium of known propagation velocity, similar to that of the specimen, and a second photograph is taken, by double exposure on the same film. The difference between the two transit times is then measured from the photograph. The distance between the transducer and the reflector, and the propagation velocity in the com-

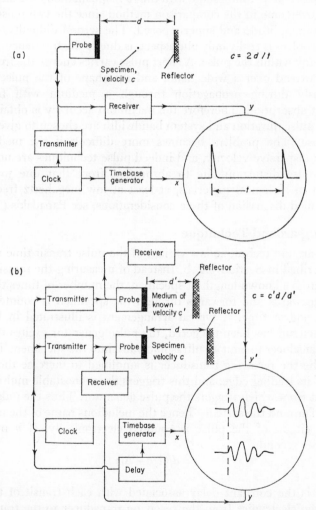

FIG. 4.2 Determination of velocity by pulse transit time measurement. (a) A-scope system (Pelham and Galt, 1946); (b) comparative system: d' is adjusted so that the transit time in the medium with known propagation velocity c' is equal to that along d in the specimen.

parison medium, are both accurately known; the velocity in the specimen may be calculated with only a small error due to uncertainty in the time-base velocity, as this is being used to measure a small difference in transit times.

Measurements made using pulse techniques suffer from two principal problems. Firstly, it is difficult to determine exactly the time-position of the beginning of the pulse, since it does not have a sharp leading edge. This is particularly troublesome with the A-scope method, but the problem is largely overcome in the comparison method since the two pulses can be matched in amplitude and superimposed. The second difficulty, of which the first problem is really only one aspect, is due to the frequency spectrum of the energy within the pulse. A short pulse carries energy the frequencies of which extend over a wide band, and the shape of the pulse changes continuously during propagation through a medium with frequency dependent absorption. Therefore the maximum accuracy is obtained only when the pulse duration and system bandwidth are chosen to give the best compromise. The problem becomes more difficult if the medium has frequency dispersive velocity, and indeed pulse techniques are not able to separate pulse distortion due to absorption from that due to velocity dispersion in biological materials, at least at low megahertz frequencies. For a detailed discussion of these considerations, see Papadakis (1972).

4.2.c Sing-around Technique

The sing-around technique is a variant of the pulse transit time measurement described in Section 4.2.b. Instead of measuring the transit time of a pulse across a known length of specimen, the number of times that pulse travels backwards and forwards through the specimen is counted over a known period of time. A typical arrangement is illustrated in Fig. 4.3. Once the circuit has been triggered, the pulse generator excites the transmitting transducer to emit an ultrasonic pulse into the specimen. The pulse detected by the receiving transducer is amplified to increase the rate-of-change of its leading edge, and this triggers the monostable multivibrator, the output from which triggers the pulse generator. Thus the pulse travels round and around the system—hence the melodious name of the method—and each circuit of the pulse is counted electronically. If n pulses are counted per second,

$$c = d/(1/n - \Delta_t) \qquad (4.1)$$

where Δ_t is the constant delay associated with each transit of the pulse through the electronics from the receiving transducer to the transmitting transducer. In order to determine Δ_t, it is necessary to calibrate the system in a medium of known propagation velocity. Although the method suffers from the difficulties inherent in all pulse techniques (see Section 4.2.b), it can have quite a high degree of accuracy. For example, the instrument constructed by Greenspan and Tschiegg (1957) is capable of the same accuracy as the comparative transit time method. The technique is particularly suited to the measurement of small changes in velocity, such as occur as a result of small changes in sample temperature.

4.2.d Velocity Difference Method

This method has been used to measure velocity dispersion in biological materials. As shown in Fig. 4.4, a test vessel is divided into two compartments by a plastic film window. One compartment is filled with water

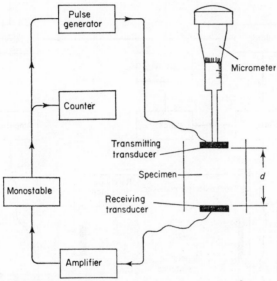

FIG. 4.3 A "sing-around" system for velocity measurement. (Based on Venrooij, 1971.)

(which is free from velocity dispersion, since it does not exhibit relaxation phenomena), and the other, with the liquid under investigation. The transmitting and receiving transducers are mounted on an assembly which can be translated horizontally: one transducer is in the water, and the other, in the sample. The separation between the transducers is fixed, and the distance moved by the assembly may be accurately measured.

If the velocities in the water and the sample differ, a phase change occurs in the received signal as the transducer assembly is moved horizontally. Effectively free-field conditions can be obtained even in a small test vessel, by pulsing the transmitted ultrasound; and the use of long pulses avoids the difficulties associated with the frequency bandwidth of short pulses (see Section 4.2.b). For example, a pulse with a duration of 10 ms contains 500 cycles at 0·5 MHz, and the half-width of the effective frequency band of such a pulse is about 1% of the nominal frequency. At 10 MHz, the situation is more favourable, the half-width being less than 0·1% of the nominal frequency.

In order to measure the phase of the received signal, the output of the receiving transducer is added to a reference signal derived from the oscillator. This sum has a minimum value when the signals are in antiphase.

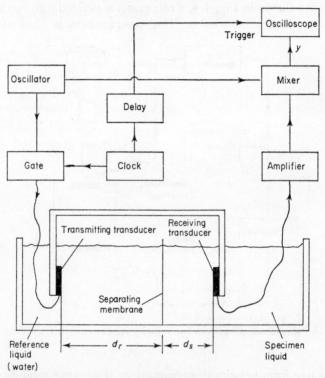

FIG. 4.4 Apparatus for velocity difference measurement by phase comparison. (Based on Carstensen, 1954.)

The phase of the received signal depends, among other things, on the number of wavelengths n which separate the transducers. Now

$$n = d_r/\lambda_r + d_s/\lambda_s \qquad (4.2)$$

where d_r and d_s are the path lengths in the reference liquid (water) and the sample respectively, and λ_r and λ_s are the corresponding wavelengths. If the transducer assembly is moved along the axis of the test vessel a distance Δ_z so that the received signal undergoes a phase change of 360°, then, if $\lambda_s > \lambda_r$, the number of wavelengths in the ultrasonic path is increased so that

$$n+1 = (d_r + \Delta_z)/\lambda_r + (d_s - \Delta_z)/\lambda_s \qquad (4.3)$$

Substracting Eqn. 4.3 from Eqn. 4.2 and substituting velocities for wavelengths, it follows that

$$c_s = c_r^2\{1/(f\Delta_z - c_r)\} + c_r \qquad (4.4)$$

where f is the frequency and c_r and c_s are the velocities in the water and the sample respectively. If c_r is frequency-independent, variation in the quantity $f\Delta_z$ is due to velocity dispersion in the sample.

The quantity $f\Delta_z \gg c_r$. Since f may be measured with any required precision, errors related to the assumed value of c_r and the measurement of Δ_z determine the accuracy of the method. A basic limitation is due to uncertainty in the value of c_r: a table of values for water has been compiled by Grosso and Mader (1972), who claim an accuracy of about 1 part in 10^5. In order to match this accuracy, it is necessary to maintain the working temperature with an accuracy of around 2 parts in 10^5 at 37°C (when the velocity in water is 1523·618 m s^{-1}) (see also Fig. 1.6).

The velocity difference method was developed by Carstensen (1954) and it has been used to determine the velocity, and velocity dispersion, in the frequency range 0·3–10 MHz, in various biological materials including aqueous solutions of haemoglobin (see Section 4.5.c).

4.2.e Reflexion Coefficient

The relationship between the characteristic impedances of the media on each side of a boundary, and the reflectivity of the boundary, is given in Eqns. 1.47 and 1.49. Since the characteristic impedance of a material is equal to the product of its density and propagation velocity (see Section 1.6), the latter may be calculated from a measurement of reflectivity if the sample (of known density) is immersed in a medium of known characteristic impedance. The method has been used by Dunn and Fry (1961) in order to determine the velocity in lung (see Section 4.7.a).

4.3 METHODS OF ATTENUATION MEASUREMENT

4.3.a Pulse Techniques

Pulse techniques may appear at first sight to offer an easy solution to the measurement of ultrasonic attenuation. There are three distinct methods. First, the pulse may be propagated through the specimen from a transmitting transducer to a receiving transducer. Second, the pulse may be propagated through the specimen from a transmitting transducer to a reflector, and then back along the same path to the same transducer which also acts as a receiver. In both these methods, the attenuation of the pulse resulting from travelling over a known length of the specimen may be measured. Third, the pulse may be emitted into the specimen by a transmitting transducer which then receives echoes from uniformly or quasiuniformly distributed discontinuities in characteristic impedance within the specimen, making it possible to measure the rate of decay of echo amplitude with distance. This is the method described by Mountford and Wells (1972).

In all three of these methods, many practical variants of which can be conceived, it is possible to measure the relative pulse amplitude in decibels (see Appendix 2) by means of a calibrated attenuator. Such instruments are both accurate and inexpensive, for they find wide application in communications engineering.

The major difficulty with all pulse systems of attenuation measurement arises as a result of the frequency dispersive characteristics of most materials, including almost all those of biological origin. Short pulses contain energy spread over a wide frequency spectrum: this is responsible also for several problems in medical diagnostics (see, for example, Chapter 6). Namery and Lele (1972) proposed a method of attenuation measurement, based on frequency spectrum analysis, which depends on the wide energy frequency spectrum of short ultrasonic pulses. The idea was taken up by Holasek *et al.* (1973), who constructed an automatic system in which discrete frequency measurements of attenuation were calculated from the effects on the frequency spectrum of a pulse transmitted through samples of material. Likewise Chivers and Hill (1975) have obtained useful results from spectral studies.

Fortunately, except in the echo method it is not generally necessary to use a very short ultrasonic pulse for attenuation measurement—unless the specimen is very small—and monotonic conditions may be assumed except close to the beginning and the end of a long pulse. The maximum usable pulse length is limited only by the need to avoid superimposition of signals, the time durations of which are determined by the thickness of the specimen and the decay of reverberations. These considerations do not apply, however, to the echo methods, in which long pulses (or narrow bandwidths) introduce errors due to uncertainty in target range.

In considering published data on attenuation, it is as well to remember that the restrictions just explained have often been overlooked.

The fixed path length instrument described in Section 4.2.d is particularly suited to the making of comparative measurements of attenuation. The changes in the received pulse amplitude resulting from changes in d_1 and d_2 can be measured by a comparison technique, and related to the attenuation in the specimen if that in the other compartment is known.

The type of pulse instrument which is best for the measurement of attenuation in any particular specimen depends upon the characteristics and quantity of the specimen. Some methods are clearly only suited to measurements in liquids, whereas others may be used to determine the attenuation of specimens the dimensions of which are outside the control of the investigator.

A simple and useful instrument for the measurement of attenuation using the pulse–echo method has been described by Hueter (1958). It consists of a C-shaped frame, on one end of which is mounted a flat reflecting surface, and on the other, a transducer attached to a micrometer drive. The axis of the ultrasonic beam is directed towards the reflector, which is normal to the beam. In use, the sample is held between the transducer and the reflector, and the echo amplitude from the reflector is compared with that obtained when the sample is replaced by a medium (usually a liquid) of known attenuation. Since the distance between the transducer and the reflector is known, it is possible to calculate the attenuation of the sample.

The development of instruments to measure attenuation in liquids is relatively much better advanced. Methods of temperature control are mentioned by Andreae *et al.* (1958) and Edmonds (1966); the particular difficulties experienced at higher frequency are discussed by Hunter and Dardy (1964); and automatic systems are described by Andreae and Joyce (1962), Edmonds *et al.* (1962) and Kessler *et al.* (1971).

4.3.b Thermocouple Probe

The time rate of change of temperature recorded by a thermocouple embedded in an absorbent medium subjected to a long ultrasonic pulse is proportional both to the ultrasonic intensity and to the absorption co-efficient of the medium. The relationship is given in Eqn. 3.27. This relationship may be used to determine the absorption coefficient of biological materials. Measurements made in this way by Dunn and Fry (1961) and Dunn (1962) of the absorption coefficient in spinal cord and in lung respectively are included in the data quoted in Section 4.4.

4.3.c Spherical Resonator

A spherical vessel containing a low-loss liquid and supported with the minimum of damping has a high Q-factor. Hueter (1958) has described such a system, consisting of a 3 litre hollow glass sphere filled with water. The resonator is shock-excited into oscillation by an electrostatic displacement of a broad band around its outer surface. The vibrations of the resonator are detected by means of a piezoelectric pickup. The system has a resonance frequency of about 8 kHz. The rate of decay of the vibrations of the resonator provides an index of the Q-factor of the system. The introduction of an absorbent specimen at the centre of the sphere lowers the

Q-factor, and consequently reduces the reverberation decay time, by an amount which depends on the absorption coefficient of the specimen. The method is very suited to the measurement of the low-frequency absorption coefficients of small samples of solid biological materials.

4.4 DATA FOR BIOLOGICAL MATERIALS

The results of many measurements of attenuation and velocity in biological materials have been published in the literature. Disappointingly, it is not possible to build up from these results a comprehensive set of data which could be used either to test relevant theories, or accurately to guide the ultrasonic instrument designer. Experiment and theory can only be compared for a limited number of materials, such as aqueous solutions of macromolecules like polysaccharides, polypeptides, and proteins, and "idealized" tissues such as homogenized liver, and a few separated tissue constituents.

Another disappointment is that often in the literature confusion arises between the terms *attenuation* and *absorption*. Absorption refers to the conversion of ultrasonic to thermal energy; attenuation refers to the total propagation loss, including absorption. In this respect—and no doubt in others—the purist may be able to criticize this book; it is hoped that both he and the ordinary reader, being aware of the problem, will allow the author a little license.

The experimental data are so sparse that it is not realistic to limit attention to tissues from man. Similar mammalian tissues are here grouped together, regardless of species. It is seldom possible to take much account of the temperatures at which the measurements were made. At least in the temperature range 7–35°C, and the frequency range 0·4–10 MHz, haemoglobin solutions of normal physiological concentration exhibit decreasing values of $\alpha\lambda$ with increasing temperature (Carstensen and Schwan, 1959b). Although it is far from being linear, the relationship at 5 MHz is approximately -1% degK^{-1}. Similar relationships occur in other protein solutions (El'piner *et al.*, 1970). This behaviour is comparable with that of polyatomic associated liquids. In contrast, Dunn (1962) has shown that, at least in the temperature range 2–28°C and at a frequency of 1 MHz, the value of absorption coefficient for tissue from the central nervous system (spinal cord of young mouse) increases with increasing temperature: at 25°C, the temperature coefficient is $+1\cdot8\%$ degK^{-1}. This behaviour is comparable with that of polyatomic unassociated liquids. The absorption coefficient of tissue (again from the central nervous system) is independent of intensity up to at least 200W cm^{-2} at a frequency of 1 MHz (Dunn, 1962; and see Section 4.8). At high intensities, this independence is valid only for short durations of irradiation, since otherwise the characteristics of the specimen may be irreversibly changed by heat. A factor which is still largely unresolved is the "freshness" of the tissue: although Hueter (1958) found that the absorption coefficient of liver fell by a factor of two at 4 MHz, 20 h post-mortem, Pauly and Schwan (1971) did not seem to notice any change in absorption in liver due to ageing. The data for absorption are

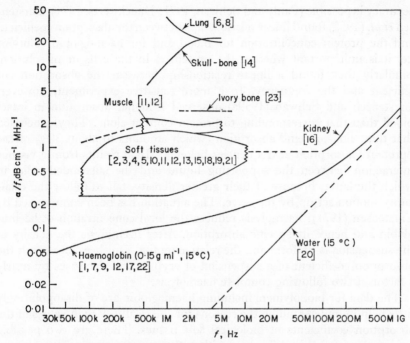

FIG. 4.5 Attenuation in biological materials, expressed in terms of α/f: collected data. Data sources: [1] Carstensen and Schwan (1959); [2] Chivers and Hill (1975); [3] Colombati and Petralia (1950); [4] Danckwerts (1974); [5] Dunn (1962); [6] Dunn (1974); [7] Dunn et al. (1969); [8] Dunn and Fry (1961); [9] Edmonds et al. (1970); [10] Esche (1952); [11] Goldman and Hueter (1956, 1957); [12] Gramberg (1956); [13] Hueter (1948); [14] Hueter (1952); [15] Hueter (1958); [16] Kessler (1973); [17] Mayer and Vogel (1965); [18] Mountford and Wells (1972); [19] Pauly and Schwan (1971); [20] Pinkerton (1949); [21] Pohlman (1939); [22] Schneider et al. (1969); [23] White and Curry (1975).

presented in Fig. 4.5. It is immediately apparent that, for biological soft tissues in the frequency range 0·1–50 MHz,

$$\alpha \simeq af^b \qquad (4.5)$$

where a and b depend upon the characteristics of the particular tissue and the conditions of measurement (such as temperature), and have fairly constant values over limited ranges of frequency. The value of b is generally only a little greater than unity. It is impossible to separate the results in the literature for different soft tissues, except to note that the absorption in muscle seems to be rather greater than that in other soft tissues. There is also some suggestion of anistropic absorption in muscle (Hueter, 1948). The data for liver, in the frequency range 1–10 MHz, are deduced from those obtained with homogenized tissue, and a relatively high degree of accuracy is possible (Pauly and Schwan, 1971; Danckwerts, 1974). Carstensen *et al.* (1953) found linear relationships between the absorption coefficient and the protein concentration for blood and for haemoglobin solution: i.e. it is unimportant whether the protein is in the cells or in solution. Similarly they found a linear relationship between the absorption coefficient and the frequency. In a more sensitive experiment, however, Carstensen and Schwan (1959a) observed a higher absorption in intact blood than that corresponding to protein content alone. They concluded that this "non-protein" absorption (which amounts to about 30% of the "protein" absorption at frequencies below 4 MHz) results from a viscous interaction between the supporting liquid and the suspended cells, in which the latter, because of their greater density, fail to follow the oscillatory motion set up by the wave. The situation has been summarized by Carstensen (1971): haemolysis reduces the local concentration of haemoglobin and hence its specific absorption. After haemolysis the density of the suspension is uniform and the relative motion vanishes. As a result the absorption coefficient of a suspension of erythrocytes decreases by nearly a factor of two following complete haemolysis.

The data for biopolymers including haemoglobin are of disappointingly little help in understanding the reasons for the relatively high values of the absorption coefficients of biological soft tissues. There are two possible explanations for this difference: either the specific absorption of tissue proteins must be considerably greater than those of blood and similar proteins, or tissue absorption must be due to some process other than relaxation at the macromolecular level. In an attempt to resolve the matter, Pauly and Schwan (1971) have discussed the mechanism of absorption in liver. They used fresh beef and lamb liver, obtained from an abattoir and stored at 4°C. The approximate composition by weight of liver is: water, 70%; protein, 20%; total lipid, 5%; carbohydrates and metabolites, 2·5%; ash, 1·5%; and nucleic acids, 1%. The absorption in minced liver, which can be considered to represent "idealized" liver tissue of random orientation of cells and unaffected by major structural disturbances, has a value $\alpha = 0.70f^{1.17}$, where α is expressed in dB cm^{-1}, and f in MHz, for the frequency range 1–10 MHz. At any frequency within this range, $\alpha \propto$ (concentration of liver material). The absorption coefficient of homogenized liver has a value $\alpha = 0.56f^{1.12}$. Thus, it has nearly the same frequency dependence as minced liver, which indicates that neither cells nor subcellular organelles contribute significantly as structural units to the total absorption. Its absolute value is about 20% less than that of solid or minced liver. Hence the major part of the total absorption seems to arise on a level of organization smaller than that defined by cells, cell nuclei and mitochondria.

Different molecular components were found to have different values of specific absorption (α per g solid per 100 ml). The supernatant (which consists of soluble proteins, microsomes and a small fraction of mitochondria) has a specific absorption comparable with that of haemoglobin. For the separated fractions of a sample of homogenate, the α values for supernatant, homogenate, and sediment are approximately in the ratio 1:2:4. According to Smith and Schwan (1971), the specific absorption of liver nuclei is about three times greater than that of haemoglobin, and five times greater than that of gelatin. It seems reasonable to suppose that at least some other tissue proteins have specific absorption values comparable with that of liver nuclei, and that tissue absorption can be explained on a macromolecular level.

Ultrasonic velocities are shown in Fig. 4.6. It is difficult to draw conclusions from these data, for the reasons that make it hard to analyse the absorption data. It can be seen from Fig. 4.6(a) that lung and bone have velocities which differ considerably from those of all other biological tissues, the restricted velocity range of which is shown in more detail in Fig. 4.6(b).

It is interesting to note that the velocity in postmenopausal breast, which contains a high proportion of fat, is only a little faster than the velocity in fat alone; whereas the velocity in premenopausal breast, which contains substantially more glandular tissue, is significantly higher. The velocity in lactating breast is greater than that in milk; there seems to be no obvious explanation for this.

4.5 RELEVANT THEORIES

4.5.a Classical Absorption

It is explained in Section 1.12 that the classical mechanism of absorption of ultrasound in fluids is due to the frictional forces which act to oppose the periodic motion of the particles in the medium. The effect is expressed mathematically in Eqn. 1.60. The absorption for which this mechanism is responsible is proportional to the square of the frequency, and it is consistent with absorption in water (see Fig. 4.5). It is not the relationship which is found experimentally to occur in biological tissues, in which the absorption coefficient has a lower power dependence (approaching unity) on the frequency. Also, the classical mechanism would give an absorption coefficient of only about 0·01 dB cm^{-1} at 1 MHz, taking tissue viscosity to

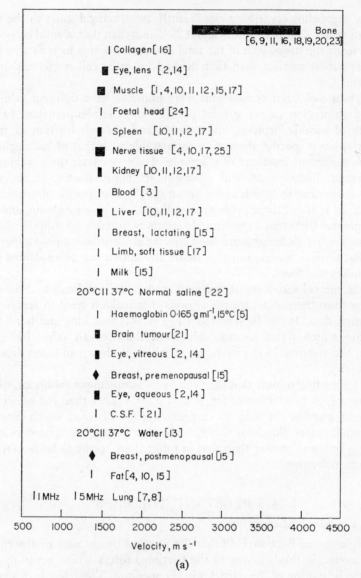

(a)

FIG. 4.6 Velocity in biological materials: collected data. (a) Including lung and bone; (b) data for soft tissues, and symbol key. Data sources: [1] Bakke and Gyfre (1974); [2] Begui (1954); [3] Bradley and Sacherio (1972); [4] Buschmann *et al.* (1970); [5] Carstensen and Schwan (1959); [6] Craven *et al.* (1973); [7] Dunn (1974); [8] Dunn and Fry (1961); [9] Floriani *et al.* (1967); [10] Frucht (1953); [11] Goldman and Hueter (1956, 1957); [12] Goldman and Richards (1954); [13] del Grosso and Mader (1972); [14] Jansson and Sundmark (1961); [15] Kossoff *et al.* (1973); [16] Lees (1971); [17] Ludwig (1950); [18] Martin and McElhaney

be 15 Pa s. In an attempt to explain how a linear relationship between the absorption coefficient and the frequency might come about, Fry (1952) hypothesized that biological soft tissue absorption might be explained in terms of viscous forces acting between a suitably chosen distribution of suspended particles or structure elements and the suspending liquid. This theory, however, has received no experimental support.

A comprehensive report from this era is that of Hueter (1958). He presented a mass of data, and a great deal of theory, including a thorough analysis of viscoelastic losses and the possible role of suspended particles.

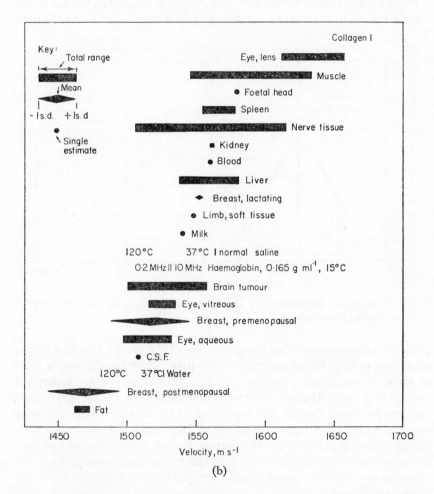

(b)

(1971); [19] Rich *et al.* (1966); [20] Thiesman and Pfander (1949); [21] Venrooij (1971); [22] Vigoureux (1952); [23] Wells (1966); [24] Willocks *et al.* (1964); [25] Wladimiroff *et al.* (1975).

4.5.b Relaxation

Relaxation is the term used to describe the behaviour of media in which the bulk modulus has one value for slow processes, and another for fast processes. A descriptive treatment of the phenomenon is given in Section 1.12. In the present Section, the discussion is restricted to basic principles and concepts, and does not deal with detailed calculations which are complicated and may even be rather tentative. For thorough treatment of the subject see, for example, Markham *et al.* (1951), Hertzfield and Litovitz (1959), Litovitz (1959) and Bhatia (1967).

If the energy stored within part of a system is suddenly changed by an outside influence, the energy is subsequently redistributed to equilibrium

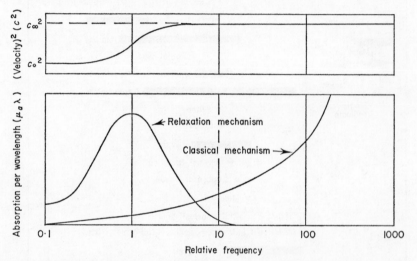

Fig. 4.7 Frequency dependence of absorption and velocity in a medium with a single relaxation frequency.

within the energy-containing compartments of the system by a sharing, or relaxation, process which occupies a finite time. The energy in one or more of these compartments changes practically instantaneously during the passage of a wave. If there were no coupling between the compartments, the energy stored during any particular phase of each cycle would be returned without loss at some later phase. In practice, however, the excess energy is shared between the compartments, and the transfer of energy is associated with time delays which give rise to changes in the phase of the returned energy. This out-of-phase energy interferes with the wave, and absorption occurs.

Figure 4.7 illustrates the relationship between both the absorption per wavelength ($\mu_a\lambda$) and the square of the velocity (c^2), and the relative frequency (f/f_r), for a medium with a single relaxation frequency f_r. At low frequencies, even though energy is transferred between system compartments, the sharing process occupies times which are short compared with the period of the wave. The associated energy phase differences are small, and the absorption per wavelength is low. As the frequency is increased, however, the wave period becomes closer to the time constant of the relaxation process, and $\mu_a\lambda$ has a maximum value $(\mu_a\lambda)_{max}$ when the two times are equal. The magnitude of $(\mu_a\lambda)_{max}$ depends on the proportion of input wave energy which is shared between the various compartments of the system. As the frequency is further increased, a decreasing proportion of the wave energy is coupled between compartments because the time available for sharing to occur is reduced. At these higher frequencies, the classical absorption mechanism due to viscosity becomes important, and μ_a increases with a quadratic dependence on frequency.

It can also be seen from Fig. 4.7 that the velocity increases in the relaxation region from a low-frequency value c_0 to a high-frequency value c_∞. The phenomenon is called *dispersion*. It is consistent with the concept that the energy-sharing between compartments becomes less significant with increasing frequency, with the result that the medium behaves as if it has an increased stiffness.

In the case of a medium with a single relaxation frequency, it may be shown (see, for example, Markham *et al.*, 1951) that:

$$\mu_a\lambda = 2(\mu_a\lambda)_{max} \frac{(\omega/\omega_m)}{1+(\omega/\omega_m)^2} \qquad (4.6)$$

and

$$c^2 - c_0^2 = (2\pi/)\{(\mu_a\lambda)_{max}\}c_0c_\infty \frac{(\omega/\omega_m)^2}{1+(\omega/\omega_m)^2} \qquad (4.7)$$

where $\omega_m = 2\pi f_m$, and f_m is the frequency at which $(\mu_a\lambda) = (\mu_a\lambda)_{max}$. Hence, approximately,

$$c - c_0 \propto \mu_a \qquad (4.8)$$

The principal relaxational mechanisms which can occur are as follows:

(i) Thermal relaxation

This is the chief cause of ultrasonic loss in gases, and it is also of majoi importance, along with shear viscosity, in contributing to the absorption in many non-associated non-polar liquids. Thermal relaxation may be due to the rise in temperature acocmpanying adiabatic compression, and the time lag for the transfer of energy from external to internal degrees of freedom. Thermal relaxation may alternatively be due to a vibrational mechanism which is a binary collision process in which, at any instant in time, one molecule interacts exclusively with only one other molecule, and the time constant depends upon the molecular size and the mean free path length. In yet another type of mechanism, thermal isomeric relaxation, the molecules of the medium can exist in different isomeric forms. The wave perturbs the equilibrium between the isomers, either by direct transfer of translational energy by a collision process, or through coupling with other internal degrees of freedom of the molecule, such as vibrational modes.

(ii) Structural relaxation

In associated liquids, such as water, thermal relaxation is not the dominant cause of ultrasonic loss. This is because the large intermolecular forces in such liquids are associated with very short relaxation times. This group of liquids exhibits a certain degree of structural order, typically extending over groups of 5–50 molecules. This short-range order is incomplete, however, and there are "holes" in the liquid "lattice". Absorption is due directly to volume changes: the wave changes the packing density of the lattice. This process of structural rearrangement occupies a finite time, and so the volume is not in phase with the pressure. For a complete treatment of this situation see Andreae and Lamb (1959).

(iii) Heat conduction relaxation

This process is concerned with the direct transfer of heat from high-pressure regions into low-pressure regions. It is relatively unimportant in biological materials.

(iv) Heat radiation relaxation

This process is concerned with the radiant transfer of heat. It is relatively unimportant in biological materials.

4.5.c Absorption and Dispersion in Biological Materials

The observed dependence of absorption coefficient on frequency can be explained neither by the classical viscosity theory nor by a mechanism involving a single relaxation frequency. Indeed, viscosity may be excluded as a significant factor at low megahertz frequencies, because as pointed out in Section 4.5.a, the contribution which this mechanism could make to absorption is far less than that which is found in practice. Hysteresis (see Hueter, 1958; and Section 1.12) can give rise to frequency independent values of $\alpha\lambda$, but this cannot account for the velocity dispersion which has been observed in haemoglobin (Carstensen and Schwan, 1959), and which is illustrated in Fig. 4.8.

The existence of dispersion, however, is good evidence of relaxation. Fry (1952) pointed out that relaxation effects, for materials with single relaxation frequencies, yield a quadratic dependence at low frequencies, a constant value at high frequencies, and no intermediate band which would correspond to the experimental data on tissues. With characteristic thoroughness, however, he mentioned that absorption in tissues might be due to a distribution of relaxation frequencies; but he did not investigate this possibility. It was H. P. Schwan (quoted by Fry and Dunn, 1962) who explained that a variation of as little as 20% in the value of $\alpha\lambda$ over a frequency decade could be accounted for by the existence of two relaxation processes, one relaxation frequency occurring near the lower end of the frequency range, with the other at a much higher frequency. This is illustrated in Fig. 4.9.

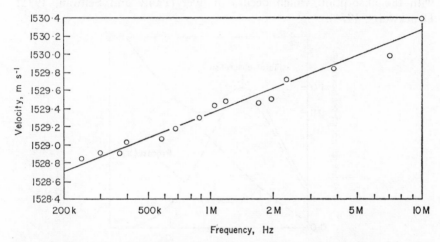

FIG. 4.8 Frequency dependence of velocity in an aqueous solution of human haemoglobin, concentration 0·165 g ml^{-1}, at 15°C. (Data of Carstensen and Schwan, 1959.)

Whilst this simple model, based on two relaxation processes, is helpful in giving an insight into the role of relaxation in absorption, it is inadequate to match the accuracy of the measurements which have been made of the absorption in aqueous solutions of haemoglobin, for which representative data are given in Fig. 4.5. The model can be extended (Carstensen and Schwan, 1959) to take account of N relaxing elements with associated frequencies ω_m equal to $\omega_1, \omega_2, \ldots, \omega_N$, so that

$$\mu_a\lambda = \int_{\omega_1}^{\omega_N} 2(\mu_a\lambda)_n {}^*f(\omega_n) \frac{(\omega/\omega_n)}{1+(\omega/\omega_n)^2}\, d\omega_n + B^*\omega \qquad (4.9)$$

and

$$c^2 - c_0^{*2} = \int_{\omega_1}^{\omega_N} (2/\pi)(\mu_a\lambda)_n {}^*c_0 c_\infty f(\omega_n) \frac{(\omega/\omega_n)}{1+(\omega/\omega_n)^2}\, d\omega_n \qquad (4.10)$$

where $(\mu_a\lambda)_n{}^* = \omega_n c(\mu_a\lambda)_{max}/2\pi$ and $B^*\omega$ represent all those absorption processes which are proportional to the square of the frequency; $f(\omega)$ is a function describing the distribution of the relaxing elements. The function $f(\omega)$ which best fits the experimental data is a "logarithmic box" distribution of relaxation times (Edmonds, 1962), with the frequency spectrum extending up to at least 300 MHz. Dunn *et al.* (1969) have quoted measurements made at 270 and 470 MHz which give further support to these conclusions. A report of minor errors in the data of Edmonds (1962) (Edmonds *et al.*, 1970) does not give cause for modification of the theory. A similar distribution of relaxation times has been shown to be compatible with the absorption which occurs in liver (Pauly and Schwan, 1971; Danckwerts, 1974).

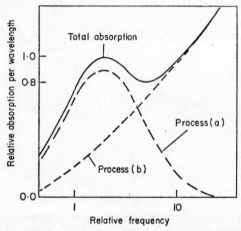

FIG. 4.9 Relative absorption per wavelength in a medium with two relaxation frequencies. (Based on Fry and Dunn, 1962.)

The data for absorption in haemoglobin reveal a high-frequency asymptotic value of specific absorption $(\alpha/f^2)\lim\limits_{f\to\infty} = 2{\cdot}87 \times 10^{-15}$ dB s^2 cm^{-1} (Schneider *et al.*, 1969). The corresponding excess absorption per wavelength

$$(\alpha\lambda)_{excess} = \{\alpha - f^2(\alpha/f^2)\lim\limits_{f\to\infty}\}\lambda \qquad (4.11)$$

is shown in Fig. 4.10 for the entire frequency range over which data are available. These results can be explained in terms of only four relaxation frequencies, as indicated on the graph. This explanation is more acceptable in physical terms than the continuous relaxation spectrum distribution proposed by Edmonds (1962), for it is difficult to imagine that more than a few relaxation processes could occur even in such a complex situation as an aqueous solution of haemoglobin. Note the value of $(\alpha/f^2)\lim\limits_{f\to\infty}$ for haemoglobin solution is greater than that of α/f^2 for water ($2\cdot60 \times 10^{-15}$ dB s^2 cm^{-1}); this indicates either that there are further relaxation processes operating at frequencies around 1 GHz, or that the water structure is altered by the presence of the macromolecule. This latter possibility has been proposed by Hammes and Lewis (1966) in connexion with absorption in polyethylene glycol solutions.

Rough analysis of the data of Carstensen and Schwan (1959) for haemoglobin reveals a linear relationship between velocity dispersion and absorption. Quantitatively,

$$c_{10} - c_1 \simeq 10\alpha_1 \qquad (4.12)$$

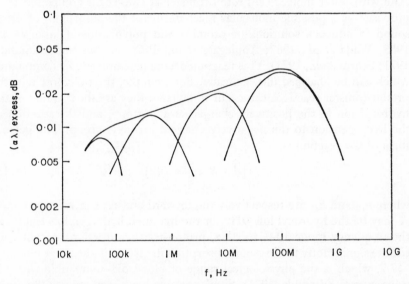

FIG. 4.10 Excess absorption per wavelength for haemoglobin ($0\cdot15$ g ml^{-1}), showing that the experimental data may be closely approximated by assuming only four relaxation frequencies. (Based on Schneider *et al.*, 1969.)

where c_1 and c_{10} are the velocities (in m s^{-1}) at 1 and 10 MHz respectively, and α_1 is the absorption coefficient (in dB cm^{-1}) at 1 MHz. This is in agreement with Eqn. 4.8 for relaxation phenomena. Assuming that the same constant of proportionality applies to soft tissues (and to some extent this is justified by the direct proportionality between absorption and concentration: see, for example, Él'piner *et al.*, 1970; Hammes and Lewis, 1966; Schneider *et al.*, 1969; and by the similarity between the high-frequency asymptotic values for haemoglobin and soft tissues: Kessler, 1973), the velocity at 1 MHz would be about 10 m s^{-1} less than that at 10 MHz for a typical value of $\alpha/f = 1$ dB cm^{-1} MHz^{-1}. This corresponds to a velocity dispersion of about $0\cdot7\%$ per frequency decade, which is negligible in comparison with the experimental ranges and errors of measurement for "solid" tissues, as illustrated in Fig. 4.6(b).

4.6 RELAXATION PROCESSES IN BIOLOGICAL MATERIALS

Biological soft tissues are very complex structures, and at the present time little is known of the relaxation processes responsible for absorption and dispersion in these materials. When a biological molecule is in aqueous solution, a certain amount of the solvent becomes an inherent part of the molecule, since the polymer possesses ionic and polar groups which associate with water molecules. Proton transfer at side-chain groups has been proposed as a possible molecular mechanism for the absorption of ultrasound in aqueous solutions of proteins and polypeptides (Burke et al., 1965; Wada et al., 1967; Applegate et al., 1968; Hussey and Edmonds, 1971; Sturm et al., 1971). This reaction occurs in simple model compounds which can be analysed ultrasonically. For example, the two most relevant proton-transfer reactions can occur in glycine: they are the addition of the hydroxyl ion to the positively charged amino group, and the addition of the hydrogen ion to the negatively charged carboxyl group. The general form of the reaction is

$$(1)A + X \underset{k_{21}}{\overset{k_{12}}{\rightleftharpoons}} B(2) \qquad (4.13)$$

where k_{12} and k_{21} are respectively the forward and reverse rate constants; X may be the hydroxyl ion OH^-, or the hydrated hydrogen ion H_3O^+. In the frequency range 10–130 MHz, proton-transfer reactions do not contribute significantly to ultrasonic absorption in glycine in the range $6 \cdot 8 \leqslant pH \leqslant 7 \cdot 7$, which is the physiological range of blood pH compatible with life (Hussey and Edmonds, 1971). Similar results have been reported by Zana and Lang (1974) for amniotic fluid in the frequency range 1–14 MHz. It has been shown by Schneider et al. (1969) that the absorption in haemoglobin is independent of pH in the range $4 \leqslant pH \leqslant 9$. Similarly, the absorption in DNA has a maximum value at $pH = 11 \cdot 9$, which corresponds to the midpoint of the denaturation of the protein molecule; but there is no evidence that proton transfer reactions occur at physiological values of pH (Sturm et al., 1971). Again, Pauly and Schwan (1971) have shown that the absorption in 25% gelatin has maximum values at $pH = 2 \cdot 5$ and $11 \cdot 5$, and that the absorption in liver has a maximum value at $pH = 11 \cdot 5$. Although it is difficult to separate effects due to proteins from those due to lipids, it seems likely that the contribution of lipids to total absorption is small. Amino and carboxyl groups on haemoglobin and plasma proteins are exchanged at pH values remote from the physiological range (Kessler and Dunn, 1969; O'Brien and Dunn, 1972), and so it may be concluded that they are not involved in relevant relaxation processes. The histidine residue is thus the only group which might take part in proton transfer reactions in the physiological pH range, but this can be excluded on the basis of known values of k_{12} and structural volume change.

The absorption coefficients of nearly all aqueous solutions of structurally ordered biopolymers of equivalent concentrations are of the same order of magnitude, and they exhibit similar frequency dependence (O'Brien and Dunn, 1972). Consequently, the absorption mechanisms, within the physiological pH range, are quite likely to be the same. There seems little reason to suppose that proton transfer reactions which, accordingly to the available evidence, operate at non-physiological values of pH, are involved in the absorption and dispersion processes in living tissues.

In solutions, structuring is at the molecular level. It has been pointed out by Zaretskii *et al.* (1972), in analysing data of Hawley *et al.* (1965a, b) that for aqueous solutions of dextran, $\alpha/f^2 \propto$ (molecular weight) at constant concentration and frequency. Serum albumin and haemoglobin, however, which have similar molecular weights, have considerably different values of α/f^2, whereas that of gamma globulin is quite close to that of haemoglobin. Therefore, it seems possible that the α-helicity of proteins may have an influence on absorption. Thus, "coiling agents" such as sodium dodecyl-sulphate, which increase protein α-helicity, increase the absorption; whilst disintegration of α-coils under the action of urea or guanidine hydrochloride, which "fuse" the protein α-structure, results in appreciable reduction in absorption. In contrast, O'Brien and Dunn (1972) concluded that proton-transfer reactions were likely to be more important than conformational changes (Kessler and Dunn, 1969) in contributing to absorption in aqueous solutions of haemoglobin. Also, O'Brien *et al.* (1972) mentioned that the absorption of DNA solution is unaffected if the molecule is denatured. Furthermore, the frequency-free ultrasonic absorption per unit concentration, defined as $(\mu_a \text{ solution} - \mu_a \text{ solvent})/cf^2$, of haemoglobin is closely similar to that of DNA. This implies that the absorption mechanisms may be the same.

The only other possible mechanisms of absorption in living soft tissues which are presently worthy of further consideration are solvent–solute interactions, and protein H-bond processes (Michels and Zana, 1969). The relaxation mechanism in aqueous solutions of polyethylene glycol is almost certainly due to perturbation of the hydrogen-bonding equilibrium between polymer and solvent (Hammes and Lewis, 1966). In view of this, it is interesting to note that a suspension of erythrocytes fixed in acrolein has an absorption coefficient which is greater by a factor of five at 30 MHz than that of an unfixed suspension (Kremkau *et al.*, 1973). The fixing process cross-links macromolecular hydrophobic groups. In proteins, H-bonds can occur between residues bearing carboxyl, hydroxyl and amino groups.

These groups are hydrophilic, and hydration processes which involve H-bonds between water and the hydrophilic residues would compete with intraprotein H-bonding equilibrium (Zana *et al.*, 1972).

4.7 CHARACTERISTICS OF OTHER TYPES OF TISSUE

4.7.a Lung

As shown in Figs. 4.5 and 4.6(a), in comparison with other tissues, lung has a high absorption coefficient and a low velocity (Dunn and Fry, 1961; Dunn, 1974). In making these measurements, freshly excised specimens of inflated lung tissue from dog were used, and the attenuation was calculated from the results of transmission measurements made at a temperature of 35°C. The results over a range of frequency are not consistent with an attenuation mechanism based on re-radiation of energy by pulsating gaseous structures (Devin, 1959). They are in broad agreement, however, with the data reported by Bauld and Schwan (1974). The very significant dependence of velocity on frequency in lung is also of interest: this may be an aspect of Dunn's (1974) experimental method, rather than a manifestation of dispersion.

4.7.b Bone

The attenuation rate in bone differs considerably from that in soft tissues. The results of Hueter's (1952) measurements on skull bone indicate that the attenuation is roughly proportional to the square of the frequency, up to about 2 MHz; above this frequency, there is a lower power dependence on frequency. The attenuation coefficient, about 13 dB cm^{-1} at 1 MHz, is an order of magnitude greater than that of soft tissues. The attenuation mechanisms are certainly more complicated than those in soft tissues, and scattering and conversion to shear waves of short range are likely to be important factors. It may be that the change in frequency dependence at about 2 MHz occurs because scattering ceases to be important at higher frequencies. The behaviour of compact ivory bone, which has been studied by White and Curry (1975), seems to be free from these complexities, presumably because of its simpler structure.

Although there seem to be no published values for attenuation and velocity in cartilage, it is probably reasonable to assume that the characteristics of this material would be similar to those of muscle.

4.8 FINITE AMPLITUDE EFFECTS

The generation, growth and decay of harmonics in a wave of finite amplitude propagating in a non-linear medium is mentioned in Section 1.14. In addition to causing the Oseen force, the breakdown of the linear wave equation may also result in changes in the absorption coefficient from that measured at very small amplitudes. Near to a source radiating finite amplitude sinusoidal waves, α is close to that for small amplitudes; beyond this region, α has a maximum value; but at larger distances, where absorption has so reduced the wave amplitude that the waveform returns to the sinusoid, α again tends to the value for small amplitudes. For example, Fox (1950) demonstrated that the absorption coefficient of water at a frequency of 10 MHz is independent of intensity below about 40 mW cm^{-2}, but is increased by a factor of five at an intensity of about 5 W cm^{-2}. It had originally been supposed that this effect might be due to cavitation, but Fox (1950) was unable to demonstrate any definite relationship between absorption and the quantity of dissolved gas, nor did he find any sudden change in the magnitude of the effect as the intensity was increased, such as might be expected at the onset of cavitation. Fox and Wallace (1954), however, were able to show that a theory based on the non-linear elastic properties of the medium is able to satisfy the experimental data. This theory has been further tested by Ryan *et al.* (1962).

The situation is more complicated in the case of finite amplitude waves of a frequency similar to that of the relaxation frequency of the supporting medium. It seems likely that intensity-dependent absorption, if it does occur at all, is associated with irreversible processes, the effect of which increases with increasing amplitude. This theory is supported by the statement of Zarembo and Kasil'nikov (1959) that the finite wave amplitude absorption coefficients of certain polymers are time-dependent during irradiation.

Dunn (1962) has measured the effect of intensity on the absorption coefficient of the spinal cord of the young mouse. At a frequency of 1 MHz, α is independent of intensity in the range 5–200 W cm^{-2}. Presumably, the same value of α applies at lower intensities. It seems reasonable to suppose that other soft tissues, possessing similar values of α/f, also have values of α which are, for most practical purposes, independent of intensity at levels which are not sufficiently high to cause irreversible damage.

4.9 CHARACTERISTIC IMPEDANCES OF BIOLOGICAL MATERIALS

Table 4.1 gives typical values of density for several biological materials, and the corresponding values of characteristic impedance (see Section 1.6) calculated from the data in Fig. 4.6. The characteristic impedance of normal liver (1.64–1.68×10^6 kg m^{-2} s^{-1}) is significantly greater than the value of 1.54×10^6 kg m^{-2} s^{-1} reported for cirrhotic liver by Gregg and Palagallo (1969).

The reflectivities of some plane biological boundaries (calculated from

TABLE 4.1
Densities and characteristic impedances of some biological tissues

Material	Density g ml^{-1}	Characteristic impedance 10^6 kg m^{-2} s^{-1}
Blood	1·06	1·62
Bone	1·38–1·81	3·75–7·38
Brain	1·03	1·55–1·66
Fat	0·92	1·35
Kidney	1·04	1·62
Liver	1·06	1·64–1·68
Lung	0·40	0·26
Muscle	1·07	1·65–1·74
Spleen	1·06	1·65–1·67
Water	1·00	1·52

TABLE 4.2
Reflectivities of some plane biological boundaries, expressed in decibels below the level from a perfect reflector

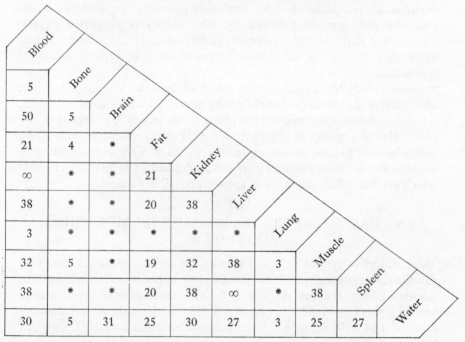

* Indicates that the corresponding boundary is unlikely to be of practical interest.
Based on data from Table 4.1.

the data given in Table 4.1) are set out in Table 4.2. It is important to realize that the data given in this table apply in the case of normal incidence on an extensive flat boundary and that the values differ for other angles of incidence, and for surfaces which are not flat (see Sections 1.8 and 5.2). The simple concept of a plane boundary representing a sudden transition between media of differing characteristic impedance does not bear close scrutiny in relation to practical, biological situations. The problem of reflexion from a region of continuous impedance change has been discussed by Wright (1973).

5. SCATTERING BY BIOLOGICAL MATERIALS

5.1 INTRODUCTION

The general concept of scattering is introduced in Section 2.5. Single-target scattering may be classified into three broadly different groups:

  (i) obstacle $>$ wavelength: $S=1$;
  (ii) obstacle $<$ wavelength: $S \propto k^4 a^6$; and
  (iii) obstacle $\simeq$ wavelength;

where S is the scattering cross-section, a is the radius of the scatterer, and $k=2\pi f$.

Biological targets can fall into any of these three categories, although small obstacles seldom exist in isolation. The large-obstacle situation corresponds to the extensive boundaries of major structures and organs. The small-obstacle situation is represented in ensembles in subcellular, cellular and tissue structures. The third situation lies between these two extremes.

The analysis of model systems can give some insight into the interactions which are observed experimentally in biological materials, but reproduction here of the elaborate mathematics would not be justifiable. An excellent review is that of Chivers (1973). The present Chapter is limited to a discussion of some of the rather sparse experimental data.

5.2 THE LARGE-OBSTACLE SITUATION

In pulse-echo diagnostics (see Chapter 6), the extensive boundaries between organs and major structures act as specular reflectors at frequencies at which surface irregularities are very small in relation to the wavelength. One result of this is that the echo amplitude backscattered from such a surface is small except at normal or close-to-normal incidence: compound scanning may be used to increase the chance of achieving normal incidence. As the frequency is increased, however, the surface seems to become "rougher" as the wavelength decreases and becomes comparable with the irregularities (Senapati *et al.*, 1972). This is illustrated in Fig. 5.1, which shows experimental results obtained for the angular dependence of echo amplitude from the surface of muscle, at several frequencies. Similar results have been reported for surfaces of differing roughness—in particular, normal and diseased mitral valve cusps—examined at the same frequency. The rougher surface exhibits the smaller variation in echo amplitude with changing angle of incidence (Reid, 1966).

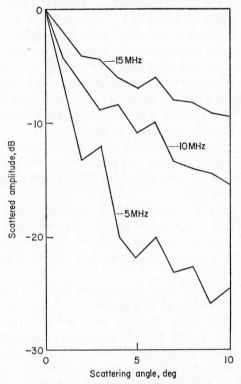

FIG. 5.1 Angular dependence of the echo amplitude from the surface of muscle, at several frequencies. (Data of Senapati *et al.*, 1972.)

5.3 THE SMALL-OBSTACLE SITUATION

The mechanisms of scattering by large concentrations of obstacles, small in relation to the wavelength, such as occur in physiological blood (which contains approximately 10^6 particles mm^{-3}) have been discussed by Twersky (1964). The subject is complicated, and it is necessary to make assumptions concerning the geometry, density and compressibility of the particles. Experiment reveals that the echo backscattered from blood irradiated by a quasi-monotonic pulse from a transducer which also acts as the receiver, fluctuates in amplitude as a function of time delay and lateral displacement of the transducer (Atkinson and Berry, 1974). (The time-dependent nature of echo amplitude has also been noted by Sigelmann and Reid, 1973.) This granular echo is not due to any structure in the blood on the scale observed, but probably arises from fluctuation scattering by the random distribution of the red cells. According to Reid *et al.* (1969), the red cell has a scattering cross-section at a frequency of 5 MHz which is about 10^{-4} times the average geometrical projected area. The scattering from the platelet is about a factor of 10^{-2} less than that of the red cell, and the contribution of platelets and white cells is negligible in whole blood. The dimensions of the ultrasonic pulse determine the scale of the fluctuation which is detected. Atkinson and Berry (1974) developed a statistical diffraction theory which accounts quantitatively for the observed variations in echo amplitude in time and space. By making assumptions concerning the properties of blood, and the dimensions of the ultrasonic beam, they predicted a value of echo amplitude which is in error by a factor of 13 in relation to the measured echo amplitude. The discrepancy may be due to errors in these assumed factors. An alternative analytical approach has been proposed by Sigelmann and Reid (1973), but they have not yet reported experimental data.

At 5 MHz the red cell is about $\lambda/10^6$ in diameter. At frequencies in the range 4–16 MHz, the scattering has an approximately fourth power dependence on frequency (Reid *et al.*, 1969). The increase in scattering with frequency, for a given particle size, has also been demonstrated by Waag and Lerner (1973).

According to Reid *et al.* (1969), the scattered wave (i.e. the backscattering cross-section per unit volume) is about 47 dB below the incident wave, for whole blood at 5 MHz. Another measurement, reported by Wells (1974), sets this level at -74 dB. The scattering is approximately proportional to the haematocrit in the range 7–40%, but with increasing haematocrit the scattering reaches a maximum value and then decreases (Reid *et al.*, 1969; Sigelmann and Reid, 1973). The physical reasons for this are obvious.

5.4 SCATTERING FROM SOLID TISSUES

The scattering from permanent structures, in which the relative positions of the elements remain constant, is a deterministic quantity (Sigelmann and Reid, 1972). This condition may be satisfied by biological soft tissue which is stationary—dead, for example—and sometimes by living tissue if it is not distorted by physiological movement.

Mountford and Wells (1972a) noted that the echo wavetrain received from liver tissue irradiated by a short ultrasonic pulse consists of cycles quite regularly spaced in time at a frequency corresponding to that of the ultrasonic pulse. This is probably due to the restricted bandwidth of the ultrasonic system. The oscillation of the wavetrain seems to be reinforced continuously (although by an amount which is exponentially decreased with increasing range) by the in-phase components of the echoes. Super-imposed on this generally decaying echo wavetrain is a granular variation in echo amplitude, in which the mean peak-to-trough envelope separation is a function of the spacing of the targets and the bandwidth of the system (Mountford and Wells, 1972b).

In diagnosis, Wild and Reid (1953) found quite large-amplitude echoes scattered from normal breast tissue at a frequency of 15 MHz, whereas

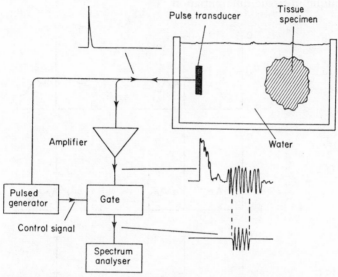

FIG. 5.2 Experimental arrangement used by Chivers *et al.* (1974) to investigate the frequency dependence of backscattering.

Howry *et al.* (1954), working with 2 MHz ultrasound, did not. Chivers *et al.* (1974) have looked into the matter of the frequency dependence of scattering by soft tissues, using the arrangement illustrated in Fig. 5.2. The ultrasound was generated at a nominal 2 MHz frequency, by a diag-nostic pulse–echo probe excited by a capacitor discharged through a thyratron (see Section 6.3). The ultrasonic pulse travelled through the water in the sound tank to interrogate the specimen of tissue. The received signals were amplified and time-gated, and Fourier transformed in the spectrum analyser. The use of a single transducer implies the measurement of backscattering spectra only. The backscattering cross-section σ_s for a particular volume is defined by the equation:

$$I_s(f) = \sigma_s(f) . I_0(f) \tag{5.1}$$

where $I_s(f)$ is the intensity of the backscattered wave, and $I_0(f)$ is the intensity of the incident wave, at frequency f. The measured backscattered spectrum $I_m(f)$ is given by:

$$I_m(f) = I_s(f) * \{\sin(\pi f \tau)\}/2\pi f \qquad (5.2)$$

where τ is the gate duration. The function $\{\sin(\pi f \tau)\}/2\pi f$ represents the Fourier transform of the gating signal, and it must be deconvolved from the measured spectrum in order to calculate σ_s. In principle, this should be possible; but to date only comparative studies of $I_m(f)$ have been undertaken, using a fixed gate duration, in order to test the likely usefulness of the technique in tissue differentiation.

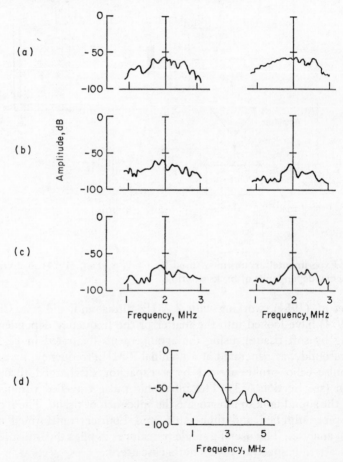

FIG. 5.3 Backscattering frequency spectra: nominal frequency$=2$ MHz; gate duration$=8$ μs. Specimens of fixed human tissue: (a) fat; (b) liver; (c) spleen; (d) transducer reference spectrum. (Based on Chivers *et al.*, 1974.)

Chivers *et al.* (1974) have presented some typical frequency spectra, some of which are reproduced in Fig. 5.3, for specimens of fixed human fat, liver and spleen. (Similar results, from Chivers and Hill (1975) are shown in Fig. 6.54, and some practical aspects of this type of study are discussed in Section 6.12.d.) In these spectra, $I_0(f)$ is complex and takes into account the characteristics of the electrical driving amplitude, the probe, and the amplifier, as represented in Fig. 5.3(d). Since $I_0(f)$ is the same in each case, however, it is valid to compare the spectra from the same and from differing tissues. The most striking characteristic is the

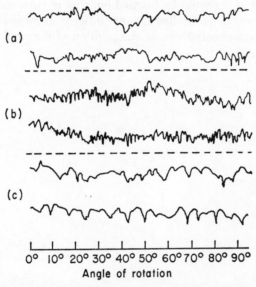

0° 10° 20° 30° 40° 50° 60° 70° 80° 90°
Angle of rotation

FIG. 5.4 Angular dependence of backscattering amplitude: nominal frequency = 1 MHz. Specimens of fresh human tissue from two individuals: (a) spleen; (b) brain; (c) liver. (Based on Hill, 1974.)

similarity of each pair of spectra for the same tissues. The amplitude of the scattering from fat is comparable with that from the spleen; the amplitude from liver seems to be significantly lower. The scattering spectra from fat are broader and more complex than those from spleen.

The use of ultrasonic spectroscopy in the investigation of biological materials is in its infancy. Much may be learned from established applications in other fields: see, for example, Gericke (1970) for a review of the technique in non-destructive testing.

Another aspect of scattering is the relationship between the organization of structure within the tissue and the directional properties of the ultrasonic beam. Hill (1974) has reported results of some experiments in which the echo amplitude of an ultrasonic pulse reflected from within various specimens of fresh post-mortem human tissue was recorded whilst the probe was rotated around the specimen. The data reproduced in Fig. 5.4 seem to reflect the existence of characteristic structural patterns of acoustically reflecting targets within each tissue, and these are presumably related to characteristic histological appearances under the microscope. In some respects, this phenomenon is analogous to *Bragg X-ray crystallography*. Nicholas and Hill (1975) have investigated the possibility that the angular frequencies of the "Bragg diffraction patterns" of different tissues might be sufficiently different to distinguish between them. The preliminary results are promising: but it should be pointed out that *in vitro* studies in which geometry can easily be controlled are very different from *in vivo* conditions with the attendant uncertainties in the position of the resolution cell (see Section 6.13.b.ii).

6. PULSE–ECHO METHODS

6.1 INTRODUCTION

6.1.a Basic Principles

The basic principles of the pulse–echo system are illustrated in Fig. 6.1. The diagrams show how an ultrasonic pulse may be used to measure the depth of an echo-producing interface. The ultrasonic probe is arranged to emit a short-duration stress wave into medium (i), in response to an electrical excitation. At the same instant, the spot on the screen of the cathode-ray tube begins to move at constant velocity from left to right. The vertical deflexion plates of the cathode-ray tube are connected to the output from an amplifier, the input of which is derived from the ultrasonic probe. The sequence of events is shown in Fig. 6.1(a–f). The spot is deflected vertically at the instant that the pulse is emitted. The pulse travels at constant velocity through medium (i), and the spot traces a horizontal line on the display. After some time, the pulse encounters the interface between media (i) and (ii): some of the energy is reflected backwards, and some travels forwards. When the reflected pulse reaches the probe, the transducer generates a voltage which is amplified to deflect the trace on the display. The transmitted wave travels on into medium (ii), some of the reflected wave is absorbed by the transducer, and the trace on the display has two vertical deflexions the distance between which is proportional to the thickness of medium (i). If the process is repeated sufficiently rapidly (at a rate of more than about 20 s^{-1}), a steady trace is observed on the display. The method can be extended to the examination of many interfaces lying along the ultrasonic beam.

Figure 6.2 is a block diagram showing the relationships between the various components of an ultrasonic pulse–echo system, such as that which might be used to obtain the display illustrated in Fig. 6.1. This particular kind of display is called an "A-scan" (see Section 6.7). The clock provides a trigger pulse for the transmitter, the swept gain generator, the bright-up pulse generator and the timebase. The minimum repetition rate is that which is required to produce a satisfactory display, in terms of brightness, freedom from flicker, time resolution and scanning rate. The maximum rate is limited by the required penetration, the reverberation decay time, the maximum speed of any associated recording system, and the increasing risk of biological damage.

Figure 6.2 also illustrates the voltage waveforms at various points in the circuitry. The transmitter, triggered by the clock, generates an electrical pulse which excites the transducer to emit a stress wave of amplitude determined by the attenuator. The signal output from the transducer is

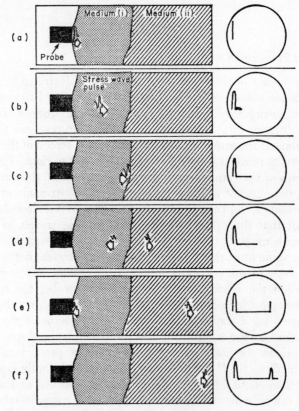

FIG. 6.1 Basic principles of pulse–echo system.

fed to the radio-frequency amplifier. The gain of this amplifier may be increased with time, to compensate to some extent for the increasing attenuation of the echoes from deeper structures. In this example, the swept gain circuits are triggered at the instant that the ultrasonic pulse is transmitted; but in the case of a variable-delay water bath scanner, it is necessary to arrange for the swept gain circuits to be triggered at the instant that the first echo returns from the patient, since the absorption in water is relatively low. Sometimes, the receiver is designed to have a logarithmic response. The bright-up pulse generator switches on the display only during the time that echo information is being received; therefore the fly-back of the timebase is not displayed. The timebase generates a voltage ramp which deflects the trace at constant velocity appropriate to the penetration. The output from the r.f. amplifier is demodulated, and the dynamic range may be restricted by suppression of the smaller echo signals, before being fed to the video amplifier. The output from this amplifier is connected to the y-deflexion plates of the cathode-ray tube to produce an

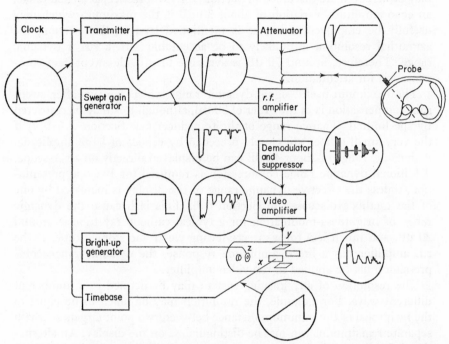

FIG. 6.2 Typical pulse–echo system. The block diagram shows an A-scope, with the probe in contact with the patient.

A-scan, or to the cathode of the cathode-ray tube to produce a B-scan (see Section 6.8).

Pulse–echo systems have many applications in medical diagnosis. Numerous variations of the circuit arrangements are possible. Some of these are discussed in this Chapter, in relation to the physical and technical aspects of the differences between the systems.

6.1.b Dynamic Range, Swept Gain and Resolution

Within the limitations imposed by noise and by the maximum transmitted power, the maximum useful dynamic range of the echoes received in conventional medical diagnostic pulse–echo systems is about 100 dB. This dynamic range is shared between the variations in echo amplitude at fixed distances, and the attenuation of echoes which increases with distance. Compensation for attenuation can be partially provided by the application of swept gain. (Swept gain is a method by which the gain of the receiver is increased with time so that the echoes from deeper structures are amplified more than those which originate nearer to the transducer, and so arrive earlier in time. Some of the methods by which swept gain compensation may be achieved are discussed in Section 6.4.) In practice, at a fixed range, an echo amplitude variation of about 30 dB is the maximum which may usefully be employed, since, as is mentioned later in this Section, the azimuthal resolution is unlikely to be acceptable with a larger dynamic range. Therefore, around 70 dB is available to provide swept gain compensation for attenuation.

The maximum useful signal dynamic range which remains after swept gain compensation is in the order of 30 dB, although this may be restricted by the limited dynamic range of the transducer (see Section 3.6.b.v) if the very small echoes are closely preceded by echoes of large amplitude. A dynamic range of about 40 dB can be displayed directly on an A-scope. Additional dynamic range compression is required for B-scope presentation, unless the effective dynamic range of the display is increased by one of the methods discussed in Section 6.6. This is because the dynamic range of brightness-modulation for a typical cathode ray tube is around 20 dB, and much less for a direct-viewing electronic storage tube. If the r.f. amplifier has a linear amplitude response, the dynamic range compression must be applied in the video amplifier.

The resolution of any imaging system may be defined in a number of different ways. For example, the resolution may be taken to be equal to the reciprocal of the minimum distance between two point targets at which separate registrations can just be distinguished on the display. An alternative definition, equivalent in concept and usually more convenient in ultrasonic diagnostic practice, is to specify the reciprocal of the distance which appears on the display to be occupied by a point target in the field. In ultrasonic systems, two different resolutions are of chief importance: these are the lateral (in azimuth or elevation) resolution, which describes the resolution along the beam diameter normal to the axis, and the range resolution, which is the resolution along the axis. Both these quantities depend on a number of factors, including the distance from the transducer. The influence of distance is particularly important in the case of the lateral resolution.

Another general concept, which it is helpful to introduce here, is that of the *resolution cell*. The resolution cell is the volume of material within which the interaction providing the data takes place. Except in the simplest and most idealized situation, the resolution cell may have several values of volume, a different value for each interaction; and for any particular interaction, it may have a volume which changes with time and frequency. Thus, there is no simple answer to the question, "What is the resolution of this ultrasonic system?"

Consider an image made up of two independent components with brightness distributions as illustrated in Fig. 6.3. Brightness is plotted on a linear scale, and as the two components are moved closer so that they overlap; the combined brightness is equal to the sum of the two contributions. Whether or not the separate components may be distinguished

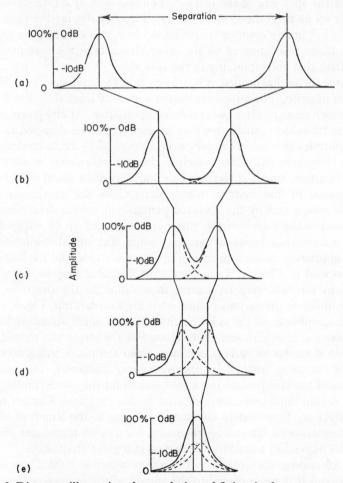

FIG. 6.3 Diagrams illustrating the resolution of finite-sized components. In this example, two components of equal brightness are shown at various separations. The maximum combined brightness is normalized to 100%.

depends on a number of factors, and particularly on the ability of the observer to detect differences in brightness. If the observer is able just to distinguish a brightness difference of 32% (i.e. 10 dB), the situation where the two components appear to coalesce is that represented in Fig. 6.3(c), and the resolution of the system may then be defined as the reciprocal of the corresponding separation.

Each of the two components in Fig. 6.3 may be considered to be a *point spread function*: this is the registration which appears on the display to be occupied by a point target in the imaged medium. The system point spread function is the combination of several image degrading processes, one of which is the spot size of the display. The spot size of a cathode-ray tube depends on its brightness, and for a good quality display the diameter of the 32% brightness contour is around 0·5 mm. No advantage is gained if the combined resolution of all the other elements of the system is made better than that corresponding to the spot size.

In pulse–echo diagnostics, it is seldom that the spot size is the limiting factor in practice. The lateral resolution is usually limited by the dynamic range which remains after swept gain compensation. At any given distance from the transducer, structures may be expected to be detected as echoes the amplitudes of which may vary over a range of 30 dB, according to the interface characteristics. In principle the dynamic range is very much larger than this: but it is restricted to not more than about 30 dB by the performance of the system, which determines the maximum overall dynamic range, and by the required penetration, which determines what proportion of the total dynamic range may be taken up by attenuation.

The relationship between dynamic range and lateral resolution is of great importance. Some aspects of the ultrasonic field and its distribution are discussed in Chapter 2; in particular, Fig. 2.2 may be found to be helpful in the following treatment, in addition to the diagrams which directly illustrate the various points in the argument. Thus, Fig. 6.4 shows how the amplitude of the echo received from a small spherical target in water was found experimentally to change as the target was moved across the beam diameter at various distances from the plane transducers for a series of operating frequencies and transducer diameters. The calculated positions of the steady-state last axial maxima for the corresponding transducers driven cophasally are indicated in the diagrams. Certain features of the data are immediately obvious; for example, the length of the near zone increases with increasing frequency, for a given transducer diameter, and with increasing transducer diameter, at a given frequency.

The ultrasonic absorption coefficient in water is 0·0022 dB cm^{-1} at 1 MHz, and it is proportional to the square of the frequency. For a path length of 400 mm (go-and-return penetration of 200 mm) at a frequency of 5 MHz, the corresponding attenuation due to absorption is 2·2 dB. This

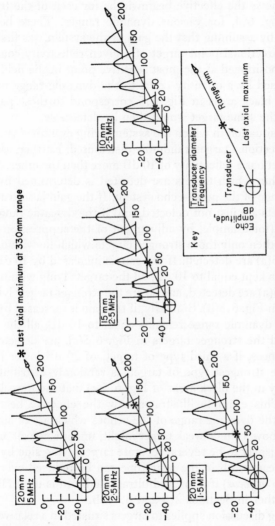

FIG. 6.4 Echo amplitude curves for pulse-echo transducers of various diameters and frequencies, plotted in water. The calculated positions of the last axial maxima for continuous wave conditions are shown. Target: steel sphere, diameter 6·3 mm. (Adapted from Wells, 1966b).

attenuation is negligible in comparison with that which would occur in soft tissues (about 200 dB), and the curves illustrated in Fig. 6.4 may be taken as being for a lossless medium, without fear of introducing qualitative errors into the discussion which follows.

Figure 6.5 shows the effective beamwidths for each of the transducers illustrated in Fig. 6.4, for various dynamic ranges. These beamwidths were calculated by assuming that the gain of the system was first adjusted so that a non-directional point target of a given reflectivity could just be detected when positioned at the most sensitive point in the field; the gain was then increased by a quantity equal to the dynamic range under consideration. The black areas in Fig. 6.5 correspond to those parts of the fields in which the same target would then be detectable.

Consider the situation in which the system being examined contains two types of non-directional target, randomly distributed. Further, assume that one type of target has a reflectivity of 10 dB more than the other. The beam distribution within which targets are detected is determined by the gain and dynamic range of the pulse–echo system. If the gain is adjusted so that the weaker targets are just not detected, and if the dynamic range is made equal to 10 dB (for example, by adjustment of the suppression level: see Section 6.4.e), then only those stronger targets which lie within the black areas of Fig. 6.5(a) are detected. If the gain is increased by 10 dB, and the dynamic range is kept equal to 10 dB, all the targets lying within the black areas in Fig. 6.5(a) are detected, and so are the stronger targets lying within the black areas in Fig. 6.5(b). Similarly, if the gain is increased by a further 10 dB, and the dyanmic range remains equal to 10 dB, all the targets in Fig. 6.5(b), and the stronger targets in Fig. 6.5(c), are detected. Under these circumstances, if a third type of target, of 20 dB lower reflectivity than that of the strongest type of target, is randomly distributed in the system, it is only in the black areas of Fig. 6.5(a) that these weaker targets are detected. This example illustrates how the effective beamwidth is determined by the dynamic range of the echoes which are of significance, and also shows how a single weak target might, under some circumstances, appear on the display to be several separate targets lying side by side.

The lateral beamwidth in the near zone can be reduced over a limited range (the *depth of focus*) if a focused ultrasonic beam is used. The matter is discussed further in Sections 2.3 and 6.10.b.

The preceding discussion applies to targets situated in a relatively lossless medium. In a medium with a constant attenuation rate, swept gain can be applied to compensate for the reduction of echo amplitude with increasing distance. Correction for dispersive absorption is quite difficult, however, in the case of a pulse observed by electronic systems of finite bandwidth. This is illustrated in Fig. 6.6. Figure 6.6(a), curve (iii), is the overall response of the receiving system in this example. Figure 6.6(b) shows the

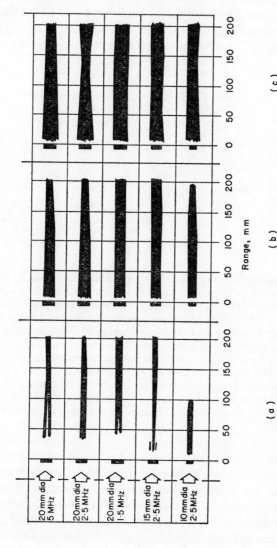

FIG. 6.5 Diagrams showing the effective beamwidths of the ultrasonic beams illustrated in Fig. 6.4. Dynamic range: (a) 10 dB; (b) 20 dB; (c) 30 dB.

various frequency spectra, each spectrum corresponding to a particular target range, which are further modified by the frequency response of the receiver before being fed to the display. The maximum amplitudes corresponding to each particular range are plotted in curve (i) of Fig. 6.6(c). On the same axes, curve (ii) shows the corresponding amplitude for continuous wave reflexion (zero bandwidth), and curve (iii) shows the linear relationship which deviates by the minimum amount from curve (i) over a 50 dB dynamic range. The maximum deviation is 4 dB, and the slope of

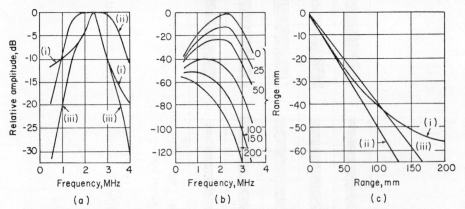

FIG. 6.6 Diagrams illustrating the effects of system bandwidth on echo amplitude with a dispersive absorber. These diagrams are for a 2·5 MHz transducer and an absorption of 1 dB cm^{-1} MHz^{-1}. (a) Curve (i) transducer receiving characteristic (redrawn from Fig. 3.18); Curve (ii) typical response of r.f. and video amplifier combination; (iii) overall response of receiving system. (b) Pulse frequency spectra after modification by the receiving system, for various target ranges (total go-and-return path length is equal to twice the range). (Spectra calculated from data in Fig. 3.17, with the addition of the curve for 150 mm range.) (c) Curve (i) relative pulse amplitudes at spectral maxima plotted against range, for a target of constant reflectivity; (ii) corresponding relationship for continuous wave reflexion. (iii) logarithmic attenuation corresponding to minimum deviation from curve (i) over 50 dB dynamic range.

curve (iii) is 3·9 dB cm^{-1}, which is the best rate of exponential swept gain in this example. (As the dynamic range is increased, so the deviation of the required compensation from an exponential increases, so that simple exponential swept gain eventually has unacceptable errors. For example, the maximum deviation is 10 dB over a dynamic range of 70 dB.)

Extending this result to other frequencies, and assuming similar shapes for the frequency response and spectral characteristics, the optimum swept gain rate for a 50 dB dynamic range is 1·6αN dB cm^{-1}, where α is the absorption coefficient for continuous waves at 1 MHz, and N is the centre frequency of the pulse in megahertz.

The situation is more complicated if, as is usually the case, various thicknesses of materials of differing attenuation rates lie in the ultrasonic path. In practice, the mean value of attenuation seems to be somewhat less than 1 dB cm^{-1} MHz^{-1} in soft tissues: this is probably due to the presence of blood and other low-loss materials. This is particularly the case in cysts, liver, heart, and the pregnant uterus. As a rough guide, a swept gain rate of about 1·3 N dB cm^{-1} is generally satisfactory, but the exact rate needs to be chosen for each individual circumstance.

As a consequence of the uncertainty in the effective value of the attenuation, the accuracy with which swept gain can be applied may be rather poor, and it becomes necessary to use a wider dynamic range than that which would be required on the basis of variations in target reflectivity alone. Therefore, it is difficult to estimate the effective beamwidth—and hence the resolution—of a system at any particular distance from the transducer because of the uncertainty in the effective value of the dynamic range. Moreover, it is pointed out in Section 2.2.c that there is a further degradation in the lateral resolution due to beam broadening resulting from the shift to lower frequencies of the distribution of energy in the pulse as it propagates through media with dispersive absorption.

The range resolution of a pulse–echo system is generally much better than the practical lateral resolution. The range resolution defines the ability of the system to separate targets spaced close together in range, and is thus equal to the reciprocal of the effective duration of the ultrasonic pulse. Consider, for example, the received echo pulse shown in Fig. 6.7. Each of the four oscillograms shows the same pulse, transmitted and received by the same transducer, but with the gain of the wideband oscilloscope on which the pulse was displayed set at different levels. This set of oscillograms could equally well have been made with the system sensitivity kept constant but with targets of different reflectivities. The zero-crossing frequency is around 1·8 MHz. Unlike the lateral resolution, the range resolution is only slightly dependent on the diameter of the transducer and the distance between the transducer and the target. Consequently the discussion which follows is quite general, and may be extended to the consideration of other situations.

Consider the situation in which the threshold level of the system is such that the amplitude of the echo signal represented in Fig. 6.7(a) is just too low to produce a registration on the display. (The same threshold level is indicated on all the oscillograms in Fig. 6.7.) If the gain of the receiver—or the reflectivity of the target—is increased by 10 dB, then the effective duration of the pulse in this example is 1·6 μs, assuming full-wave demodulation is employed (see Section 6.6.e). Similarly, the effective durations corresponding to increases of 20 and 30 dB can be seen to be 2·7 and 3·5 μs respectively. These time durations correspond to distances of about 1·2, 2·0 and 2·6 mm respectively for dynamic ranges of 10, 20 and 30 dB. The dynamic range is equal to the difference between the threshold level and the maximum amplitude of the pulse. For the same transducer, the lateral resolutions at a distance of 100 mm (see Fig. 6.4) correspond to effective beamwidths of about 10, 16 and 25 mm respectively.

The pulse waveforms illustrated in Fig. 6.7 were obtained directly from the transducer and displayed on a wideband oscilloscope. In a pulse–echo system, the pulses would normally be applied to an amplifier of limited frequency bandwidth. Nevertheless, if the bandwidths of the r.f. and video

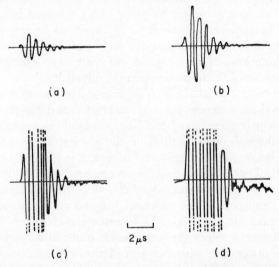

FIG. 6.7 Typical received echo pulses. Each oscillogram shows the same pulse, but for a different receiver gain. In this example, the zero-crossing frequency near the centre of the pulse is equal to 1·8 MHz. Gain: (a) 0 dB; (b) +10 dB; (c) +20 dB; (d) +30 dB.

amplifiers are each made equal to the zero-crossing frequency of the ultrasonic pulse, then the transducer is usually the most important element controlling the frequency response, and the receiver electronics only slightly degrades the range resolution. In general, a typical system has range resolutions corresponding to 1·5, 2·5 and 3·0 wavelengths with dynamic ranges of 10, 20 and 30 dB respectively, and the lateral resolutions at a range of 120 wavelengths are about 10 times worse than the corresponding range resolutions.

It is helpful at this stage to reconsider the concept of the resolution cell, which was introduced earlier in this Section. The resolution cell is the volume formed by revolving the envelope of the displayed pulse about the central axis along which the pulse–echo system is operating. This is illustrated in Fig. 6.8. The resolution cell is shaped like a shortened tear-drop, pointed at its leading surface.

The time duration of the displayed pulse is inversely proportional to the range resolution, as explained in the preceding paragraphs. This is quite distinct from the *precision* of the system in simulating the position of a reflecting surface. In Fig. 6.7, it may be seen that the position of the leading edge of the pulse is quite well defined when the dynamic range is large, because the pulse amplitude rapidly rises above the threshold. Therefore only a small error is introduced if the position of the interface is taken to correspond to the beginning of the display registration. An error of about $0 \cdot 3$ λ occurs in this example if the same criterion is used with a dynamic range of 20 dB; the error increases to about $0 \cdot 8$ λ with a dynamic range of 10 dB. If half-wave demodulation is used, there may be an additional error of $0 \cdot 5$ λ.

It might be supposed that half-wave demodulation would be preferable to full wave demodulation, because there is a possibility that, if the pulse

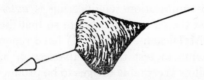

FIG. 6.8 The resolution cell of a typical pulse–echo system.

is of an appropriate shape, the range resolution may be improved by an amount corresponding to a distance of as much as a wavelength. The advantage of such an improvement is generally offset, however, by the disadvantage of less efficient demodulation. Moreover, any improvement in range resolution which may thus be obtained is at the expense of a loss in the precision of range measurement, and this may be an important disadvantage.

The estimation of range resolution on the basis of pulse shape and dynamic range becomes more difficult if the pulse is propagated in media with dispersive absorption, such as biological soft tissues. The fundamental effect is that a stress wave as transmitted contains energy spread over a wide frequency spectrum, and the higher frequency components are dissipated with distance more rapidly than those of lower frequency. The situation is made more complicated, although the magnitude of the overall effect is reduced, by the restricted bandwidth of the receiving system. In practice, it is necessary to compromise between a long pulse, which is relatively free from dispersion and noise, but which gives poor range resolution, and a short pulse, which has good range resolution, but which is stretched by dispersion and has a poor signal-to-noise ratio on account of its large frequency bandwidth. The usual arrangement is to make the bandwidth of the electronics sufficiently wide so that the transducer is the effective bandwidth-limiting component (see Fig. 3.18).

Pulse stretching due to dispersive absorption degrades both the range resolution and the precision of the system. In most practical systems, however, these quantities remain substantially better than the lateral resolution, unless strong focusing is used, and so the effects may often be neglected. On the other hand, the effective attenuation rate may be significantly modified by the spectral frequency shift which occurs in a dispersive absorber. It is shown in this Section that, as a rough guide, a pulse with a transmitted frequency of N MHz may be taken to be attenuated at a rate of $1\cdot3$ N dB cm^{-1} of penetration (target range) in soft tissues. On this basis, 50 dB of dynamic range due to attenuation corresponds to a penetration of about 250 mm at a frequency of $1\cdot5$ MHz, and this is about the maximum penetration which is possible at this frequency.

Although swept gain is used in most contemporary pulse–echo systems, it is certainly not the only method of dynamic range compression. A technique familiar in communications engineering is *automatic gain control*, which serves to adjust the gain of the system so that the larger the signal, the lower the gain. McDicken *et al.* (1974) have reported the results of preliminary experiments to test the effectiveness of a.c.g. in ultrasonic diagnostics. It does allow acceptable images to be produced, and it involves the operator in little manipulation of controls. One limitation is that information concerning the relative amplitudes of echo complexes tends to be lost; another is that the time constant of the control circuit determines the range beyond which the influence of a preceding echo complex extends.

6.1.c Interface Characteristics

The reflectivities of various biological interfaces are discussed in Section 4.8, for the rather idealized case of normal incidence on a perfectly flat boundary. The situation is much more complicated when the incidence is not normal, or when the interface is very close to the transducer. For example, Fig. 6.9 shows how the echo amplitude depends upon the angle of incidence at various target ranges with a typical pulse–echo system. In this typical situation, the amplitude is reduced by about 22 dB at an angle of incidence of 3°, irrespective of target range. At more acute incidence, the subsequent reduction increases with range. (The maxima and minima which occur with increasing angulation at short range are due to interference. It is not important in practice, because the transmission pulse, during which information retrieval is impossible, usually extends beyond this region.) There is a simple qualitative explanation for this observation. With the target in the near field, the portion of the roughly cylindrical beam which falls on the surface of the transducer is crescent-shaped, and the area of this crescent is decreased with increasingly acute angulation. On the other hand, with the target far into the far field, the transducer is in the limit uniformly excited by the portion of the reflected beam which reaches it, and the variation in echo amplitude with changing angulation is simply the diametrical distribution of intensity across the beam: this corresponds to a beam profile such as those illustrated in Fig. 6.4.

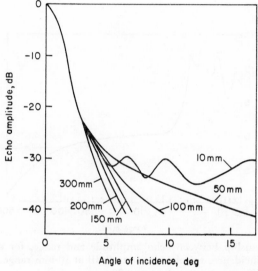

FIG. 6.9 Relationship between echo amplitude and angle of incidence, for a flat target in water at various ranges. Each curve is relative to 0 dB at normal incidence. Zero-crossing frequency, 1·7 MHz; transducer diameter, 20 mm. (Adapted from Wells, 1966a.)

Figure 6.10 shows how the echo amplitude at normal incidence depends upon the target range in water, with a typical pulse–echo system. Water has an absorption coefficient of about 0·0064 dB cm^{-1} at 1·7 MHz. A 20 mm diameter transducer operating with continuous waves at this frequency has a near field which extends for a distance of 113 mm (see Section 2.2.a). Therefore, for a target situated at 57 mm from the transducer, the echo amplitude is reduced by only 0·07 dB as the result of absorption. The amplitude is actually reduced by 1·2 dB: the excess attenuation is at least partly due to geometrical diffraction. At greater target ranges, the amplitude falls because of the divergence of the beam, which results in an increasing proportion of the reflected energy falling outside the area of the receiving transducer. (When the target is very close to the transducer, the echo amplitude exhibits a number of maxima and minima with changing range, similar to those produced by changing the angulation of a short-range target. The increase in echo amplitude associated with these fluctuations is due to the pressure amplification which occurs in a standing wave field: see Section 1.10. In clinical diagnosis, this effect is usually unimportant, because it occurs in the region occupied by the transmission pulse.)

The examples illustrated in Figs. 6.9 and 6.10 are typical of the characteristics of all pulse–echo systems. Thus, the relationships between attenuation, angulation and range depend on the frequency and dimensions of the transducer.

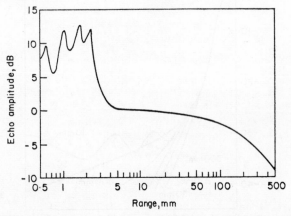

FIG. 6.10 Relationship between echo amplitude and range, for a flat target in water at normal incidence. Levels relative to 0 dB at 10 mm range. Zero-crossing frequency, 1·7 MHz; transducer diameter, 20 mm.

6.1.d Reflexion and Scattering from Biological Materials

In an unlimited lossless homogeneous liquid, the wave velocity $c =$ $(K/\rho)^{1/2}$, where K is the bulk modulus (see Eqn. 1.20). Furthermore, the characteristic impedance $Z = \rho c$, as explained in Section 1.6. Combining these two results shows that

$$Z = (K\rho)^{1/2} \tag{6.1}$$

According to Fields and Dunn (1973), the densities of soft tissues are closely similar. They stated that the density variation is 1% or less; and so concluded that it is variations in elasticity which largely account for the echoes from within soft tissue structures. (Note that ignoring density variation may not be justified if the data given in Table 4.1 are correct: here the soft tissue density range amounts to 15%.) Collagenous fibres exhibi at d.c. elastic modulus greater by a factor of about 1000 than that of other soft tissues, and Fields and Dunn (1973) hypothesized that the amount of collagen may be the dominant component in determining characteristic impedance. Thus, Fry *et al.* (1971) demonstrated that pig liver, with well-developed connective tissue between lobules, returns high-amplitude echoes, whereas those from cat liver, in which the connective tissue is poorly developed, are of low amplitude. Also, Mountford and Wells (1972) have shown that there is an increased echo amplitude from cirrhotic liver in relation to normal liver, and according to Boyett and Sullivan (1970), there may be a three-fold increase in collagen content in cirrhosis. Similarly, there is an increase in echo density in the postmeno-pausal breast (Fry *et al.*, 1972), in which there is an increase in fibrous tissue in relation to the premenopausal breast.

It is easy to find many other examples of changes in connective tissue structure which could be correlated with changes in reflectivities associated with disease. What are lacking are experimental data which could show whether the collagen content is the cause of the changes, or merely con-comitant with them.

Whatever the properties of biological materials which result in them having different characteristic impedances, the physics of the reflexion and scattering phenomena is complicated. One aspect of this, which can be mentioned here and immediately dismissed in relation to the present discussion, is that reflexion and scattering within biological materials reduce the energy which is transmitted, and so contribute, along with absorption, divergence and diffraction, to the total attenuation.

When an ultrasonic pulse encounters a boundary which is relatively extensive in relation to the wavelength—such as, for example, the boundary between perirenal fat and kidney—the situation is relatively straightfor-ward. At least to a first approximation, the reflexion is specular. The situation is more complicated when the reflector is in the form of a rough surface, or an ensemble of small scatterers. Except when nature is kind, as in the case of blood, calculation is not worth the effort, and the reflectivity is best measured experimentally. Some typical values of echo amplitude, expressed in decibels below the level from a perfect reflector in a lossless medium at the same range, are given in Table 6.1. It is important to realize that these values are approximate, and that in general there may be quite wide variations between different clinical circumstances.

Further detailed discussions of this topic may be found in Chapter 5 and Section 6.12.

6.1.e Ultrasonic Frequency

The choice of the best ultrasonic frequency for a particular diagnostic application depends on a number of factors. In general, the potential resolution under ideal conditions is improved as the ultrasonic frequency is increased. In practice, however, it is not possible (unless signal averaging techniques are employed) to increase the ultrasonic frequency above a limit which, for a given penetration, target reflectivity, and attenuation rate, is determined mainly by the signal-to-noise ratio, and also partly by the required accuracy of swept gain compensation. It is helpful to consider the ultrasonic wavelength as the factor which controls the dimensions of the imaged anatomy: thus, a shorter wavelength gives a higher resolution over a more limited penetration. If a 50 dB dynamic range of swept gain is available, a soft tissue penetration of up to around 250 mm can generally be obtained at a frequency of 1·5 MHz. The maximum penetration is inversely proportional to the frequency: consequently, at 15 MHz a penetration of 25 mm might be achieved. It is only in the most advanced

TABLE 6.1

Typical echo amplitudes for some biological materials, expressed in decibels relative to the echo amplitude from a perfect reflector at the same range in a lossless medium. Frequency = 1·5 MHz

Reflector or scatterer	Range, mm	Echo amplitude, dB
Smooth skin surface in water	100	−20
Foetal skull, 30 week gestation	80	−50
Posterior left ventricular wall	100	−50
Posterior liver surface	120	−50
Brain midline	70	−60
Cirrhotic liver structures	80	−60
Hydatidiform mole structures	80	−65
Normal liver structures	80	−65
Anterior mitral valve leaflet	70	−70
Uterine fibroid structures	80	−70
Blood	60	−100

grey-scale systems, however, that noise is at present the limiting factor which determines penetration; restricted gain, and the onset of instability, are more common problems. Moreover, in commercial equipment a dynamic range of swept gain of only 30 dB (and sometimes less) is not unusual, and this allows a compensated penetration of only 150 mm at 1·5 MHz: this is equal to 100 wavelengths.

In systems in which the swept gain dynamic range is limited to about 30 dB, it is generally difficult to do better than to select the maximum frequency which will give the required penetration, and to make the transducer diameter equal to at least 20 wavelengths. The transducer diameter may be increased slightly above this value with increasing frequency, so that it is, for example, 30 wavelengths at 5 MHz. Another practical trick is to use a focused beam, so that the echoes from a small ensemble increase in amplitude as the focus is approached from the transducer. If 50 dB of swept gain dynamic range is available, however, or if the transducer stands off from the patient in a water bath, it may be better to use a rather larger transducer.

The effects of the different attenuation rates of different tissues become more pronounced as the frequency is increased. For example, Donald *et al.* (1958) have shown that a differential diagnosis between fibroid and ovarian cyst is possible, because both are quite transonic at 1·5 MHz, whereas, under the same conditions of gain and swept gain, the cyst remains transonic at 2·5 MHz, whilst the fibroid does not. This method is very convenient if the frequency can be changed readily. In systems designed for optimum performance, however, the frequency is often fixed. This is because of the difficulty of manufacturing interchangeable probes with coaxial ultrasonic beams. Nevertheless, as far as attenuation is concerned, an equivalent diagnosis can be made by testing the effect of changing the swept gain rate. This is not the case, however, if the diagnostic information is deduced from a study of the echo amplitudes arising from within tissue masses, since scattering is frequency-dependent (see Chapter 5 and Section 6.12.d).

6.1.f Multiple Reflexion Artifacts

The basis of the pulse–echo method is the reflexion of ultrasonic energy at characteristic impedance discontinuities. Consider again the simple situation illustrated in Fig. 6.1, in which a transducer is directed normally at a plane, reflecting interface. At the instant that the transmitted ultrasonic pulse leaves the transducer, the timebase circuit associated with the display begins to operate. After a delay which depends on the range of the target and the velocity of the pulse, an echo returns to the transducer and a registration appears on the display at a position determined by the timebase. This is the process which is described in detail in Section 6.1.a. The process, however, does not end at this stage. There is an acoustic mismatch at the surface of the transducer, and although some of the energy in the reflected pulse enters the transducer to produce the registration, quite a large proportion is reflected away from the transducer, back towards the target. This pulse behaves as if it were a second transmitted pulse, of smaller amplitude than the first, delayed in time by an interval equal to the delay in the return of the first, real, echo. Consequently, in due time a second echo returns from the target, and this may be large enough in amplitude to produce a registration on the display corresponding to twice the range of the interface. Similarly, second and subsequent *artifacts* may appear, until the multiple reflexion echoes fall below the threshold level of the system (Wells, 1965).

Multiple reflexion artifacts can arise from other paths in addition to the simple, direct route. For example, multiple reflexions may occur between two surfaces lying in sequence along the axis of the ultrasonic beam. Again, under some circumstances artifacts can be caused by the reflexions of the pulse in directions which do not lie along the axis of the ultrasonic beam: if the pulse strikes a second reflector which returns the echo to the first, an artifact occurs at the corresponding position on the timebase.

In systems in which the transducer stands off from the patient in a water-bath, the patient's skin and the surfaces of the water may give rise to quite large amplitude artifacts. The problem has been discussed, for example, by Robinson *et al.* (1966). The multiple reflexion artifact which occurs between the transducer and the skin is typically some 30 dB below the first skin echo, and its appearance on the scan can be prevented by arranging for the path length in the water to be greater than the penetration into the patient which appears on the display. Multiple reflexions between the skin and the surfaces of the water may be more difficult to eliminate, however, although a substantial improvement is obtained if ultrasonic absorbers are placed at those water surfaces from which artifacts may arise.

The maximum pulse repetition rate in a system employing water bath coupling may be limited by the decay time of the reverberation echoes. This decay time can be quite long because of the relatively low ultrasonic absorption coefficient of water at low megahertz frequencies.

Contact scanning is less liable to multiple reflexion artifacts, but under some circumstances quite large amplitude artifacts which are difficult to recognize may occur. This is because echoes which arise within the patient may cause artifacts due to reflexion at the skin–air, skin–transducer, and similar interfaces, which have higher reflectivities than the skin–water interface associated with water-bath scanning.

Multiple reflexion artifacts due to gas-containing structures within the patient are perhaps the most common. Their occurrence is a fundamental limitation in ultrasonic diagnostics. Such artifacts are usually quite easily reorganized, however, and so they should seldom cause diagnostic errors.

6.2 TIMING, SWITCHING AND GATING CIRCUITS

The timing circuits in pulse–echo systems fall into three main categories: these are rate generators, delay generators (as distinct from delay lines), and timebase generators. Such circuits are described in many textbooks on electronics, and only a brief discussion of the factors which determine the choice of the circuit for each particular application is given here.

The rate generator, or clock, provides the trigger pulses which control the repetition frequency of the system. This may be fixed in the range $25–3000 \ s^{-1}$, according to the particular application. The frequency stability of the rate generator is not usually important, because all the other timing circuits are synchronized with the trigger pulse which it generates.

Most systems employ an astable multivibrator as the rate generator. It is sometimes necessary to synchronize the rate generator with a particular frequency, such as that of the mains power supply, or the patient's electro-cardiogram. Synchronization with the mains frequency can be achieved by applying a voltage derived from the mains to an overdriven amplifier, so that the output of the amplifier consists of a series of pulses at mains frequency. A trigger signal synchronized with the e.c.g. can be provided by a circuit which is itself triggered by a characteristic part of the e.c.g. signal, such as the R-wave (see, for example, Davies and Mitchell, 1960).

In two-dimensional scanners (see Section 6.8), an improvement in image quality can sometimes be obtained if precautions are taken to prevent overwriting on the display if the position of the probe remains stationary with respect to the patient. One way in which this can be done is to arrange that the repetition frequency is controlled by the displacement of the probe, so that it is related to the velocity of the probe over the skin, or to the angular movement of the probe, or to a combination of the two (Hall, 1970).

Delay generators are required to perform a number of different functions, such as the provision of gating and trigger pulses delayed by time intervals corresponding to fixed ultrasonic pulse-lengths. The choice of circuitry is governed by the precision with which the delay must be generated. For most gating purposes, the monostable multivibrator is satisfactory. Such circuits can be designed to cover at least a decade of time variation, with a maximum jitter of less than 1%. Where greater precision, time variation and freedom of jitter are required, a voltage comparator fed with an accurate sweep voltage may be used.

Timebase circuits for one-dimensional displays are based on normal oscilloscope practice. The sweep time lies within the range 25 μs (for examining small organs like the eye), to 500 μs (for the investigation of the largest abdomen). The special timebase circuits used in some two-dimensional scanned B-scopes are discussed in Section 6.8.

An ideal switch has zero "on" resistance, and infinite "off" resistance. A bipolar transistor may be used as a switch, as shown, for example, in Fig. 6.11(a). The principal disadvantage of this arrangement is that, when the gate is closed (i.e. when the transistor is "on"), the base-collector voltage, typically a few tenths of a volt, forms a pedestal on the signal line. This may be troublesome, since, even if the gate is decoupled by capacitors, switching transients are introduced in addition to those due to the transistor capacitances. This simple circuit has an on–off ratio of around 40 dB. The circuit using a field effect transistor, illustrated in Fig. 6.11(b), has a better performance. When the gate is negative with respect to the source, the drain-source resistance is typically 10 GΩ. When the gate-source voltage is increased to equal zero, the drain source resistance decreases to about 25 Ω. There is no pedestal, and the switching transients are caused solely by feedback though interelectrode and stray capacitances, since there is no charge storage effect. A single shunt FET switch may have an on–off ratio of around 50 dB.

Field effect transistors are also very convenient in application, requiring series switches. A typical circuit is shown in Fig. 6.11(c): this arrangement is particularly appropriate when the source impedance is low. In order to switch the device on—i.e. to open the gate—V_{GS} must be zero. If the turn-on drive voltage is higher than the highest positive input voltage, the diode in the gate circuit becomes reverse-biased and the high-value source-gate resistor ensures that V_{GS} is zero and the device is saturated. The switching speed is limited by the time constant formed by the load resistor

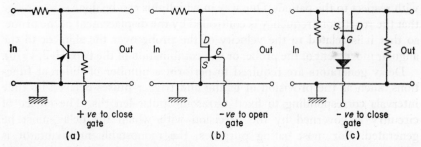

FIG. 6.11 Signal gating circuits. Shunt gates for negative-going video signals: (a) bipolar transistor; (b) field effect transistor; (c) series gate using a field effect transistor.

and the gate-drain capacitance, so higher speeds may be achieved with lower values of load resistance.

A combination of shunt and series gates may be used to achieve a better on–off ratio—say 60 or 70 dB—than that which is possible with either arrangement alone. The FET series gate is also useful in sample-and-hold circuits.

To a first approximation, the drain-source resistance in a FET is inversely proportional to the gate-source voltage. This characteristic makes the device eminently suitable as a voltage-controlled resistor: see Section 6.4.c.

6.3 TRANSMITTERS

The function of the transmitter is to excite the transducer to emit a short-duration pulse of ultrasonic energy. One of the earliest transmitter circuits, which is still in common use today, consists of a capacitor, previously

charged to a high voltage, which is suddenly discharged across the transducer by means of an electronic switch. The switching action may be
achieved by either a thyratron, a thyristor, or a transistor. A typical circuit
is shown in Fig. 6.12. The active element which energizes the transducer
is an avalanche transistor, which acts virtually as a short-circuit when the
base is made positive by the application of the trigger pulse. This discharges the capacitor C through the resistor R_1 in parallel with the series
combination of the transducer and the current-limiting resistor R_2.
Typically this transmitter produces a unipolar pulse with an amplitude
approaching that of the d.c. supply, and a rise-time of around 10 ns. In
response to this form of excitation, the transducer generates a train of stress
waves, separated in time by intervals corresponding to its thickness. This
mechanism is discussed in Section 3.6.b.v. The electrical charge available

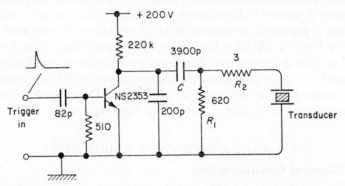

FIG. 6.12 Typical shock-exciting transmitter circuit, using an avalanche transistor.
(After Myers *et al.*, 1972.)

from the transmitting capacitor is typically 1 μC per pulse, and radiation
pressure measurements (see Section 3.7.e) can be used to determine the
corresponding power in the pulse, which might be 10 μJ. The total charge
fed to the transducer can be increased by increasing the value of the transmitting capacitor, and the energy carried by the pulse can be increased by
increasing the d.c. supply voltage. In practice, both these changes increase
the ultrasonic power, provided that the duration of pulse does not exceed
half the period of the wave. They also increase the current passing through
the switching transistor, and this must be limited by the performance of
the device.

Thyristors (and thyratrons) are generally capable of operating at higher
voltages than transistors. They cannot operate at such high speeds as
transistors, however, and care needs to be taken in the design of thyristor
circuits to ensure that the recharge rate of the capacitor is not so fast that
spurious triggering occurs.

Kossoff *et al.* (1965) have described the use of a blocking oscillator as a transmitter. Shunt and series tuning are used to increase the bandwidth, and the best results in terms of power transfer are achieved by designing the shape of the electrical pulse so that it matches half a cycle of the ultrasonic waveform.

A gated sine-wave oscillator is occasionally used as the transmitter in pulse–echo systems. The output from such a transmitter can be arranged to be symmetrical, so that there is no shift of the d.c. level at the transducer. This gives certain advantages in the design of the r.f. amplifier. The duration of the transmitter pulse is necessarily longer than in the case of shock or half-cycle excitation, however, and so the use of this type of transmitter is associated with a degradation in range resolution. The matter is discussed further in relation to pulsed Doppler techniques in Section 7.2.f.

Although in most contemporary pulse–echo diagnostic instruments the transmitter generates a short-duration, unipolar pulse, a simpler ultrasonic waveform is produced in response to a step excitation. Cheney *et al.* (1973) have developed a circuit which charges the transducer into a stressed condition, then decouples and discharges the transducer, and finally leaves the transducer decoupled from the charge source whilst echo signals are being received. The discharge is through a "totem-pole" avalanche transistor chain, producing a 250 V step discharge into a 24 pF load in 10 ns.

6.4 RADIOFREQUENCY AMPLIFIERS

6.4.a General Considerations

The range resolution of a pulse–echo system is determined, other factors being equal, by the total bandwidth and dynamic range. The bandwidth is limited by the performance of the transmitter, the transducer, the receiver and the display. The display is seldom the limiting factor as far as bandwidth is concerned, but it is important in relation to dynamic range (see Section 6.1.b).

The receiver consists of all the various circuits, some of which may be non-linear, which together process the echo signals fed from the transducer into a form suitable for presentation on the display. In general, the broader the frequency response of the receiver, the better is the range resolution. It is explained later in this Section, however, that the signal-to-noise ratio of the system depends upon the bandwidth, and that it is necessary to compromise between range resolution and sensitivity. A reasonably satisfactory arrangement is to make the r.f. amplifier bandwidth equal to the zero-crossing frequency of the ultrasonic pulse, and to arrange for the passband to be centred on this frequency. The video amplifier frequency response is often chosen to process the signal by restriction of the low-frequency gain, and this is discussed in Section 6.5.

The bandwidth of a system is normally taken to be equal to the difference between the frequencies at which the output is reduced by 3 dB from the maximum output, when the input amplitude is kept constant.

The dynamic range of the signal output from a transducer used in a typical pulse–echo system is very large. As discussed in Section 6.1.b, there are so many factors which control the useful dynamic range of the system that it may not be worth while to try to estimate its value with precision. The lower limit is ultimately determined by the equivalent input noise of the receiver amplifier (unless signal averaging is employed): the integrating properties of the system determine the minimum signal-to-noise ratio which can be accepted to give statistically reliable information about the occurrence of an echo. The upper limit is determined, for a given target range and transducer sensitivity, by the maximum amplitude of the transmitted pulse. Theoretically, it could be made quite large, simply by increasing the power of the transmitter. The risk that biologically undesirable effects may be caused, however, naturally increases as the energy is increased (see Section 9.12), and so designers should be unwilling to make changes in this direction.

The noise of a receiver arises from a variety of different sources. These include thermal agitation or resistance noise, and noise generated within the amplifying devices.

Thermal noise is due to the random nature of electron movements in a conductor. At any instant, there are likely to be more free electrons moving in one direction than the other, and this results in the appearance of a voltage across the conductor. The noise energy is uniformly distributed over the whole frequency spectrum; over the range of frequency f_1 to f_2.

$$E^2 = 4kTR\,(f_2 - f_1) \qquad (6.2)$$

where E = effective value of voltage components in the spectrum lying between the frequencies f_1 and f_2,

k = Boltzman's constant $(1.37 \times 10^{-23}$ J degK$^-)^1$,

T = absolute temperature, and

R = resistive component of impedance across which the thermal agitation noise is produced.

Thus, a resistor R may be considered as a generator of voltage E with a noiseless internal resistance R. Similarly, any source of noise voltage uniformly distributed over a frequency spectrum may be considered in terms of the equivalent noise resistance for the spectrum. For example, a resistance of 37·5 Ω at a temperature of 20°C operating in a circuit with a bandwidth of 1·5 MHz generates an equivalent mean-square noise voltage of 1 μV.

Within transistors used as amplifiers, there are three distinct noise sources. These are emitter noise and collector noise, due to fluctuations of diffusion and recombination in the base region, and base noise, due to the thermal noise of the equivalent base resistance. The contributions of both emitter and collector noise sources depend on the junction currents. The best noise performance is obtained with circuits designed to provide the optimum compromise between the conflicting goals of low current and low input impedance.

The noise figure of an amplifier is a measure of its noise performance: it is defined as the ratio of the input and output signal-to-noise ratios. An ideal amplifier would make no contribution to the noise content of a signal, and its noise figure would be unity, or 0 dB. Practical amplifiers have noise figures of greater than unity. In an amplifier consisting of several stages in cascade, the noise figure of the whole system is normally determined by the noise of the first stage. This is because the noise contribution of each succeeding stage becomes decreasingly important as the amplitude of the signal fed from the preceding stage becomes greater.

The noise figure of an amplifier depends upon the operating frequency and the bandwidth. The noise power is distributed (usually, but not necessarily, uniformly) throughout the frequency spectrum, and therefore the noise figure is improved as the bandwidth is decreased. In general, for a given bandwidth, the gain of the amplifier falls as the passband frequency is increased: this is because the losses in the system increase with increasing frequency. Consequently, the noise figure deteriorates as the operating frequency is increased, because the noise contribution from an amplifying device may be considered as a constant quantity referred to the input, independent of the stage gain.

In ultrasonic pulse–echo systems, it is rather difficult to estimate the signal-to-noise ratio at the input to the receiver. Most of the noise output from the receiver arises in the input resistance and the first amplifying stage. Therefore, in discussing the performance of a system, the noise figure is not such a useful quantity as the value of the equivalent noise voltage referred to the input. The concept of the noise figure is helpful, however, in discussing the performance of a system, particularly in consideration of the effects of alterations in operating frequency and bandwidth.

Another quantity which is often found useful in discussing the performance of an amplifier is the gain–bandwidth product. In any particular amplifier, the product of gain and bandwidth is a constant. In an amplifier consisting of N identical stages, the overall bandwidth equal to the one-stage bandwidth divided by $1.2\ N^{1/2}$.

The receiver in an ultrasonic pulse–echo system is subjected to a grossly overloading signal at the instant that the output from the transmitter is applied to the transducer. This overload is followed by a finite recovery time, during which the receiver is insensitive to small signals such as those which the transducer generates in response to echoes. A good receiver has a short recovery time. The period of paralysis following the transmission of the ultrasonic pulse is rather loosely known as the *transmission pulse*, during which information retrieval is impossible.

6.4.b Radio Frequency Amplifier Design

A radio frequency amplifier for ultrasonic pulse–echo applications needs to satisfy the following requirements:

   (i) adequate gain–bandwidth product at low noise;
  (ii) selectable centre frequency, if appropriate;
 (iii) low phase distortion;
 (iv) appropriate amplitude response;
  (v) quick recovery from overload;
 (vi) ability to withstand transmitter output; and
(vii) provision of swept gain.

A wide frequency response can be obtained by using a few (usually two) synchronously tuned stages of moderate bandwidth, the other stages being untuned, or by staggering the tuning of relatively narrow-band stages in a multistage amplifier. Indeed, the requirements (i)–(iii) in the preceding list can readily be achieved using integrated circuits designed for radio-communications applications.

The amplitude response of the radio-frequency amplifier may be linear, or it may have a signal compression characteristic to reduce the dynamic range. A detailed discussion of this matter is given in Section 6.5.c, where reference is made to the possibility of applying this process in the radio frequency, rather than in the video amplifier.

Any tendency of the receiver to paralyse is an undesirable feature, because this results in a long transmission pulse. An overloading signal can change the bias conditions of the amplifying stages, as a result of alterations in the charges stored in the coupling and decoupling capacitors. This may be due, for example, to the passage of base current in a transistor. The amplifier becomes insensitive to small signals until the biasing conditions have returned to normal. The effects of paralysis can be minimized by making the capacitors which control the biasing so large that overloading signals produce only small charges in the operating conditions, and by arranging for the gain of the system to be low at the time when the largest signals are applied to the input. To some extent, this latter protection is afforded by the swept gain by up to around 50 dB from the maximum at the time that the transmitter pulse is applied to the receiver. The transmitter pulse is the largest signal which the receiver is required to accept: it is several orders of magnitude greater than the largest echo signal.

The problem of paralysis can be reduced if some kind of limiting circuit is included at or near the input to the amplifier. Two such circuits are illustrated in Fig. 6.13. In Fig. 6.13(a), the peak input to the receiver is limited to about 1 V, being the forward voltage of the reverse-connected diodes. In Fig. 6.13(b), the unitrode diode is made to conduct just before the arrival of the transmitter pulse, and to continue to act as a short circuit until the overload conditions have ceased.

The requirements for swept gain depend upon many factors. These are discussed in Section 6.1.b. For example, in the case of an ultrasonic pulse with a nominal frequency of 2·5 MHz, the swept gain rate needs to be 3·3 dB cm^{-1} in soft tissues. This corresponds to about 0·25 dB μs^{-1}, and a 50 dB dynamic range would need to be swept in about 200 μs. It is gen-

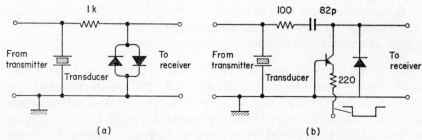

FIG. 6.13 Circuits designed to protect the r.f. amplifier from the transmitter pulse. (a) Forward biased diodes; (b) unitrode (after Myers *et al.*, 1972).

erally best for the gain to be controlled in such a way that it increases by equal fractions for equal increases in time; that is, an exponential swept gain is required. More accurate compensation in which account is taken of variations in the attenuations of different materials soon becomes unmanageable, although attempts to do this, which are useful clinically, are discussed in Section 6.4.d.

There are two methods by which swept gain can be obtained. In one method, the gains of suitable stages are controlled by the alteration of feedback or biasing conditions (for example, see Fig. 6.14). In the other method, the gain of each stage of the r.f. amplifier is kept constant, and electronically controlled attenuation (see Section 6.4.c) is introduced at appropriate points in the circuit.

In a multistage amplifier, the overall gain is equal to the product of the gains of each stage. If the gain of any stage is altered, whilst its frequency response remains unchanged, the overall gain is altered in proportion, without affecting the overall frequency response. Therefore, the points in the circuit at which gain controlled is applied to the amplifier are of no consequence to the frequency response, whether the amplifier is synchronously tuned, stagger tuned, or untuned. These points are important, however, in so far as they affect the dynamic range and noise performance of the system. The earlier stages of the amplifier are usually designed to operate most satisfactorily with small signals: distortion may be introduced if large signals are applied. Therefore, it is necessary to apply swept gain to the earlier stages, so that they do not become overloaded. It would be both difficult and uneconomic to apply swept gain at a circuit point at which the signal amplitude is already large. A compromise may be necessary when it is desirable to keep the dynamic range of control of each stage as small as possible, so as to maintain a good exponential relationship between

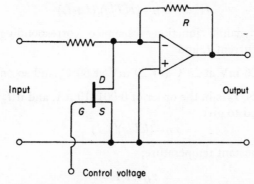

FIG. 6.14 Gain control by variable negative feedback. The resistor R and the field-effect transistor from a variable potentiometer which controls the fraction of the output voltage fed back to the input of the amplifier.

gain and controlling voltage. In such cases it may be best to include potentiometric attenuators between the early stages. Similarly, if swept gain is applied to only one stage, it is generally best if this is also the first stage.

6.4.c Electronically Controlled Attenuators

Gain control in transistorized amplifiers by variation of the d.c. bias conditions is associated with alterations in impedances so that considerable difficulties arise with this method, particularly in the case of tuned amplifiers. A better method of gain control in such amplifiers is by the use of a suitable number of variable attenuators connected between appropriate stages. Such attenuators can take the form of networks containing diodes or transistors, the a.c. resistances of which can be controlled by alteration of their d.c. conditions.

The relationship between current and voltage in a semiconductor pn junction is given, according to first order theory by:

$$I = I_s(e_q V/kT - 1) \qquad (6.3)$$

where I = forward current across the junction corresponding to an applied
  voltage V,

     I_s = reverse saturation current,

     k = Boltzman's constant ($1\cdot37 \times 10^{-23}$ J degK^{-1}),

     T = absolute temperature of junction, and

     q = electronic charge ($1\cdot60 \times 10^{-19}$ C).

From Eqn. 6.3,

$$V = (kT/q) \ln (1 + I/I_s)$$

so that

$$dV/dI = r_D = (KT/q)/(I + I_s) \qquad (6.4)$$

where r_D = dynamic junction resistance corresponding to forward
  current I, and

$(kT/q) = 26$ mV at 25°C (or 29 mV at 60°C, and so on).

In most diodes, I_s is in the order of $0\cdot001$–10 μA, and if $I_s \ll I$, Eqn. 6.4
may be simplified to give

$$r_D = (kT/q)(1/I) \qquad (6.5)$$

and hence, at constant temperature,

$$r_D \propto 1/I \qquad (6.6)$$

and from Eqn. 6.3,

$$r_D \propto e^{-cV} \qquad (6.7)$$

where c is a constant.

The relationship given in Eqn. 6.3 is based only on considerations of
diffusion current. More exact theory requires that account is also taken of
such factors as the geometry of the junction, the series resistance associated
with bulk semiconductor material, and generation and recombination in
the space charge region. Equations 6.6 and 6.7 are sufficiently accurate,
however, to indicate the proportional relationships between dynamic
resistance, current, and voltage. The resistance of a practical diode may
differ from that predicted by simple theory by as much as a factor of five,
and the characteristics of any particular type are best determined experimentally (see, for example, Fig. 6.15). It is important to appreciate the
distinction between the dynamic resistance, which is given by the slope
dV/dI of the characteristic curve, and the static d.c. resistance, which
is equal to V/I.

Transistors may be used as controlled resistors in suitable circuit configurations. For example, Morris (1965) has discussed the relationship

between the bottomed emitter-collector resistance r_T and the base current I_b of a bipolar transistor, and has shown by making certain simplifying approximations that:

$$r_T = (kT/qI_b)\{1/\beta_n + 1/(1+\beta_i)\} \qquad (6.8)$$

where β_i and β_n are respectively the inverted and normal common emitter current gains.

It can be seen from Eqn. 6.8 that r_T depends mainly on the smaller of the two current gains. In addition, if I_b and β_i are both large, then the collector-to-emitter voltage V_{ce} is given by:

$$V_{ce} = (kT/q)/(1+\beta_i) \qquad (6.9)$$

Of the two possible arrangements, it is better to operate the transistor

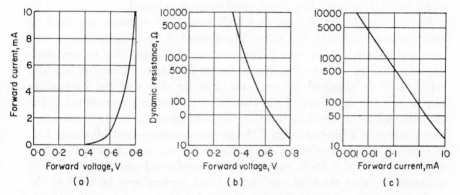

FIG. 6.15 Forward characteristics of a typical 1N916 diode. (a) Current–voltage characteristic; (b) variation of dynamic resistance with voltage; (c) variation of dynamic resistance with current.

in the inverted mode, with the base current flowing through the collector. In this situation, $\beta_i = h_{FE}$, and, from Eqn. 6.9, it can be seen that V_{ce} is quite small (typically less than 1 mV). Moreover, r_T is determined mainly by $\beta_n = h_{RE}$, which is usually of the order of 1% of h_{FE}. In practice, there is some deviation from simple theory, and it may be difficult to estimate with accuracy the value of h_{RE}. Therefore it is generally best to measure r_T experimentally.

Field-effect transistors may also be used as voltage-controlled resistors. The effective dynamic drain-to-source resistance r_{DS} can be reduced by forward-biasing the gate with respect to the source. When biased with drain-to-source voltage below pinch-off,

$$r_{DS} = V_p/\{2I_{DSS}(V_{GS} - V_p)\} \qquad (6.10)$$

where V_p = gate-to-source voltage cut-off (the "pinch-off" voltage),

I_{DSS} = zero-gate-voltage drain current, and

V_{GS} = gate-to-source voltage.

The value of r_{DS} is maximum when $V_{GS}=V_p$, and minimum when $V_{GS}=\phi$, where ϕ is the contact potential of the device (around 0·5 V). There is some deviation between the values obtained in practice and from simple theory, but over a limited range r_{DS} is inversely proportional to V_{GS}. It is interesting that the range of linear operation can be increased by arranging for a voltage to be fed back from the drain to the gate, so that this voltage is added to the controlling voltage. A remarkably good performance can be obtained if half the drain voltage is fed back to the gate (Martin, 1962). The values of the feedback resistors can be made quite large compared with the drain-to-source resistance, so that they have little effect apart from providing the desired correction signal.

Some examples of circuits in which controlled resistors are used as attenuators are given in Fig. 6.16. The control characteristics shown were obtained experimentally, and differences may be found due to variations between devices of the same types. In an L-section attenuator, a linear relationship is obtained between the loss (in dB) and the controlling function, if the resistance of the controlled element is proportional to the exponent of the controlling function. This relationship exists in the junction diode over a limited range if the device is voltage-controlled (see Fig. 6.16(b)). Constant-resistance networks, however, such as the T-section illustrated in Fig. 6.16(c), require quite complicated control functions to maintain accurate tracking, no matter what devices may be used as the controlled resistors. Similarly, the relationships between controlling function and network loss in decibels is non-linear in every case illustrated in Fig. 6.16, with the sole exception of the voltage-controlled shunt diode attenuator. Moreover, all these networks are temperature-sensitive, and methods of temperature correction or control are necessary in precision applications. Because the devices are essentially non-linear, they all introduce signal waveform distortion which increases with increasing signal amplitude across the controlled resistor. The transistor is the least satisfactory in this situation, and distortion becomes noticeable at peak amplitudes of around 10 mV; the junction diode distorts significantly at 20 mV peak; but the junction FET may be operated up to 150 mV peak before distortion becomes important.

As explained in Section 6.4.b, the positions in the r.f. amplifier at which the electronically controlled attenuators are placed are determined by considerations of signal distortion, dynamic range and noise. The largest echo signals are in the order of a few volts, and it is necessary in the case of a diode attenuator, for example, for a loss of 40 dB to be introduced

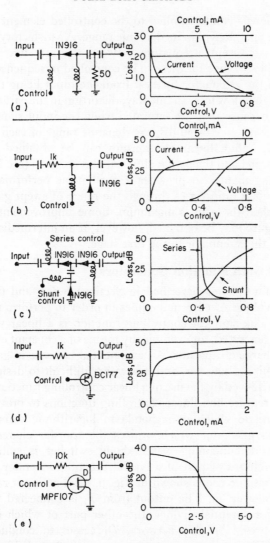

FIG. 6.16 Examples of electronically controlled attenuators. At r.f., all the inductors have high reactances, and all the capacitors have low reactances. Each circuit operates with negative control current or voltage, but the control supplies are shown in the conventional forward directions to simplify the diagrams. For the control characteristics shown, with the exception of (c), the effects of the source and load impedances are negligible. (a) Series diode attenuator; (b) shunt diode attenuator; (c) constant-resistance (600 Ω) T-section attenuator; (d) transistor shunt attenuator; (e) junction field-effect transistor shunt attenuator.

before such signals can be applied to the controlled element in the attenuator if it is to operate within its dynamic range. A satisfactory arrangement
is to insert four swept attenuators between the first five stages of the
amplifier, and to arrange for these to be controlled in sequence (by suitable
biasing), with the attenuator furthest from the input being the first to be
swept from high to low loss. In this way, distortion in the earlier attenuators
is minimized because they are saturated when the input signal is greatest.
For a swept gain range of 50 dB, the dynamic range of each attenuator is
only 12·5 dB, and a linear relationship can be obtained between the
controlling voltage and the gain if shunt diodes are used (see Fig. 6.16(b)).
Such an arrangement also provides a good noise performance, because
the signal-to-noise ratio varies through the range of swept gain to a minimum value when the gain is maximum. Some improvement in the mid-
range noise figure may be obtained, however, if an intermediate attenuator
is swept after the attenuator in the first stage.

6.4.d Swept Gain Function Generators

The swept gain systems described in Sections 6.4.b and 6.4.c require
time varying voltage or current supplies in order to perform the necessary
gain control. The simplest controlling function is a linear voltage ramp,
which can be generated, for example, by means of a constant current source
arranged to charge a capacitor. An exponential increase in gain with time
is usually required, however, and it is rather difficult to design circuits in
which this is achieved by the use of a linear controlling function. Therefore,
most circuits require non-linear controlling functions to provide the gain-
time characteristic which corresponds to logarithmic compensation. A
diode function generator which utilizes the transfer characteristic of a
resistive network containing biased diode switches is suitable for this
purpose. The circuit of part of a typical function generator designed for
diagnostic ultrasonic use is shown in Fig. 6.17. The input ramp is fed to
the emitter follower T_1. The output from T_1 is connected to R_1, which
forms part of a potential divider, the other part of which is the diode-
controlled network. In this network, D_1 ceases to conduct when the
divided voltage is equal to the first break potential, and this switches out
the resistive components adjusted by the first slope potentiometer. Similarly, the diodes D_2 and D_3 switch out in turn as the divided voltage
increases. Thus the output, which is fed through the voltage followers T_2
and T_3, consists of a voltage which increases with time as indicated in the
diagram.

If care is taken to design a swept gain system in which the gain (in dB)
is proportional to the control voltage, it is a relatively simple matter to
generate a control voltage which can tailor the gain-variation with time so
that it is especially suited to each particular clinical application or beam

orientation. Thus, Barnes *et al.* (1975) have described one way in which this can be done. Their swept gain curve is synthesized from sequentially gated analogue switches, each of which independently controls the receiver gain over a short range interval (typically 10 mm). By arranging for the gain in each distance interval to be controlled by a separate slide-adjustable potentiometer in an array, the positions of the control knobs can be made to trace out the swept gain curve. The curve can be smoothed by an integrator, to avoid sudden steps in the value of the gain. This kind of system is particularly useful in cardiological studies—and indeed it is available on some commercial instruments—since it enbales, for example,

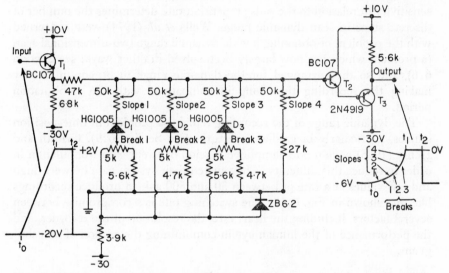

FIG. 6.17 Part of a typical diode function generator for swept gain voltage control.

the gain to be low in the regions where anterior and posterior ventricular walls are situated, and high in the region of the mitral valve leaflets. The reason that this may be advantageous is that the dynamic range of the display may be inadequate to allow these structures to be seen satisfactorily with exponential swept gain, so that either the valve echoes or the posterior wall echo can be seen, but not both simultaneously.

A method of display dynamic range expansion using system gain wobbulation has been proposed by Wells *et al.* (1974). The basis of the technique is that, within the limitation of the dynamic range of the recording material, the density of the recording of a light source of given intensity is determined by the time duration of the exposure. Consider the situation where there are three echoes of differing amplitude and spaced in time position. At low system sensitivity, only the strongest echo produces a registration on the display. At higher gain, the second echo is displayed in addition to the first; but because of the restricted dynamic range, the brightness of the registration of the first echo may be the same, or only slightly greater, than that of the second. At still higher gain, all three echoes are displayed, but again with small brightness differences. Next, suppose that the gain is wobbulated at a regular rate between the limits at which the weakest and only the strongest echoes are displayed. The relative densities of the three recordings are thus in a brightness magnitude sequence of 3 to 2 to 1. There are several methods by which this system may be realized. It is possible to wobbulate the transmitted power, or the receiver gain, or the range of swept gain variation. In each case, the rate of change of system sensitivity in relation to the pulse repetition rate determines the number of discrete steps in scan dynamic range. Wells *et al.* (1974) were concerned with the problem of obtaining a wide dynamic range two-dimensional scan (a problem which has now largely been solved in other ways: see Section 6.6), and so they arranged for the dynamic range to be continuous by making the recording time long in comparison with the wobbulation period.

The dynamic range of the recording remains a problem in time-position studies, particularly of cardiac structures (see Section 6.9). Griffith and Henry (1975) have used a simplified version of swept gain wobbulation in order to reduce this difficulty. They switch their system gain between high and low values at a rate of between 30 and 500 s^{-1}, to produce recordings like that shown in Fig. 6.18. The switching rate is a compromise between several factors, including the heart rate, the resolution of the recorder, and the performance of the human eye in combinining the section of an echogram.

6.4.e Demodulation and Suppression

The output from the r.f. amplifier consists of signals extending in amplitude over a dynamic range which is typically in the order of 30 dB. It is normally necessary to demodulate these signals so that further amplification and processing may occur in the video amplifier.

Demodulation in ultrasonic systems is usually carried out by means of suitable diode networks, such as that illustrated in Fig. 6.19(a). The characteristic of the ideal diode (Fig. 6.19(b)) is such that $R_D = R_0$ when $V > 0$, where R_D is the equivalent resistance of the diode, V is the voltage across the diode, and R_0 is the forward resistance of the diode (a constant in the ideal case). Thus:

$$v_{out}/v_{in} = R_L/(R_S + R_L + R_D) \quad \text{when } v_{in} > 0 \qquad (6.11)$$

and

$$v_{out}/v_{in} = 0 \quad \text{when } v_{in} < 0 \qquad (6.12)$$

assuming that the input impedance of the video amplifier is either very large, or is included in the value of R_L. Consequently the circuit shown in Fig. 6.19(a) provides a half-wave demodulated output signal, the amplitude of which is proportional to the instantaneous forward value of the r.f. input signal.

Practical diodes do not possess the ideal characteristics. For example, Fig. 6.19(c) shows the forward characteristics of typical germanium point-contact (OA91) and silicon junction (1N916) diodes. That of the

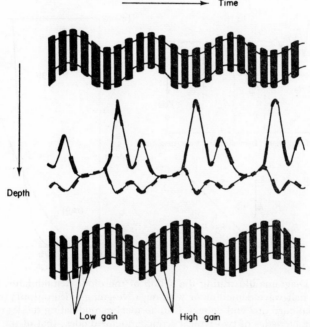

FIG. 6.18 Diagrammatic echocardiogram (see Section 6.16.b) with switched gain. The valve leaflet echoes can be seen at high gain, and the posterior ventricular wall echoes can be identified at low gain.

point-contact diode approaches more closely to the ideal, but even this device has a much higher resistance at low forward voltage than at high forward voltage. This non-linearity of the forward characteristic of the diode demodulator determines the lower limit of the dynamic range of the signals which the circuit can accept. The upper limit is controlled by the maximum output voltage available from the r.f. amplifier, provided that the forward current and reverse voltage maxima of the diode are not exceeded.

Consider, for example, a r.f. signal the maximum amplitude of which is

10 V peak, and a type OA91 diode demodulator. Figure 6.20 shows how
the insertion loss of such a demodulator varies with the forward input
voltage, for various values of $R = R_L$, with $R_S = 0$. (Curves of the same
shape correspond to situations in which $R_S > 0$, but for which $(R_S + R_L) =$
R; R_S and R_L simply form a potential divider to share that part of the
input voltage which does not appear across the diode, and the curves are
shifted by an additional insertion loss which is independent of the input
voltage.) The effect of demodulator amplitude non-linearity is to expand
the dynamic range of the video signal. Thus, if the input to the demodu-

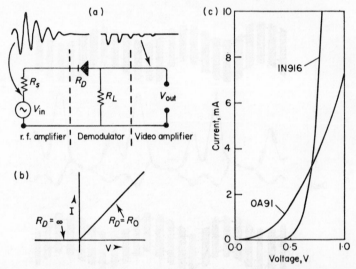

FIG. 6.19 Diagrams illustrating the action of the diode demodulator. (a) Circuit
diagram of half-wave demodulator with negative-going video output; (b) relationship between current I and voltage V in an ideal demodulating diode; (c) current/
voltage characteristics of two typical semiconductor diodes: that of the type OA91
(point contact) diode approaches more closely to the ideal.

lator has a dynamic range of 30 dB, and a maximum amplitude of 10 V
peak, then the minimum input signal is 320 mV peak. The dynamic range
of the demodulated output (video) signal depends upon the total value of
$(R_S + R_L)$; in this example, it increases from about 32 dB with 100 kΩ, to
38 dB with 1 kΩ.

Although the effect of the non-linearity of the demodulator can be
reduced by increasing the total value of $(R_S + R_L)$, there are in practice
factors which limit this improvement. The input impedance of the video
amplifier is generally in the order of 1 kΩ, and this sets an upper limit on
the value of R_L. Moreover, R_L must be kept quite low so that the effects of
the stray capacitances do not become significant. R_S can be increased, for

example by means of a series resistor, but R_S and R_L form a potential divider which reduces the amplitude of the signal fed to the video amplifier. In addition, the reverse current of a typical point-contact diode is around 0·1 μA at 0·5 V, and the efficiency of the device as a rectifier is reduced if it is operated in a high impedance circuit. In practice, these considerations limit $(R_S + R_L)$ to around 10 kΩ.

It follows from this discussion that, even if the r.f. amplifier is able to supply 10 V peak into a 10 kΩ load, the effect of the diode demodulator is to expand a 30 dB input dynamic range by about 5 dB. The effect can be compensated if a video amplifier with a logarithmic characteristic is used, because such an amplifier performs the reverse function of dynamic range

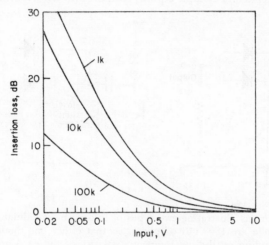

FIG. 6.20 Insertion loss of type 0A91 half-wave demodulator similar to that illustrated in Fig. 6.19(a). Each curve is for a different total value of resistance $(R_S + R_L)$.

compression (see Section 6.5.c). Another way around the difficulty is to introduce dynamic range compression before demodulation.

A very small improvement in the performance of the demodulator can be obtained if the diode is biased in the forward direction in the absence of an input signal. The difficulty with this arrangement is that the efficiency of the diode as a rectifier is thus reduced, and the output signal contains an increasing fraction of the undemodulated input signal. Another possible solution is to incorporate the diode in the feedback loop of an operational amplifier, but here the problem is that the slew rate of available devices is hardly fast enough to function at ultrasonic frequencies.

Full-wave demodulators, typical examples of which are illustrated in Fig. 6.21, are more efficient than half-wave demodulators. Such circuits have the additional advantage that the demodulated output accurately conveys the information contained in the input (apart from degradation due to dynamic range expansion). Therefore there is less possibility of error in estimating the time–position of the echo: an error equal to about half the period can occur in the case of half-wave demodulation when the phase of the signal is such that the diode is open-circuit to the first half-cycle.

In practice, the dynamic range expansion of the conventional diode demodulator may not be a serious problem. This is because the dynamic range window of the input signals which is eventually fed to the display is usually deliberately restricted. This is the case, for example, when only the signals which exceed some particular amplitude are considered to be of clinical significance. Perhaps equally important, the resolution becomes

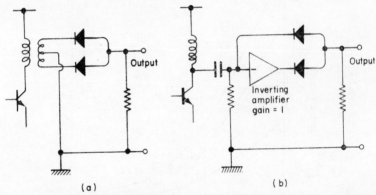

(a)   (b)

FIG. 6.21 Diagrams illustrating two types of full-wave demodulator. The signals fed to each diode are 180° out of phase, so that either one diode or the other conducts, depending on the instantaneous polarity of the r.f. signal. The phase change is achieved (a) with a centre-tapped transformer; (b) with an inverting amplifier.

rather poor when a wide dynamic range is displayed (see Section 6.1.b), and a system input dynamic range (after swept gain compensation) of as little as 10–20 dB may represent the best compromise, in which case a diode demodulator is perfectly satisfactory. The process of dynamic range restriction is known as *suppression*, or *rejection*. It is important to realize the distinction between suppression and dynamic range compression. Suppression is equivalent to the action of a non-linear demodulator, because such a demodulator expands the dynamic range so that the small-amplitude signals become relatively even smaller. Variable signal suppression can be introduced by reverse-biasing either the demodulator, or by a separate reverse-biased diode connected in the forward direction in the video signal path. The use of a separate diode is generally preferable, because the demodulator can be designed to give the minimum dynamic

range expansion, and the suppression diode can be forward biased when
zero suppression is required.

6.5 VIDEO AMPLIFIERS

6.5.a General Considerations

The demodulated output from the r.f. amplifier consists of video signals
with a useful dynamic range in the order of 30 dB and a maximum amplitude of around 1 V peak. It is necessary for these signals to be amplified
to a level suitable for driving the particular display which is being used.
Usually, the display is a cathode-ray tube arranged as an A-scope or as a
B-scope. In most cases, the maximum small-signal gain required in the
video amplifier is around 50 dB, and it can often be very much less.

The video amplifier must be designed to meet the following requirements:

(i) adequate gain to drive the display when the input signal is of the
smallest value of clinical significance;

(ii) adequate bandwidth to maintain the pulse characteristics, unless it
is deliberately intended to process the signal, for example by
differentiation; and

(iii) dynamic range compression to avoid overdriving the display with
large amplitude signals: this may be achieved by limiting the
maximum value of the output of an otherwise linear amplifier, or
by logarithmic amplification.

Some aspects of this matter have been discussed by Wells (1974). The
degree of dynamic range compression which is required depends on the
dynamic range of the signals of clinical significance at the input to the
video amplifier, and upon the type of display which is being used. An
A-scope display normally has a dynamic range of around 40 dB, and in any
event overloading signals do not confuse the interpretation of what is
displayed, and so it may not be necessary to apply any compression. The
dynamic range of a cathode-ray tube used as a B-scope, however, is not
greater than around 20 dB, and dynamic range compression by limiting
in a linear amplifier is not ideal, unless the dynamic range is deliberately
restricted to improve the resolution. In other cases, a logarithmic video
amplifier provides a satisfactory characteristic.

Brinker (1966) and Brinker and Taveras (1966) have mentioned the use
of a video amplifier in which the output dynamic range is effectively zero.
Such an arrangement is used on several commercially available instruments. A video-activated monostable multivibrator generates a short pulse
(typically 0·4 μs) for every echo which is greater in amplitude than some
fixed threshold. The monostable cannot be retriggered by another video

signal until an additional time (say 4 μs) has elapsed, so that the resulting B-scan consists of a large number of appropriately positioned bright spots, all of equal size. The method is convenient when the display is a bistable direct-view storage tube, and in tissue mapping applications produces a picture made up of thin lines which may be aesthetically pleasing, but it has little else to commend it.

An alternative method of zero dynamic range processing, which retains the amplitude information in the input signal, is pulse width modulation in which the duration of the output pulse is proportional to some function of the amplitude of the input (Railton and Hall, 1975). This has some potential advantage in brightness-modulating a cathode-ray tube (see Section 6.6) because the deflexion circuits operate with a constant electron beam density, and it is employed in at least one commercial scanner.

6.5.b Linear Video Amplifiers

The various aspects of the design of linear video amplifiers are discussed in many textbooks on communications engineering. The simplest and most commonly used type of video amplifier is made up of several amplifying stages coupled together by resistor-capacitor networks, or constructed into an integrated circuit. At low megahertz frequencies, the passband of frequency response (3 dB down from the mid-band gain) is conveniently made equal to the zero-crossing frequency of the ultrasonic pulse. For operation at higher frequencies, a somewhat narrower bandwidth may be satisfactory.

Difficulties can arise if the video amplifier response cuts off at a frequency in the range 10–100 kHz. Such a response results in serious degradation of long pulses, and the recovery time following large signals becomes excessive. Therefore, unless differentiation associated with time constants of a microsecond or so is required, it is necessary for the low frequency response to extend to about 1 kHz.

If sharp limiting of the video output signal is required, it is often achieved by driving an appropriate amplifying stage or biased diode into saturation. It is best to include the limiter in an early part of the amplifier, so that the following stages are protected from overload.

6.5.c Logarithmic Video Amplifiers

Amplifiers in which the output voltage is proportional to the logarithm of the input voltage have been used in anticlutter systems since the earliest days of radar. In pulse–echo ultrasonic diagnostics, logarithmic video amplifiers are used to compress the dynamic range of the useful signals into that of the display. One way of obtaining this characteristic is to arrange for each stage in the amplifier to operate logarithmically over a limited range and in sequence, as illustrated in Fig. 6.22. The logarithmic

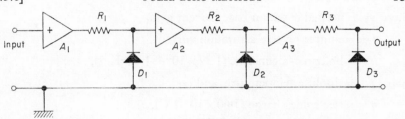

Fig. 6.22 Logarithmic amplifier with sequential operation, for negative-going video input.

characteristic can be obtained by means of diodes connected in the forward direction across the signal path, coming into operation as the signal voltage exceeds the corresponding junction voltage. Over a limited range, the characteristic is such that, to a first approximation, the forward voltage is proportional to the logarithm of the input voltage (see Fig. 6.19) if the diode is used as part of a potential divider of which a fixed impedance, or constant source impedance, forms the other part. In Fig. 6.22, A_1, A_2 and A_3 are linear video amplifiers. When the input signal is small, diode D_3 acts as the logarithmic component of a potential divider with resistor R_3. As the input signal amplitude is increased, the resistance of D_3 tends to a constant value, but D_2 begins to conduct and, in combination with R_2, acts so that the overall response continues to be logarithmic. In principle there is no limit to the number of stages, and in this example R_1 and D_1 come into operation when R_2 and D_2 begin to become linear. In this circuit, silicon junction diodes are satisfactory although rather temperature-dependent.

It is rather more satisfactory to use a transistor (or a diode) as the negative feedback element in an operational amplifier, in order to obtain a logarithm response. The basic principles are illustrated in Fig. 6.23. Provided that $V_e > 0\cdot1$ V,

$$I_c = \alpha_n I_{ES} e^{qV_e/kT} \qquad (6.13)$$

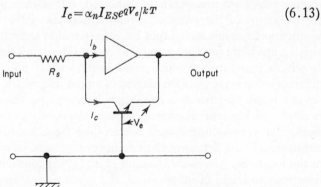

Fig. 6.23 Arrangement of a transistor to apply negative feedback to an amplifier, resulting in a logarithmic amplitude response.

where α_n = normal common base current gain,

I_{ES} = emitter reverse saturation current,

k = Boltzman's constant $(1 \cdot 37 \times 10^{-23}$ J degK$^{-1})$,

T = absolute temperature, and

q = electronic charge $(1 \cdot 60 \times 10^{-19}$ C$)$.

An accurate conversion device requires that α_n is independent of the current, so that feedback degeneration increases with the exponent of the output. This condition is almost perfectly satisfied by silicon diffused transistors of the mesa or planar types, and such devices exhibit logarithmic behaviour over extremely wide ranges. For example, Lunsford (1965) has described a pulse amplifier in which a 2N2219 transistor is used as the feedback element, and in which an input range of 10 mV–10 V (60 dB) is compressed into an output range of 2–10 V (14 dB), within a conformity of about 2·5%. The rise-time of this amplifier is less than 0·1 μs, and high thermal stability is achieved by maintaining the critical transistors at constant temperature.

The nature of the logarithmic characteristic makes it difficult enough to adjust the level of the input, let alone to apply swept gain, in a logarithmic amplifier. Therefore swept gain must be applied before logarithmic compression in a conventional arrangement. As far as the signal levels are concerned, in effect the input noise level is adjusted by the gain of the r.f. amplifier, and the system output, by the video amplification which follow logarithmic compression.

6.5.d Other Processing Arrangements

The positional information in an ultrasonic wavetrain may be emphasized by differentiating the signals (Wells, 1967), because the positions of the leading edges are preferentially displayed, rather than information about the durations of the echoes. Differentiation also introduces some signal suppression, because the output is proportional to the rate of change of the signal amplitude: for a given pulse shape, this becomes smaller as the signal amplitude is reduced. Another consideration which applies particularly in differentiating systems is the degree of smoothing which is necessary after demodulation to generate a suitable video envelope shape. Differentiation is employed in many diagnostic systems, especially in those in which the display is a two-dimensional B-scan (see Sections 6.8 and 6.9), but unfortunately the details of the circuit arrangements are seldom described in the literature. Moreover, Kossoff et al. (1965) consider that differentiation leads to a loss of information, and gives no real improvement in the quality of the scan. This is possibly because their system employs a logarithmic video amplifier, which makes good use of the echo information.

In systems using linear amplification, the improvement in the clarity of the scan which results from differentiation is generally more important than the loss of information. This information loss seems to arise mainly from the suppression, and partly from the small shift in system threshold which is associated with the recovery, of the differentiating network. This matter has been discussed by Reid (1968). Thus, although these aspects of logarithmic compression had been discussed by Kossoff *et al.* (1968), it was not until four years later that the Australian group described the combination of this form of processing with the differentiate-and-add circuitry which revolutionized two-dimensional scanning by the reintroduction of grey-scale images. This form of processing had apparently been in use in his laboratory for a few years before it was first described by Kossoff (1972). The rationale behind this technique is that, in many examinations, a situation is encountered in which a large amplitude and relatively long duration echo is received, which shows small and slowly changing modulation. For example, in obstetrics the echo from the foetal surface has this characteristic. In these circumstances, it may be desirable to emphasize *changes* in the amplitude, rather than to display the *absolute* value of the amplitude. In this way, the observer notices sudden changes, without losing sight of the overall amplitude as he would do if the signal were merely differentiated with respect to time. Kossoff's (1972) circuit is shown in Fig. 6.24. The waveform from the detector follows two paths, in proportion under the control of the designer (or the operator). Along one path, the shape of the waveform is unchanged, along the other, it is differentiated. The ratio of the differentiated to the undifferentiated signal is typically 0·2–0·3. The time constant of the differentiating circuit is chosen to have no significant effect on very short echo signals of the type obtained from single, flat interfaces, normal to the beam. Since the majority of echoes resembles this ideal pattern, this method of signal processing does not affect the general character of the image.

The process of taking the video signal, differentiating it, and adding an appropriate fraction of the original, undifferentiated signal has also been discussed by Ide (1974). He called images formed from differentiated signals, "contour" images; and those formed from both differentiated and added signals, he called "contour emphatic" images.

Inverse filtering, which is the process of compensating for the restricted bandwidth of a system by appropriate shaping of the gain-frequency response, can bring about some improvement in the range resolution. It has been pointed out by McSherry (1974) that the improvement is limited by the signal-to-noise ratio, the bandwidth of the initial data, and prior non-linear processing. Similarly, it might be supposed that deconvolution could compensate for the width of the ultrasonic beam, thus improving the resolution in azimuth. This was first proposed by Howry (1955). Unfortunately, it seems unlikely that this process could be successful, despite the apparently optimistic view of Kossoff *et al.* (1968), because the ultrasonic beam may be deflected from its geometrical central axis within the body during the scanning process. This is another limitation which arises from the uncertainty in the position of the resolution cell. Thus, Hubelbank (1972) has attempted to improve the azimuthal resolution of a conventional two-dimensional scanner, using digital processing which closely resembled a matched filter, matched both to the spatial response and the angle of the

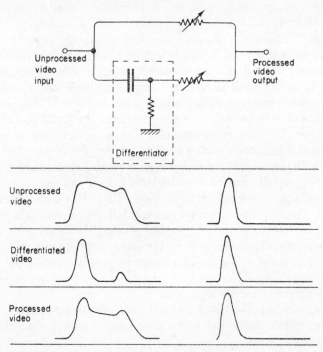

FIG. 6.24 Circuit arrangement and signal processing characteristics of the "differentiate-and-add" network. (After Kossoff, 1972.)

transducer. Radiologists were asked to comment on sets of pictures showing both the original and the processed scans. They were asked to point out the differences, advantages and disadvantages of the two groups of pictures. In almost all cases where measurements of the size of structures were involved, the processed pictures were preferred. Processing was of little advantage, however, and often even degraded the result, when only a subjective interpretation (such as locating the placenta) was required.

It has been suggested by Mars (1974) that it might be possible to obtain improved ultrasonic two-dimensional scans of the brain, if the degrading effects of the skull could be eliminated by deconvolution. Deconvolution could be achieved by inverse filtering, if the pulse and directivity function were known. The presence of the skull, however, makes this impossible; but the situation might be improved by homomorphic filtering techniques.

6.5.e First Echo Swept Gain Trigger Circuits

In systems in which the transducer is in direct contact with the patient, the swept gain circuit is triggered by the same pulse as is used to trigger the transmitter. This arrangement is not satisfactory, however, in systems in which the transducer is separated from the patient by a variable length water delay path. The attenuation of the ultrasonic pulse travelling in

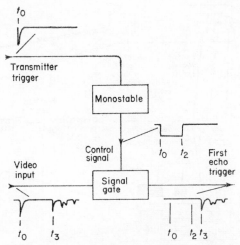

FIG. 6.25 Block diagram illustrating the derivation of a trigger pulse corresponding to the skin echo. The signal gate is closed during the interval t_0–t_2, during which time the video signal consists of the transmission pulse; the gate opens before the time of the earliest occurrence of the skin echo, shown here at t_3.

water may generally be neglected, and swept gain is only required from the instant that the first echo returns from the patient. Because the distance between the transducer and the skin surface is not fixed in a scanning system, it is necessary to derive this trigger pulse from the echo signal corresponding to the skin.

Although quite complicated methods of doing this have been described (see, for example, Wells and Evans, 1968), all that is necessary is a simple gating circuit in the video line, the gate being closed during the transmission pulse. As shown in Fig. 6.25, the first signal which passes through the gate is then the skin echo, and this can be arranged to trigger the swept gain generator.

6.6 DISPLAYS

6.6.a Conventional Cathode-ray Tubes

Cathode-ray tubes are extensively employed for the presentation of ultrasonic pulse–echo information. Modern cathode-ray tubes are precision devices possessing linear deflexion sensitivity, and are capable of providing excellent resolution. Their design is a specialized subject, and only a brief account of the most important considerations is given here.

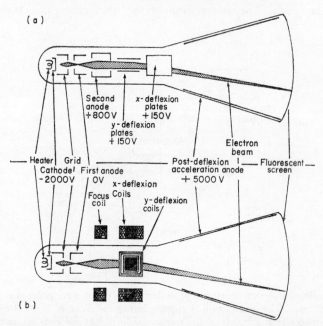

FIG. 6.26 Diagrams illustrating the constructions of typical post deflexion acceleration cathode ray tubes. (a) Electrostatic; (b) electromagnetic. Typical electrode voltages are shown.

Cathode-ray tubes are classified into two groups, according to their deflexion systems, which may be either electrostatic or electromagnetic. The principal features of the two types are illustrated in Fig. 6.26. Arrangements are normally made to prevent the control grid from being driven positive with respect to the cathode. The grid-cathode cut-off potential is typically around −40 V. In the electrostatic tube, focusing is accomplished by variation of the second anode potential, and the deflexion sensitivity is around 100 V for one screen radius. The coils of a typical electromagnetic tube draw 20 mA for focusing, and 50 mA to produce a deflexion of one screen radius. Electromagnetic deflexion is associated with less defocussing than electrostatic deflexion, and for this reason it is generally preferable where a large display is required.

The accelerating voltage is made as high as possible in order to develop the maximum energy at the screen for conversion to visible radiation. The most economical arrangement is to accelerate the electron beam after it has been deflected. In this way, the high deflexion sensitivity of a low energy beam is obtained together with the high brightness of a high energy beam. Post-deflexion acceleration is obtained by means of a conductive coating on the inside of the front part of the tube, which is kept at a high voltage relative to the final anode in the electron gun. The ratio of these two voltages may be as much as 10:1, but with high ratios the field from the postdeflexion acceleration anode tends to penetrate behind the deflexion plates and thus to accelerate the beam before deflexion. In some tubes, this effect is minimized by forming the postdeflexion acceleration electrode into

TABLE 6.2

Characteristics of some common phosphors used in cathode ray tubes

Type	Colour	Decay time to 10% brightness	Typical application
P1	Yellow-green	22 ms	General purpose
P11	Blue	65 μs	Photography
P31	Green	40 μs	General purpose
P33	Orange	6 s	Long persistence

a helix, which acts as a potential divider and reduces the accelerating field as the distance from the screen increases.

A disadvantage of postdeflexion acceleration is that if the beam is deflected off the screen it may strike the postdeflexion acceleration electrode and generate secondary electrons: these secondaries produce large areas of fluorescence on the screen, which tend to obscure the trace and to spoil photography. The effect can be minimized by careful selection of operating voltages. Because of the rather low duty cycle in many ultrasonic diagnostic applications, however, the advantage of high brightness makes postdeflexion acceleration *de rigueur*.

The screen is formed by coating the inside surface of the tube with a suitable phosphor, which emits luminous radiation under the impact of the electron beam. The best type of phosphor depends upon the particular application. The characteristics of some common phosphors are given in Table 6.2. Type P31 is about three times more efficient in terms of light conversion than type P1. Long persistence phosphors, such as type P33, can be used in displays from which, for example, the operator can gain an impression of a complete scan as a preliminary to photographic recording.

The useful resolution, in terms of the number of separate lines which can be displayed across the screen, is determined by the relationship between the size of the screen and the diameter of the luminescent spot. In practice, imperfections in the electron optics distort the shape of the spot, especially near the edge of the screen. Moreover, the brightness of the spot also decreases towards the edge of the screen. The spot has no sharp boundary, but its edge is defined as the contour at which the brightness has fallen to some specified (or implied) fraction of the maximum brightness. This fraction is usually chosen so that if the centres of two spots are one spot diameter apart, the spots can just be resolved. The spot diameter is conveniently measured by the "shrinking raster" method. A series of, say, 100 lines is drawn on the screen by means of two timebases as in a television raster. Under conditions of optimum focus and stigmatism, the lines are brought closer together, by decreasing the amplitude of the slower timebase, until the separate lines cannot be distinguished. The height of the raster divided by the number of lines then gives the line width, which is equal to the spot diameter.

The measurement of spot size is further complicated by non-linearity in the relationship between brightness and beam current, which causes variation in the spot diameter as previously defined. As a general guide, however, the spot diameter is typically about 0·5 mm for a display tube with a diameter (or diagonal) of about 150 mm. When other screen sizes are used, it is reasonable to assume that the ratios of the spot sizes are proportional to those of the screen diameters for similar electron gun assemblies.

The spot size not only determines the maximum potential resolution of a diagnostic ultrasonic system, but also to some extent controls criteria, such as the maximum useful scanning speed, upon which the designs of complete systems are based.

In ultrasonic scanning, the echo information is often displayed on a brightness-modulated cathode-ray tube. There are two characteristics which are especially important in such applications. Firstly, the dynamic range of the display system, which is determined by the linearity of the phosphor as a luminescent source, limits the signal dynamic range which can be accepted from the video amplifier. This is typically in the order of 20 dB. This is much less than the dynamic range of vision, which is normally at least 50 dB, and considerably more if time is available for adaptation. The video signal may be applied either to the cathode or to the grid of the cathode-ray tube. Cathode drive has the advantage that this electrode is readily accessible by capacitive coupling but this method of coupling is suitable only for low-duty-cycle, short duration pulses, as the time constant of the circuit is typically around 100 μs. Another difficulty with cathode modulation in electrostatic tubes is that the effective deflexion sensitivity and the focusing field are directly dependent on the cathode potential: these effects limit the maximum cathode drive to about 20–30 V. Grid modulation is relatively free from these disadvantages, and direct coupling is normally possible. In brightness-modulated display, it is often most convenient to apply the echo information in the form of negative-going pulses to the cathode, whilst the grid is controlled by the bright-up pulse. These factors do tend to limit the dynamic range of the display, however, and one method which has been used to overcome this difficulty is to use pulse width modulation of the electron beam, rather than pulse amplitude modulation. The problem with this is that the time available for modulation control is very short when displaying ultrasonic echoes, and the range resolution is degraded with large amplitude signals.

The second characteristic of the cathode-ray tube which is important in ultrasonic scanning is the extent to which it contributes to the integration of the echo information. Video integration is dependent upon the signal-to-noise ratio and the scanning variables (beam width, speed of scanning, pulse repetition rate, and timebase velocity), and it is also affected by the dynamic range of the display system, and the integrating characteristics of the screen of the cathode-ray tube, and of the observer or the recording process. It is important to realize that the storage which can be accomplished in the eye and mind of an observer is extremely effective, and, at least in high-speed scanners, it may be substantially better to use a directly observed display than to present the image on an electronic storage tube, or even to record it photographically. Visual integration by the observer, however, is not satisfactory over long periods of time.

6.6.b Direct View Electronic Storage Tubes

The need frequently arises in ultrasonic pulse–echo diagnosis for the storage of information presented on a cathode-ray tube display, either for subsequent study or as part of an integrating process. This kind of storage can generally be achieved photographically; but the photographic process suffers from disadvantages, either in time delay or expense, or both. It is possible, however, to record many of such data quite adequately on a direct-view electronic storage tube, and thus to avoid the disadvantages of photography.

Two types of direct-view storage tube are in common use. They differ in the method of modulating the viewing beam: this may be achieved either by transmission control, or by bistable landing-velocity control. Storage tubes of either of these types generally have resolutions which are about half as good as those of conventional cathode-ray tubes of the same screen sizes.

Figure 6.27(a) is a diagram showing the main features of a transmission-control electronic storage tube. The operation of this type of device has been described by Knoll and Kazan (1956). The writing gun deposits a charge pattern on the storage surface, which consists of an insulator coating a metal mesh backing electrode. The quantity of charge deposited depends on the writing beam current and the speed and number of the superimposed scans. Low velocity electrons from the flood gun (which must be operating during the writing process in order to avoid runaway charging) approach the storage mesh normally at constant current density. These electrons penetrate the mesh in those areas on which the charge pattern has been written, and are accelerated to the viewing screen where they produce an image. The brightness of the image is determined by the

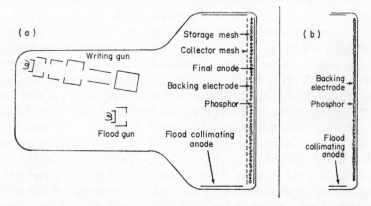

FIG. 6.27 Diagrams illustrating the construction of typical direct-view electronic storage tubes. (a) Transmission-control type: for simplicity, certain electrodes, particularly those associated with the collimation of the flooding electron beam, have been omitted from the diagram; (b) construction of the target area of the bistable type: the electron gun arrangements are similar to those shown in (a).

stored information, and so this type of tube is capable of displaying several shades of grey: the dynamic range is typically around 10 dB. The image can be completely erased by the application of a small positive pulse (about 1 s duration) to the backing electrode. Such a pulse produces an instantaneous rise in the storage mesh potential as a result of capacitive coupling, and this allows the flood beam electrons to land on the entire surface of the storage mesh. The potential of the storage mesh is consequently reduced to near flood gun potential, so that the stored charge pattern is erased. The flow of flood beam electrons to the screen is cut off at the end of the erasing pulse, and the tube is then ready for the next writing operation. Varying degrees of display persistence can be obtained by the application of a continuous train of short pulses of appropriate duration to the backing electrode.

A typical transmission-control direct view storage tube* has a screen diameter of just over 100 mm, and gives a viewing time of at least 10 min. Storage times of several days can be obtained by cutting off the flood beam. The maximum writing speed is about 25 mm μs^{-1}, which is adequate for ultrasonic displays of life-size or smaller.

The bistable direct view storage tube differs from the transmission-control type chiefly in the construction and performance of the target area. The target of a bistable tube (Anderson, 1967) is shown diagrammatically in Fig. 6.27(b). The writing gun forms a charge image on the dielectric storage layer which controls the transmission of flood current to the storage screen. Where the target background is unwritten the screen is at low potential, and the flooding electrons bombard the target at low velocity: this results in a secondary emission ratio of less than unity, and these areas become negative. Conversely, the areas of the target which have been written on are at increased potential: the flooding electrons cause secondary emission with a ratio of more than unity, and these areas become positive. Thus, the target has bistable properties, and can be charged in opposite directions by bombardment from a single source. The image can be erased by reducing the voltage applied to the backing electrode.

The performance of a bistable storage tube is largely dependent on the design of the target area. The phosphor is deposited in the form of a porous layer with a semicontinuous surface. The useful storage time is limited by the migration of charge across the dielectric layer, and it is up to about 1 h under optimum conditions. Writing speeds of more than 0·25 mm μs^{-1} are quite common, and some specially selected tubes† are capable of writing speeds of more than 1 mm μs^{-1}. The fastest writing speed, however, corresponds to a maximum display size in ultrasonic diagnosis of only just slightly more than the dimensions of the soft-tissue structures being examined. Moreover, the performance deteriorates with age.

The dynamic range of a bistable storage tube is effectively zero, as the image is either stored or not stored.

6.6.c Scan Conversion Memory Tubes

The scan conversion memory tube is almost ideal as a storage device in two-dimensional ultrasonic scanning. In its simplest form, the device contains an electron gun which serves alternately for writing, reading, and erasing. The construction of a typical tube is illustrated in Fig. 6.28. The cathode of the electron gun may be kept at a low potential, and the target voltage is adjusted so that either a positive or a negative charge may be deposited according to the degree of secondary emission. The position of the electron beam on the target is controlled by electromagnetic deflexion.

---

* Type E702C: English Electric Valve Co. Ltd., Chelmsford, UK.

† Type T5640–201: Tektronix Inc., Beavertron, Oregon, USA.

The target is a silicon–silicon oxide wafer of about 25 mm diameter, divided up into a matrix of elements of around 10 μm square on a 15 μm grid.

The detailed mechanisms of the various processes in a conventionally operated scan conversion memory tube* are illustrated in Fig. 6.29. The first stage is to erase any charge pattern which may be stored on the target, and this is done by fixing the backplate potential at $+20$ V with respect to the cathode: the potential of the dielectric is shifted to 0 V (cathode potential) because the secondary emission ratio with the unfocused beam is less than unity. At the beginning of the writing process (Fig. 6.29(b)i), the target potential is shifted to $+200$ V, and the storage surface potential

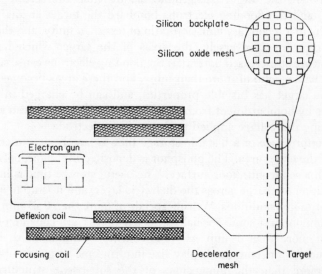

FIG. 6.28 Diagram illustrating the construction of a typical single-ended scan conversion memory tube.

moves to $+180$ V by capacitive coupling. When the electron beam modulated by the video signal scans the storage surface, corresponding positive charges are deposited because the secondary emission ratio is greater than unity. The maximum writing speed is typically 50 μs per line. The charge pattern can be read by shifting the backplate potential to $+10$ V, so that the target current provides the output signal when the storage surface is scanned with an unmodulated beam. The read-out is essentially non-destructive, and continuous viewing times of around 10 min are satisfactory. The resolution is typically equivalent to 800 lines per diameter with orthogonal writing and reading at 50% modulation.

Operated in this conventional mode, a scan conversion memory tube

* For example, type TME 1238: Thomson-CSF, Paris, France.

integrates the input signal in a similar way to the integration provided by a direct-view storage tube, or a conventional cathode-ray tube with photographic recording. In two-dimensional ultrasonic scanning, this is undesirable, because if the ultrasonic beam is stationary, or it is moved irregularly, the brightness of the image is not related to the distribution of the echo-producing characteristics of the tissues being studied. As explained

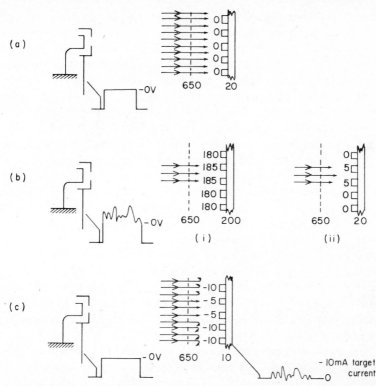

FIG. 6.29 Operation of a single-ended scan conversion memory tube. The numbers on the diagrams are voltages relative to the cathode, except where otherwise indicated. (a) Erasing; (b) writing (i) conventional mode, (ii) equilibrium writing mode; (c) reading.

in Section 6.6.e, various methods have been used to solve this problem. One such method depends on operating a scan conversion memory tube in an equilibrium writing mode. The erasing and reading processes are the same as in conventional operation. During the writing process (Fig. 6.29(b)ii), the target potential is kept at +20 V, and the storage surface is scanned with a focused electron beam modulated by the video signal. Thus the storage surface has its potential distribution clamped to the corresponding voltages of the cathode, and the final potential of any point on the storage surface is equal to the lowest potential reached by the cathode whilst the electron beam was in that position during the writing process. Therefore video integration does not occur, apart from that associated with the time constant of the voltage clamping circuit.

There is at least one commercially available unit built around a single-ended scan conversion memory tube operating in the equilibrium writing mode designed specifically for ultrasonic and similar image storage*. This instrument has virtually solved the problem of achieving perfect storage of two-dimensional ultrasonic scans. The stored image can be reproduced in television format on an inexpensive monitor, and television accessories, such as character generators, can readily be incorporated in the system. Moreover, the stored image is in a form which is easily processed by analogue methods, such as by colour-coding, and it is also conveniently interfaced to a computer. The method has only one important limitation. This arises from the use of a single-ended tube, in which the writing and reading processes cannot take place simultaneously. It is necessary to switch from the reading to the writing modes during the periods when echoes are being received, and this happens typically 10 times during a single frame. Consequently the read-out displayed on a standard television monitor is split up into bands during the time of scanning the patient. This irritating difficulty can be circumvented by blanking the monitor during scanning, and using a direct-view storage tube to ensure proper scan coverage. Alternatively, a monitor with a long-persistence phosphor at least eliminates the flicker. A complete solution to this problem would be afforded by the use of double-ended scan conversion memory tube, in which separate guns are used for writing and for reading. Such devices are available commercially,† but they do not seem yet to have been used for ultrasonic image storage with equilibrium writing.

In summary, the scan conversion memory tube has four major advantages as a storage device for two-dimensional ultrasonic scanning. These are:

(i) The writing timebase may be randomly orientated, whilst the reading timebase may be in a regular TV compatible format: this makes it possible to use inexpensive picture monitors, and accessories such as character generators.

(ii) The stored dynamic range is better than that even of a direct-view non-storage cathode-ray tube, and adjustment of contrast and brightness controls of the reading minotor allows different parts of the dynamic range of the image to be examined without the need to rescan the patient.

* Type PEP-400: Princeton Electric Products, New Brunswick, New Jersey, USA.

† For example, Type TME 1496: Thomson-CSF, Paris, France.

(iii) There is negligible overwriting when operated in the equilibrium writing mode; and

(iv) The resolution is much better than that of a conventional direct-view storage tube, and indeed it is at least as good as most non-storage display tubes; consequently storage does not degrade the image if the full-screen capability is used, and an acceptable quality can be obtained if only part of a stored image is magnified for display (this is a "zoom" facility), or if several complete serial images are stored, and displayed one at a time.

Scan conversion memories are now available with the systems of at least four commercial manufacturers. The excellence of the resolution may allow several scans to be stored simultaneously. A scan conversion memory is about four times more expensive than a conventional storage system using either a bistable or a transmission control cathode-ray tube. The convenience of use (not least the ability of the method to tolerate poor scanning techniques), the variable dynamic range, and the facility to use cheap television accessory instruments, such as monitors and character generators, frequently justify the extra cost.

6.6.d Photographic Recording

Although the diagnostic information available from an ultrasonic investigation may often be studied directly on the cathode-ray tube, the need frequently arises for a photographic recording to be made. This may be required as a step in the process of video integration, or for subsequent reference or publication. Single events or transients which occur in a very short time interval can only be studied in the form of recordings, and photography is frequently the best method.

The most convenient cameras for oscilloscope photography generally employ either 35 or 70 mm film, or Polaroid–Land material. The Polaroid* process (Land, 1947) is invaluable where a positive print (or a negative) is required very rapidly. With type 47, 87 and 107 films, which have speeds of 3000 ASA, the print is ready only 10 s after the exposure has been completed. No darkroom facilities are required.

In ultrasonic diagnostic applications employing brightness modulation of the display, the dynamic range of the photographic recording process may be a limiting factor controlling the system resolution. The effect is similar to the non-linearity of the brightness modulation of the cathode-ray tube. In general, higher speed emulsions produce images of higher contrast, or smaller dynamic range. For example, a film with a speed of 3000 ASA might

---

* "Polaroid" is a registered trade-mark of Polaroid Corpn., Cambridge, Massachusetts, USA.

have a dynamic range of 15 dB, whilst a speed of 2 ASA might correspond to 50 dB.

Photographic recording depends upon a change being produced by light in the photographic emulsion to form a latent image which can be developed by suitable chemicals. The action of light on the emulsion may be considered in terms of the statistical probability that it will produce such a change. For a given light intensity, the probability that a latent image will be formed increases with the exposure time. This property of photographic recording gives rise to a theoretical possibility of resolution improvement in certain ultrasonic scanning systems. Thus, due to the finite width of the scanning beam, the registration of a small target may appear as a series of lines in a two-dimensional compound sector B-scan. These lines ought to intersect at the point corresponding to the true position of the target on the display. If the conditions of exposure were carefully chosen, a latent image would only be formed on the photographic emulsion at the intersection of the crossed lines, because it is only there that there would be sufficient light to produce a chemical change. In practice, however, errors in registration (see Section 6.13.c prevent this theoretical advantage from being realized.

The conditions which determine the dynamic range of the photographic recording are discussed further in Section 6.6.e. It is not possible to state the exposure times for every diagnostic application. As a rough guide, however, and using 3000 ASA material, an A-scan of normal brightness can be photographed with an exposure of 1/25 s at f8; a two-dimensional abdominal B-scan made up of about 1000 lines and displayed on a conventional cathode-ray tube during the scanning process requires an aperture of around f4 for satisfactory recording. Other conditions of brightness and film speed require exposures calculated on a proportional basis.

6.6.e Grey Scale and Colour Displays

Conventional two-dimensional ultrasonography is a tissue-mapping process which indicates structure boundaries. From the earliest use of ultrasound in medical diagnosis, the possibility of identifying neoplastic tissue (Wild and Reid, 1952), and more generally of identifying tissues of all kinds, has often been proposed. The first routine application of such a method was in placentography, where the area of the placenta "fills in" with echoes as the system sensitivity is increased, whereas the amniotic fluid remains transonic (see Section 6.16.f). Likewise hydatidiform moles may be identified. A similar technique, known as the "sensitivity graded method of ultrasonotomography", has apparently proved to be accurate in the differential diagnosis of breast tumour (Kobayashi et al., 1974). The method of "sensitivity-graded tomography" referred to in Japanese publications is exactly the same as the technique of McCarthy et al. (1967) whereby several scans are made of the same section using differing system sensitivities. Recently, the so-called "grey scale" display has become popular. In this method, the dynamic range of the image is sufficient to give some indication of the amplitudes of the echoes arising from within tissue structures, whilst simultaneously showing the stronger echoes from organ boundaries (Kossoff and Garrett, 1972; Taylor *et al.*, 1973).

The brilliance control sets the level on the transfer characteristic relating output brilliance to the amplitude of the Z-modulation. Operating at a lower level of brilliance suppresses the smaller echoes. It has been pointed out by Hall and Railton (1975a) that the best grey-scale rendition is obtained by operating at the highest brilliance and the smallest aperture which are possible to obtain a satisfactory photograph. Generally this can most easily be achieved by increasing the brightness (which is a d.c. control which shifts the threshold of the display, and which is equivalent in function to the suppression control if the brightness is such that the unmodulated timebase is invisible) until the timebase is just visible on the CRT, and by then closing the aperture so that the timebase almost disappears from the photograph. This ensures that the smallest echo signals reaching the display do intensify the brightness; and, because the aperture is as small as possible, the available range of photographic density is spread over the largest range of signal amplitude.

Even under these conditions, the transfer characteristic of the tube–film combination is somewhat sigmoid. The effect of this is relatively to suppress very small signals and to compress very large signals. Compression of large signals is in any case usually desirable, and is assisted by logarithmic amplification. Logarithmic amplification has the effect of emphasizing the small signals, and thus improves the grey-scale rendition. Some further improvement can be obtained by incorporating a gamma-correction network to compensate for the low-amplitude tail of the sigmoid transfer characteristic.

In practice, the scan conversion memory tube (see Section 6.6.c) is very suitable for grey scale scanning. Because of its wide dynamic range, it is quite tolerant to the setting of the gain control of the scanning instrument. The dynamic range of the stored image which is displayed can be selected by the contrast and brilliance controls of the television monitor.

The scan conversion memory tube has two disadvantages when used to store ultrasonic images. The first is that, with a single-ended tube, the reading and writing processes cannot take place simultaneously, so that the television display needs to time-share between ultrasonic wavetrains during the scanning process: this gives rise to an irritating "banding". The second is that there is some tendency to integrate, even when the tube is operated in the equilibrium writing mode. The only method which promises completely to solve the probelm of overwriting is that proposed by J. Satrapa and D. Lavichi, and described by Kossoff (1974). The scan is divided up into a matrix of separate elements by means of a computer, and the magnitude of the echo corresponding to each matrix element is compared with the value already existing in the store, during the scanning process. If the new value is greater, the computer stores it in place of the old value. Thus, only the highest values of echo amplitude are stored, and this is achieved without integration.

In another application of the computer, due to D. E. Robinson, and also described by Kossoff (1974), the echoes corresponding to each element in the matrix are summed and a count is made of the number of times the element is updated. When the scanning has been completed, these two quantities—the sum and the number of updatings—are multiplied for each element, and the result is displayed as a normalized image.

If the echogram is divided into a coarse grid, the display has a mosaic appearance. Ito *et al.* (1974) have smoothed this type of display by taking into account the values of the neighbouring elements to interpolate into the final image.

The number of shades of grey which can be identified on a scan is rather dependent on the pattern of the display. A simple illustration of this is given in Fig. 6.30. It has been pointed out by Hall and Railton (1975b) that, no matter what criterion is adopted in defining the minimum detectable difference between grey shades, ultimately the number of shades is determined by the range of brightness from black to white levels. If a $2:1$ variation can be appreciated, for example, and the range from black to white is $32:1$ (which is typical for a paper print), then five shades can be perceived, since $2^5 = 32$. Similarly, the range of transmission of light transmission through emulsion on a transparent base may extend from 0.09 to 99%, so that 10 shades can be perceived, since $2^{10} = 1000$. In this connexion, it is relevant that a cathode-ray tube display adjusted to match the input dynamic range of Polaroid print material is insufficiently "contrasting" for direct viewing, and therefore it is desirable to have separate monitors for photographing and viewing the output of a scan converter. The problem of restricted dynamic range occurs in many branches of imaging. It can in some circumstances be solved by inverting the grey scale (so that the display becomes darker as the echo amplitude is increased), or by combining deflexion and brightness modulation (Baum, 1970), or by recirculating the grey scale several times across the dynamic range, or by colour coding. In some applications, such as in nuclear medicine images, contrast can be very effectively enhanced by recirculating grey scales, or by allocating sharply different colours to neighbouring amplitudes. In this way, contrasting colours have been used to code ultrasonic scans (see, for example, Ito *et al.*, 1974; Bronson and Pickering, 1975; Flinn, 1975). It has been pointed out by Milan and Taylor (1975), however, that this has two serious disadvantages. Firstly, there is no obvious relationship between colour and amplitude, so the coding scheme has to be learnt before a scan can be interpreted. Secondly, the eye cannot average the plethora of colours which are presented in areas where there are rapid variations in amplitude. In order to overcome these limitations, Milan and Taylor (1975) used a colour coding corresponding to the temperature scale (red–orange–yellow–white).

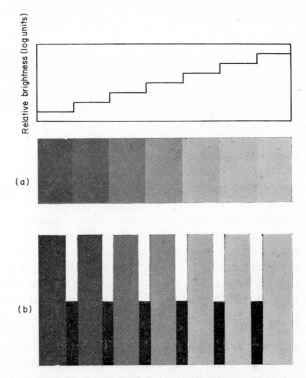

FIG. 6.30 Grey scales. In (a) it is quite easy to distinguish the different shades of grey, but in (b), which is an identical grey scale, but interrupted by black or white bands, it is more difficult, or even impossible, to recognize these differences.

The red scale was adjusted to be equivalent to the grey scale of a monochrome display. At higher amplitudes, green was added to produce the orange tones, and finally blue was added to produce yellow and white. In this way, 16 separate levels could easily be distinguished, as compared with 8 on a conventional grey-scale display. Although a computer was used to store the two-dimensional scan in a 96×96 matrix before colour coding, this function has perhaps better, and certainly more conveniently, been performed by a scan conversion memory (Ide, 1974).

6.6.f Other Display Methods

(i) Hard copy instruments

The use of a storage display, either direct-view or scan conversion, allows the image to be scanned at a relatively slow speed in a regular raster. Various commercially available systems* make use of this to reconstruct hard copies on dry silver paper with tolerable degrees of grey-scale reproduction, which compare favourably both in cost and convenience with photographic methods (Lee, 1975).

(ii) Fibre-optic recorders

The light output from a cathode-ray tube can be collimated by means of a fibre-optic faceplate, thus greatly increasing its effective brightness. Such is the efficiency of this technique that the output from an ultraviolet phosphor may be great enough directly to produce a recording on bromide paper, without any need for chemical development. Alternatively, full chemical processing may be used to enhance the contrast and to ensure archival permanence. Instruments based on this system are available from several manufacturers,† and writing speeds can be sufficiently high to allow direct intensity-modulated signals to be recorded at ultrasonic rates in real time. This is of great importance, particularly in echocardiography. In some designs of instrument, there is some difficulty due to the sampling rate being chosen to allow optimum recording of phonocardiograms, so that a recirculating shift register needs to be used to change the recording rate of the ultrasonic signals. This degrades the quality of the recording according to the number of bits per word, and the number of words per line, so that the best results are obtained when this complication is avoided.

(iii) Pen recorders

When it is necessary to display the relationship between two variables—for example, time and position, as in the study of the motion of a single structure isolated by gating circuits—a pen recorder may be used, either with orthogonal drive or with a constant velocity drive on one axis. The frequency response of the recorder is generally of prime importance, apart from considerations of cost and convenience. Most pen recorders using ink styli or heat-sensitive paper operate satisfactorily at frequencies of a few tens of hertz. For higher frequencies, of up to around 10 kHz, mirrors drvien by galvanometers can be used to deflect a beam of light on photographic paper. When a response of up to around 1 kHz is required, how-

---

* For example, Type 4601: Tektronix Inc., Beavertron, Oregon, USA.

† For example, Cambridge Medical Instruments Ltd., Cambridge, UK; Honeywell Test Instruments Division, Denver, Colarado, USA; Medelec Ltd., Old Woking, Surrey, UK.

ever, probably the most convenient instrument is the ink-jet recorder*, in which the inertia of the pen in a conventional recorder is eliminated, and which produces dry, and permanent tracings in real time on cheap paper. Moreover, the ink-jet recorder can be intensity-modulated if it is modified to incorporate an electrostatic ink control system (Hertz *et al.*, 1967: Hertz and Simonsson, 1969; Lindström *et al.*, 1973).

6.7 THE A-SCOPE

The basic principles of the A-scope are described in Section 6.1.a. The modern ultrasonic A-scope is fitted with a number of manually operated controls. There is considerable variation in this respect between different instruments. The minimum requirement is generally that the system should be sufficiently sensitive for echoencephalography (see Section 6.16.a), and that its range measuring axis should be calibrated, either in time or in distance. Some instruments have an electronic pulse generator which constructs a distance-measuring scale, in millimetres and centimetres, on the display, so that changes in timebase velocity are matched by corresponding changes in calibration.

For many years, the A-scope was the most important ultrasonic diagnostic instrument. Books were virtually exclusively devoted to its use (see, for example, Schiefer *et al.*, 1968).

Nowadays, the A-scope is only of limited clinical usefulness: it has its main applications in echoencephalography and, at higher frequencies, in ophthalmology for distance measurements within the eye. It has some value in distinguishing between cystic and solid lesions. Its principal usefulness, however, is as an aid in operating two-dimensional scanners and time–position recording systems. Thus, some manufacturers use their basic A-scope as the ultrasonic system within a complete instrument, and others supply modules to allow pulse–echo data, observed on the A-scope, to be displayed in various ways.

6.8 THE B-SCOPE

6.8.a General Considerations

The information obtained by a pulse–echo system is a combination of range and amplitude data. It may be presented in the form of an amplitude-modulated timebase on an A-scope. The information may, in principle, be displayed equally well on a brightness-modulated timebase, in such a way that the brightness is proportional to some function of the echo amplitude. This kind of display, called a *B-scope*, is compared with the A-scope in Fig. 6.31.

* For example, the *Mingograf*: Elema-Schönander AB, Stockholm, Sweden.

Practical B-scope displays have certain limitations in comparison with their corresponding A-scans. The dynamic range of brightness-modulation (see Section 6.6) of a conventional cathode ray is around 20 dB, and it may be between 0 and 10 dB in a direct-view electronic storage tube. A typical A-scope is capable of displaying around 40 dB. Dynamic range compression is often necessary to obtain satisfactory results with a B-scope

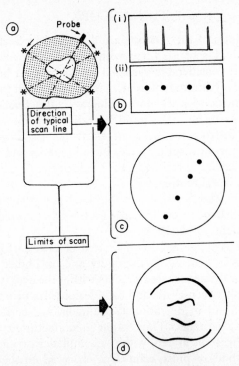

FIG. 6.31 A-scope and B-scope methods for displaying ultrasonic pulse–echo information. (a) Schematic representation of a section through a patient; (b) (i) A-scope presentation of a typical scan line, (ii) B-scope presentation of the same scan line; (c) B-scan as in (b) (ii) but with the direction and position of the timebase linked to those of the ultrasonic beam across the patient; (d) two-dimensional B-scan, integrated from many individual scans, each one similar to (c).

in ultrasonic diagnostics, and it is difficult to make quantitative measurements of echo amplitude. Brightness-modulation is associated with some degree of spot degradation, and so the display resolution is rather worse in the B-scope than the A-scope. All these limitations are minimized, however, if a scan conversion memory tube is used as the storage device.

The B-scope forms the basis of several important diagnositc displays, some of which are described in the following Sub-sections.

6.8.b The Two-dimensional B-scope

The B-scan illustrated in Fig. 6.31(b) corresponds to pulse–echo information obtained along a single line. Its interpretation requires a knowledge of the possible anatomical and pathological situations which it might represent, so that at least some of the echoes may be identified as arising from particular structures. Thus, it is a one-dimensional display which can only be recognized and used by a skilled observer with *a priori* information.

It is a simple matter in principle to link the direction and position of the timebase across the display to the direction and position of the ultrasonic beam across the patient, as shown in Fig. 6.31(c). The B-scan then represents the space–position of each echo-producing interface, and not simply its range from the transducer. If the probe is moved over the patient, and all the separate B-scans (each one similar to that in Fig. 6.31(c), but corresponding to a different transducer position and beam direction) are stored, then an image such as that in Fig. 6.31(d) is produced. This represents a two-dimensional section through the patient in the plane of the scan.

The angles of incidence and reflexion of an ultrasonic beam are equal at a flat surface. The maximum echo amplitude is detected at normal incidence, since only then does the echo return directly to the transducer. Consequently, in visualizing extensive and fairly flat surfaces, an improved image (a *compound* two-dimensional B-scan) is obtained if the probe is oscillated as it is moved around the patient, because this increases the likelihood of the occurrence of normal incidence with specular reflectors. Complete information can only be obtained in this way, however, if all the surfaces are normal to the scan plane, and it is possible to scan in a complete circle. The problem can be reduced if a wide aperture transducer is used (Kossoff *et al.*, 1968). It is important also to realize that echoes originating from within tissues tend not to be dependent in amplitude on the orientation of the beam, and it is these echoes which are displayed in grey-scale echography (see Section 6.6.e). In these circumstances, compounding the scan may be disadvantageous.

Various two-dimensional scanning systems are possible. As a matter of convenience, such scanners are often considered to be divided into two main groups, according to whether the transducer scans the patient through an intervening water bath or by direct contact with the patient's skin. This division is somewhat arbitrary, and the pattern of scanning, for example, is really just as important as the coupling system.

The various scanning systems which have been described in the literature are illustrated in Fig. 6.32. Methods a, b, c, j, k, l and m are simple scanning systems in which each interface is examined only from one direction. This severely restricts the capability of the technique when

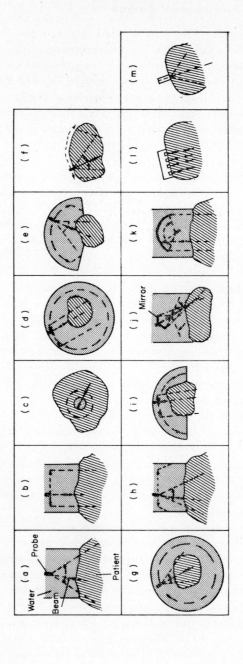

specular reflectors are to be visualized. The likelihood of detecting the
presence of any given interface is increased if the ultrasonic beam is arranged to scan in a compound fashion from many different directions, as
in methods d, e, f, g, h and i. Even the most complete two-dimensional
scanning system, however, cannot detect the maximum echoes from interfaces which are curved out of the plane of the scan.

Water-bath scanners can be arranged so that the part of the patient which
is being examined is either actually immersed in the water, or is in acoustic
contact with the water by transmission through a thin membrane and some

FIG. 6.32 Two-dimensional B-scanning systems. The table gives references to
some articles in which the systems are described.

Diagram	Principal diagnostic site	Reference
a	Breast	Wild and Reid (1952a, b)
	Miscellaneous	Howry and Bliss (1952); Brown and Greening (1973)
b	Breast	Wild and Reid (1954)
	Breast and abdomen	Kikuchi et al. (1957)
c	Rectum	Wild and Reid (1957)
	Liver and heart	Kimoto et al. (1964)
	Heart	Bom (1972); Eggleton et al. (1970)
d	Miscellaneous	Howry (1957)
e	Eye	Baum and Greenwood (1958); Filipczyński et al. (1967)
	Uterus	Kossoff et al. (1965)
	Breast	Wells and Evans (1968)
f	Abdomen	Brown (1960); Holmes et al. (1965); Wells (1966); Filipczyński and Groniowski (1967); Holm and Northeved (1968)
	Brain	de Vlieger et al. (1963); Greatorex and Ireland (1964)
g	Miscellaneous	Gordon (1962)
	Brain	Makow and Real (1966)
h	Brain	de Vlieger et al. (1963)
	Abdomen	Evans et al. (1966)
	Blood vessels	Tomey and Reid (1969)
i	Miscellaneous	Howry (1965)
j	Heart	Hertz and Olofsson (1963)
	Miscellaneous	Fry et al. (1968)
k	Miscellaneous	Krause and Soldner (1967)
l	Heart	Bom (1972)
m	Brain	Somer (1968)
	Heart	McDicken et al. (1974); Griffith and Henry (1974); Thurstone and von Ramm (1974); Holm et al. (1975)

kind of coupling medium. Coupling problems are eliminated by immersion, but the method is not always acceptable to the patient, and the water may become contaminated. The useful life of the water can be extended, both in immersion and non-immersion scanners, by the addition of a sterilizing chemical*.

A major difficulty with water-bath scanners is due to the occurrence of artifacts which arise from multiple reflexions between the transducer and the patient's skin. It is necessary to make the water path length equal to at least the required penetration into the patient. The difficulty can be minimized by gating the bright-up pulse so that the timebase only appears when useful echoes are being displayed. Multiple reflexions within the water bath may take a substantial time to decay. This is particularly so if the echoes arise from primary reflexions at the walls of the tank, or at air boundaries, and so have large amplitudes. The maximum repetition rate may be limited by the decay time of these reverberations.

In general, scanning may be either by mechanical movement of a single-element transducer, or by an array (see Section 6.10.c). Probes designed to be introduced into the patient's body, as in Fig. 6.32(c), need to be quite small and special constructional techniques are necessary. Such a single-element probe may consist of an unbacked transducer (Kimoto et al., 1964), or it may be a miniature version of a full-sized conventional probe (Wells, 1966). It has been pointed out by Kossoff (1966) that the sensitivity and range resolution of an unbacked transducer can be improved by matching its characteristic impedance to that of the loading medium (see Section 1.11). The lateral resolution of a miniature probe is rather poor on account of the wide divergence of the beam, and this also results in low sensitivity.

The mirror system illustrated in Fig. 6.32(j) is described in Section 2.3.c. Originally developed for heart scanning, it never achieved popularity, and has largely been superseded by high-speed contact scanners and arrays (Fig. 6.32(l, m)). A high-speed system giving a linear scan is illustrated in Fig. 6.32(k). In a commercial version† of this system, two transducers are mounted back-to-back within a cylindrical housing which rotates at a constant rate, and each transducer is switched into circuit as it comes to face the parabolic mirror at whose focus it is situated. This gives a frame rate of 16 s^{-1} at a pulse repetition rate of 2000 s^{-1}, with 140 lines across an aperture of 140 mm (Pätzold et al., 1970). A similar system but with an elliptical mirror would give a radial scan.

The direction and position of the timebase on the display can be coupled to that of the ultrasonic beam across the patient either by an electrical or a

* For example, chlorhexidine gluconate 1.5% w/v, cetrimide B.P. 15% w/v ("Savlon": Imperial Chemical Industries, London, UK), diluted 1 in 5000.

† "Vidoson" model 635ST: Siemens Aktiengesellschaft, Erlangen, West Germany.

mechanical system. It is necessary for the display to be related by some fixed scale factor to the dimensions of the scanned anatomy. The x-and y-scale factors are usually (but not necessarily) equal. For example, the display might be one-fifth actual size in the case of an abdominal scan presented on a cathode-ray tube with a 100×80 mm screen. Thus, a movement of the transducer through a distance of 50 mm would produce a corresponding displacement of 10 mm in the position of the timebase. The angular direction is not altered by the scale factor. In order to maintain the correct spatial relationships, it is necessary to choose the timebase velocity (in the direction of the scan line) so that the scale factor remains constant. Thus, in the example of the one-fifth actual size display, the timebase velocity would need to be about $(1500/2) \times (1/5) = 150$ m s^{-1}. This is equal to $0 \cdot 15$ mm μs^{-1}. The exact timebase velocity must be adjusted to match both the actual propagation velocity and the scale factor, so as to obtain satisfactory registration (except in the case of simple scanning systems such as those illustrated in Fig. 6.32(a, b, c, j, k, l and m), in which error in the timebase velocity simply distorts the scan without spoiling the registration).

Two factors which may limit the registration in water-bath scanners are due to the differences in the velocity in water and in tissue. Such differences may typically be as much as 4%. At an angle of incidence of 30°, a 4% velocity change refracts the ray by $1 \cdot 5°$ from its original direction. This corresponds to an error of $2 \cdot 5$ mm for a target at a range of 100 mm beyond the skin surface. Similar velocity variations occur at the interfaces between soft tissues of different kinds, and in practice such variations constitute a fundamental limitation in the registration accuracy. The mean value of velocity in soft tissue is 1540 m s^{-1}, and this is equal to the velocity in water at 50°C. This temperature is rather too high to be comfortable for the patient, and the temperatures of most water-bath scanners are maintained at 37°C (normal body temperature): this corresponds to a velocity in water of 1520 m s^{-1}. An alternative approach to this problem is to arrange for the timebase velocity to be shifted to a new value at the instant that the first echo returns from the patient's skin (i.e. by the first echo swept gain trigger pulse: see Section 6.5.e). In this way, the optimal velocities in both water and tissue can be used. This technique has been applied to breast scanning by Jellins and Kossoff (1973).

Water-bath scanners are generally motor-driven. This ensures a uniform scan pattern. Best results are obtained if the transducer moves at constant velocity (as in the scanners of, for example, Krause and Soldner, 1967; Tomey and Reid, 1969), and in the case of reciprocating angular motion special mechanical systems are necessary to satisfy this condition. The motors need to be chosen so that they do not generate electrical interference which could confuse the echo information. In at least one research instrument, the scanner is under computer control (Fry *et al.*, 1968).

Contact scanners may be either motor or hand driven. Manual drive has the disadvantage that the uniformity of the scan depends at least to some extent on the skill of the operator. In some scanners, only one of the available motions is motor driven (e.g. Holmes *et al.*, 1965; Holm *et al.*, 1975): this allows the operator to concentrate on obtaining better uniformity in the movements which he is controlling.

Although contact scanning is undoubtedly more convenient than the use of water-bath coupling in most examinations particularly of the adult abdomen, the water-bath method does have several advantages:

(i) The structures being examined are not displaced by the probe;

(ii) It can provide coupling into awkward corners and sharply curved surfaces which are inaccessible with contact scanning;

(iii) The patient does not feel the movement of the probe;

(iv) It provides an acoustic delay line which allows the transducer to stand off from the patient so that the scanned anatomy may be in the optimum region of the ultrasonic beam; and

(v) The movements of the transducer are easily mechanized.

Those advantages numbered (i)–(iii) can be obtained by attaching a water bath to an ordinary contact scanner. This has been done by Fleming and Lyons (1974), who have used their system to scan the kidneys of infants, and eyes.

(i) Electrical coupling

The coordinates of the transducer (either its position or its direction, or both, according to the scanning system) are measured by means of resolvers. (It may be possible not even to use resolvers, if stepper motors and pulse-counting circuits are used: see, for example, Holasek and Sokollu, 1972.) Potentiometers are widely used in this application. Linear potentiometers can be coupled mechanically to the probe to give information about linear movements in rectangular coordinates, and about angular movements; sine/cosine potentiometers can be used to give angular information in polar coordinates. Some typical systems are illustrated in Fig. 6.33.

High-precision potentiometers of both the wire-wound and conducting-film types are commercially available. Nowadays, conducting-film types are almost exclusively used in ultrasonic scanners, since they have much longer lives than wire-wound potentiometers.

In the arrangements shown in Fig. 6.33(b, c), timebase voltages are applied directly to the sine/cosine potentiometers. This may not be entirely satisfactory because potentiometers are designed to be accurate with d.c. signals. The effects of capacitive loading can be minimized, however, by using a low resistance potentiometer, and by having high input–impedance voltage followers mounted within the scanner. A sine/cosine potentiometer is in any case designed to maintain accurate conformity only when it is driving a specified load impedance. This impedance is usually chosen to be as high as possible, so as to minimize the current drawn through the brushes of the potentiometer. A typical sine/cosine potentiometer might have a resistance of 20 kΩ per quadrant and so its output is susceptible to interference from external fields (such as mains-induced hum voltages).

The electronic system illustrated in Fig. 6.33(d), which could also be used with the scanner in Fig. 6.33(e), avoids the necessity for the timebase voltage to be applied directly to the potentiometers. The potentiometers operate at d.c., and the x and y timebases are generated from the d.c. information by means of feedback integrators and adding circuits.

The use of sine/cosine potentiometers, and the need for wires and pulleys, can be avoided by means of sine/cosine function generators. This is illustrated in Fig. 6.33(f). A typical analogue function generator* has an accuracy of rather better than 1% in this application. Although this may seem to be rather a large error, it should be remembered that very accurate linear potentiometers are relatively inexpensive, and that wire and pulleys (which are far from being accurate) are eliminated from the measuring system on the scanner. Moreover, acceptably low errors may be achieved by the use of diode function generators to convert small angles to their sines and cosines: for example, Holasek and Sokollu (1972) have described circuits which have errors of less than 0·2% for angles of up to 30°. It is also possible to use digital techniques in this application. The output from an analogue resolver may be digitized, or a digital resolver may be used, to drive a read-only digital memory arranged as a sine function generator. Cosines can be obtained by appropriate logic circuits. A typical look-up table† using a bipolar read-only memory with 10 bit precision can convert angular information in increments of 0·1% with an access time of 150 ns.

The x, y, θ coordinate information is processed in the systems described here in such a way that the x, y position defined on the display is the centre about which θ rotates. No further difficulty arises if the ultrasonic probe is placed so that its centre of rotation passes along a diameter of the front face of the transducer. Unfortunately, this cannot always be so arranged in practice. The problem can be solved by positioning the front face of the transducer at some fixed radius (say 50–100 mm) from the centre of rotation corresponding to the x, y coordinates. The correct spatial relationships of the display are maintained by delaying the triggering of the transmitter until the timebase generators have been running for a period equal to the time corresponding to the radial distance. It is necessary for this delay to be generated quite accurately, to avoid distortion of the spatial information.

* Model 4301: Burr-Brown Research Corporation, Tucson, Arizona, USA.
† Type MM5086: Monolithic Memories Inc., Sunnyvale, California, USA.

9

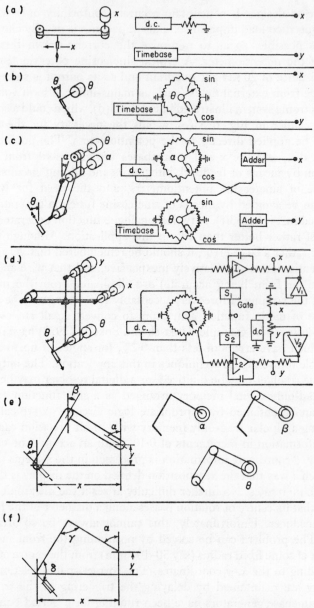

FIG. 6.33 Systems for electrical coupling of the probe coordinates to the display. (a) Simple linear scan. The voltage developed by the potentiometer is proportional to the x-coordinate of the probe. The timebase velocity is chosen to match the scale factor. (b) Simple radial scan. Balanced, antiphase timebase ramps are applied to the sine/cosine potentiometer. (c) Compound sector scan (water-bath scanner). Balanced, antiphase timebase ramps are applied to the θ sine/cosine potentiometer.

(ii) Mechanical coupling

It is possible by means of a mechanical linkage to couple a movable cathode-ray tube (or camera) to the ultrasonic probe in such a way that a B-scan in a fixed position on the screen of the tube is related by a suitable scale factor to the position and direction of the ultrasonic beam in space. This method of generating a compound B-scan was proposed by Gordon (1962), who described the construction of a water-bath scanner based on the principle. Figure 6.34(a) shows the main features of his instrument. A similar arrangement was used by Filipzcyński and Groniowski (1967) in an abdominal contact scanner; their machine employed a pantograph constructed from articulated arms, as illustrated in Fig. 6.34(b). Again, Filipczyński *et al.* (1967) used a system of articulated linkages in a water-bath scanner for examining the eye.

As an alternative to moving the cathode-ray tube in this type of scanner, McDicken (1970) has described a system in which a stationary cathode-ray tube has its light output transferred along a series of flexible fibre-optic pipes arranged so that the other ends of the pipes are in a linear array which is moved by the mechanical linkage with the ultrasonic transducer.

Mechanical coupling avoids some of the complications of electrical systems, and essentially operates without distortion. The principal disadvantage is its lack of versatility. Although Gordon's (1962) scanner has provision for adjustment of the scale factor of the scan, this is necessarily a much more complicated procedure than the simple alteration of deflexion amplifier gain which is all that is required in an electrically coupled system. Again, it may be difficult to arrange for alteration of the plane of the scan on account of the unwieldy nature of the combined electromechanical system, and it is often much easier—although maybe inappropriate—to move the patient than the machine. The electronic and scanning systems must be constructed as an integrated unit if mechanical coupling is em-

---

The d.c. supply to the α sine/cosine potentiometer is adjusted to match the scale factor. (d) Compound sector scan (contact scanner). The potentiometers are supplied with d.c. The x and y timebases are generated by feedback integrators I_1 and I_2, controlled by the clamps S_1 and S_2 respectively. The outputs from these integrators, which are equal to zero volts at zero time, are shifted to the appropriate d.c. levels corresponding to the x and y coordinates, by adding circuits driven from voltage followers V_1 and V_2. (e) Compound sector scan (contact scanner). Conversion of x and y coordinates from polar to rectangular form is carried out by the sine/cosine potentiometers measuring the angles α and β. The appropriate outputs from these potentiometers are added together to give $x \propto \sin \alpha + \sin \beta$ and $y \propto \cos \beta$ $- \cos \alpha$. (f) Compound sector scan (contact scanner). Linear potentiometers are used at each joint. In this arrangement, the angles indicated in diagrams (e) can be derived by adding networks, since: $\alpha = \alpha$; $\beta = \gamma - \alpha$; and $\theta = \pi + \alpha - \gamma - \delta$. Function generators can then be used to calculate $x \propto \sin \alpha + \sin (\gamma - \alpha)$, $y \propto \cos (\gamma - \alpha) - \cos \alpha$, and the sines and cosines of θ.

ployed, whereas they can be physically separated with electrical coupling. Therefore, it may be possible to effect substantial economy with electrical coupling by using the same electronic system with several different scanners, each designed for a particular diagnostic site.

Although mechanically coupled scanners are simple in principle, in practice their registration performance depends to a large extent upon the

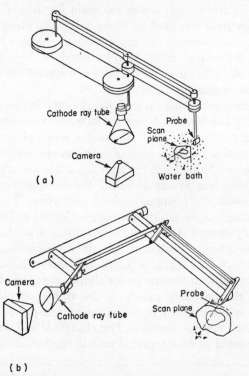

FIG. 6.34 Systems for mechanical coupling of the probe coordinates to the display. (a) Water-bath scanner for compound sector scanning (Gordon, 1962); (b) contact scanner for compound sector scanning (Filipczyński and Groniowski, 1967.)

precision of their mechanical construction. Modern electrically coupled instruments are almost always better.

(iii) Scan uniformity

One of the most difficult skills which it is necessary for the novice to master if he is to produce good two-dimensional B-scans with a manually operated machine is the art of moving the probe in a regular fashion, whilst maintaining good contact with the skin. Probably it is the ability to do this really well, which, more than any other expertise, distinguishes the doyens of ultrasonic diagnostics from the common herd.

Ultrasonography cannot become a science whilst its practice depends on art. Several developments aimed at eliminating this limitation have been described. Some depend on arrays (see Section 6.10.c), others on scan conversion memory tubes (see Section 6.6.c). The Sub-section is concerned with the following techniques:

(i) Automatic probe movement. The first successful contact scanner (Brown, 1960) had its probe mounted in a sphere, which climbed around the patient, oscillating as it went, the movements being controlled by pressure sensitive switches. The pioneers soon found that their manual skills produced equally good, or even better,

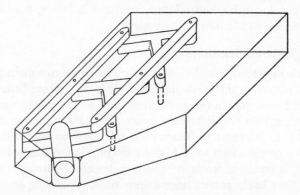

FIG. 6.35 Semiautomatic probe system for contact scanner. The linkage system sets the centre of rotation of the probe beyond the transducer, in the region of the plastic window. The casing is filled with oil. (Mountford *et al.*, 1974.)

pictures, without risk of hurting the patient should the sensing devices fail.

(ii) Semi-automatic probe movement. A compromise was developed by Holmes *et al.* (1965), in whose machine the probe oscillation was motor-driven to compound the scan, whilst the whole probe assembly was moved by hand around the patient. The difficulty of maintaining contact between the probe face and the skin remained. In a refinement of this arrangement, illustrated in Fig. 6.35, Mountford *et al.* (1974) placed a plastic window between the probe and the patient, so that the beam might be rocked whilst the contact with the patient remained stationary apart from movements of translation. The space between the probe and the plastic window, which was inclined in such a way as to minimize multiple reflexions, was filled with oil. The isocentric method of mounting the probe

allowed its centre of rotation effectively to be within the patient.
A difficulty with this arrangement is that multiple reflexions do
occur if the plastic window comes out of contact with the patient's
skin.

(iii) Velocity controlled line display rate. In two-dimensional scanners
in which the display system allows overwriting (see Section 6.6),
non-uniform scans are obtained if the scanning times devoted to
the inspection of each individual target element are not equal. This
is particularly troublesome with manually operated contact scanners.
To some extent the nuisance can be reduced by linking the line
display rate to the movement of the probe. The movement which is
sensed can be x or y displacement, or rotation, or some combination
of these (Hall, 1970). Either the pulse repetition rate, or the bright-
up pulse, can be controlled; the former is better, because it minimizes the irradiation of the patient.

6.8.c High-speed Scanners

In ultrasonic diagnostics, real-time visualization has three main advantages.
Firstly, it allows rapid physiological events to be studied. Secondly,
physiological movements (such as those due to the cardiac pulse, or to
foetal breathing) do not distort the image. Thirdly, it allows the operator
more quickly to interpret the anatomical relationships within the patient.

For real-time visualization, a high image rate is necessary. In ultrasonic
diagnostics, a compromise is necessary between the image rate and the
number of lines in the frame, since a finite time, depending on the penetration, is required for each line. For example, a penetration distance of 100
mm is associated with a time of 133 μs. A time of, say, 250 μs must be
allowed to elapse between pulses, so that the signals from the previous
pulse are of low amplitude before the next pulse is transmitted. Consequently, the maximum repetition rate is around 4000 s^{-1}, and this is
equal to the product of the frame rate and the number of lines per frame.
For example, at a frame rate of 20 s^{-1}, there would be 200 lines per frame.
There would have to be fewer lines if a greater penetration was required.

The application of arrays to beam steering is discussed in Section 6.10.c.
High-speed scans can also be obtained by rapid mechanical scanners, such
as those illustrated in Fig. 6.32(h, j, k, m). Thus, McDicken et al. (1974)
have constructed a scanning system, primarily for cardiac studies, in which
a conventional probe is oscillated at a sufficiently high speed effectively to
generate a real-time display. The instrument executes eight complete
oscillations per second, giving a frame rate of 16 s^{-1} with a 60° sector.
Coupling to the patient is through a very thin layer of oil in a small tank
with a thin polyethylene window. The method combines the advantages of
the good resolution of a relatively large transducer (2·5 MHz, 15 mm

diameter), and simple electronics, with real-time imaging and the capability of making conventional time-motion recordings of structure motion. A somewhat similar system has been constructed by Griffith and Henry (1974), but with a 30° sector and a frame rate of 30 s⁻¹. Another design uses four transducers operated in sequence as a turret on which they are mounted rotates at constant speed (Holm *et al.*, 1975).

6.8.d Gated Displays

Moving structures are generally best studied by two-dimensional ultrasonography by means of a real-time scanner. Clinically useful scans of structures which move cyclically (such as the heart) can often be obtained by building up an image corresponding to any particular phase in the cycle, by gating a conventional slow-speed scanner. This is discussed further in Section 6.16.b. Two approaches are possible. Either the transmitter can be triggered by a signal derived from the physiological movement (such as the R-wave of the e.c.g.), or the same signal can be used to gate the display of a continuously running scanner. A variant of the later system has been described by Hussey *et al.* (1973): they used a gated closed-circuit television system to select the required times from a conventional, non-storage, two-dimensional scanner.

6.8.e Considerations in Choosing a Scanner

Blackwell *et al.* (1973) have enumerated a number of design features which, in their opinion, are important in making one instrument preferable to another. They did this in relation to the requirements for obstetric investigations (particularly the measurement of biparietal diameter and placentography), and on the basis of experience gained in the use of seven different models of commercially manufactured scanners. No one instrument satisfied all their requirements, but some came closer to this objective than others. Their criteria were:

(i) The transition of scanning plane from the longitudinal to transverse should be achieved with a minimum of effort, and certainly without having manually to shift the scanning gantry around the examination couch;

(ii) The arms holding the probe should be of sufficient length, and the constraints so adjusted to allow adequate compounding of the scan at both flanks of a patient with a large abdomen;

(iii) The probe mounting should be sufficiently compact to allow scans to be made in a plane lying at an acute angle to the surface of the abdomen;

(iv) Scales should be provided to indicate the orientation of the plane of scan relative to the patient and to register the angle of the probe to the vertical;

    (v) The controls should be arranged so that the risk of unintentionally adjusting the wrong control is minimized, especially as instruments are often operated in semi-darkness;

    (vi) The display screen (or screens) should be capable of displaying a stored image, a long persistence image, and an image having a good grey scale (say 20 dB dynamic range);

    (vii) The instrument should have an attenuator to control the ultrasound output intensity over a range of at least 30 dB;

    (viii) It should be possible to display graphically on the screen the effect on the sensitivity of the receiver produced by adjusting the swept gain controls;

    (ix) An A-scan presentation relating to any chosen line on the B-scan should be immediately obtainable; and

    (x) An electronic caliper generating markers on both A- and B-scans should be provided;

Naturally different or additional criteria need to be applied in considering the specification of instruments for examining other clinical areas.

6.9 TIME–POSITION RECORDING

Pulse–echo information is a combination of time and amplitude data. The instantaneous position of a moving reflector can be determined from the time data. This can be presented in the form of a recording, in which a waveform represents the variation with time in the position of the reflector.

Probably the most usual method by which this type of recording is obtained nowadays is that illustrated in Fig. 6.36. The recording is made up of separate B-scans, lying side-by-side: they merge together if the repetition rate is sufficiently great. The timebase velocities are chosen according to the clinical application, the ultrasonic timebase being determined by the depth of penetration, and the slow-sweep timebase, by the period over which observation is required. A disadvantage of the method is that the photograph must be developed before the recording can be assessed. This difficulty can be eliminated by the use of an electronic storage tube, rather than a photographic film, to integrate the display.

The slow-sweep method suffers from the serious limitation that only a rather short period of observation can be accommodated on a single recording. There are three ways around this difficulty. The slow sweep timebase is omitted, and time (as opposed to range) is obtained on the recording by means of a continuous strip of recording material moving at constant velocity, as explained in Section 6.6.f. The convenience and versatility of the fibre-optic recorder has led to the present popularity of this device.

Before the widespread introduction of the fibre-optic recorder, a time-to-voltage analogue converter was often used to study the movements of single, isolated structures such as heart valve cusps. The method is still in use today, although to a limited extent in cardiology, but also increasingly in studying blood vessel wall movements, cerebral structure pulsations, and foetal breathing. Wells and Ross (1969) have described a time-to-voltage analogue converter which has some significant advantages in comparison with earlier systems. A block diagram is given in Fig. 6.37. This circuit produces signals which allow spurious triggering to be recognized, and which enable the operator to be certain that the circuit is tracking the structure of interest. It does require a high-speed recorder, such as an ink-jet or ultraviolet system. In some applications (see, for example, Hokanson *et al.*, 1970), satisfactory results can be obtained with a slow-speed recorder by smoothing the output waveform.

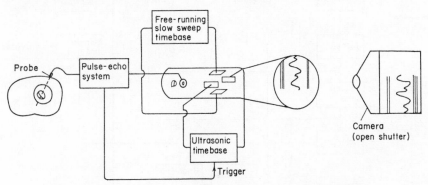

Fig. 6.36 Time-position recording system using two timebases.

In radar, the basic moving target indicator procedure accomplishes isolation of moving target information by comparing echo information subsequent to a transmit pulse with the echo information which arose from the preceding pulse. By subtracting one wavetrain from the other, stationary echoes are eliminated, leaving only echoes which are moving and which consequently do not appear in the same position on the two timebases. Barnes and Thurstone (1971) have applied this method in an attempt to enhance echocardiograms, and time position recordings of arterial wall movement. They used an acoustic delay line of 2·5 ms, with a bandwidth of 5 MHz, and stored wavetrains of 500 μs duration at a pulse repetition rate of 400 s^{-1}. Although there may be a marginal improvement resulting from the type of processing, it is not surprising that it is rather disappointing. Almost every signal, including artifact and noise, moves in an echocardiogram, and there are probably no stationary echoes from real structures which the system could eliminate.

6.10 OTHER SYSTEMS

6.10.a The C-scope

The C-scope is a brightness-modulated display in which the x-deflexion corresponds to the bearing in azimuth, and the y-deflexion, to the elevation. It is thus a two-dimensional image in a plane perpendicular to the two-dimensional B-scan. Kimoto *et al.* (1964) used a modified form of this display, in which the y-deflexion is proportional to the vertical position of the probe, to demonstrate an atrial septal defect by means of a small ultra-

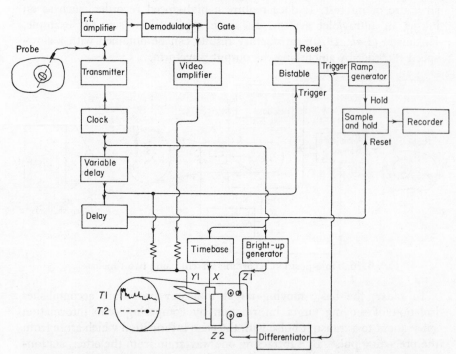

Fig. 6.37 Time-position recording system using time-to-voltage analogue conversion. The clock triggers the transmitter which excites the probe. The clock also triggers a variable delay generator, the timebase and the bright-up pulse generator. The output from the variable delay generator causes a step deflexion on the A-scan display, triggers the bistable and a fixed delay generator, and opens the gate. The first echo to pass through the gate resets the bistable. The duration of the square wave from the bistable is converted to a voltage by the ramp generator and the sample-and-hold, and the trailing edge of the bistable pulse is differentiated to produce a bright marker on the second beam of the cathode-ray tube. The sample-and-hold is reset after an interval equal to half the pulse repetition period, by a signal generated by a fixed delay. The output from the sample-and-hold is an approximately square wave, the amplitude of which is proportional to the distance between the "position" of the gate opening and the tracked echo-producing target.

sonic probe introduced under X-ray control into the right atrium. (The scan resembles a radiograph, because it presents the data as a plan, rather than as a section: the thickness and depth of the plane can be adjusted by changing the range-gate.) The ultrasonic pulse generator was triggered by the R-wave of the e.c.g. Using this method, Omoto (1967) demonstrated atrial septal defects in six out of seven patients.

McCready and Hill (1971) have studied some of the problems and possibilities of C-scanning using an external ultrasonic probe. Their probe had an ordinary 2 MHz transducer arranged for pulse–echo work, but fitted with a plastic lens to give a sharp focus at a range of 50 mm. The probe was moved in a raster pattern near the surface of a water tank within which a specimen (a sheep's kidney) was immersed. Quite encouraging results were reported, as a result of which Hill and McCready (1975) developed a contact scanner which describes a spiral scan, and from which C-scans can be reconstructed. Northeved *et al.* (1974) have described a similar scanner which, from a single position of the surface of the patient, by means of an automatic spiral movement makes possible the registration of 60° spherical sections at any desired range in planes perpendicular to the axis of the spiral. The spiral movement is obtained by means of a system consisting of a spindle, a nut, a gearwheel, a gear rim and a stepping motor with an axis and a carrier. When the motor is started, the carrier with the spindle rotates and makes the rear end of the ultrasonic probe describe a circular arc. At the same time the gear-wheel, which is connected to the spindle, starts rotating in mesh with the fixed rim. When the spindle rotates along its axis, the nut moves along the spindle and thereby alters the inclination of the transducer, since the rear-end of this is fastened to the nut by means of a bearing. The front-end of the transducer is mounted through a flexible membrane into a cavity containing glycerine and distilled water, and the ultrasound travels across this cavity and through a rubber membrane the outer surface of which is in contact with the patient. The outside diameter of the casing of the instrument is 90 mm, and its overall length is 180 mm. The transducer operates at a nominal frequency of 2 MHz, and has a diameter of 12 mm. A single scan is completed in 60 s.

Carson *et al.* (1975) have described similar apparatus and results to those of others who have studied the usefulness of the C-scope in medical diagnostics. The method is interesting but does not seem to have any particular advantages over two-dimensional B-scanning in the display of amplitude data. It may yet prove its worth when other tissue properties (see Section 6.12) are visualized.

6.10.b Strongly Focused Systems

The lateral resolution of a pulse–echo system may be improved over a limited part of its range by the use of a highly focused ultrasonic beam. The focusing need not necessarily be applied to both the transmitting and receiving transducers.

At any particular focal length, it is the diameter of the transducer in relation to the wavelength which determines the sharpness of the focus. This may be expressed another way: in a focused field at any particular frequency, the focus becomes smaller as the diameter of the transducer is increased. Kossoff (1972) uses the terms "weak", "medium", and "strong" to describe the degree of focusing. Using the notation defined in Section 2.3.a,

$$h/\lambda = a^2/2\lambda A \qquad (6.14)$$

where A is the radius of curvature of the transducer and $a < A$; the focusing is classified as weak if $h/\lambda < 3$, medium if $3 < h/\lambda < 10$, and strong if $h/\lambda > 10$. As the focusing becomes stronger, other factors being equal, the depth of focus becomes smaller and the effect of target surface inclination becomes less.

Von Ardenne and Millner (1962) seem to have been the first to use a strongly focused beam in ultrasonic diagnostics. Their system employed a curved 5 MHz transducer. The transducer was mounted at one end of a water-filled column, which also contained an aperture and a lens, arranged so that the focal length was at a convenient distance from the end of the column. The echo information was displayed on a linear B-scope. The display was time-gated by means of a slit mask placed in front of the screen of the cathode-ray tube. This mask was moved in synchrony with the transducer, so that only echoes which returned from the focus appeared on the scan.

Thurstone and McKinney (1966a) have developed the method (apparently without knowing of the work of von Ardenne and Millner, 1962). They used reflectors instead of a lens, and an electronic system to gate out the focal echoes. At a frequency of 2·25 MHz, the time-gate was 1 μs, and the corresponding volume had a diameter of 0·75 mm. The improvement in resolution in comparison with B-scanning is obtained at the expense of increased scanning time. Nevertheless, the encouraging results of Thurstone and McKinney (1966b) in visualizing a brain specimen (removed from the skull) seem to have been confirmed by Fry (1968) (see Section 6.16.e.iv).

There have been various other attempts to use strongly focused beams in order to improve azimuthal resolution. These being conventional arrangements all have limited depth-of-focus (which may, or may not, be a disadvantage). As an aid to the interpretation of two-dimensional scans, produced using focused transducers, Kossoff (1972) has described how it may be arranged that the position corresponding to the focus of the beam may be indicated on the scan by brightening the timebase except where echoes are being received. The method applies only to water-bath scanners;

if the swept-gain generator has been triggered, it appears from the published scans that the brightness circuit associated with the focus is inhibited.

In optics, a collimated beam of light of circular cross-section may be focused over an extended interval of range—which is equivalent to operating with a large depth of focus—by means of a conical lens known as an axicon. Each ray is deflected through an equal angle, so that the rays nearest to the axis on the incident side of the lens intersect the axis closest to the axicon, and those at the edge of the beam intersect the axis furthest away. Therefore, along the length of the axis between the lens and the point of intersection of the outermost rays, there is a cylinder of high-intensity light, surrounded by a lower intensity.

Burckhardt *et al.* (1973) have applied this principle to an ultrasonic system, as illustrated in Fig. 6.38. Ultrasound pulses from a conventional

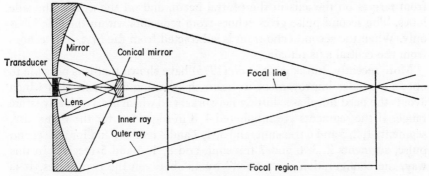

FIG. 6.38 The ultrasound axicon. In a typical arrangement, the focal line extends from a range of 200–400 mm from the edge of the front surface of the curved mirror. (Based on Burckhardt *et al.*, 1973.)

probe are focused by a plastic lens and are then reflected by a small conical mirror. This mirror reflects the ultrasound to a large mirror, which acts as the ultrasonic analogue of the optical axicon. Since the incident ultrasonic beam is divergent, the surface of the mirror is in the form of a combination of a cone and a sphere, its surface being generated by rotating a circle around the axis of the device, the centre of the generating circle being off-axis. Measurements on an experimental system operating at 2 MHz, with a large mirror of outer diameter equal to 100 mm, revealed at 6 dB beam-width of about 2·5 mm over the range interval 200–400 mm. The principal difficulty in the application of the system in medical diagnostics seems likely to be the rather large amplitude of the side-lobes; the first of these, about 3·5 mm off-axis, is only 16 dB below the central axial echo amplitude.

Burckhardt *et al.* (1974) have since described a simplified arrangement in which an annulus with an outside diameter of 100 mm and consisting of 12 piezoelectric segments is mounted so that the ultrasound beam covers a distance of between 200 and 400 mm on the central axis. The division of the annulus into segments allows a cunning method to be used to reduce the sidelobe amplitudes. For a first pulse of ultrasound, all the segments transmit and receive in phase. These received echoes are digitized, delayed by digital shift registers (8 bit resolutions) and converted back to analogue form. Meanwhile, for a second ultrasonic pulse, the phase of the pulse transmitted by each segment is made to be proportional to the angular position of the segment in the annulus. The corresponding signal which is received by each segment is multiplied by a phase factor equal in magnitude but opposite in sign to the phase factor of the transmitted pulse. These processed signals are subtracted from the signals received from the first pulse, as they emerge from the delay lines. In physical terms, the method suppresses side lobes as follows. The echoes received by the first pulse are from targets on the axis in the central beam, and off the axis in the side lobes. The second pulse gives echoes from reflectors within the side lobes only. When the second echo train is subtracted from the first, only echoes from the central axis remain.

More recently, Burckhardt *et al.* (1975) have shown that it is possible to obtain a similar improvement in beam shape using a modification which avoids the need for phase shifting networks, and which has a wider dynamic range. If the segments are numbered 1–8 in sequence, for the first pulse, segments 1, 2, 5 and 6 transmit, and 3, 4, 7 and 8 receive; and for the second pulse, segments 2, 3, 6 and 7 transmit, and 8, 1, 4 and 5 receive. In this way, the configuration is "rotated" by 45° between the two pulses. It is easier to switch segments between transmitting and receiving operations, than it is to introduce phase shifts. Even more important, in the new method the echo trains from the first and second pulses are added (instead of being subtracted), and the dynamic range is maintained since the output is no longer the small difference between two large signals.

Initial experimental results have apparently been most encouraging. The azimuthal resolution is similar to the range resolution over what is a practically very useful depth-of-focus. No doubt the method will find important applications where water-bath scanning is possible, since it avoids the need for the swept delay lines of the alternative processing scheme described in Section 6.10.c.iii.

6.10.c Arrays

(i) General considerations

This Section deals with some aspects of the use of several transducers in a single system. Arrays may be broadly separated into two kinds. Thus, an array of transducers consists of several transducers separated in space, the signals from which are processed incoherently, without account being taken of the phase. A transducer array, on the other hand, consists of a transducer separated into elements the signals from which are processed coherently, either all together or in groups, to shape and steer the beam by taking account of the phases of the signals from each element.

(*ii*) *Linear arrays*

It is possible to obtain real-time visualization of a two-dimensional section by the use of a large number of small transducers arranged in a row, functioning in rapid sequence as separate transmitter–receiver elements. Such a system has been constructed by Bom *et al.* (1971, 1973). A detailed description of this system has been given by Bom (1972). Twenty transducers are used, in a line of 66 mm length, as shown in Fig. 6.39. Overall,

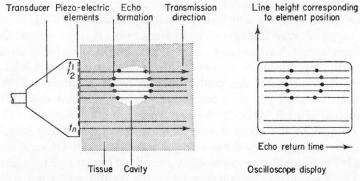

FIG. 6.39 Schematic drawing of a multi-element probe and the corresponding oscilloscope display. (Based on Bom *et al.*, 1971.)

the probe face is 80 mm long and 10 mm wide. Operating at a nominal frequency of 3 or 4·5 MHz according to the construction of the probe, and with a diameter of 3 mm (more recent models, including those in a commercial instrument*, are rectangular, and operate at 2·25 or 4·5 MHz; in this connexion, see Adams and McCutcheon, 1973), each transducer in sequence transmits a pulse of ultrasound and receives echoes from within the patient. The duration of a complete frame is 6560 μs, corresponding to 150 frames per second. A time of 230 μs is allocated to each transducer in turn; upon completion of a sequence, the electrocardiogram is sampled and displayed for 460 μs, and this is followed by a 1500 μs period during which characters which identify the scan are displayed.

Although the original impetus for the development of this type of real-time imaging system was the desire to solve cardiological problems, similar

* Echo-Cardiovisor: Organon Technika, Oss, The Netherlands.

instruments can be used to examine other parts of the body. Such instruments are commercially available, and a typical system* has 64 transducer elements operated in groups of four to produce 61-line scans at a frame rate of 40 s⁻¹: the scanned anatomy is typically 170 mm wide and 200 mm deep at a frequency of 2·25 MHz, and proportionally smaller at higher frequencies.

The number of elements is chosen to give the best compromise between resolution and line density. Once this compromise has been made, the performance of the system in terms of sensitivity to inclined specular reflexions may be estimated.

In order to complete this review, mention should be made of the somewhat similar system of W. Buschmann, who constructed an arc of 10 transducers to scan the eye, and the instrument of R. Uchida *et al.*, who used 200 closely spaced transducers with overlapping groups of 20 small elements switched electronically to provide better resolution. Both these systems are described in a little more detail by Bom *et al.* (1973).

This type of array of single-element transducers is quite distinct from a transducer array. A transducer array allows the beam to be steered, and focused by appropriate combination of the signals associated with each element. An example of this is illustrated in Fig. 6.40. Somer (1968) has reviewed the subject of electronic beam steering, and has described the construction of a 1·3 MHz, 21 element array with dimensions 10 × 11 mm. Each element of the array is energized by a separate transmitter; each transmitter is triggered by the same pulse applied through separate voltage-controlled monostables acting as delay circuits. Thus, the phase across the array can be adjusted by altering the main control voltage, a different proportion of which is applied to each delay circuit according to the position in the array of the corresponding transducer element. Alteration of the phase distribution causes the ultrasonic beam to swing through a sector: the instantaneous value of the main control voltage is related to the beam direction, and may be used to control the timebase direction on the display oscilloscope, and in a conventional two-dimensional B-scope (see Section 6.8). The receiving beam may likewise be steered (to coincide with the transmitting beam) by the introduction of delay lines (see Section 6.10.c. vii) in the signal paths from each element in the array, so that the appropriate phase relationships at the summing point are maintained.

Unfortunately, electronically steered beams with simple addition of the element signals have rather large side-lobe amplitudes, which restrict the dynamic range in a practical diagnostic system. Somer and van Dael (1972) have shown that both the calculated and measured directional patterns are greatly improved if the signals from each element are multiplied, rather

---

* Advanced Diagnostic Research Corpn., Tempe, Arizona, USA.

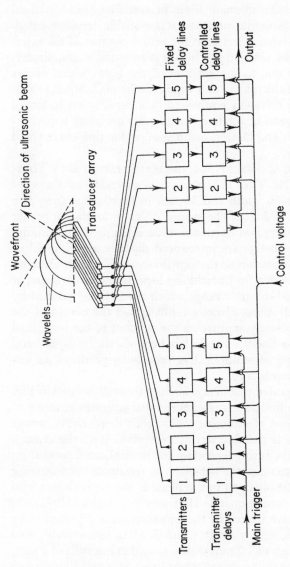

Fig. 6.40 Beam steering with a phased array. In this example, the array has five elements. A separate transmitter is associated with each element, and each transmitter is triggered in sequence by a pulse delayed in time from the main trigger pulse, by a monostable multivibrator. For the direction of the beam illustrated here, element 1 has the shortest delay, and 5, the longest. The delays are determined by the control voltage, alteration of which changes the direction of the transmitted beam. Delay lines capable of handling ultrasonic signals are inserted into the receiver paths from each element. Controlled delay lines determine the direction of the received beam. Since negative delays cannot be achieved, it is necessary to swing the beam from one end of the array, rather than from its centre; therefore fixed delay lines are connected in series with the controlled delay lines. For the direction of the beam illustrated here, the delay associated with element 1 is shortest, and that with 5, longest. The beam can be steered through a sector by the use of a staircase control voltage.

than summed. This form of non-linear processing greatly increases the angular resolution. There is one *caveat*: it remains to be determined whether or not the "multiple target problem" is disastrous.

With sector scanners, the ultimate limit to scanning speed is fixed (provided that adequate ultrasonic information is available despite the high scanning speed) by the deviation between the actual position of the echo-producing interface and the position at which it is recorded on the display. This deviation, which is due to the rotation of the beam which occurs during the propagation of the pulse—and which can be made equal to zero by the use of a staircase drive—is equivalent to a degradation in lateral resolution. For a given speed of rotation, the angular deviation is proportional to the target range: and clearly, compensation for this effect could be provided electronically.

A similar system to that of Somer (1968) has been constructed by Thurstone and von Ramm (1974). They use an array, 25 mm wide, consisting of 16 elements each 0·7 mm in width and 14 mm in length, operating at a resonance frequency of 2·25 MHz. The system differs from that of Somer (1968) in that swept focusing (see Section 6.10.c.iii) is used, in addition to beam steering, and the delays are introduced digitally after individual analogue logarithmic compression of the signal received by each element. An immediate, practical reason for introducing logarithmic compression at this stage is that the signal dynamic range which needs to be handled by the delay lines is reduced. A less obvious result is that the output of the summing amplifier more closely approaches the product of the individual received signals than their linear sum. As has been shown by Somer and van Dael (1972), this type of multiplicative processing produces an improvement in azimuthal resolution.

Kossoff (1973) has suggested that arrays such as those illustrated in Fig. 6.41 could overcome the limitations of conventional scanners in terms of lateral resolution and speed of scanning. With both these arrays, swept focusing in the long axis is possible during reception. With the crossed array, the focus is also swept during reception, and multiplicative processing from both arrays is used to make the out-of-plane resolution for scattering targets nearly equal to that obtained in the plane of the scan. Others who have tried this kind of approach include Hottinger and Meindl (1973).

Havlice *et al.* (1973) have described the construction and performance of two 30-element arrays, operating at 4 and 5 MHz respectively. The 5 MHz system had elements of 1·2 mm width, spaced at intervals of 2 mm, and was capable of imaging slots approximately 1 mm wide and 2 mm apart, at a range of 200 mm. Two-dimensional scans were made by mechanical translation of the array. Clearly the concept could be developed to generate two-dimensional images by electronic scanning of appropriate arrays, either using reflexion or transmission systems. By scanning the transmitting and receiving arrays at right angles, it should be possible to obtain an image with N^2 resolvable spots using a total of only $2N$ elements.

A logical and almost certainly worthwhile development would be the combination of the advantages of a linear array operated with groups of elements, each group performing an electronically steered sector scan. Moreover, the system could incorporate swept focusing (see Section 6.10.c.iii) in the plane of the scan. Some work along these lines has been reported by Whittingham and Evans (1975).

(iii) Annular arrays

As explained in Section 6.1.b, in two-dimensional ultrasonic scanning the effect of the relatively poor lateral resolution is to generate roughly elliptical

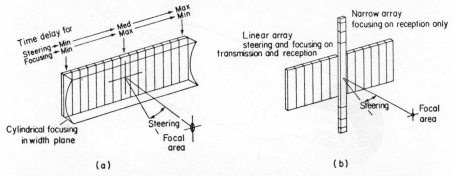

(a)   (b)

FIG. 6.41 Two types of linear phased array. Both allow beam steering in the plane of the long axis of the array, and focusing during reception. (a) This array has a cylindrical lens for focusing in the width plane over a fixed depth-of-field; (b) this arrangement with a subsidiary crossed array improves out-of-plane focusing for diffuse scatterers. (After Kossoff, 1973.)

registrations of point targets. In practical terms, this may make it difficult or impossible to visualize details of structures situated close together across the ultrasonic beam.

At any particular range, this limitation can be minimized by the use of a lens (or curved transducer) to focus the beam. The target is "in focus" where the ultrasonic disturbances originating from the entire surface of the transducer arrive simultaneously at the target, and the echoes from the target arrive simultaneously at every point on the transducer. In the absence of focusing, this does not occur, because the transit time between the transducer and the target depends on the radial position of the transducer element. Viewed in this way, the lens achieves its focusing action by introducing into each ray path a thickness of high-velocity material which increases with radius to compensate for the increasing delay due to the corresponding increase in path length.

The depth-of-focus limitation can be eliminated by a system in which the focus is swept along the axis of the ultrasonic beam so that it always coincides with the instantaneous position of the target (Brown and Haslett, 1963). This can be achieved by means of a probe, such as that illustrated in Fig. 6.42, similar in size and method of use to that of a conventional two-dimensional scanner, but in which the transducer has separate elements— a small central disc and several coaxial annuli. These elements are electrically and acoustically isolated. The arrangement allows a focus to be synthesized at any desired range along the central axis by introducing delays in the electrical signal paths for each element, such that the differences between the delays correspond to the accelerations which would be introduced by a lens in a fixed focus system.

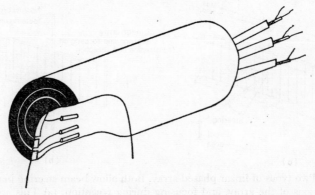

FIG. 6.42 Construction of an annular transducer array for electronic focusing of the ultrasonic beam.

Figure 6.43 illustrates the principles of the arrangement. The master clock is the repetition rate generator for the imaging system. It triggers the transmitter, which simultaneously excites all three elements in the array via the three series diodes. The array generates an unfocused transmitted beam. At any instant in time, an echo is being received from a particular point target on the central axis. This echo arrives at different times according to the path lengths to each element in the array. First to arrive is that received by the central disc, element 1. This is followed by those at elements 2 and 3 in sequence. The signal from element 3 is fed directly to a summing point, and those from elements 2 and 1 are fed to the same summing point through separate delay lines, so that the echo signals from the target arrive simultaneously for summing.

The position of the focus can be swept out with time from the surface of the array so that it coincides continuously with the changing position of the resolution cell along the central axis, by appropriately changing the time

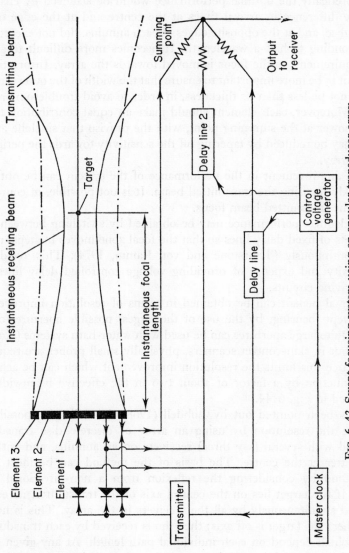

FIG. 6.43 Swept focusing system using an annular transducer array.

delays introduced by the delay lines. In order to achieve this, voltage controlled delay lines (see Section 6.10.c.vii) are driven by a control voltage generator triggered by the master clock.

Theoretically the optimal performance would be achieved by ensuring that the difference in arrival times at the centre and at the edge of the central disc, and at the opposite edges of each annulus, did not exceed that corresponding to half a wavelength. It becomes more difficult to satisfy this requirement, as the focus is moved towards the array. In practice, it turns out to be more important to ensure that the width of the outer annulus should not be less than its thickness, in order to avoid troublesome resonances. Moreover, each element should make an equal contribution to the signal power at the summing point, with the proviso that sidelobe amplitudes may be reduced by tapering off the sensitivity towards the periphery of the array.

Some improvement in the performance of the system can be obtained by weakly focusing the transmitted beam. It is not possible, of course, to sweep the transmitted beam focus.

An adequate performance may be obtained by switching between, say, three sets of fixed delay lines so that the focal zone moves in steps, rather than continuously (Thurstone and von Ramm, 1974). This avoids the complexity and expense of providing voltage controlled delay lines and their driving circuits.

Maximal benefit can be obtained in terms of resolution improvement with swept focusing, by the use of the largest possible aperture for the array. Quite large apertures can be used with water-bath systems (Kossoff, 1973), but in skin-contact scanners, physically small probes are required. In practice this limits the resolution improvement which can be achieved to a reduction by a factor of about two in the effective beamwidth, as illustrated in Fig. 6.44.

It has been pointed out by Lobdell (1968) that it is also possible to improve the resolution by using an array of discrete disc transducers arranged with several (say three) receivers on an annulus, and with one transmitter at the centre. The basis of the method can be most easily understood by considering the reflexion from a non-directional point target. If the target lies on the central axis of the transmitter, its echo is detected simultaneously by all the receivers in the array. This is not the case where the target is off axis: the echo is received by each transducer at times which depend on each individual path length. At any given target range, the period of time during which the echo is being received depends upon the distance that the target is off the axis. The output from the receiver at which the echo arrives first is arranged to trigger a gate; and unless the echo from the target is detected by all the other receivers in the array during the gate time, no output is passed on to the display. In

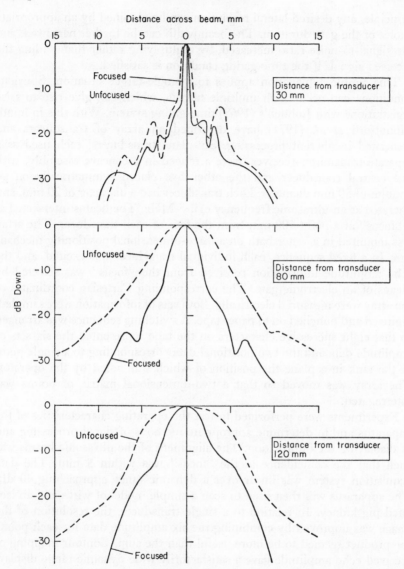

FIG. 6.44 Comparison of beam profiles with an annular transducer array, operating as a plane unfocused transducer, and with swept focusing applied during reception. The array used for these measurements has a central disc and two annuli, and an outside diameter of 20 mm. The frequency was 2.5 MHz. (Data of E. J. Guibarra.)

principle, any desired lateral resolution can be obtained by an appropriate choice of the gate duration. The beamwidth can be further narrowed, and the signal-to-noise ratio increased, by multiplying rather than adding the received signals if the time-gating condition is satisfied.

This simple explanation applies to a single-target situation. Spurious conditions can occur with multiple targets, which can give rise to false registrations with Lobdell's (1968) time-gating system. With this in mind, Mountford *et al.* (1974) have described an array of transducers and associated incoherent processing. Six plane transducers, each used as a separate transmitter-receiver, were arranged in a concave assembly, with one central transducer and the other five placed symmetrically on an annulus of 50 mm diameter. Each transducer had a diameter of 20 mm, and operated at an ultrasonic frequency of 1·5 MHz. The beams intersected at a "focus" at a point 100 mm from the face of each transducer. The array was mounted in a water bath on a three-dimensional positioning mechanism. In a fixed sequence, each individual transducer was excited, and the echo amplitude information received from the "focus" was selected by means of an electronic gate. The corresponding Cartesian coordinates of the array were measured electrically. Both sets of information were sampled, digitized and punched on to paper tape. A switching sequence was arranged so that eight successive characters on the tape represented the six sets of amplitude data and the two positional data corresponding to a single point in the tank in a plane the position of which was noted by the operator. The array was moved so that a two-dimensional matrix of points was interrogated.

Experiments were performed to test the operating characteristics of the apparatus and to determine appropriate methods of signal processing and of displaying the information. The alignment of the ultrasonic beams was such that the coincidence at the "focus" was within 5 mm. The data acquisition system was linear over a dynamic range approaching 40 dB. The apparatus was then used to scan a simple model of wires and an isolated pig kidney. In relation to a single transducer, the resolution of the image was improved by combining the six amplitude data for each point; the product seemed to be more useful than the sum. Contour mapping of received echo amplitude gave a satisfactorily wide dynamic range display.

This arrangement with multiplicative processing has the advantages over a simple plane transducer of increased aperture, improved resolution, large dynamic range display, and improved sidelobe suppression albeit at the expense of signal-to-noise ratio. It is slow, however, although this limitation could be overcome if magnetic tape or solid state store was used. Moreover volume scanning is possible. In this case, for each raster point, and each transducer, the ultrasonic waveform over an entire range interval, say 0–300 mm, would be continuously sampled and recorded. After a completed array movement, each point within the scanned volume would have been interrogated by all six transducers. Suitable processing could be performed on the six data corresponding to each point in the volume. These points would be stored as a three-dimensional matrix. Any two-dimensional scan plane could be extracted from this matrix and displayed; or maybe the whole matrix could be displayed as a three-dimensional image. Thus improved azimuthal resolution could be achieved without restrictions in depth of focus. In practice, however, the situation would be rather less favourable, because of physiological movements and other factors causing uncertainties in resolution cell placement.

Further development could lead to a synthetic aperture device utilizing only one transducer free to move in any direction. The returned signals would have to be processed by a phase sensitive detector to realize a true synthetic aperture (see Section 6.10.c.vi).

(iv) Circular arrays

Single-element catheter-mounted transducers are discussed, *inter alia*, in Section 6.8.b. Rotation of such a probe can be made to produce a circular two-dimensional B-scan, analogous to the plan-position-indicator display familiar in radar. There is an alternative possibility of eliminating the need to rotate the probe, by replacing it with an array of transducers arranged to scan outwards along radii. Thus, Eggleton *et al.* (1970) constructed a probe with four disc transducers spaced 90° apart in a plane normal to the axis of the catheter, and used these transducers in sequence to measure two diameters of the left ventricle, practically at right angles. Martin *et al.* (1974) have described a catheter-borne array of six transducers, constructed from a single cylindrical element. Undoubtedly the most advanced project along these lines, however, is that of Bom (1972). He described an arrangement whereby several small elements are electrically connected in parallel to give a narrower beam. His catheter-mounted probe has 32 elements mounted on the surface of a cylinder of 3 mm diameter, so that the width of each element is about 130 μm. The length of each element is about 4 mm. Phase compensation is used with subgroups of eight elements operated at any one time. The frequency is about 5 MHz, giving a 6 dB beamwidth of about 10° in the main lobe, the principal sidelobe having a maximum sensitivity of about -6 dB at angles of 60° from the main axis. A kind of plan-position-indicator display is obtained by fast electronic scanning, stepping around the array by one element at a time to give 32 lines with a line separation of 11·25°.

Before leaving this topic, mention should be made of a spherical catheter-mounted transducer described by Manoli (1974). He has claimed to be able to measure the diameter and length of the left ventricle simultaneously, since separate echoes of large amplitude are alleged to be obtained from the surfaces of the ventricle "normal" to the spherical ultrasonic beam. The method assumes that the catheter tip is situated at the centre of the circular horizontal section through the ventricle, and that the ventricular walls are smooth and ellipsoidal. It is difficult to imagine that these conditions could often be satisfied in practice.

(v) Two-dimensional arrays

This Sub-section is limited to a discussion of two-dimensional arrays used particularly for pulse–echo reflexion ultrasonography. It is not concerned with arrays for transmission or holographic imaging, which are dealt with in Chapter 8.

Meindl et al. (1974) were set the task of identifying priorities for research into ultrasonic transducers, signal detection and preprocessing. They concluded that the development of arrays capable of generating images generally comparable to those which are produced by high resolution radar should be the most important research objective. Ultrasonic diagnostic system designers might aim to achieve: average ultrasonic intensity of less than 100 mW cm^{-2}; sensitivity better than 0·1 μW cm^{-2}; operating frequency from 1 to 10 MHz; field of view larger than 250 mm cube; resolution better than 1 mm cube; range greater than 250 mm; frame rate higher than 30 s^{-1}; A, B, C and T-P displays; real-time operation; flexible signal processing; full system dynamic range of more than 100 dB; 10 level grey scale with hard copy; and extremely simple system operation.

The technological difficulties in constructing piezoelectric arrays immediately become much greater on moving from one to two dimensions. The major problems to be solved include electrical interconnexions or access to the elements of the array using low cost batch fabrication techniques, elimination of acoustic and electrical cross-talk, aliasing creating sidelobes, the achievement of adequate bandwidth and sensitivity, and a high degree of uniformity in both amplitude and phase characteristics. Apparently the only practical solution to the problem of designing the electronics associated with an array of a very large number of elements is to integrate the circuits with the transducers.

The use of integrated circuit techniques has allowed Maginness et al. (1974) to construct several elegant two-dimensional arrays with various degrees of complexity up to 32×32 elements on 1 mm centres, operating typically at 3·5 MHz (see Fig. 6.45). The multiplexing switches used with these arrays are constructed as an integral part of the array, and consist of field effect transistors arranged so that access to any element may be obtained by the application of two address signals. These transistors are required to control, in the transmit path, signals of 100 V at peak currents of up to 500 mA, whilst retaining sufficiently low leakage to isolate the transducers which are supposed to be inoperative.

The transducer material, lead metaniobate, enables very substantial bandwidths to be achieved without the addition of backing and matching layers such as are necessary with lead zirconate titanate.

This array has been mounted in an assembly with an f4·5 acoustic lens. Each element in the array is addressed in sequence, and operated in the pulse–echo mode: this generates a C-scan display. Alternatively, one row of elements is used to produce a B-scan. In a system with a large number of elements, a complication arises because the time required to transmit and receive echoes by one element limits the maximum number of elements which can be used in a "real-time" display. Maginness *et al.* (1974) propose to overcome this difficulty by simultaneously accessing several elements. Alternatively, they propose to time share by transmitting from

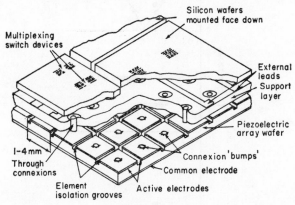

FIG. 6.45 Construction of two-dimensional array based on integrated circuit technology. (After Maginness *et al.*, 1974.)

several elements in rapid sequence, then readdressing the successive elements for the correspondingly delayed echoes from the same depth: but this method might suffer from ambiguity.

(vi) Synthetic aperture arrays

The synthetic aperture antenna was one of the major radar developments of the 1950s (Cutrona, 1970). The basis of the method is the synthesis of an array by the movement of a single element (antenna or transducer) to each of the points in turn which would be occupied by an element in a real array, so that the performance of a wide-aperture system may be realized by combining coherent recordings.

A wide aperture focused system has the advantages, in relation to a conventional ultrasonic beam, that the lateral resolution and the detection of tilted specular reflectors are both improved. Unfortunately, with a system of fixed focal length, the improvement in lateral resolution is achieved only over a limited depth of field. As explained in Section 8.2, the depth-of-focus problem is solved in ultrasonic holography where the operations of recording the ultrasound and of focusing are performed separately. There are, however, serious—probably insuperable—difficulties in the application of holography to medical diagnostics.

Burckhardt *et al.* (1974) have described a synthetic aperture system which is a hybrid between the conventional B-scan and holography. It combines the advantages of both methods. The synthetic aperture system

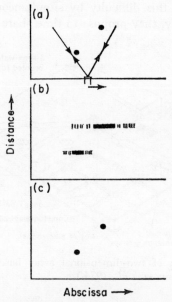

Fig. 6.46 Synthetic aperture sonar. (a) Recording arrangement; (b) recording; (c) processed image. (After Burckhardt *et al.*, 1974.)

measures range by the pulse–echo method, and azimuth, by holography. A thin, flat beam of wide angular divergence is used, and the phase information is preserved by a detector in which the echoes are multiplied by a continuous wave reference signal which is coherent with the transmitted pulse. The recording which results from the scanning process illustrated is in Fig. 6.46. The registration corresponding to a point target is extended in azimuth, and modulated in intensity according to the phase relationship between the echo and the reference signal. This modulation is a one-dimensional Frésnel zone plate—whereas the recording obtained in conventional holography is a two-dimensional Frésnel zone plate. The image is obtained by optical processing of the interference pattern: this is analogous with the reconstruction process in holography. The design of the processor needs to take into account the variation with distance of the focal lengths of the zone plates.

The principles of the method have been tested using a 2 MHz experimental system, designed to scan a useful depth extending in range from 200 to 400 mm, with a width of 300 mm. The resolution was fixed 1·5 mm at a range of 200 mm. The transducer was a standard commercial pulse–echo probe, fitted with a plano-convex polymethylmethacrylate lens of 20 mm radius of curvature. The reference frequency was offset by 100 Hz from the ultrasonic frequency: the effect of this was to modulate the zone plate on a spatial carrier frequency, thus eliminating the difficulties which would otherwise occur due to the two focal points of the zone plates, one real and one virtual. The recording of the signals was made by a high-resolution camera translated past a focused, intensity modulated time-base on a cathode-ray oscilloscope: this was necessary since the zone plate spatial frequency was beyond the limitation of the spot size of the display. In the area of the image with the worst resolution, wires spaced at 3 mm intervals could be distinguished.

Several problems would be encountered in the application of the method to medical diagnostics. Thus, object motion would lead to a degradation in resolution—in the experimental system, a movement of more than about 0·1 mm would be intolerable. Also, the resolution perpendicular to the plane of the scan is the same as that of a conventional B-scan. Another effect of unknown importance is the speckling which occurs in the image of a diffusely reflecting surface when its illumination is spatially coherent.

In summary, it seems unlikely that this type of synthetic aperture system could offer an adequate performance for clinical diagnostics. The method might be developed for laboratory use, however, to investigate inanimate objects, possibly of microscopic size if the frequency could be sufficiently increased.

An ultrasonic imaging system using optical pulse compression has been described by Sato *et al.* (1972). The basic idea is to illuminate a point object with a linear frequency modulated ultrasonic pulse, and to let a pulse of coherent light pass through the ultrasonic waves reflected from the object at the instant that these waves form a portion of a phase zone plate whose centre lies at the object. The image of the object is reconstructed by the light diffracted by the ultrasonic waves, and the range is discriminated either by shifting the timing of the optical pulse, or by changing the index of modulation of the linear f.m. signal. In principle, the method gives a high resolution in both range and azimuth. It may thus be considered to be an application of pulse-compression techniques, used in chirp radar, to ultrasonic imaging, but it has image-forming as well as range-discriminating capability. Preliminary experimental results have confirmed that the method indeed has these capabilities, but that it is limited to some extent by the restriction on the frequency range of the chirp imposed by the bandwidth of the ultrasonic transducer. With some development, however, it might become useful in medical diagnostics.

(vii) Address circuits

In some systems using arrays of transducers, it is necessary to address each element in the array in sequence. This can be done with switches (see, for example, Suckling and Hendrickson, 1969), and in some applications this simple method is satisfactory. Sometimes it is not, however, and then the ingenious solution described by Havlice et al. (1973) may be appropriate. Their basic receiving system is illustrated in Fig. 6.47. It consists of a linear

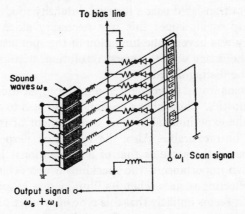

FIG. 6.47 System for combining the signals from the separate elements in an array. (After Havlice et al., 1973.)

array of a large number of piezoelectric detectors, on to which an image is cast, for example by means of a lens, either by reflexion or transmission from an object irradiated by a separate transducer. An acoustic surface wave delay with an appropriate number of equally spaced taps is used as the electronic scanning device. The output signal from each tap is mixed with the output from the corresponding element in the array. If the signal inserted onto the delay line has an angular frequency ω_1, and the frequency of the ultrasound forming the image is ω_S, the output signals from the individual mixers have frequencies of $\omega_S + \omega_1$ and $\omega_S - \omega_1$. The mixer outputs are added, and either the sum or difference frequency is passed through a filter into the output circuit.

If a short pulse of frequency ω_1 is injected into the delay line, then as this pulse travels past each tap, the instantaneous output from the adder is that from the corresponding element in the array. Thus, as the pulse travels along the delay line, it scans each element in turn so that the output may be used to intensity modulate a display corresponding to one line of the ultrasonic image.

The electronic scanning system retains both amplitude and phase information. By an appropriate signal injected into the delay line, it is possible to use the phase information to synthesize a focal plane within an object at any chosen distance from the array. This eliminates the need for a lens. Havlice *et al.* (1973) have shown that the appropriate signal to focus at a distance z is a linear frequency sweep of instantaneous frequency $\omega = \omega_1 + \mu t$, where $\mu = \omega_s v^2/zc$, and v is the velocity of the wave along the array. Thus, changing the sweep rate is equivalent to changing the focal length of the array.

Because there is a finite number N of elements in the array, there are sidelobes at a distance $d_S = z\lambda N/L$ from the main image, where L is the length of the array. These sidelobes correspond to an additional 2π phase shift between rays reaching neighbouring elements. Thus, the number of resolvable spots is approximately equal to the number of elements in the array.

(viii) Delay lines

Save in the simplest applications of arrays, a key component is the delay line. Lumped LC delay lines, distributed electromagnetic delay lines, and switched capacitor delay lines, are all attractive since they make use of components which are readily available. On the other hand, they are expensive (prohibitively so if large numbers are required), large in size and limited in performance. The surface acoustic wave delay line is not electronically variable, nor can it be used directly at ultrasonic frequencies. Digital delay lines cannot operate on very low-level signals, and it is difficult to achieve the required high sampling rate.

It is possible to control the delay introduced by an LC delay line, by using a varactor diode as the capacitive element. A varactor diode is a semiconductor device in which the thickness of the depletion layer, and hence the capacitance, is controlled by changing the value of the reverse bias. Unfortunately, the range of capacitive variation which can be obtained with such a device is rather small, and a large number of diodes is needed in a delay line in which a range of time delay of 5–10 μs is required.

A delay line consisting of a series of capacitors into which consecutive samples of the input signal are deposited, and from which these samples are subsequently read out, has been developed by Doornbos and Somer (1972). The basic principle is illustrated in Fig. 6.48. The input signal is sampled by switches 1 to N, and the samples are stored in capacitors C_1 to C_N respectively. Subsequently the signal is read out by switches $1'$ to N'. At any instant, the signal is being stored in C_n, whilst the delayed signal is being read out of C_{n+1}. The capacitors are commutated consecutively, and the delay is equal to $(N-1)\tau_S$, where $1/\tau_S = f_S$, the sampling frequency.

In their system, Doornbos and Somer (1972) used series FET switches similar to those described in Section 6.2. The voltages across the storage capacitors (150 pF) were sampled by FETs arranged as voltage followers. With a delay line of six sections, the time delay in the range 0·5–2·0 μs was linearly related to the clock frequency (20–5 MHz). The dynamic range

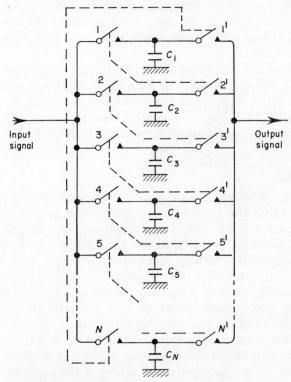

FIG. 6.48 Consecutively commutated capacitors arranged as a delay line. (Based on Doornbos and Somer, 1972.)

was 45 dB at $f_S = 6$ MHz, and increased to 55 dB at $f_S = 20$ MHz, when delaying a signal of 1·4 MHz with an output bandpass filter with cut-off frequencies of 0·5 and 3·0 MHz. This filter was required to smooth the output waveform, which, in its unsmoothed state, would consist of a series of steps at the sampling frequency. In theory, the maximum signal frequency is equal to one half of the sampling frequency, and this is a further limitation of the system.

Integrated circuit versions of the consecutively commutated capacitor delay are available commercially*. The input and output switches are controlled by shift registers operated as ring counters. These shift registers are stepped at equal rates, and the stored sample in each capacitor is read out serially, immediately prior to a new sample being read in. In the serial analogue memory device, there is a single array, typically of 64 capacitors. In the serial analogue delay device, there are two delay lines each typically with 50 capacitors, which are operated in parallel: each register is clocked at half the sampling frequency, with one clock staggered by a quarter cycle behind the other. Moreover, the serial analogue delay devices incorporate reset clocks. Typically, these devices can operate at sampling frequencies of up to 12 MHz, giving video bandwidths of up to 6 MHz according to the sampling frequency; signal-to-noise ratio is 50–70 dB.

Another kind of delay line which seems promising for ultrasonic applications, although it is not yet commercially available for this purpose, is the charge coupled device. In this type of device, charge proportional to the instantaneous value of the analogue signal is stored and transferred as minority carriers in the inversion layers of an array of MOS capacitors (Thompsett and Zimany, 1973). A linear array of MOS electrodes is pulsed in sequence to move potential wells for minority carriers along the surface of the silicon. These wells contain packets of electrons. Once a charge packet of a size related to the instantaneous value of the analogue input signal has been fed into one of the potential wells, it is transferred, essentially intact, from under one electrode to the next and so moved across the device. A typical charge coupled delay line might have 250 elements, and would be capable of delaying signals for times of down to around 1 μs, according to the clocking frequency. The signal-to-noise ratio might be 60 dB or better with a charge packet size of 0·05 pC and 500 transfers.

A fairly recent development of this type of delay line is the peristatic charge-coupled device (Esser, 1974). This device has a profiled structure, which effectively reduces the distance from the stored charge to the transfer electrode. As a result, the charge transfer efficiency approaches 99·995%, in comparison with the 99·990% efficiency of the conventional charge coupled device, and the maximum data rate is greater by a factor of 20–40.

In consecutively commutated capacitor delay lines and similar devices, the time delay is proportional to the control voltage, if the period of the clock frequency is arranged also to be proportional to the control voltage. Snoeck (1972) has developed a circuit, shown in block diagram in Fig. 6.49, which has this characteristic. The clock pulse frequency—that is, the frequency of the voltage controlled multivibrator—is fed to the pulse-width-to-voltage converter, which produces a voltage proportional to the

* For example, types SAM-64 and SAD-100: Reticon Corpn., Sunnyvale, California, USA.

clock period. This voltage is compared with the control voltage input, by the differential amplifier, thus forming a closed negative feedback loop. The accuracy of the arrangement is determined by the characteristics of the pulsewidth-to-voltage converter. In a practical arrangement, the output clock frequency may be divided in the feedback loop; in Snoeck's (1972) circuit, this division is by 16: the pulsewidth-to-voltage converter operates at a maximum frequency of 1·5 MHz, and the clock frequency is in the range 5–20 MHz with a linearity of better than 1%.

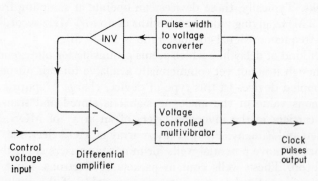

Fig. 6.49 Block diagram of clock pulse generator for controlling sampled delay lines. (Based on Snoeck, 1972.)

6.11 DISPLAY OF THREE-DIMENSIONAL DATA

Conventional two-dimensional scans contain only information about single planes, albeit of finite thickness. This represents a substantial improvement in comparison with a single A-scan, and in many situations the information contained in such a scan is adequate for an accurate diagnosis to be made. It often happens that a satisfactory diagnosis cannot be made from a single two-dimensional scan, however, and it is then necessary for several scans to be made, each in a different plane. The most usual method is to scan in parallel planes, either in transverse or in longitudinal section. An experienced observer can form a three-dimensional impression of the structures visualized in such a series of two-dimensional scans, and is thus able to arrive at a diagnosis. Some doctors become very good at this, others never learn. It is particularly to help those who find it difficult to perceive three-dimensional data that techniques have been tried aimed at presenting what is essentially a three-dimensional matrix of data in simpler ways.

Baum and Greenwood (1961) prepared a series of photographically reversed (i.e. the higher the echo amplitude, the blacker the registration) scans on transparent plates. By stacking these plates with appropriate spacing they constructed a three-dimensional model. Such a model enables even a relatively unskilled observer to appreciate ultrasonic information in a three-dimensional form. However, the deeper parts tend to be visible only poorly because they are obscured by structures closer to the edge of the model. Redman *et al.* (1969) have to some extent overcome this difficulty by making a hologram in which the serial scans are recorded in sequence. When the hologram is reconstructed, each scan is quite clearly visible because it is self-illuminated. (This method is a development of the holographic multiplexing technique of Leith *et al.*, 1966.)

The problem of transferring data from serial two-dimensional scans to a computer for subsequent three-dimensional reconstruction has been solved by Rasmussen *et al.* (1974) by the use of a pencil follower, and the involvement of the clinician at this stage in the process. On scans made in standardized planes, the outlines of the patient and the organs of interest are traced out with the pencil follower, and the computer stores the co-ordinates of every point which is thus interrogated. If the clinician is only concerned, for example, with the liver, he digitizes only the contour of that organ; if he desires a projection of the body surface and a tumour, he digitizes the skin and the tumour outlines. Once the scans have been digitized, the data can be transferred to computer cards or tape, and may be kept as part of the patient's record.

Several modes of display are possible. The three-dimensional matrix of data points are first entered on the computer's bulk storage. The viewing position is then specified as degrees of rotation about the spatial axes. The composite image may then be projected on to the computer monitor screen, with a perspective correction such that points further away from the viewer are in smaller scale. If appropriate, a plane may be selected, data originating from beyond which are not displayed (see also Howry *et al.*, 1956).

Visualization of this type of perspective image in three dimensions, although requiring some concentration and practice, is possible by most observers. With experience, it is apparently quite easy properly to orientate various structures in their correct relationships. The greatest problem associated with such images is multistability, or the spontaneous and in-voluntary shift of viewpoint. When the perspective image is inadequate for a three-dimensional effect, a simple modification of the computer program can generate an image with a horizontal shift of the viewpoint of 80 mm. Photographs of the two images form a true stereo pair which can be studied in any suitable viewer (see also McDicken *et al.*, 1972). A scanner particu-larly designed for stereoscopic display is that of Brown and Greening (1973).

The computer program may easily be modified to suit individual needs. The options include rotation about all three axes, provision for using oblique scanning sections as input data, and the selective elimination of data points. Thus, it would be possible to display only data from a particular plane of any chosen orientation. It would be a simple matter to impose additional contours, such as those necessary for radiotherapy treatment planning (see Section 6.16.g).

According to Rasmussen *et al.* (1974), digitizing a complete set of scans requires 15–20 min, depending on the number of sections and the experience of the operator. The method has the advantage of simplicity, but the data reduction which occurs at the digitization stage is necessarily very considerable. If the clinician fails to notice an important feature on the two-dimensional scans, the information is lost. This difficulty does not arise with the method of Robinson (1972), who has described a technique to input data from conventional serial two-dimensional scans to the computer, without the involvement of a clinician in what is essentially a data-reduction process as in the method of Rasmussen *et al.* (1974). He used a flying spot picture scanner with a resolution of 1024×1024 points and 8-bits (256 level, or 48 dB dynamic range) to generate digital signals for direct input to a computer. In his experimental work, he used a set of 14 echograms made at 13 mm intervals across the abdomen of a woman in late pregnancy. A point spacing of 1 mm on the echogram was used, and the grey scale was reduced to 6 bits (64 levels, 36 dB) to allow the data to be packed with three points to a single 18-bit word. He was able to generate a variety of different displays, but he did not attempt a three-dimensional reconstruction. (There is no reason to suppose that such a reconstruction would be useful, for there is far too much information to allow this type of image to be interpreted, particularly since weakly echoing structures often lie inside those which reflect ultrasound strongly.) Pictures regenerated in planes perpendicular to those of the original scans are of quite acceptable quality. Oblique planes are often more easily interpreted than the original scans. The possibility of consolidating from scans made in two mutually perpendicular sets of planes on to a single set of serial sections was also demonstrated by Robinson (1972).

Although it is unlikely that this technique will find wide application with the present generation of pulse–echo diagnostic machines, it may prove to be useful in specialized examinations of complicated anatomical situations.

A three-dimensional impression is experienced if serial scans are photographed in sequence and projected like an ordinary ciné film. The effect is similar to that experienced when travelling through fog: structures seem to emerge, become clearer and then disappear again. The film can be arranged in a loop, alternately with reverse and forward sequences, so that the "motion" is continuously in and out of the three-dimensional volume. The scanning time necessary to obtain a very large number of scans situated close together renders the method impracticable as a routine with manually operated scanners. If only a limited number of scans is projected in strict sequence, the result is both jerky and rapid. Under such circum-

stances, the best effect is obtained by projecting in a sequence such as
. . . 1112122232333 . . .

Szilard (1974) has developed an ingenious method to view serial two-dimensional scans made in parallel planes, rapidly in sequence to present a three-dimensional image. The scans are projected in sequence on to separate screens, each screen being at an appropriate distance from the observer: the screen on which appears the scan at one extremity of the series is closest, and that from the other end, is farthest away. By cunning arrangement of wheels and pulleys, each of the screens is at the same position in space, except for the position in depth, at the instant when the corresponding image is displayed. Moreover, all the images in the series are presented in 1/15s, thus giving a flicker-free impression of a three-dimensional object. The image may be viewed through quite wide angles, thus enhancing the three-dimensional advantages; colour may be used to give better discrimination between layers at different depths; and the brightness of layers at different depth may be controlled independently of each other.

In an attempt to overcome what may occasionally be a disadvantage in the use of a two-dimensional scanner to obtain three-dimensional data in the form of serial scans, Dekker *et al.* (1974) have constructed a scanner with five degrees of freedom. They have used this instrument for investigating the heart. The video signals from a conventional 2·25 MHz ultrasonic pulse–echo system were fed to a PDP-12 computer through a 2-bit (4 level, 12 dB dynamic range) analogue-to-digital converter operating at 1·85 MHz. Seven other sets of data—one set from each of the five resolvers in the scanner, one from a respiration transducer, and one from an e.c.g. amplifier —where digitized at 55 kHz, and also input to the computer. All this information was stored on a fixed disc, the size of which limited the scanning time to 5 min at a p.r.f. of 10 Hz. The data were transferred from the PDP-12 to an IBM 360/50 ACME computer.

The data processing consisted of calculating the xyz spatial coordinates of the leading edge of each echo, so that this information could be stored according to the time after the R-wave. Thirty-five files were compiled, each corresponding to a 20 ms interval during the cardiac cycle. All data taken during inhalation were discarded.

The data were processed to reconstruct two-dimensional cross-sections using the ACME computer and a video display unit. The operator could select the position, thickness and orientation of the viewed slice, and the time in the cardiac cycle. Timing of events occurring just before R-waves— such as the closing of the mitral valve at the beginning of ventricular systole —was made by counting back in time from the following R-wave, rather than by counting on in time from the preceding R-wave: this is in general a more accurate process, less liable to introduce errors due to arrhythmias.

Apparently the system can be used by a relatively unskilled operator. A superficial look at the published results, however, does not prove to be particularly exciting in comparison with those obtained with other, two-dimensional, imaging techniques. Maybe this is because of the small dynamic range. The potential importance of the system seems to be that, with the four-dimensional data (i.e. time and three-dimensional space) stored on the computer, it should be possible to develop programmes to determine such properties as ejection fraction, wall thickness, aneurysms, defects, valve motions, structure velocities, and cardiac power. Image enhancement routines should also be applicable.

6.12 ANALYSIS OF PULSE–ECHO DATA

6.12.a General Considerations

Present-day "conventional" methods of displaying pulse–echo information enable many conclusions to be reached concerning the structure and function of the scanned anatomy and related biological systems. Under some circumstances, analytical methods can be applied to the echo data, which enhance the image, identify tissue, or quantitate physiological function.

Kelsey *et al.* (1974) have pointed out that a "signature library" consisting of representations of the echoes obtained from particular tissues and organs under different conditions of frequency and focusing, etc., would be extremely useful and allow a designer to make an optimal choice of parameters. Such a library could exist on three subject levels:

(i) *The scan picture*: scan atlases for existing machines would be of great clinical utility, but, because the signal processing is so different from machine to machine, such atlases would only have limited value to designers;

(ii) *The time response of a bandwidth limited pulse*: such responses would be functions of frequency, transducer aperture, tissue range, pulse length, and system bandwidth: they would be useful to designers using transducers of similar or relateable performance; and

(iii) *The time response to an impulse*: such responses could be used to calculate the response to any wave form, by the use of convolution techniques.

Since the frequency domain curve of reflexion is the Fourier transfer of the time–domain impulse response, these forms of data are interchangeable.

A preliminary to the implementation of many analytical techniques is the acquisition and recording of the ultrasonic signals. This can be done by analogue or digital methods.

An example of the use of a video-tape recorder to store ultrasonic data is in the study of pulsations in echoencephalography as described by de Vlieger *et al.* (1974). This particular application does not necessitate the recording of the video signals, but merely the time–positions of the leading edges of each of the echo envelopes exceeding a threshold level. The system allows the recording to be replayed to display the movements in range either of all structures simultaneously in a two-dimensional time–position format, or of one selected structure on a paper strip recorder with a timing resolution of 10 ns. Taken overall, the measurement uncertainty is ± 70 ns, corresponding to about ± 0.05 mm. The advantage of the video-tape recorder is that it allows the movements of many structures to be studied, both in isolation and in relation to others, without inconvenience to the patient.

Ide and Masuzawa (1975) have described the application of a domestic, 525-line, 30 frame per second, video-tape recorder with a helical track, as a store for ultrasonic pulse–echo data. The principal difficulty is the different scan formats and rates of the ultrasonic and television systems. One way around this is to use a scan conversion memory tube (see Section 6.6.c). Ide and Masuzawa (1975) used another approach: they synchronized the ultrasonic system to a clock operating at television frame rate.

Several different methods have been described for converting ultrasonic signals to digital form. Possibly the simplest is to use a light-pen manually to trace along a projected A-scan (Trier and Reuter, 1973; Fields *et al.*, 1975). This is a tedious process, however, and generally automatic methods are preferable. Of these, the simplest in principle is to take the video output from the pulse–echo system, and to feed it to a sample-and-hold circuit, controlled by a triggering signal delayed from the transmission pulse by a time corresponding to the target range. The output from the sample-and-hold, which may be arranged to correspond to the peak input amplitude during the gate time, is fed to an analogue-to-digital converter; and the output from this may be recorded, for example, by a paper-tape punch. The punch speed limits the rate of data acquisition, and the flag signal from the punch is arranged to initiate the next ultrasonic pulse sequence. The character capacity of the paper tape limits the dynamic range of the data and determines the resolution required of the analogue-to-digital converter. Thus, 6 bits correspond to a dynamic range of 36 dB, 8 bits to 48 dB, 10 bits to 60 dB, and so on.

An alternative method (Milan, 1972) uses a fast analogue-to-digital converter, with direct input to a digital computer using the data-break facility. The minimum sampling time is equal to the cycle time of the computer memory (typically 1.5 μs for a modern mini-computer).

Single-point-per-pulse digitization has been used to record the envelope of echo variation with range, using a system of incremental delay and repeat transmission (Erikson and Brill, 1970). The technique depends on pulse-to-pulse reproducibility, and is inapplicable if the patient moves, or if the echoes are stochastic.

Serial-point digitization is possible by means of a transient recorder (Wells, 1974). A transient recorder consists of a high-speed analogue-to-digital converter and a recirculating shift register memory, which can transfer data asynchronously. The output may be fed to a digital computer or to a digital recorder; or a digital-to-analogue converter may be arranged to allow the contents of the memory to be displayed on an oscilloscope or chart recorder. In general, information theory requires that the sampling frequency should be at least twice the signal frequency. The specification of the most advanced instrument at present available commercially* is: sampling frequency, 100 MHz; capacity, 2000 words; precision, 8 bits. The output rate of the transient recorder must be chosen to suit the data store. If this is paper tape, it might be less than 20 words per second. Magnetic tape typically works at 10000 words per second. Direct input to an on-line computer might be at 500000 words per second. The role of the transient recorder is thus twofold: it digitizes and slows down the data.

Goldstein *et al.* (1975) have designed a system to digitize the ultrasonic data obtained from a conventional pulse–echo scanner, and to input these to PDP-15 computer (64 k of core, two 250 k word fixed head discs and two 10·2 M word disc pack drives). One of their output devices was a display with a matrix of 128×128 elements, coded in up to 16 colours or grey levels. This powerful system does not yet seem to have been used for research.

A system of digitization of ultrasonic data for direct storage in a computer has been described by Kay *et al.* (1975). The video signals from a conventional two-dimensional abdominal scanner are applied to 10 voltage comparators arranged for multi-threshold parallel analogue-to-digital conversion. A 750 kHz clock is used to define time periods of 1·33 μs, which correspond to distances of approximately 1 mm in soft tissues. At the end of each 1·33 μs period, the maximum levels attained in the 10 comparators are binary coded and stored in shift registers as 4-bit words. When four such 4-bit words are stored in each shift register, the data are transmitted to the computer (Varian 620 L) as a series of 16-bit words.

This particular arrangement does not make full use of the 4-bit word capability—which corresponds to 16 separate levels, or a 24 dB dynamic range—since the digitization is only to 10 levels, or 20 dB dynamic range. This type of analogue-to-digital converter, however, does have the advantage that the digital output may be arranged to bear any desired relationship to the analogue input, by a suitable choice of the reference voltages fed to

* Model 8100: Biomation, Palo Alto, California, USA.

the comparators. In common with all real-time systems, its usefulness as a part of an image processing system would be limited by the capability of the computer to accept and manipulate data at ultrasonic frequencies. There is only a restricted range of such processes which can be performed by small computers, and it would be difficult to justify the dedication of a large computer in this type of application. Therefore, at the present time, it seems sensible to devote more effort to the development of off-line systems.

6.12.b Image Enhancement

Hirsch *et al.* (1973) have used a transient recorder to digitize the ultrasonic (video) echo signals originating from within the heart during the time-range interval 90–130 μs. The sampling rate was 5 MHz, and 256 samples were taken. The echoes corresponding to one out of every 10 transmitted pulses were digitized, generating 256 6-bit words every 10 ms. The four most significant bits of each of the 256 words were packed into 64 16-bit words by hardware, and transmitted to an H-P 2100 computer. The computer collected these data into buffers, and transferred it to an H-P 7900 moving head disc. Ninety-six seconds of digitized echocardiogram could be stored in a single disc pack.

The system was used to analyse echoes from the aortic wall. The basis of the analysis was the detection of the leading edge of each echo complex, and the exclusion of other data from the display. This was done by defining a peak to be a sample point of greater amplitude than the preceding point, but less than the following point. Next, the computer was used to track the posterior aortic root echo automatically. This was done after the beginning of the aortic root echo had been identified on a storage tube display by a clinician: the computer then tracked the indicated structure throughout the recorded echocardiogram. In order to do this, two assumptions were made: firstly, that there were no strong echoes in the vicinity of the echo of interest, and secondly, that the aortic root velocity was less than 50 mm s^{-1}. Then, for each new sample—10 ms after its predecessor— a search was made for the echo within the range change ± 0.5 mm. The most anterior echo within this interval was considered to be the echo from the aortic root: in this way, the system tracked the inner wall of the posterior wall. If no peak was found within the permitted range, the range was extended to the next set of samples, and the permitted range was increased to ± 1.0 mm, and so on until the aortic root was again located. The permitted range was then returned to its original size. Finally, the tracking signal was smoothed by a 6.5 Hz low-pass digital filter: this removed sampling irregularities and noise. The tracking signal was then recorded, using all the columns of an electrostatic printer: this gave a rather distinct line against a background of the other echoes, which were printed in alternate columns. Also, the velocity and acceleration of the smoothed tracking signal were calculated by the computer and printed out on the recording, together with a matrix of markers at 10 mm and 100 ms spacings.

Hirsch *et al.* (1973) commented that recordings obtained in this way revealed subtleties previously unnoticed in motion of the aortic root. They considered that the method might be developed to track the left ventricular diameter, and so to calculate the stroke volume and cardiac output (see Section 6.16.b). Moreover, if the leading edges of the echoes were identified by analogue preprocessors, the computer necessary for the tracking calculations might be sufficiently small to allow an economic system to be constructed to operate in real time.

Automatic echo-tracking systems such as that just described depend for their success on there being a reliably distinctive characteristic in the nature of the echo to be studied. In echocardiograms this is often not the case. Pai *et al.* (1974) showed how this difficulty can be circumvented by having a skilled interpreter tracing along the echo waveform with a pencil-follower, thus digitizing the time–position data and making computer analysis possible.

Once ultrasonic signals have been digitized, it is possible to apply a great variety of signal processing methods without the need to build special apparatus. The potential of this has hardly yet been explored. One technique which has been tried, however, is that of frequency bandpass filtering (McSherry, 1974): thus, filtered echocardiograms more clearly reveal the thicknesses of valve cusps, and layers of calcification.

Rather an empirical approach to the possibility of improving two-dimensional ultrasonic scans has been adopted by King and Wong (1972). They worked on a scan of the brain made through the intact skull—and, nowadays, this might not be thought to represent an urgent clinical problem, in the light of the discussion in Section 6.16.e. They began by digitizing what was considered to be a "good" scan, into a matrix of 256×256 data points, with a dynamic range of 48 dB (256 levels). A computer was then used to perform various processes. Firstly, a high threshold filter was used: this is equivalent to restricting the displayed dynamic range by suppressing small-amplitude echoes, and offers no advantage over its analogue equivalent. Next, the computer was arranged to find those areas of echoes expected in the scan—the skull and the midline—and then to search the remaining areas for abnormalities. This is easier said than done! According to King and Wong (1972), "The procedure used to enable the computer to detect the abnormal echo follows, basically, that used by the human". Many people think that this kind of interpretation by a human observer is so unreliable that it is useless. It seems certain that this approach cannot succeed in the investigation of the brain. Programming a computer for pattern recognition might be worthwhile, however, to assist in the analysis of scans of organs, such as the kidney, where quite high reliabilities are presently obtained by skilled observers.

6.12.c Amplitude Analysis

(i) Amplitude measurements

The interpretation of A-scans and two-dimensional B-scans is generally left to the judgement of the observer. Differential diagnosis based on careful inspection of the A-scan, both in respect of its pattern and its amplitude, has been quite thoroughly developed by Ossoinig (1974). The method depends on the use of an instrument with standardized characteristics, so that comparisons are valid. Likewise, Rettenmaier (1974) estimated both echo amplitude and attenuation from two-dimensional grey-scale hepatic scans, and found that echo amplitude is generally increased in diffuse disease in comparison with the normal, and that slightly fatty liver has lower attenuation; the attenuation becomes increasingly greater in chronic hepatitis, severe and moderately fatty liver, and cirrhosis.

The first quantitative approach to the interpretation of A-scans seems to be that of Wild and Reid (1952), in connexion with the diagnosis of breast disease. Subsequently Schentke and Renger (1964) reported that both the mean echo amplitude and the echo (spatial) frequency increased in various abnormalities of the liver including cirrhosis. Wells *et al.* (1969) applied the original method of Wild and Reid (1952) to study the echo amplitudes in a series of patients with various liver abnormalities. They calculated an index

$$\sum_i h_i / T$$

where h_i is the amplitude of the ith internal echo and T is the duration of the echo train subjected to analysis. For each individual, they made two demodulated A-scans made along different paths through the liver, and they standardized the system operating conditions, including swept gain rate and sensitivity. The positions of the A-scans were marked by intensifying the corresponding lines on two-dimensional B-scans used in the same subcostal planes, and echoes of large amplitude—supposed, probably often erroneously, to arise from the concave inferior surface of the liver—were "identified" on the B-scans, and the corresponding echoes were somewhat arbitrarily excluded from the A-scan analyses. The mean index for each abnormal liver was compared with the value for a corresponding normal, and found to be greater in 25 out of 32 patients with cirrhosis.

A somewhat similar method of analysis was used by Czarnecki and Kubicki (1970), who not surprisingly found that the diagnosis was more reliable in patients with more advanced disease. Having likewise localized an area for analysis on a two-dimensional B-scan, Fields *et al.* (1975)

photographed a series of separate A-scans through this area. From the illustrations of their article, it appears that the demodulated A-scan was used. An image of this was projected on to a screen, and the positions and amplitudes of the maxima were digitized with a pencil follower. In this research, however, only six A-scans per patient seem to have been analysed, and the results had rather large standard deviations. Very similar methods have been applied by Decker *et al.* (1973) to the analysis of A-scans for ophthalmic diagnosis.

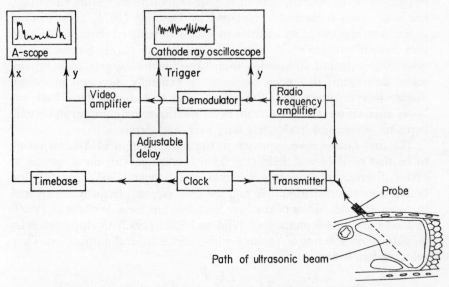

Fig. 6.50 Block diagram of the apparatus used by Mountford and Wells (1972a, b) to study hepatic echo amplitude. The position of the ultrasonic probe is illustrated by a longitudinal section through the right side of the patient, who is viewed from the left.

Mountford and Wells (1972a, b) used a refinement of earlier methods of quantitatively analysing the A-scan to determine variations in the echo amplitudes in normal liver and in cirrhosis, and to estimate the effective attenuation of ultrasound in the liver assuming a random spatial distribution of intrahepatic targets. They also investigated the effects of variations in the characteristics of the anterior abdominal wall, since it had been suggested by Wells *et al.* (1969) that the muscle and fat layers might significantly influence the amplitudes of intrahepatic echoes detected transcutaneously.

A block diagram of the measuring apparatus is shown in Fig. 6.50. Provision was made for standardizing the system sensitivity, using techniques discussed in Section 6.13. The pulse repetition rate was 1000 s^{-1}, and the transducer had a diameter of 20 mm, a zero-crossing frequency of 1·67 MHz, and a 20 dB bandwidth of 1·2 MHz. The field was resonably regular at ranges beyond 50 mm. The waveform displayed on the cathode-ray oscilloscope corresponded to echoes selected by the adjustable delay to have originated from the range interval commencing at 50 mm and extending to approximately 100 mm. The circuitry which processed this signal was linear. The conventional demodulated A-scan was presented on a second display, and by studying this it was possible to be certain that the ultrasonic beam was passing through the liver, and that the range interval 50–100 mm lay entirely within the liver.

For each individual examined, the oscilloscope display was photographed 30 times, each with a new position of the probe. These photographs were analysed by measuring the amplitude of each cycle from the peak to the succeeding trough. The measurements were begun at the graticule line corresponding to a range of 50 mm, and were repeated sequentially for 100 cycles. Generally these cycles were regularly spaced, and occupied a range interval of about 47·5 mm (the frequency being about 1·67 MHz). Each amplitude was measured to the nearest millimetre. (Ultimately these measurements could be related to the corresponding backscattering co-efficients of the examined tissue volumes: see Section 5.4.) The maximum amplitude which could be contained on the photograph was 56 mm, so that the maximum measurement precision was equivalent to a word length of between 5 and 6 bits. There were 3000 data-points for each individual.

Thus, each scan consisted of 100 data-points. These data-points may be regarded as samples of echo amplitude y at regular intervals of distance x. Therefore, for each individual, there were 100 x-values, each with 30 data-point estimates of y. The analysis was based on the assumption that these echoes originated from targets within the liver, randomly distributed spatially.

Since the echo amplitude might be expected *a priori* as a first approximation to decay exponentially with range, then the regression of the logarithm of the mean values of the 30 data-point estimates of y for each value of x (i.e. ln $\bar{y}$) against x should be linear. Moreover, the slope of this regression line should reflect the attenuation of ultrasound within the liver.

Thirty individuals with normal livers were studied (Mountford and Wells, 1972a). Pooling the results for the whole group revealed a very good linear relationship between ln y and x (see Fig. 6.51). Echo amplitude was approximately log normally distributed about this line. The apparent attenuation rate was 1·76 dB cm^{-1}, corresponding to 1·05 dB cm^{-1} MHz^{-1}. Investigation of the echo amplitude values failed to confirm the anxiety of Wells *et al.* (1969), referred to previously in this Sub-section, concerning the possible importance of variations in the characteristics of the body wall according to somatotype. On the contrary, individuals with high meso-morphy ratings tended to have higher echo amplitudes.

The results obtained with normal livers were compared with corres-ponding measurements in 13 patients with cirrhosis (Mountford and Wells, 1972b). The differences between the slopes of the regression lines were not significant (although generally the attenuation was lower in cirrhotics than in normals), but the echo amplitudes in cirrhotics were always greater than those in normals, the separation being greatest when the amplitudes corres-ponding to the ln y intercepts of the regression lines mid-way through the sampled tissue were compared. This separation, illustrated in Fig. 6.52, is equivalent to 6 dB.

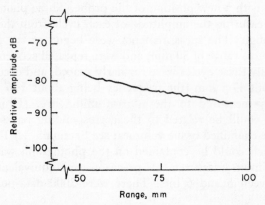

FIG. 6.51 Variation in echo amplitude with range in normal liver at 1·67 MHz. The relative amplitude is derived from the mean value of echo amplitude in a pooled group of 30 individuals, and is expressed in decibels below the echo ampli-tude from a perfect reflector at normal incidence in a lossless medium. (Data of Mountford and Wells, 1972a.)

For each individual set of data, the effect of the exponential regression was removed by adding the appropriate factor to each value of ln y. Con-secutive values of ln y may be regarded as equidistant samples of the envelope. Averaging all the data in the normal group and in the cirrhotic group allowed the mean envelope shapes to be compared. In relation to the normals, the cirrhotics had significantly faster rise-times, and signifi-cantly fewer peaks and troughs.

It has been pointed out by Chivers and Hill (1975) that the extent of the information which it may be possible ultrasonically to obtain from a volume of tissue cannot yet be defined, because so little is known of the interactions yielding the information. Moreover, experimental data are also sparse. It seems that, besides breast and liver, it is only for heart muscle that any characteristics relating echo amplitude to pathology have been obtained. Thus, in stylized measurements on *in vitro* samples of normal and infarcted myocardium, Namery and Lele (1972) have shown that the normal muscle has the higher impedance; according to their data, the echo amplitude from infarcted tissue is about 1·3 dB greater than that from normal tissue. This difference is so small that it seems impossible that echo amplitude measurements alone could be used to distinguish between normal and infarcted myocardium *in vivo*, where the orientation of the myocardial surface with respect to the ultrasonic beam would vary from point to point, and even at the same point during the cardiac cycle.

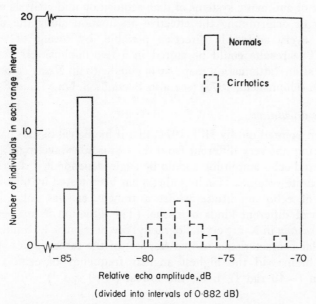

Relative echo amplitude, dB

(divided into intervals of 0·882 dB)

FIG. 6.52 Histogram showing the distribution of mid-way echo amplitudes for 30 individuals with normal livers, and 13 with cirrhosis. Relative amplitude expressed as in Fig. 6.51. (Data of Mountford and Wells, 1972b.)

(ii) Automatic methods

Manual methods of analysing pulse–echo data, such as those described in Section 6.12.c.i, are tedious. Fortunately techniques which avoid most of the drudgery of manual work have been developed.

Grossmann (1971) has constructed an instrument, using analogue circuits, in which the number of echoes occurring along a gated section of the A-scan is counted automatically. The clinical value of this instrument does not seem to have been reported.

Mountford *et al.* (1973) automated the manual method used previously by Mountford and Wells (1972a, b). A 128-word, 6-bit transient recorder was used to digitize a 20 mm range interval at a sampling frequency of 5 MHz, and the captured waveform was dumped on paper tape.

It is of interest that the most successful application of ultrasonic pulse–echo techniques to the study of breast disease is due to the shadowing, or "antishadowing", of tissues lying beyond suspect areas visualized on non-compounded two-dimensional scans (see Section 6.16.g). This phenomenon seems to be due to differences between the attenuation rates in the normal breast tissue and in the lesion. Extremes are cysts, which have low attenuation, and calcified tumours, which have high attenuation. The development of automatic systems of data acquisition and analysis opens the possibility of determining the effective attenuation along the ultrasonic beam for every accessible direction possible, by means of regression analysis. The results could be stored in a two-dimensional matrix and displayed as an "attenuation map" analogous with an X-ray computerized tomograph (Hounsfield, 1973) (see also Sections 8.1.a.vi and 8.1.b.iii).

(iii) Tissue orientation

It has been pointed out by Hill (1974) that if biological tissues have structure ordering not very different from the ultrasonic wavelength, then the backscattered echo amplitude should be angle-dependent if the resolution cell has a finite volume. This hypothesis has been tested by measuring the variation of echo amplitude whilst a transducer was rotated around specimens of different kinds of tissue. (The situation is analogous with *Bragg diffraction* in X-ray crystallography: see Section 5.4.) Similar tissues have similar characteristics in this respect; of the three tissues studied at 1 MHz, brain had the highest angular frequency of echo amplitude fluctuation (~ 40 rad^{-1}), liver, the lowest (~ 10 rad^{-1}), with spleen, in between.

Unfortunately, uncertainty in the position of the resolution cell when examined from different directions (see Section 6.13.c.ii) make it seem unlikely that the angular dependence of scattering would be worth investigating clinically. Except in the simplest and most idealized situation, the resolution cell may have several values of volume, a different value for each type of interaction: and for a given interaction, it may have a volume which changes with time and with frequency. Also, there may be uncertainties in the position of the resolution cell, in range due to velocity variations in different propagation paths, and in azimuth and elevation due to beam distortions resulting from refraction and transverse attenuation changes, and in any aspect due to physiological movements. These factors make it difficult to imagine how it could be possible to examine the same resolution cell from different directions, and why it is that compounded two-dimensional B-scans are sometimes less informative than linear or radial scans. Expressed simply, it may be better to know *what* something is, whilst not knowing exactly *where* it is, than to emphasize the uncertainty in the position of something the structure of which is also in doubt.

(iv) Fluctuation measurements

The echo amplitude received from blood (or plasma) fluctuates with time (see Section 5.3). The dimensions of the ultrasonic pulse determine the scale of the fluctuation which is detected. Shung *et al.* (1975) have used this phenomenon to measure blood coagulation time. Fluctuations in the amplitude of a backscattered 15 MHz pulse of 4 μs duration persist until a fibrin clot forms, when the fluctuations generally are rather suddenly greatly reduced in amplitude.

6.12.d Frequency Analysis

Strictly speaking, measurements of frequency characteristics cannot be made using short pulses of ultrasound assumed to have associated with them a particular value of frequency, since such pulses contain energy spread over a wide frequency spectrum. This situation has been exploited by Namery and Lele (1972) in experiments designed to confirm that frequency spectrum analysis may be used to measure the dependence of attenuation on frequency over a wide range. They used a transducer with a wide-band frequency response, excited by a fast step voltage, and observed the effect on the echo received from a flat surface when a specimen of tissue was placed in the ultrasonic beam. In this situation, the tissue may be considered to behave like a frequency selective filter, the frequency characteristics of which depend on the attenuation of the ultrasound. Convoluted with this is the frequency response of the measuring system, which determines the frequency spectrum measured with a "lossless" medium.

The experimental results obtained with a slow-sweeping frequency spectrum analyser showed that there are substantial differences in the frequency dependences of attenuation in normal and infarcted myocardium; infarcted tissue attenuates higher frequencies more than does normal tissue. The application of the method to *in vivo* diagnostics, however, would present several problems due to the continual movement of the heart (making spectrum analysis by a slow-speed technique impossible in real time), and to the lack of a standardized reflector on the distal side of the myocardium. Namery and Lele (1972) suggested that the former problem might be overcome by the use of a transient recorder (see Section 6.12.a), but they offered no solution to the latter.

The most detailed and careful study of the frequency characteristics of ultrasound backscattered by biological tissues which has yet been undertaken is that reviewed by Chivers and Hill (1975). The basic experimental apparatus is illustrated in Fig. 6.53. Transducers with nominal frequencies of 1·0, 1·5, 2·0 and 4·0 MHz were used. The duration of the gate opening time determined the depth of the volume of tissue from which back-scattered energy was collected. This is another way of stating that the gate duration affects the frequency spectrum of the echo signals (unless the duration of the echo is less than the gate duration, which may be the case if the reflector is, for example, a flat plate). Therefore, only comparative and rather empirical studies could be made of volume scattering. In these experiments, the gate duration was 8 μs. The typical results illustrated in Fig. 6.54 should be considered with this in mind. The spectra are also convoluted with the frequency response of the transducer. Clearly, and disappointingly, there are no simple criteria for distinguishing the spectra

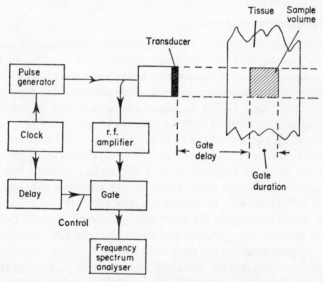

FIG. 6.53 Experimental arrangement for backscattering measurements. (Based on Chivers et al., 1974; Chivers and Hill, 1975.)

from different tissues. Moreover, the comparison of spectra from different tissues, whilst being experimentally convenient, is of little relevance to clinical situations. Another possible application, however, is quite promising: this is in the grading of known types of tissue. Thus, Freese and Hamid (1974) have shown that the frequency dependence of the energy backscattered from fish muscle depends upon the lipid content of the tissue.

These results must lead to caution in considering the value of the ingenious method of Holasek et al. (1975) for colour-coding two-dimensional B-scans according to the frequencies of the echo signals. It must be accepted that tissue characterization on the basis of frequency spectrum analysis is a long way off. Many problems remain to be solved, not the least of which is the uncertainty in the position of the resolution cell, mentioned in Section 6.12.c.iii. Another major difficulty, in common with other methods of tissue characterization by ultrasound, is that of pattern matching; but here, computer-based techniques now being developed in geophysics (Pace, 1975) may hold the key.

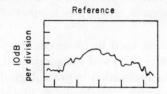

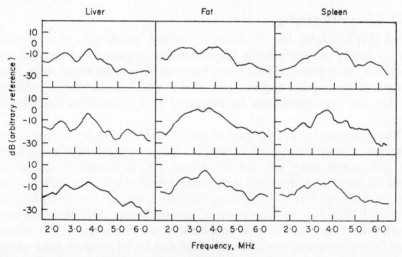

FIG. 6.54 Backscattering spectra from fixed liver, spleen and fat. The reference is the spectrum reflected from a plane surface. Filter width, 300 kHz; gate duration, 8 μs; transducer, "4 MHz". (From Chivers and Hill, 1975.)

6.12.e Signal Averaging

In a conventional pulse–echo system, the equivalent noise level at the input is equal in amplitude to that of the smallest echo signal which is detectable. This is one of the factors which determines the highest frequency which may be used to obtain signals from a particular type of target at any given range (because attenuation increases with frequency). Other things being equal, the frequency is proportional to the resolution (see Section 6.1.b).

It is possible to extract from a wavetrain a signal which is lower in amplitude than the noise, by means of signal averaging. This process, well known in communication theory, depends upon the random nature of noise and the repetitive nature of the signal. Wavetrains obtained with successive ultrasonic pulses are recorded and added together in the correct time relationships: a simple way of doing this is to store sequential samples of the wavetrains in an array of capacitors. The noise signals integrate to zero; the echo signals integrate to produce a noise-free wavetrain equal in amplitude to n times the amplitude which would be produced by a single noise-free echo wavetrain applied to the integrator, where n is number of wavetrains actually captured.

Signal averaging has apparently not yet been used in ultrasonic diagnostics, although it is mentioned by Lees *et al.* (1973) and Furgason *et al.* (1975). One factor which militates against its application is physiological movement, which may disturb the pulse-to-pulse reproducibility of the time–position of the echo signals.

6.12.f Impediography

Jones (1973, 1975a) has described a method which uses time-domain deconvolution of appropriately shaped acoustic impulses and their echoes to obtain the impulse response as a function of acoustic travel time. The integral of the impulse response is related to the characteristic impedance, so that the impedance may be measured as a continuous function of position.

The basic principles of the method are illustrated in Fig. 6.55. The source generates a short broad-band pulse, and the receiver, which detects both the transmitted wave $x(t)$ and the echoes $y(t)$, is located in the initial medium. Now the output $y(t)$ is the convolution of the input $x(t)$ and the impulse response $h(t)$ of the system. Therefore, since $x(t)$ and $y(t)$ may be measured, $h(t)$ may be calculated by deconvolution. The deconvolution process which seems to be most suitable is in the time domain. The effects of additive noise are minimized by the use of an initial pressure pulse which is unipolar, although no doubt algorithms suitable for conventional pulses could be developed. The mathematical analysis is based on the assumption that the media under investigation are arranged in parallel planes, and it is not clear how the results are affected in the study of irregular structures. Nevertheless, some interesting pictures have been published by Jones (1975b).

6.12.g Correlation Techniques

As explained in Section 6.1.a, in a conventional pulse–echo system the transmitted pulses are identical, and in order to avoid range ambiguity it is necessary for the echo from the most distant target to be received before the next pulse is transmitted. Hence

$$T \geqslant 2R_{max}/c \qquad (6.15)$$

where T is the period between pulses and R_{max} is the range of the most distant target. The range resolution ΔR is given by

$$\Delta R = c\Delta\tau/2 \qquad (6.16)$$

where $\Delta\tau$ is the duration of the transmitted pulse. From Eqns. 6.15 and 6.16, the ratio of the peak to the average transmitted powers may be expressed as

$$P_{pk}/P_{av} = T/\Delta\tau \geqslant R_{max}/\Delta R \qquad (6.17)$$

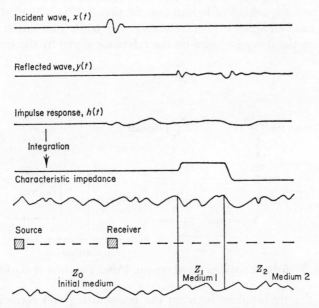

FIG. 6.55 A simple example showing how the characteristic impedances of media may be determined. $Z_2 < Z_0 < Z_1$. (After Jones, 1975a.)

In a practical system, $R_{max}/\Delta R$ is of the order of 100, and so the peak power is at least 100 times greater than the average power.

In medical diagnostics, the peak power (which is directly related to the average power) must be kept as low as possible, in order to minimize the hazard of the procedure. It is self-evident that noise considerations determine the maximum range at which echoes can be detected for a given transmitted power; and noise is related to the bandwidth of the system. Thus

$$SNR_{out}/SNR_{in} = B_{in}/B_{out} \qquad (6.18)$$

where SNR_{out} and SNR_{in} are respectively the signal-to-noise ratios at the output of the system and at the output of the echo-receiving amplifier, and B_{out} and B_{in} are approximately equal (in order to maintain range resolution); and consequently the received echo must be larger in amplitude than the thermal noise of the echo amplifier.

It has been pointed out by Furgason *et al.* (1975) that the input signal-to-noise ratio can be greatly increased by the use of time-averaging techniques which effectively reduce the output bandwidth (see Section 6.12.e). They have also used noise as the transmitted signal: detection involves correlation, and resolution is independent of signal duration. Consequently the peak-to-average transmitted power may be close to unity, and this is relevant to the question of hazard (see Section 9.12). A block diagram of the basic random signal system is shown in Fig. 6.56. The output is a maximum when the delay imposed on the reference signal by the delay line is

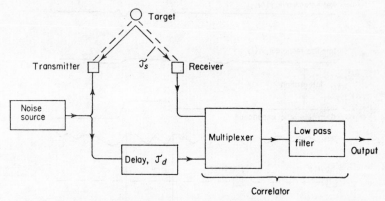

FIG. 6.56 Basic random signal system. (After Furgason *et al.*, 1975.)

equal to the transit time between the transmitting and receiving transducers via the target. (Under these circumstances the two inputs to the correlator are identical, so that it produces its maximum output.) Analysis shows that

$$\Delta R \simeq c/2\pi B \tag{6.19}$$

where B is the bandwidth of the transmitted noise spectrum. This is an important result, since it demonstrates that the resolving power depends on bandwidth and not on the time duration of the transmitted signal. Furthermore, it can be shown that the range resolution does approach a minimum value equal to one-quarter wavelength of the maximum transmitted frequency.

Furgason *et al.* (1975) have described an experimental system and its performance. They used bursts of 4·8 MHz sine waves, and bursts of noise of 2 MHz bandwidth. Their results confirmed that the range resolution does not depend on the signal duration, but only on the bandwidth. The improvement in signal-to-noise ratio was achieved both with sine waves and with noise: the enhancement ratio was 8000 with a mark-to-space ratio of 0·05 and an integration time of 0·1 s.

In principle, several aspects of the operation of this type of system are relevant to its application to medical diagnostics. Firstly, it depends on a time-invariant target situation in order that the correlation process may be completed: it is clear that this condition cannot be totally satisfied in practice. Secondly, although echoes from targets outside the range cell are uncorrelated with those from within, they do increase the effective input and output noise: therefore, they affect the mean value of the output signal corresponding to the target under observation. One solution to this second difficulty would be to use narrow transmitting and receiving beams, over-lapping only in the region under investigation: but see Section 6.13.b.ii for a discussion of the factors affecting the estimation of the position of the resolution cell.

6.13 SYSTEM PERFORMANCE

6.13.a Introduction

The performance of an ultrasonic pulse–echo diagnostic system depends on many factors. This Section is concerned primarily with the performance of the ultrasonic signal path and the registration accuracy.

The overall response of the system is determined by the responses of each of the many individual components in the signal path. It is often necessary to be able to maintain the overall sensitivity of a particular instrument at a constant level, so that the comparison of different scans may have a diagnostic significance. It is desirable to use uniform standards of calibration to allow results to be interchanged. In this connexion, Lypacewicz and Hill (1974) have recommended that on the grounds of comparability with human tissue targets, appropriate absolute target strength and general convenience of use, a steel ball target in the diameter range 4–12 mm should be considered as an intercomparison standard.

6.13.b Signal Path Performance

(i) Ultrasonic frequency

The ultrasonic frequency is determined by the thickness of the transducer (unless it is deliberately driven at an odd harmonic) and its mounting arrangements. This frequency is most easily estimated by measuring the zero-crossing frequency in a received echo–pulse displayed on a calibrated oscilloscope. It is important to realize that it is not strictly correct to describe the pulse as having any particular frequency, because the pulse energy is actually distributed over quite a wide frequency spectrum (see Section 3.6.b.v).

(ii) Transmitted pulse shape and energy

These quantities are rather difficult to measure. The shape of the transmitted pulse may be observed by a wideband detector, such as a capacitor microphone (see Section 3.7.d.i); but it must be remembered that the shape of the pulse propagated in a medium with dispersive absorption changes with time and position. The pulse energy may be calculated by dividing the average (space–time) power (measured, for example, by radiation pressure: see Section 3.7.e.i) by the pulse repetition rate. If radiation pressure is used, corrections may be necessary for the vector directions of divergent or convergent beams.

(iii) Overall voltage transfer function of the transducer

This quantity depends on the bandwidth and sensitivity of the transducer. Its importance and measurement are discussed in Section 3.6.b.v.

(iv) Transducer diameter, beam shape, and intensity

The transducer diameter can be directly measured, but the beam shape depends on many factors. Most plane transducers operating with pulses generate beams which are similar in shape to those which can be calculated for continuous wave excitation, but with changes at the beginning and end of the pulse (see Section 2.2). The distribution of focused beams is more complicated (see Section 2.3). For most practical purposes, it is best to plot the beam distribution by measuring the echo amplitudes received from a small spherical target as it is moved about in the field (see Section 3.7.1).

Given the beam shape and P_{av}, the average (space-time) power, it is quite easy to calculate $\hat{I}_{av}$, the peak spatial-average–temporal intensity. The diametrical distribution of the relative intensity of a typical beam is illustrated in Fig. 6.57. Since all the energy flows along the beam, the ratio of the peak (space–time) intensity to the peak (space–time) power (which is equal to the ratio of the average (space–time) intensity to the average (space–time) power) is given by $\hat{I}_{rel}$ divided by the volume (V) formed by rotating the area under the beam profile provided that these quantities are expressed in compatible units. Therefore

$$\hat{I}_{av} = (\hat{I}_{rel}/V) . P_{av} \tag{6.20}$$

The relationship between $\hat{I}$, the peak (space–time) intensity, and $\hat{I}_{av}$, the peak-spatial average–temporal intensity, depends on the shape of the transmitted pulse and the pulse repetition rate. It is the determination of the pulse shape which poses the most difficult experimental problem. The

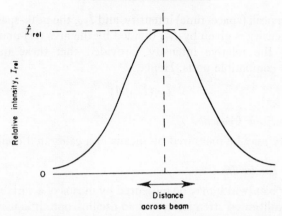

FIG. 6.57 Diametrical distribution of the relative intensity of a typical beam at the temporal peak of an ultrasonic pulse, represented on a linear scale. $\hat{I}_{rel}$ is the relative peak (space–time) intensity.

simplest way of approaching this is to reflect the pulse back into the transducer by which it was generated, and to make the assumption that the voltage waveform thus detected is proportional to the pressure pulse. It is not: but it may be accurate enough, particularly in relation to a clinical situation in which the pulse is transmitted through biological tissues with dispersive absorption, which act as a low-pass filter. A better method, adopted by Kossoff (1969), is to use a receiving transducer with a resonance frequency several times greater than that of the pulse being studied. The next step is to square this voltage waveform: this produces a representation of the intensity oscillation in the pulse, as illustrated in Fig. 6.58. Now the

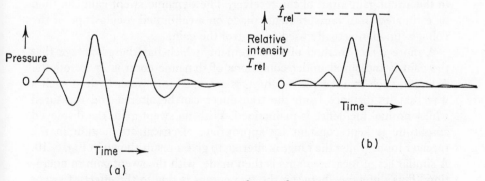

FIG. 6.58 Graphical steps in calculation of $\hat{I}$ from, $\hat{I}_{av}$ for, a typical transmitted pulse. (a) Pulse pressure waveform detected by a wideband receiving transducer; (b) pulse intensity waveform, calculated by squaring the pressure waveform. (After Kossoff, 1969.)

ratio of $\hat{I}$, the peak (space–time) intensity, and $\hat{I}_{av}$, the peak-spatial average–temporal intensity is given by $\hat{I}_{rel}$ divided by the area (A) under the curve representing the relative intensity, provided that these quantities are expressed in compatible units. Hence

$$\hat{I} = (\hat{I}_{rel}/A) \qquad (6.21)$$

(v) Pulse repetition frequency

This quantity may be measured by means of a calibrated oscilloscope.

(vi) Receiver bandwidth

The receiver bandwidth may be measured by means of a variable frequency oscillator, a calibrated attenuator, and an oscilloscope. It is usually best for the input amplitude to the receiver to be varied so that the output remains constant as the frequency band is covered, so that the demodulator threshhold does not introduce any error.

(vii) Maximum receiver gain

This quantity may be determined under pulse conditions by means of a calibrated attenuator at the input to the receiver, and a calibrated oscilloscope at its output, using an echo signal of measured amplitude obtained from a convenient target with the transmitter and transducer normally used in the equipment.

(viii) Swept gain rate

The swept gain is usually controlled by a time-varying voltage. It is possible to measure the receiver gain using the same apparatus as is used to measure the maximum receiver gain, for several values of d.c. control voltage applied to the swept gain input of the receiver. The dynamic swept gain can then be estimated from measurements made on a calibrated oscilloscope of the voltage function actually used to control the gain.

A more direct method of measurement, which has the advantage that the gain is measured under conditions of dynamic control, is as follows. A target, such as a flat plastic sheet, is arranged in a water bath in such a way that its distance from the transducer can be altered and measured whilst normal incidence is maintained. With no swept gain, the displayed amplitude is kept constant by appropriate electrical attenuation in the receiver input whilst the range is altered, to give a result shown in Fig. 6.10. A similar set of measurements is then made, with the swept gain in operation. This difference between the two curves is due to the effect of swept gain.

A somewhat similar method employs an electrical pulse generator triggered by a variable delay (Wells, 1971). The variation in pulse amplitude necessary to maintain constant amplitude at the display as the delay is altered corresponds to the swept gain characteristic. The circuit of the test instrument is indicated in Fig. 6.59. The monostable is triggered by a pulse derived from a precision variable delay circuit, which might conveniently be a comparator fed with a linear voltage ramp. (The timing of the delay generating circuit might be adjusted by reference to the transmission of an ultrasonic pulse across a known distance in water.) The output from the monostable switches off the transistor T. Whilst T is switched on, current flows through L: this current is interrupted when T is switched off, and oscillation occurs in the resonant circuit formed by L and C. The first positive-going oscillation to occur after T has been switched on again is rapidly damped. A proportion of the voltage developed across L is fed to an amplifier which is asymmetrically loaded by D so that the positive and negative half-cycles are of equal amplitudes. The final

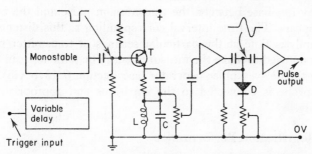

FIG. 6.59 Outline diagram of delayed pulse generator. (From Wells, 1971.)

amplifier provides an output of a suitable impedance to feed a standard calibrated attenuator.

In connexion with the adjustment of the swept gain characteristic, Blackwell (1972) has described an ingenious method of generating a sequence of pulses exponentially decaying in amplitude. Such a sequence should be displayed with uniform amplitude by a system with an appropriately adjusted exponential swept gain. The basis of the method is that a pulse generator is arranged to produce a continuous sequence of short-duration square waves; typically these pulses might have durations of 2 μs, and their leading edges might be separated in time by 13 μs (corresponding to a range interval of about 10 mm). These pulses are multiplied by a second waveform consisting of an exponential decaying voltage with a time constant of perhaps 75 μs. Consequently the output of the multiplier consists of a train of 2 μs pulses, at a repetition frequency of 75 kHz, decaying exponentially in amplitude with time at around—in this particular example—1·5 dB cm^{-1}.

(ix) Signal processing arrangements

An accurate specification of the signal processing arrangements may be very complicated. The amplitude and frequency characteristics of the receiver are particularly important.

(x) Overall dynamic range

The amplitude of an input signal derived from a standard target, or for example from the delayed pulse generator mentioned in connexion with swept gain rate measurement, is adjusted to determine the range over which variations in the output signal may be detected. This is the overall dynamic range.

(xi) Overall paralysis time

Buschmann (1965) has described how the paralysis time may be measured by moving the transducer towards a flat target until the disturbed part of the display timebase between the transmission pulse and the echo signal just disappears. The time interval corresponding to this distance is equal to the paralysis time at the particular settings of transmitter power and receiver gain used to make the measurement. The same test can be carried out using the delayed pulse generator (see Section 6.13.b.viii), provided that the probe is connected to the apparatus and appropriately loaded acoustically.

6.13.c Registration Performance

(i) Timebase circuits and geometrical adjustment

It is easy to check the range calibration of an A-scope designed for echo-encephalography, by means of a plastic rod of appropriate length, grooved at its centre to give an echo corresponding to the midline (Hudson and Bradley, 1973). A polystyrene rod of 190 mm length is suitable, with slabs of polytetrafluorethylene of 9·5 mm each end to simulate the skull. This thickness of p.t.f.e. gives an apparent skull thickness of five times normal, but it has a realistic attenuation at a frequency of 2 MHz.

The diagnostic value of time–position recording frequently depends upon accurate calibration. Fixed-range targets can be used for distance calibration, and an ordinary stopwatch for time-calibration. A convenient method which provides calibration of both distance and time has been described by Wells and Ross (1969). A block diagram of the arrangement is shown in Fig. 6.60. The multivibrator provides trigger pulses at a rate of 2 s^{-1}: the two outputs from the bistable are antiphase square waves with "on" times of 0·5 s. These pulses switch reed relays which connect either one or other of two transducers into circuit. One transducer provides an echo delayed by a time corresponding to a distance of 50 mm in blood, and the other, to 70 mm. Reed relays are suitable in this application because of their fast switching time, long life, and small open/closed signal ratio. The reflexions from each of the two transducers are matched in amplitude by the preset attenuators.

Fleming and Hall (1968) have discussed the various factors which control the display registration accuracy in two-dimensional electrically coupled scanners. They defined the registration accuracy as the accuracy with which a point reflector is represented as a single point on the display when viewed ultrasonically from a number of different positions, assuming a system with zero beamwidth and perfect range resolution. Within the terms of this definition, the registration is limited by the precision of the mechanical and electrical parts of the scanning system. Although primarily concerned

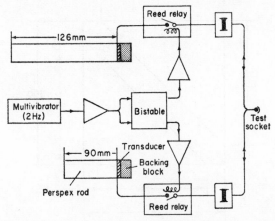

FIG. 6.60 Block diagram of instrument for distance and time calibration of time–position recording system. (After Wells and Ross, 1969.)

with a scanner such as that illustrated in Fig. 6.33(d), much of the discussion in their article is relevant to other arrangements. They considered the effects of imperfections in the sine/cosine and linear potentiometers, and of errors in the mechanical alignment of the measuring axes, in the timebase generators and deflexion amplifiers, and in the adjustment of the transmitter delay and the timebase velocity. They concluded that, in the system which they analysed, there was more than a 90% probability that the spot would fall within three spot diameters (1·5 mm) of the true position, at a range of 200 mm on a one-fifth actual size display. This is an acceptable performance in relation to the lateral and range resolutions which can be achieved in practice.

A phantom for testing the accuracy of both the timebase delay and velocity of two-dimensional contact scanners is available commercially, and has been described by Blackwell (1972). As shown in Fig. 6.61, it consists of a block of polymethylmethacrylate, 300 mm square and 40 mm thick. Two cuts parallel to the diagonal are made, and the pieces glued together again with an impact adhesive. The dimensions are such that if both the transmitter delay and the time-base velocity are correct, the result of scanning around the three accessible faces of the block is an image of a 300 mm square with a central cross. This is because, no matter what may be the position of the probe save at the corners enclosed by the diagonals, the path length of the pulse in the plastic is constant (261 mm), since the diagonal cuts act as reflectors. The dimensions are chosen so that the associated delay is equal to that which would be experienced in a tissue-

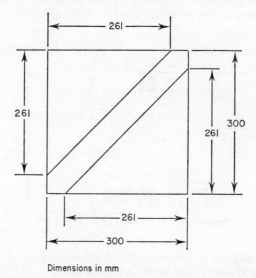

Dimensions in mm

FIG. 6.61 Phantom for testing the adjustment of the resolvers and timebases of two-dimensional scanners. (After Blackwell, 1972.)

equivalent material with a central cross reflector: that is, the velocity in the plastic is taken to be 1·74 times that in soft tissue. On the other hand, if the instrument is incorrectly calibrated, two crosses appear near the centre of the display.

Another method of testing the registration accuracy of two-dimensional contact scanners has been described by Hall and Fleming (1975). It depends on the use as an accurate timing reference of a PAL chrominance delay line. This is an acoustic delay line which produces echoes separated by 63·943 + 0·005 μs over the temperature range 20–50°C: it is a cheap, commercially available device, manufactured primarily for the domestic television market. This time delay corresponds to a distance of 49·23 mm at a velocity of 1540 ms^{-1}, so that the third (i.e. second multiple reflexion) echo is produced at a range of 147·69 mm. The calibration method consists of replacing the transducer with a linkage, fixed to a bearing at one end, which allows the position normally occupied by the face of the transducer to rotate around a circle with a radius of 147·69 mm, with the centre of the circle on the line normally occupied by the ultrasonic beam. The pulse–echo system is connected to the delay line. When the probe housing is rotated, a series of arcs is drawn on the display, with the third arc appearing as a single point in a correctly adjusted instrument. If the instrument is incorrectly adjusted, a small arc is registered near the position of the centre of rotation, according to the error giving rise to the misalignment.

Test targets, consisting of grids of fine, parallel wires, which can be immersed in water and scanned, are popular with many people as aids in checking and adjusting the registration of two-dimensional scanners. One such target is illustrated in Fig. 6.62. It would be wrong to seem to be enthusiastic about this type of test. It is unnecessarily complicated for the checking of alignment, and anyway the velocity in water does not necessarily match that in tissue. As a method of estimating resolution, it can be misleading, since gain and swept gain adjustments which are correct in tissue are inappropriate in water.

(ii) Registration errors due to inhomogeneous propagation

The various phenomena which lead to errors in registration—or, to express the matter more generally, to uncertainties in the position of the resolution cell—have been considered, particularly in relation to the effects of the skull and the brain, by White et al. (1969a, b), and, in relation to soft-tissue structures, by Halliwell and Mountford (1973) and Mountford and Halliwell (1973). In principle, these phenomena include:

(i) Spatial compression or extension of the ultrasonic beam along its axis, due to differences in velocity in different tissues (causing errors in range estimation);

(ii) Refraction at boundaries across which velocity changes occur (causing errors in azimuth and elevation due to deviation of the axis of the ultrasonic beam);

(iii) Deformation of the beam, which may be in the form of changes in direction, profile or divergence. Thus the beam may be deviated if it travels through a region across which there is a uniformly changing attenuation. The deviation may amount to a change in beam profile if the change in attenuation is non-uniform. Finally, the divergence of the beam may change, due either to refraction at non-planar boundaries, or to the downward shift in the centre frequency of the pulse resulting from dispersive absorption; and

(iv) Physiological movements (see Taylor and Hill, 1975).

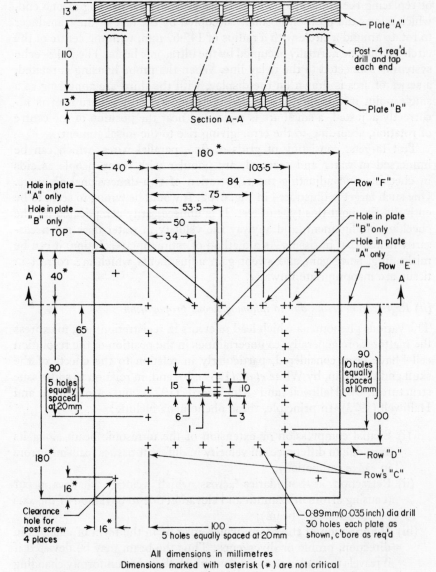

All dimensions in millimetres
Dimensions marked with asterisk (∗) are not critical

FIG. 6.62 "Standard 10 cm Test Object" recommended by the American Institute of Ultrasound in Medicine, for checking and adjusting the alignment of two-dimensional ultrasonic scanners. The target is used by scanning it immersed in a water bath.

In the skull, the effects of beam deformation may be so severe as to make transcranial investigations virtually useless, except possibly for measurements of the position of the midline structures, or visualization of the ventricles in hydrocephalics. In soft tissues, deviation and divergence changes are small, but the deformation of the beam could lead to registration errors of the order of 20 mm in abdominal scans, and proportionate errors at higher frequencies in smaller structures. This may make compound scanning most unsatisfactory.

In considering the quality of an echogram, one of the factors with which the clinician is concerned is the minimum spacing at which he can distinguish separate structures as separate registrations on the display. In two-dimensional scans, particularly of the foetus, certain structures are quite regularly spaced, and Garrett and Kossoff (1975) have proposed that the minimum detectable rib or vertebra spacing, might be taken as the reciprocal of the resolution. As test objects, foetuses are freely available in places where ultrasonic scans are routinely made for obstetric purposes; moreover, since the scans are required for patient care, ethical difficulties do not arise. This approach is convenient nowadays, when resolutions of up to about 0.5 mm^{-1} are being achieved, but may become unduly coarse in the future.

6.14 MEASUREMENT OF PATIENT IRRADIATION

The data concerning the irradiation conditions used in pulse–echo diagnosis are sparse indeed. Once in a while, an article on a diagnostic procedure includes some estimate, more or less reputable, of the intensity of the ultrasound. It is well known, however, that the intensities of different instruments may be very different. Thus, Hill (1971) measured the ranges quoted in Table 6.3 for commercially produced pulse–echo systems. Even where the irradiation conditions at the surface of the probe (or in a lossless medium) are known, it is difficult to predict the "dose" which will be

TABLE 6.3

Operating conditions of output for some commercial pulse–echo instruments

Quantity	Value
Nominal frequency, f	0.5–6.0 MHz
Pulse duration	0.2–2.0 μs
Pulse repetition rate	480–1200 s^{-1}
Average ultrasonic power, P_{av}	<0.3–21 mW
Peak (space–time) intensity, $\hat{I}$	1.4–95 W cm^{-2}

From Hill (1971).

received by a volume of tissue irradiated within the patient. For example, Bang (1972) has reported a surprisingly low value of apparent attenuation (2·5 dB) in the transmission of 2·25 MHz pulses from the abdominal wall to the uterine cavity.

Practitioners of ultrasonic diagnostics are well advised to be cautious lest the method may be hazardous. This possibility is discussed in Section 9.12. Being aware that more data are necessary, some users of ultrasonic diagnostic systems have constructed instruments which record the "dose" received by the patient during an examination.

Thus, Whittingham (1973) has described an instrument which indicates a number related to the worst-case "dose" which could have been received by the patient, assuming perfect ultrasonic coupling. Likewise, Hutchison (1974) has described a circuit which derives a voltage proportional to that applied to the transducer, and generates a signal with a frequency which is proportional to the square of this voltage. This frequency is proportional to the "intensity" of the ultrasound produced by the transducer. At a fixed interval (30 μs) after the transmitter has been triggered, a gate is opened (for 270 μs), and if echoes are received during the time that this gate is open, a second gate is opened which allows the pulses from the voltage-to-frequency converter to be fed to a digital counter. This second gate is held open for a time in excess of the longest pulse repetition period. The presence of echoes indicates that the probe is in contact with the patient, and that ultrasound is being delivered. Therefore, the number integrated by the counter is proportional to the total ultrasonic energy received by the patient.

In "dosemeters" of this type, a major source of inaccuracy is inadequate coupling between the probe and the patient: this leads to overestimation of the energy delivered. Even with perfect coupling, however, errors of 10% or so can occur due to variations in the characteristic impedances of differing tissues (see Section 4.8).

6.15 AIDS FOR TRAINING OPERATORS

It cannot be overemphasized that really satisfactory scans can be obtained with two-dimensional contact scanners only if the operator has mastered the art of scanning. Aids like the velocity-controlled timebase (see Section 6.8.b.iii) and the scan conversion memory (Section 6.6.d) only go part of the way towards replacing the skill of the operator. In addition, operators need to learn how to adjust the various controls.

To a limited extent, novices can gain experience by scanning phantoms instead of patients. Some suitable phantoms have been described by Holmes and Williams (1973). Their so-called "training tank" consists of a barrel-shaped chamber approximately 300 mm in diameter and 360 mm long, made from a flexible plastic tube with rigid end plates, and filled with water. Various test objects can be inserted through holes in the end plates, and supported at appropriate places within the tank.

A training tank has three main advantages. These are:

(i) The trainee can compare his scan with the shape of the phantom;
(ii) The need to practise on patients is reduced, thus avoiding mutual embarrassment; and
(iii) Patients are not unnecessarily exposed to ultrasound.

Presumably a difficulty in the use of this type of training tank is due to the attenuation of ultrasound in water being very much less than in soft tissues, so that reverberation may be troublesome, and the swept gain and sensitivity controls need special adjustment.

In addition to two-dimensional contact scanning, operators must learn the arts of A-scanning and time–position scanning. When the preliminaries are over, there is no substitute for practising on patients under the supervision of an expert. The extent to which the novice needs to become competent before he can begin to examine patients independently depends upon the degree of isolation with which he has to cope. If he is to work side-by-side with friendly physicists and helpful radiologists, on the average a couple of weeks of training in the clinic is all that is required by a person with a reasonable knowledge of anatomy, pathology, and the basic physical principles of echography. If he is to be single-handed in some distant hospital, the apprenticeship must be longer.

It is very helpful to the newcomer to be aware of the mistakes which are commonly made, so that he may try to avoid them. In this connexion, papers by Hall *et al.* (1972) and Holm *et al.* (1972) deal with many of the salient points.

In places where ultrasonic diagnostics is well established, satisfactory schemes generally exist for describing and labelling scans in relation to the corresponding anatomical sections. Difficulties can arise when comparison is to be made of scans from different centres, labelled in different ways. Standardization is desirable here, and Holm *et al.* (1971) and McDicken and Evans (1975) have proposed how this might be done.

A number of courses for training operators are running in different parts of the world. No doubt the number will increase as more patients demand this type of investigation, and more doctors come to depend on it. The content of the course must be chosen to suit the needs of the trainee— technicians require to be taught physics, anatomy and pathology, radiographers and doctors need more physics than anatomy and pathology, and physicists, vice versa. Reading is an essential element of training, and the book edited by Wells (1977) may be helpful here. As the number of people involved in providing ultrasonic diagnostic services increases, so will the need for their examination and certification. This operational problem already threatens to inhibit the introduction of this powerful aid in patient care.

6.16 CLINICAL APPLICATIONS

6.16.a Angiology

(*i*) *Angiography*

Studies of the abdominal aorta have been made using the A-scan (Segal *et al.*, 1966; Evans *et al.*, 1967; Leopold, 1970), and the two-dimensional B-scan (Goldberg *et al.*, 1966; Evans *et al.*, 1967; Laustela and Tähti, 1968; Leopold 1970; Holm, 1971; Kristensen *et al.*, 1972; Birnholz, 1973; Winsberg *et al.*, 1974). The patient is examined in the supine position. Both direct-contact probes and water-bath coupled instruments have been used, although the former are generally the more convenient. In up to about half of the patients, it is impossible to visualize the aorta because of the intervention of gut containing gas. In such circumstances, satisfactory results can sometimes be obtained later, possibly after the patient has taken a mild laxative.

The examination of the aorta is best begun by making a number of longitudinal two-dimensional B-scans parallel to, and extending as far as possible from the xiphoid to the symphysis. A typical scan is shown in Fig. 6.63. Although the tortuosity of the aorta may preclude the visualization of its entire length on a single scan, it is possible to see—particularly in grey-scale displays—such features as intraluminal thrombus, dissections, false aneurysm, teflon grafts, and aneurysmal involvement of the iliac arteries (Winsberg *et al.*, 1974). If the aorta is more than 30 mm in diameter, it is likely to be abnormal.

Conventional radiological investigations of the aorta have several disadvantages. Thus, although computerized tomography is likely to be as reliable as ultrasound, it is not widely available and in any case it cannot be used to scan a patient repeatedly on account of the radiation hazard. Although calcification may allow the aorta to be visualized on a plain film, it is more usual for contrast aortography to be required. Ultrasonic aortography is useful in patients in whom contrast aortography is contraindicated. The comparative results of Birnholz (1973) indicate that it is more informative than scintigraphy, which in any case reveals only the lumen of the vessel.

Although the aorta is the abdominal vessel which has received most attention in ultrasonic scanning, other arteries and veins can be visualized. According to Taylor (1975), the terminal portion of the inferior vena cava can be demonstrated by two-dimensional scanning in every patient, and in cases of obstruction it is possible either directly or indirectly to deduce the cause. Leopold (1975) has discussed the visualization, in addition to the aorta and vena cava, of the mesenteric and renal arteries, and the portal, mesenteric and renal veins. Visualization of the portal vein should lead to better guidance in percutaneous portal venography. It may soon become possible to measure flow in these vessels by range-finding Doppler methods. Moreover, visualization of vessels enables neighbouring structures to be identified; for example, the portal vein may be used as a landmark for the pancreas.

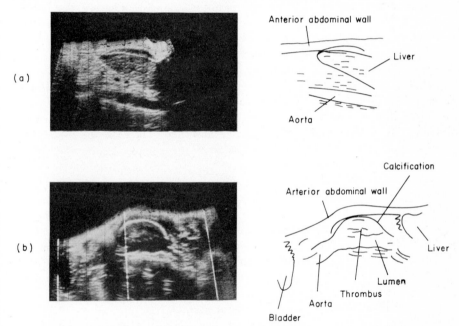

FIG. 6.63 Longitudinal sections through the abdominal aorta. (a) Normal; (b) aortic aneurysm. (Courtesy F. G. M. Ross.)

Pulse–echo techniques have also been used in evaluating aneurysms of the femoral artery (Holm *et al.*, 1968), and in estimating the diameter of the thoracic aorta and of the right pulmonary artery, with the probe in the suprasternal region (Goldberg, 1971).

(ii) Arterial wall properties

Atherosclerosis is a disease which involves the arterial system in an irregular fashion. It results in hardening of the arteries—arteriosclerosis—and in an irregular narrowing of the arterial lumen which results in impaired flow. Atherosclerosis of the coronary arteries is the cause of most heart attacks and sudden cardiac deaths; disease of the carotids is a common cause of stroke; and involvement of the arteries of the leg can cause intermittent claudication, and gangrene of the limb.

Present diagnostic methods depend on X-ray angiography (involving an injection of contrast medium). When the blood supply to the heart is impaired, the e.c.g. may be suspect.

Ultrasonic echoes from an artery exhibit pulse-synchronous displacements as well as variations in amplitude. Kristensen *et al.* (1971) found that these pulsations in the internal carotid artery tended to be reduced in carotid artery disease. The method is not easy to use, however. A variant of it has been described by Buschmann (1973), who used an A-scope instrument, designed for ophthalmology, to study on a time–motion display the movements of the anterior and posterior walls of the common carotid artery. The probe had a diameter of 5 mm, and a nominal frequency of 5–8 MHz. Direct coupling was used. Successful recordings were obtained in 20 out of 38 volunteers. The adjustment of the probe position is of crucial importance. The best procedure is to find the middle of the artery using the minimum possible sensitivity, and then to increase the sensitivity slightly to allow continuous recording of the echoes despite the small movements of the arterial walls.

Skelton and Olson (1972) have described how it is possible to obtain echoes from the walls of the pulmonary artery, using an ultrasonic probe positioned in the oesophagus. The probe could be rotated, and the transducer could be tilted (using a remote control at the far end of the probe) to adjust the direction of the ultrasonic beam to the optimum position. It is difficult to obtain this information by any other method, on account of the short length, thin wall, low intraluminal pressure, and inaccessible position of the artery. In dogs, it was found that the pulmonary artery expands by $20 \pm 7\%$ of its diastolic diameter during systole.

Preliminary experiments carried out by Lees *et al.* (1969) have indicated that the diameter and the wall thickness of a blood vessel may be measured to within 0·1 mm, using a pulse–echo system excited with a transient of 7 ns duration.

Atherosclerosis, in its fully developed form, is associated with structural changes in all layers of the arterial wall. The changes alter its viscoelastic properties. As new methods for the treatment of lipid disorders are developed, it becomes more urgent to have a better knowledge of the natural history of the disease. Mozersky *et al.* (1972) have used the ultrasonic echo-tracking method of Hokanson *et al.* (1972) to study changes in the diameter of the artery, and for recording wall movement. Since the instrument operates transcutaneously, the procedure may be repeated as often as may be desired.

An ultrasonic probe is positioned on the skin, to which it is coupled through an acoustic gel, to receive echoes from both the proximal and distal walls of the artery. Typically, the ultrasonic frequency is 5 MHz, and the pulse repetition rate is 60 s^{-1}. The echoes are displayed on an A-scope: echoes from the vessel walls can be distinguished from those arising from other interfaces, since they move synchronously with the cardiac pulse. In order to track an echo, a gate is opened for about 100 ns at a selected time interval after the transmitter trigger. This allows one half-cycle of the echo to be received. When the arterial wall moves, the phase of the echo alters. A feedback circuit is arranged to move the time–position of the gate, thereby preserving the original phase relationship. Thus, the gate locks out a single half-cycle of the echo and tracks its movement. The use of two gates enables the proximal and distal echoes to be tracked simultaneously, and the delay between the two gates corresponds to the diameter of the artery. Time is converted to distance by the use of a digital timer-counter.

Mozersky *et al.* (1972) obtained the following data from 68 common femoral arteries in 36 normal patients, divided into three groups according to age: mean diastolic diameter (D), maximum change in diameter (ΔD), and pulse pressure (ΔP). They calculated the corresponding values of E_p, the pressure–strain elastic modulus, from the relationship

$$E_p = (D/\Delta D).\Delta P \qquad (6.22)$$

In this calculation, D is considered to be the external diameter. Although there is some uncertainty about the actual parts of the walls from which the tracked echoes arise, the maximum error is unlikely to exceed 10%. Summarizing the results, for the age group under 35 years, $E_p = (2\cdot64 \pm 0\cdot26) \times 10^{-7}$ N m^{-2}; for the 35–60 year group, $E_p = (3\cdot88 \pm 0\cdot43) \times 10^{-7}$ N m^{-2}; and for the group over 60 years, $E_p = (6\cdot28 \pm 1\cdot03) \times 10^{-7}$ N m^{-2}; the ranges indicated are the standard errors of the means. This is in agreement with the widely held opinion that even in the absence of significant arteriosclerosis, the arteries become less distensible with age. It is only fair to point out, however, that there was considerable variation within the groups, and there was a quite substantial overlap in E_p values for individuals in the oldest group, into the range of the youngest group.

Finally, it has been shown by Hartley and Strandness (1969) that the presence of calcified plaques may be detected by an increase in the attenuation of ultrasonic pulses transmitted through aortic and iliac vessel walls. At 5 MHz, this attenuation is 100–130 dB cm^{-1}, compared with up to 15 dB cm^{-1} for normal vessel walls and non-calcified plaques.

(iii) Detection of gas bubble formation within tissues due to decompression

When people are decompressed—for example, on returning to normal pressure after diving, or working in caissons, or on flying to high altitudes— bubbles of oxygen may form within the tissues of their bodies. The immediate result is localized pain; and subsequently, permanent damage, particularly to bones, may result. In order to minimize these risks, quite strict procedures are enforced in occupations where the dangers are recognized. It has long been realized, however, that merely to rely on the individual complaining of pain as a yardstick in controlling the rate of return to normal pressure is not good enough. A method is needed to warn that bubbles have formed in the tissues, before they are noticed by the person being decompressed. In this application, ultrasound seems to offer the best chance of success. There are five methods which have been tested:

(i) Attenuation of ultrasound in traversing an accessible sample of tissue: Powell (1972) has reported that, in rats, the transmission through the feet or thigh muscles may be reduced by up to 25 dB at 6 MHz, during experimental decompression;

(ii) Reduction in the echo amplitude from an anatomical interface of controlled geometry: Walder *et al.* (1968) reported that the echo from the surface of a skin-fold opposite a pulsed ultrasonic probe is reduced if gas bubbles form within the tissue;

(iii) Distortion due to non-linear response of tissue containing gas bubbles: this method, proposed by Tucker and Welsby (1968), depends on the detection of second harmonics in a wave transmitted through gas-containing tissue, but in practice it has turned out to be unreliable;

(iv) Visualization of bubbles by a high-speed, high-resolution two-dimensional B-scanner: it has been shown by Rubissow and MacKay (1974), using such an instrument operating at an ultrasonic frequency of 7·5 MHz, that bubbles tend first to appear in blood in fatty tissue, except after short dives, when they appear in muscle; and

(v) Detection of Doppler shifts in ultrasound backscattered by bubbles moving in blood: this is discussed in Section 7.3.a.vi.

6.16.b Cardiology

The possibility that clinically useful information about cardiac structure and function might be obtained from pulse–echo ultrasonic measurements was first proposed by Edler and Hertz (1954). They showed that echoes can be obtained transcutaneously from within the heart. In a series of elegant experiments, Edler (1961) identified many of the structures which gave rise to these echoes.

It would not be appropriate, in this book, to present anything more than a rather superficial review of the clinical applications of pulse–echo ultrasonic diagnostics in cardiology. For a more detailed description of the subject, reference should be made to a specialized work, such as the excellent monograph by Feigenbaum (1972). In addition, a collection of recent articles and abstracts dealing with various aspects of echocardiography may be found in White (1975), pp. 1–109.

The anterior of the heart is normally covered by lung and pleura, save for a small triangular area in the left parasternal region. It is only through the intercostal spaces of this area that the heart can be examined by ultrasound without interference by gas-filled lung or by ribs. Echocardiography

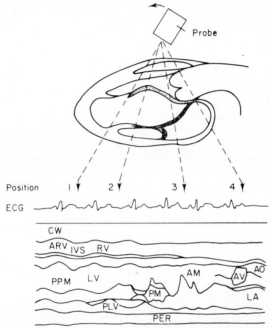

Fig. 6.64 Time–position arc scan of the left heart. The diagram of the heart shows the mitral valve in its closed position (black) and its fully opened diastolic position (stippled). The various structures identified in the scan are: ARV, anterior right ventricular wall; RV, right ventricle; IVS, interventricular septum; LV, left ventricle; PPM, posterior papillary muscle; PLV, posterior left ventricular wall; PM, posterior mitral valve cusp; AM, anterior mitral valve cusp; PER, pericardium; AV, aortic valve cusps; LA, left atrium; AO, aortic outflow tract; CW, chest wall. Note that the scan is distorted spatially by the increasing distance corresponding to a given angular change at increasing range.

may not be possible in patients with emphysema, and in those in whom the ribs have been disturbed by previous surgery.

(i) Heart valve studies

Echoes can generally be received from the anterior leaflet of the mitral valve, if the probe is placed over an intercostal space in the left parasternal region, as shown in Fig. 6.64. In the average adult, the anterior cusp lies

58–83 mm from the anterior surface of the chest, depending on various factors including the phase of the cardiac cycle.

The examination of the mitral valve is based on techniques reviewed by Edler (1966). The method of investigation can be understood by reference to Fig. 6.65, which shows a time–position arc scan of a normal left ventricle. This is obtained by slowly changing the direction of the ultrasonic beam from the apex of the heart to the aortic root, whilst simultaneously making a time–position recording of the received echoes, together with the e.c.g. and phonocardiogram. In this application, an ultrasonic frequency of

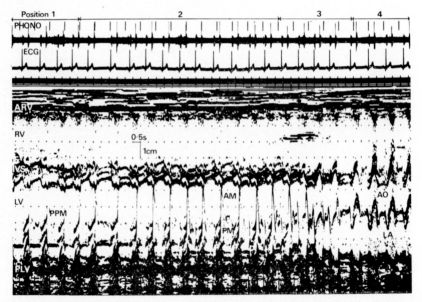

FIG. 6.65 Time–position arc scan of the normal left heart. (Courtesy Ö. Feizi.)

2–3 MHz is generally used, at a pulse repetition rate of 1000 s⁻¹. Suitable instrumentation is described in Section 6.9.

When the ultrasonic beam passes through the edge of the anterior cusp of the mitral valve, a recording such as that shown diagrammatically in Fig. 6.66 is obtained. This is called the "mitral valve echocardiogram". During left atrial systole, the mitral valve opens and the echocardiogram moves upwards to point A, which occurs just after the P wave of the e.c.g. This is followed by a rapid deflexion downwards through B to C, produced by the closing of the valve at the beginning of systole. Point C coincides with the first heart sound. This is followed by a slow rise of the trace to D, corresponding to the forward movement of the whole valve and its ring during ventricular systole. In order to be completely satisfactory from a technical point of view, it is necessary simultaneously to record the motion of both the anterior and the posterior mitral valve leaflets. The posterior leaflet normally moves with a similar pattern to that of the anterior leaflet, but in the opposite direction and with a smaller amplitude. The first component of the second heart sound, due to closure of the aortic valve, occurs 10–50 ms before point D. As the ventricle relaxes in diastole, the valve cusps swing wide open and the echocardiogram rises steeply upwards to point E. The ventricle fills rapidly with blood from the left atrium, and the anterior mitral valve cusp is forced backwards whilst the valve ring also moves in the same direction. During this phase, the echocardiogram may transcribe a two-stage downward slope, sometimes called the "diastolic

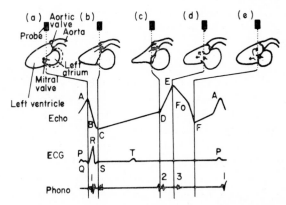

FIG. 6.66 The normal mitral valve echocardiogram, showing the time-relationships to the e.c.g. and the phonocardiogram. The arrows indicate the directions of the blood flow in the diagrams of the left side of the heart. On the echocardiogram, increasing downward deflexion of the trace corresponds to increasing depth of the anterior cusp of the mitral valve (i.e. closing of the valve). (a) Atrial systole; (b) early ventricular systole; (c) late ventricular systole; (d) ventricular diastole: rapid filling phase; (e) late ventricular diastole. (After Ross, 1972.)

slope", through point F_0 to point F, the first part of the slope being less steep than the second part; these two stages are often merged into one. After point F, the trace may remain level during slow ventricular filling, particularly if the heart rate is slow. Occasionally a low amplitude rise may be seen shortly after point F, but usually the trace moves directly to the next A-wave. In sinus arhythmia, which in the young is normal during respiratory inspiration, the A-wave disappears.

The normal mitral valve echocardiogram may be quantitated in terms of the diastolic slope (the slope of the E–F line, even if F_0 ispresent) and the amplitude of its excursion (the distance C–E): typical values are given in

TABLE 6.4

Speed and amplitude of movement of the anterior cusp of the mitral valve in various clinical conditions

Clinical condition	Diastolic slope, mm s^{-1}		Amplitude, mm	
	Mean	Range	Mean	Range
Normal	114	70–160	22	14–33
Stenosis	19	6–40	17	8–32
Regurgitation	198	120–280	33	22–55
Regurgitation with dominant stenosis	20	10–36	16	10–22
Stenosis with dominant regurgitation	77	55–90	24	20–30

Data of Ross (1972).

Table 6.4. This table also lists corresponding values in disease, the relevance of which is discussed in the following paragraphs.

The characteristic pattern of the mitral valve echocardiogram is modified when the valve is diseased. Some examples are given in Fig. 6.67. In mitral stenosis, the anterior cusp cannot move rapidly backwards during early diastole, because of the raised left atrial pressure. The backward movement is slower than in the normal, and it continues for a longer time. The amplitude of the excursion of the valve is also reduced. Typical values are given in Table 6.4. Although the A-wave is often absent, multiple A-waves may appear when the interval between contractions is long.

In the early days of echocardiography, it was thought that a slow rate of posterior movement of the anterior mitral valve cusp following the E wave was diagnostic of mitral stenosis. It is now clear, however, that this abnormal motion may also be found in atrial myxoma, primary pulmonary hypertension, aortic stenosis, aortic insufficiency, and hypertrophic cardiomyopathy. Some aspects of this are mentioned later in this Sub-section. Thus this slope is a measure of the rate of ventricular filling, and in the absence of mitral valve obstruction it has been shown by Quinones et al. (1974) to be due to alteration in the diastolic properties of the left ventricle.

In pure mitral regurgitation, the echocardiogram is similar in form to that in the normal, but increased in both diastolic slope and excursion amplitude, as indicated in Table 6.4. The clinical significance of this has been discussed by Segal et al. (1967b). Some caution in interpretation is necessary, since similar echocardiograms may be found in patients with high flow-rates through the mitral valve, such as may occur in congenital heart disease (Ultan et al., 1967), and even in normals.

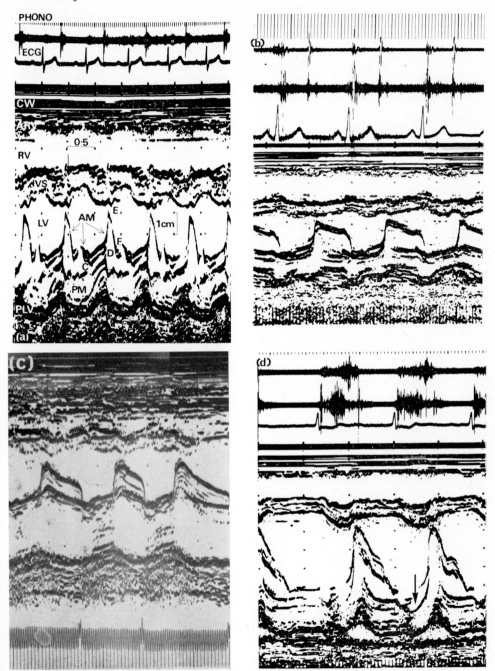

FIG. 6.67 Echocardiograms of the mitral valve. (a) Normal mitral valve; (b) mitral stenosis; (c) combined mitral stenosis and regurgitation; (d) mitral prolapse: the arrow indicates the characteristically abnormal movement. ((a), (b) and (d), courtesy Ö. Feizi; (c), courtesy F. G. M. Ross.)

In patients who have combined mitral stenosis and regurgitation, the shape of the echocardiogram depends on which lesion is dominant. If stenosis is dominant, the tracing resembles that in pure mitral stenosis, as indicated in Table 6.4. On the other hand, if regurgitation is dominant, the early diastolic slope is greater than that in pure stenosis, and a more gradual slope continues for the next phase of diastole (Segal et al., 1967a).

Mitral valve prolapse may be diagnosed from the mitral echocardiogram by the appearance of an abrupt posterior displacement of the anterior leaflet during systole (Dillon et al., 1970).

Duchak et al. (1972) seem to have been the first to report the erratic motion of the anterior leaflet of the mitral valve during diastole in patients with torn anterior chordae; the fluttering is much coarser than that seen in aortic regurgitation. With torn posterior chordae, the posterior mitral valve leaflet remains posterior throughout systole and returns anteriorly during ventricular diastole. Prolapse of the mitral valve, on the other hand, does not affect the posterior leaflet motion in early systole.

Hypertrophic cardiomyopathy (HC), with or without obstruction, is a condition in which there is asymmetrical hypertrophy of the interventricular septum and the left ventricular wall. The echographic aspects have been discussed by Feizi and Emanuel (1975). Mitral valve echocardiography (Popp and Harrison, 1969; Shah et al., 1969) reveals, as shown in Fig. 6.68, that the normal gradual anterior systolic movement (C–D) is replaced by a more pronounced deflexion which begins after the onset of ejection from the ventricle and continues to the end of systole. Kingsley and Segal (1969) seem to have been the first to demonstrate that this is because the anterior mitral valve leaflet and the interventricular septum come into contact during systole in patients with hypertrophic obstructive cardiomyopathy (HOCM). Clinically it is often difficult to distinguish these patients from those with coronary artery disease. In addition there may be a reduced diastolic (E–F) slope due to the reduced rate of filling resulting from the low compliance of the ventricle. Even in the presence of fixed left ventricular outflow obstruction, Chung et al. (1974) were able to find abnormal systolic anterior movement of the anterior mitral valve leaflet, on retrospective examination of the echocardiograms of patients who subsequently proved to have HOCM.

A myxoma of the left atrium is a pedunculated soft tissue mass which arises from the interatrial septum. It may enlarge sufficiently either to grow, hour-glass fashion, through the mitral valve orifice, or it may move into the left ventricle during diastole, returning to the left atrium during systole. The tumour may be diagnosed from its echocardiogram (see Fig. 6.69) which is reminiscent in shape of that which occurs in mitral stenosis, and which is characterized by multiple echoes in the left atrium particularly in diastole (Edler, 1965; Wolfe et al., 1969).

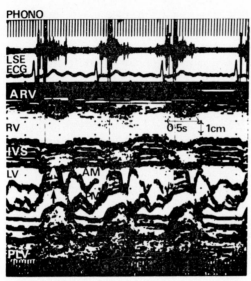

FIG. 6.68 Mitral valve echocardiogram in hypertrophic cardiomyopathy. LSE: left sternal edge. (Courtesy Ö. Feizi.)

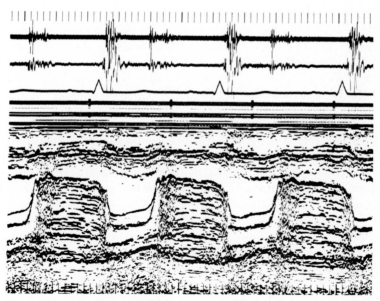

FIG. 6.69 Mitral valve echocardiogram in left atrial myxoma. Note anechoic space posterior to anterior leaflet in early diastole, preceding the movement of the tumour into the orifice. (Courtesy Ö. Feizi.)

In the presence of aortic regurgitation, an apical diastolic rumbling murmur is often heard: this is the so-called "Austin Flint murmur". In the presence of this murmur, it is not possible to determine, using conventional methods of diagnosis, whether or not the mitral valve is diseased. Echocardiography of the mitral valve can quickly resolve this problem. Moreover, in this situation Pridie *et al.* (1971) have described the occurrence of small-amplitude fluttering of the anterior cusp during diastole. Fortuin and Craige (1972) have concluded, from analysis of the phonocardiograms, apexcardiograms and mitral valve echocardiograms of patients with aortic regurgitation, that the Austin Flint murmur is probably due to antegrade flow across the mitral valve. The rumble seems to occur during rapid closure of the valve as the flow velocity is increasing although the actual volume of flow may be decreasing.

The movements of mitral valve prostheses have been studied by echocardiography. Although studies of this kind may be helpful in patient care, it should be pointed out that they are often not definitive. The Starr–Edwards valve gives rise to a pattern which resembles that seen from a natural valve in mitral stenosis (Gimenez *et al.*, 1965; Winters *et al.*, 1967; Reid and Bor, 1969; Siggers *et al.*, 1971). The ball remains in the fully open position throughout diastole, and any movement which is seen during this phase is due to movement of the cage. There seems always to be some regurgitation at the beginning of systole; more serious regurgitation can also be diagnosed (Miller *et al.*, 1973). Malfunction of a mitral ball valve prosthesis is a rare but serious situation. It may be caused by fibrous overgrowth on the valve ring as well as on the atrial and ventricular struts in the Cutter–Smeloff prosthesis, so that the ball tends to stick in a partially closed position. Thus at any instant the ball is likely to be in one of three distinct situations, and this can be seen in echocardiograms of the ball motion (Belenkie *et al.*, 1973). Some indication of the effective area of a stunted fascia lata mitral valve graft, and its changes with time, can be obtained in terms of the E–F slope of the corresponding echocardiogram (Mary *et al.*, 1974).

The recording in man of the aortic valve echocardiogram was first reported by Edler (1961) and Effert *et al.* (1964). The position of the probe is adjusted to obtain the mitral valve echocardiogram, and, with this as a reference, the beam is directed medially 10–15° towards the sternum and slightly superiorly towards the right shoulder. In this orientation, the anterior echoes from the aortic valve originate from the right coronary cusp, whilst the posterior echoes are due either to the left coronary or to the posterior cusp. This is illustrated in Fig. 6.65. According to Feizi *et al.* (1974), who used a focused probe and examined their patients in the left lateral position, satisfactory recordings can be obtained in more than 80% of those with normal aortic valves and in the majority of those with diseased valves. In the most favourable circumstances, the normal aortic valve echocardiogram is seen within the aortic root as slender cusp echoes producing a box-like configuration during systole and a single, nearly central, line in diastole. More often, however, the cusps are visualized only in systole and early diastole. In disease, the density of cusp echoes correlates well with the assessment of valve calcification found at operation, but the presence of these echoes makes it impossible to measure the movements of the cusps. Moreover, Feizi *et al.* (1974) disagreed with the statement of Gramiak and Shah (1970) that the density of the aortic cusp echoes is an indication of the degree of aortic stenosis. Consequently, aortic echocardiography is not very helpful in grading the severity of aortic stenosis. In the rare absence of calcification, the expected reduction in the separation of the aortic valve cusps in stenosis is not seen if the valve is domed so that the orifice is displaced superiorly beyond the ultrasonic beam, as with a biscuspid aortic valve. In aortic regurgitation, however, the valve separation is generally greater than in the normal: if the separation is increased, regurgitation is almost certain to be present. False negatives, however, do occur.

Dissecting aortic aneurysm may be diagnosed from the appearance on the echocardiogram of normal aortic valve leaflets within two anterior and two posterior echoes which correspond to the dilated aortic root and the false lumen of the aneurysm (Yuste *et al.*, 1974).

The identification in man of the echoes from the tricuspid valve was first reported by Edler (1961). The procedure for obtaining the tricuspid valve echocardiogram has been described by Joyner *et al.* (1967b), using the mitral valve recording position as a starting point. It is easier, however, first to locate the aortic valve, and then to redirect the beam medially and inferiorly. Qualitatively, echocardiograms of the tricuspid valve are similar to those of the mitral valve. Moreover, the tricuspid valve may flutter during diastole in patients with pulmonary regurgitation, just as the mitral valve may do in aortic regurgitation. According to Gramiak and Shah (1971), the diastolic slope of the tricuspid valve echocardiogram may be significantly decreased in the absence of stenosis, by restrictive processes involving the right ventricle and pericardium, and so caution in interpretation is necessary.

The pulmonary valve is not easily accessible to ultrasonic examination. Although Edler (1964) mentioned having observed echoes from this valve, it was not until eight years later that Gramiak *et al.* (1972) described their procedure for detecting the valve. Taking the position of the probe for visualizing the aortic valve as the starting point, the probe is moved one interspace superiorly: the beam then passes through the supravalvular portion of the aorta. The beam is redirected in a lateral and superior direction. As the echoes from the aortic walls disappear, the pulmonary artery becomes visible as a transonic space lying superficially near the aorta with its anterior wall with 10–20 mm of the inner surface of the chest. The posterior wall is characterized by a thick echo complex which may lie 20–40 mm behind the anterior echo. Valve cusps appear as thin lines which move between the margins of the pulmonary artery. The procedure is difficult and often impossible. The use of a focused probe increases the possibility of success; but even so, the detection rate is lower than 60% in children less than 14 years of age, and only 25% in adults.

According to Nanda *et al.* (1974), the pulmonary valve echocardiogram may be of value in assessing pulmonary hypertension. In comparison with the normal, in hypertension the pulmonary valve opens more rapidly, the pre-ejection period is longer, and the posterior displacement following atrial systole (the A-wave) is smaller or even absent. Some caution is necessary, because the A-wave amplitude is also affected by respiration, so that its amplitude must be measured during the inspiratory phrase of quiet respiration. Weyman *et al.* (1974a) reported similar findings in respect of diastolic slope (but with less confidence) and A-wave amplitude, and also mentioned that mid-systolic fluttering is commonly seen in pulmonary hypertension. Moreover, in some of their patients, they observed a negative E–F slope: this was never seen in normals. The effect of pulmonary hypertension may also be apparent in the mitral valve echocardiogram, which may mimic mitral stenosis (McLaurin *et al.*, 1973).

In pulmonary stenosis, Weyman *et al.* (1974b) have reported that the amplitude of the A-wave is greater than that in the normal.

(ii) Diagnosis of congenital heart disease

In congenital heart disease, the paediatric cardiologist is frequently required to investigate seriously ill patients who have complex abnormalities. The value of echocardiography in this situation has been reviewed by Chesler *et al.* (1971). When right ventricular enlargement is present, as in atrial septal defect or complete transposition of the great vessels, the septum is located more posteriorly than normal, and so is the position of the anterior cusp of the fully open mitral valve. Discontinuity in the echoes from the mitral valve and the aortic root indicates the presence of a double-outlet right ventricle. Congenital mitral valve disease is associated with abnormalities in the movement of the anterior cusp. If the absence of an interventricular septum is demonstrated by echocardiography, differential diagnosis becomes much easier because it excludes many conditions in which two atrioventricular valves and two ventricles are present. Stop-action (e.c.g.-gated) two-dimensional scans have been reported to be capable of visualizing the transposition of the great vessels (King *et al.*, 1971).

Atrial septal defects have been demonstrated in radial ultrasonic two-dimensional scans produced by rotating small transducers mounted at the tips of catheters introduced through the external jugular or the femoral veins into the right atrium (Kimoto *et al.*, 1964; Omoto, 1967). The method is neither convenient nor safe, and so it has not come into general clinical use. Transcutaneous echography, however, may give a clue to the presence of atrial septal defect, if the mitral valve is found to be unusually posterior (as already mentioned), or if the motion of the interventricular septum is abnormal (Diamond *et al.*, 1971). In some patients it is possible to visualize the atrial septum, and defects if present, using stop-action (e.c.g.-gated) two-dimensional scanning (Matsumoto *et al.*, 1975).

In those patients in whom it is possible to obtain echocardiographic recordings of the pulmonary valve, Weyman *et al.* (1974b) have reported that with increased pulmonary blood flow due to left to right shunt, both the C–D and E–F slopes are greater than in the normal.

Two-dimensional real-time or stop-action (e.c.g.-gated) ultrasonic imaging may be very helpful in determining anatomy in congenital heart disease (Tanaka *et al.*, 1971; Sahn *et al.*, 1974).

An excellent review of the subject has been published by Murphy *et al.* (1975).

(iii) Measurements of left ventricular volume and function

A technique for measuring stroke volume (and hence cardiac output) non-invasively by ultrasound has been described by Feigenbaum *et al.* (1967a). They demonstrated good correlation between the stroke volume and the product of the amplitudes of the mitral ring movement and the distance between the anterior and posterior heart walls. In clinical practice, it is easier to measure the left ventricular internal dimension (minor axis) in diastole ($LVID_d$) and in systole ($LVID_s$), and to calculate the stroke volume ($LVSV$) by substitution in the empirical formula of Feigenbaum *et al.* (1969):

$$(LVSV) \simeq (LVID_d)^3 - (LVID_s)^3 \qquad (6.23)$$

This method was used by Pombo *et al.* (1971) to study patients suspected of having myocardial infarction. Measurements could only be satisfactorily made in 9 out of 14 patients, but good correlations were found between ultrasonic and dye-dilution results. It was pointed out by Redwood *et al.* (1974) that the ultrasonic method is unreliable in patients with abnormally contracting segments of the left ventricular wall. They also pointed out, however, that this limitation is not too serious in the study of acute serial changes in left ventricular volume, and they estimated from experiments on volunteers in which tilt was changed, atrial fibrillation was observed, and nitroglycerin and phenylephrine were administered, that it should be possible to detect a change of 8–10 ml in stroke volume.

Left ventricular dimensions determined by echocardiography (see also Section 8.1.a.i, in which a transmission method is mentioned) have been compared with biplane angiographic measurements, by Fortuin *et al.* (1971), Murray *et al.* (1972), and Gibson (1973). The latter study involved 50 patients: the correlation coefficient was 0·91, and the standard error of the estimate was 61 ml. In 32 patients, duplicate determinations were made by both methods: lack of fit was found when the left ventricular cavity shape was abnormal. The ultrasonic method has two great advantages: it is non-invasive, and it can be used repeatedly on the same patient.

Echocardiographic diagnosis of hypertrophic cardiomyopathy may generally be made by the observation of abnormal mitral valve motion. These patients, however, represent only one subgroup of a cardiac disease in which the characteristic anatomical abnormality is asymmetric septal hypertrophy (ASH). In most patients with ASH, left ventricular outflow is unobstructed and cardiac dysfunction is presumably due to widespread left ventricular myocardial abnormality; a few patients exhibit HOCM. Henry *et al.* (1974) have demonstrated by echocardiography, and subsequent post-mortem examination, that the interventricular septum is thickened in obstructive ASH. Moreover the thickening of the free wall behind the posterior mitral leaflet appeared to regress after surgery for the relief of outflow obstruction.

In favourable circumstances, it is possible echographically to measure the thickness of the posterior left ventricular wall. This has been used to measure stress–strain relationships (Gibson and Brown, 1974), and to estimate preload and after-load (Ratshin *et al.*, 1974) in man; the results are possibly more interesting to the physiologist than to the clinician. Sjögren (1974) measured diastolic left ventricular wall thickness in 219 patients with ischaemic heart disease. Statistically, it was found to be significantly increased in comparison with the healthy heart.

The velocity of circumferential fibre shortening (VCF) may be measured from ultrasonic recordings of the posterior left ventricular wall during systole. Thus Paraskos *et al.* (1971) found a mean VCF of 1·45 circumferences per second (standard error 0·08) in 23 patients with normal left ventricular function. Mean VCF was significantly depressed (0·91 circumferences per second, standard error 0·09) in 38 patients with non-localized impaired left ventricular function. Data have been obtained by Sahn *et al.* (1974) for the VCF in normal newborns: the mean value was 1·51 circumferences per second, with a standard error of 0·04, in the age range up to 150 h.

Results of experiments with pigs (Paulev *et al.*, 1973), in which the posterior left ventricular wall echo movement was recorded whilst the ventricular pressure was measured, confirmed that the echographic method accurately determined the myocardial contraction velocity. These measurements were made with apparatus of Paulev and Pedersen (1973), who had constructed an electronic circuit to differentiate the time–position pulse–echo recording of the posterior wall movement. They related their measurements to work rate in normal individuals. Similar instrumentation could be used for the study of disease.

A few years ago, two reports appeared in the literature which indicated that measurements of posterior left ventricular wall movements (PWM)—both of velocity and amplitude—might be of diagnostic value. Wharton *et al.* (1971) found that both measures of PWM were reduced after acute myocardial infarction, and Carson and Kanter (1971) reported similar changes in heart failure. Experiments with dogs (Kerber and Abboud, 1973) have shown that the posterior wall motion of the left ventricle was not affected by infarction of the apex, whereas with posterior wall infarction there was a large initial posterior displacement—aneurysmal bulging—during isometric contraction, followed by a slow anterior movement during ventricular ejection, and then by a rapid anterior recoil motion during isometric relaxation. It was concluded that the changes in PWM following posterior infarction were due to dyskinesis of the infarcted area, rather than to generalized changes in ventricular function. The posterior wall velocity seemed not to provide a reliable index of left ventricular performance when localized dyskinesis, as indicated by abnormal PWM, was present. The same conclusion was reached by Ludbrook *et al.* (1974) in a study of patients with coronary artery disease.

Measurements of the maximum and mean velocities of the posterior heart wall, the amplitude of the excursion of the left ventricular wall, and estimates of the ejection fraction, were made by Kisslo *et al.* (1973) in patients with occlusive coronary artery disease, before and after aortocoronary saphenous vein grafting. All these parameters seemed to be increased following successful surgery: but it is now clear that this observation needs to be applied with caution in clinical situations.

In view of the difficulty of interpreting PWM in myocardial infarction, anterior left ventricular wall motion, which is more difficult to record and to interpret due to the proximity of the myocardium to the thoracic wall, is likely to be of limited clinical value. A brave attempt at clinical interpretation has been made, however, by Corya *et al.* (1974).

The ultrasonic methods of assessing left ventricular performance in man have been discussed in relation to other non-invasive methods by Weissler (1974).

(iv) *Two-dimensional imaging of the heart*

Although conventional echocardiography is a two-dimensional (space–time) imaging process, this Sub-section is concerned with imaging in two spatial dimensions.

Despite the movement of the heart, it may be possible to visualize

abnormalities by means of a conventional two-dimensional scanner producing an image integrated over several cardiac cycles. Thus Kratochwil
et al. (1974) reported that ultrasonic scanning was helpful in the diagnosis
of one patient with a pericardial cyst, and another with a right atrial
tumour. Subtle details cannot be seen in this way, however, due to blurring
and superimposition of signals. In terms of available instrumentation, this
difficulty is probably most easily overcome by gating the display of a
conventional scanner from the e.c.g. signal, so that only echo signals
obtained during a particular phase of the cardiac cycle are integrated over
many cardiac cycles to produce a stroboscopic image. Descriptions of the
technique and its clinical value have been given by, for example, Tanaka
et al. (1971), Hussey *et al.* (1973) and King (1973). Under favourable
circumstances, characteristic abnormalities can be visualized in hypertrophy, cardiac enlargement, valvular disease, atrial and ventricular defects,
and the alignment of the great arteries. Moreover, the cross-sectional image
of the left ventricle is very comparable with that obtained by angiography.
The design and performance of a commercially available instrument* for
e.c.g.-gated stop-action scanning of the heart has been described by
Hileman *et al.* (1975).

The use of an e.c.g.-gated scanner has several practical limitations. Apart
from early systole, *R*-wave triggering may not be a good index of cardiac
phase in patients with arhythmias. Also the method wastes most of the
information which is available, because only one (or at most a few) images
are constructed although the transmitter normally is arranged to operate
continuously. An ingenious way of getting around this later limitation has
been demonstrated by Gramiak *et al.* (1973). The method is illustrated in
Fig. 6.70. The images thus constructed are distorted since they represent
sectors, but appear to be linear scans. The tedium of manual work has now
been eliminated by the use of a computer (Waag and Gramiak, 1974).

None of the methods of two-dimensional imaging so far described in
this Sub-section operates in real time. Apparently Åsberg (1967) was the
first to demonstrate a scanner fast enough to operate in real time, but his
instrument was bulky, used a water-bath coupling, and produced only
seven frames per second; it does not seem to have been used clinically.
There are now three types of real-time scanner, however, which are finding
clinical applications.

Firstly, there are conventional scanners which operate at high speed.
For example, Griffith and Henry (1974) have developed an instrument,
described in more detail in Section 6.8, in which an ordinary pulse–echo
probe is held in contact with the skin whilst it is oscillated through an arc
of 30°, 15 times per second. This produces a 66-line image at a frame rate

* Cardioniner: Unirad Corporation, Denver, Colorado, USA.

of 30 s^{-1}. Another single-probe instrument, also described in Section 6.8, produces a linear scan by means of curved mirror and a water-bath coupling*.

Secondly, arrays of transducer operating at high switching speeds have been constructed. For example, the multiscan system, developed by Bom *et al.* (1973) as described in Section 6.10.c, is primarily useful because it

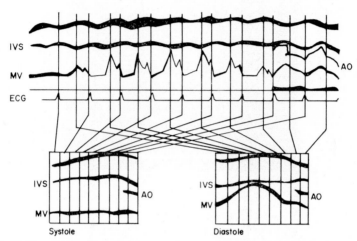

FIG. 6.70 Reconstruction of cross-sectional images of the heart from a time–position arc scan. A portion of the arc scan is removed at the time of each simultaneously recorded R-wave, and many such portions are assembled into an image of the entire area under study at the beginning of systole. Similarly a diastolic image can be constructed by sampling in mid-diastole, and so on. If sufficient samples are available in each cardiac cycle, a motion picture can be produced. (After Gramiak *et al.*, 1973.)

produces a real-time image of the moving heart in two dimensions. The clinical value of this has been discussed by Roelandt *et al.* (1974). The patient is examined in the supine position, with the head of the bed raised about 20–30°. The cross-section of the heart obtained with the probe in the oblique position corresponds with the time–position arc scan described in Sub-section (i) of this Section. According to the position of the probe, in suitable patients, it is possible to visualize the aorta, the aortic root, the left atrium, the mitral valve, the posterior papillary muscle and chordae, and the left and right ventricles. A typical scan—a single frame from a ciné film—is shown in Fig. 6.71. The rate of structure recognition has been

* "Vidoson" model 635ST: Siemens Aktiengesellschaft, Erlangen, West Germany.

analysed by Bom *et al.* (1974), from results obtained in four different clinical cardiology centres. The study involved 580 patients. The recognitions of the aortic root, anterior mitral valve leaflet and the left ventricular posterior wall, were excellent or good in 75, 66 and 66% respectively of all the patients. The recognition rate of any specific cardiac structure became constant after a brief period of experience. More experience was necessary

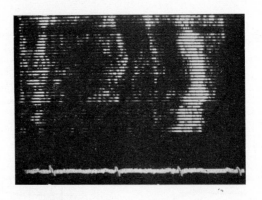

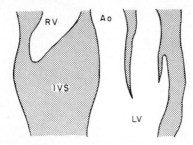

FIG. 6.71 Two-dimensional scan of left heart: hypertrophic cardiomyopathy. Single frame from a real-time movie. (Courtesy N. Bom.)

to recognize dynamic ventricular abnormalities. In this initial series, most confidence was felt in diagnosing patients with congenital, valvular, or myocardial diseases, or with pericardial effusions.

With at least one commercially available apparatus* it is possible to record with a time–motion system (see Section 6.9) the echo signals received by any selected transducer in the array, whilst simultaneously studying the real-time two-dimensional display. This combines the advantages of positive structure recognition with conventional echocardiography.

Arrays of transducers suffer from the limitations imposed by the neces-

* ECHO-cardio-VISOR 01, Organon Teknika, Oss, Holland.

sity to compromise between the number of transducers (which is equal to the number of lines) and the directivity (which is a measure of resolution) and sensitivity. These limitations can in principle be overcome by the use of transducer arrays, in which a number of small elements are arranged to operate together as the equivalent of a single transducer. Groups of elements can be used to produce a linear scan. Alternatively, all the elements in the array can be used to produce a sector scan, by appropriate phasing to steer the beam. This technique is discussed in more detail in Section 6.10.c, and its clinical application in cardiology has been described by Kisslo *et al.* (1975) and von Ramm and Thurstone (1975).

(v) Ultrasonic contrast studies

In a series of elegant experiments, Gramiak *et al.* (1969) positively identified several important echo sources within the heart, using as a marker a contrast medium injected during catheterization of various cardiac chambers. They used indocyanine green, and in this connexion Kremkau *et al.* (1970) demonstrated that the echo enhancement to which the injection gives rise is due to cavitation at the tip of the catheter. According to Ziskin *et al.* (1972), however, cavitation is not necessary for echo enhancement if there is a sufficient number of air bubbles already present in the liquid from the mixing process in its preparation. Moreover other agents can also act as ultrasonic contrast media. Water saturated with carbon dioxide is particularly effective since it contains numerous bubbles, and gas embolization is not a problem as the bubbles are rapidly absorbed in blood. Ether is the most effective agent yet tested: it boils vigorously at body temperature. In large quantities (20 ml in 9–18 kg dogs) it is lethal; but doses of 0·3 ml are regularly used in man for the measurement of circulation times. A volume of 0·1 ml is generally sufficient to produce an effective ultrasonic contrast.

Both mitral and aortic regurgitation can be confirmed by ultrasonic contrast studies during cardiac catheterization. Thus Kerber *et al.* (1974) detected contrast echoes in the left atrium after left ventricular injection of indocyanine green or normal saline in 14 of 16 patients with mitral regurgitation, and in the left ventricle after aortic root injection in 13 of 16 patients with aortic regurgitation. Valvular regurgitation as small as 10% by angiographic determination was detected ultrasonically. Likewise it may be possible to detect atrial and ventricular septal defects, patent ductus arteriosus, and tetralogy of Fallot.

(vi) Pericardial effusion

In the normal heart, the two layers of the pericardium are in close proximity, and it is not possible by echocardiography to separate the echoes from the chest wall or the posterior pleura and the walls of the heart. If fluid collects in the pericardial space, however, it may separate the heart from the chest wall or the pleura, and these structures can then be identified by echocardiography since the pericardial fluid is echo-free. Therefore, ultrasound provides a quick, safe and fairly reliable method of diagnosing pericardial effusion (Feigenbaum *et al.*, 1967b; Pridie and Turnbull, 1968). A typical recording is shown in Fig. 6.72.

Once it has been detected, it may be considered to be desirable to aspirate a pericardial effusion. This can easily be done under ultrasonic guidance with the aid of a probe which has a central axial hole through which the pincture needle may be inserted. A most useful phenomenon is

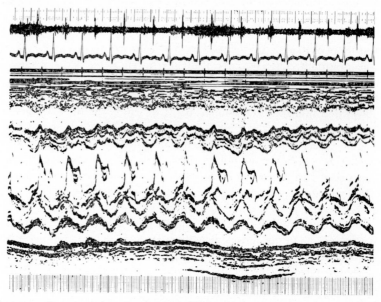

FIG. 6.72 Echocardiogram through mitral valve region: pericardial effusion. The effusion appears as an anechoic space posterior to the epicardium. (Courtesy Ö. Feizi.)

the return of an echo from the tip–liquid interface as the needle is advanced into the effusion. This was first described by Goldberg and Pollack (1973). It allows the position of the needle tip to be seen in the liquid on an A-scope display during aspiration, so that there is no need constantly to look from the display to the needle in order to avoid an accident. It has been suggested by Goldberg and Ziskin (1973) that this rather remarkable phenomenon may be due to the sudden change in the area of the beam when the ultrasonic pulse travels past the tip of the needle.

(vii) Pleural effusion and pulmonary embolism

Examination of the lungs is discussed here because of their anatomical proximity to the heart. The A-scope (Pell, 1964), the two-dimensional B-scope (Taylor, 1974), and time–position recording (Joyner *et al.*, 1967a) have all demonstrated the value of ultrasound in the diagnosis of pleural effusion. The clinical problem is that the differential diagnosis of large opacities in a chest radiograph can be very difficult. In this situation, a liquid collection is anechoic and transonic, and ultrasound can resolve the anatomical structures, demonstrate the movement of the diaphragm, and visualize liquid. Therefore the presence of a pleural effusion may be confirmed, and subphrenic collection may be excluded.

In patients suspected of having pulmonary embolism, the diagnosis can sometimes be made by scintigraphy. If this fails, arteriography may be necessary: this is a difficult and potentially hazardous procedure. The interpretation of ultrasonic echoes obtained transcutaneously from lung is very difficult because transmission is attenuated rapidly, whilst at the same time reverberation gives rise to artifacts. It has been reported by Miller *et al.* (1967) that the length of the timebase on an A-scope occupied by echoes when the probe (2 MHz) is in contact with the chest is much greater over areas of ischaemia than over normal lung. Ross *et al.* (1968) concluded that the effect is due to decreased ventilation following interruption by pulmonary emboli in the perfusion of a lung segment. A similar conclusion was reached by Gordon (1974), who mentioned the possibility that changes in the thickness of the alveolar walls resulting from oedema might be important. Moreover, he has developed a simple instrument with a yes–no display and which generates an audible signal the pitch of which increases with increasing "penetration". Using this device, it is apparently a simple matter to scan the lungs and thus to identify suspect areas.

6.16.c Endocrinology

(i) Adrenal glands

The normal adrenal is seldom seen in two-dimensional ultrasonic scans in adults, but it can often be visualized—particularly on the left side—in children (Lyons *et al.*, 1972). Mass lesions of the adrenal were first visualized ultrasonically in children by Damascelli *et al.* (1968), and subsequently by Hunig (1971), Goldberg *et al.* (1972) and Bearman *et al.* (1973). The method may also be successful in disease in the adult: thus, Holm (1971) described the diagnosis of adrenal tumours in two patients, and Birnholz (1973) found that a mass of 30 mm in size can usually be seen in either adrenal. Davidson *et al.* (1975) confirmed these results, and stated that ultrasound is useful as a preliminary to venography, or to exclude suspected false positive radiological results.

None of these authors used grey-scale displays. Doubtless better results could be obtained more easily with this advantage.

(ii) Thyroid gland

The thyroid gland is situated just below the skin with no overlying air or bony structure, and so it is readily accessible for ultrasonic examination. It is possible to distinguish between solid and cystic lesions (Blum *et al.*, 1971; Rasmussen *et al.*, 1971; Thijs *et al.*, 1972; Miskin *et al.*, 1973; Ramsay and Meire, 1975), and this is particularly useful since both may appear to be "cold" in scintiscans. Moreover it is possible to compare functional and structural volumes of the thyroid, by means of isotope and ultrasonic scans (Tanaka *et al.*, 1966). The structural organization of the tissues may be revealed by grey-scale echography (Jellins *et al.*, 1975), but there are as yet insufficient data to place the distinction between different types of lesion on a quantitative basis. In general, however, malignant tumours are distinguishable from both normal thyroid, which returns echoes of higher amplitude, and cysts, which are less reflective (Taylor *et al.*, 1975).

6.16.d Gastroenterology

(i) Teeth and mouth

In the developed world, one of the main sources of exposure of the population to ionizing radiation is in the dental surgeries. Moreover, for the individual patient, the time required to process the films may involve delays and return visits. Therefore social advantages would be gained by the development of safe and rapid ultrasonic diagnostic techniques in dentistry, provided that the clinical results were as reliable as X-radiography and the apparatus was economical to purchase and to operate.

One early report (Smirnow, 1966) was rather discouraging: it was not possible to distinguish between fillings and caries on scans made with a 15 MHz two-dimensional ophthalmological instrument. Kossoff and Sharpe (1966), however, showed that under favourable circumstances both transmission and reflexion ultrasonic methods are capable of detecting degenerative pulpitus. They used probes of 1 mm diameter, operating at 18 MHz. The transmission method, which depends on the attenuation of the ultrasound by the gas associated with the disease, is the more reliable, and it is not affected by the inclination of the surfaces; but it does require access to both sides of the tooth.

The positions of the dentino-enamel junction and the pulp chamber wall have been demonstrated on an A-scope by Lees and Barber (1971). They used an aluminium rod between the transducer and the tooth, so that the echoes from the tooth surface could be detected: aluminium has a similar characteristic impedance to that of dental enamel. The results of the preliminary experiments suggested that it may be possible to estimate the thickness of water film between an amalgam filling and the dentin: since most restorations are radio-opaque, this might be clinically useful. It may also be possible to detect changes due to demineralization of the enamel. Thus it might be feasible to locate a subsurface carious lesion, before it became evident by other means. In all these possibilities, it has been pointed out by Lees (1972) that the chief technical problem is to inject ultrasound into the tooth and to recover echoes from the substructure. Some advance in this direction has been reported by Lees *et al.* (1973), who succeeded in measuring the demineralization of the dental enamel of teeth being etched in hydrochloric acid.

Daly and Wheeler (1971) have claimed that it is possible to measure the thickness of the oral mucosa with an accuracy of better than 1% in the range 0·5–10 mm. This might have clinical applications in the discovery of likely areas of trouble in prosthetic fittings, in mapping bony defects, and as a periodontal probe.

The salivary glands may be visualized by two-dimensional transverse scanning through the upper neck. This has been reported by Macridis *et al.* (1975), who found it possible to distinguish between solid and cystic lesions of the gland.

(*ii*) *Stomach and intestine*

Apart from examination of the teeth—which presently is of academic rather than practical interest—ultrasonic diagnosis in gastroenterology is limited primarily to parenchymal organs of the upper abdomen, and the biliary system. There are a few exceptions; for example, it is possible to visualize omental cysts (Mittelstaedt, 1975). Generally studies of these structures are made more difficult by the gas which tends to exist in the alimentary canal. Moreover, many abnormalities of the alimentary tract can be examined safely (apart from the hazard of ionizing radiation) if disagreeably by contrast radiography. According to Lutz and Rettenmaier (1973), however, real-time two-dimensional ultrasonic imaging can reveal bowel tumours as having almost non-reflecting outer layers with dense echoes in their centres. This preliminary report does not seem yet to have had a sequel.

(*iii*) *Liver*

Howry and Bliss (1952) were the first to publish two-dimensional ultrasonic scans of the liver. They used a water-bath scanner. It was not until more convenient scanners, such as the direct contact type of instrument, became available that the possibility of obtaining clinically useful information began to be investigated.

Much of the liver is accessible to transcutaneous ultrasonic investigation. Caution is necessary, however, in analysing scans obtained through ribs; and parts of the liver near the diaphragm may be obscured by lung. Within

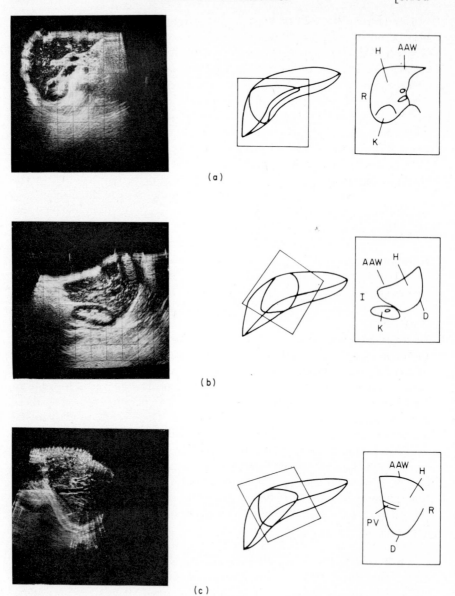

FIG. 6.73 Normal liver scans. (a) Transverse; (b) longitudinal oblique; (c) sub-costal oblique. AAW, anterior abdominal wall; D, diaphragm; H, liver; I, inferior; K, right kidney; PV, portal vein.

these limitations, ultrasonic scanning can provide most useful information about the structure of the organ.

The anatomical orientations of the planes in which the liver is usually scanned are illustrated in Fig. 6.73, together with corresponding scans of a normal liver. Good results are almost always obtainable with the oblique subcostal approach (McCarthy *et al.*, 1967), except when the patient is very obese, or the colon contains gas which interferes with the transmission of the ultrasound. To some extent this latter problem may be minimized by scanning during the inspiratory phase of quiet respiration. In some circumstances, however, it may be appropriate to scan the liver in transverse or longitudinal planes (Holm, 1971; Rasmussen *et al.*, 1973). For example, Rasmussen (1972) has estimated liver volume by making a series of longitudinal sections placed as a fan around the vertebral column; using the method of computation developed by Stigsby and Rasmussen (1971), he achieved a median difference 94 ml between the calculated and the actual volumes, with 95% confidence limits in the range 149–235 ml. One example of the clinical value of this method of estimating liver volume is in following changes resulting from portal decompression surgery (Rasmussen *et al.*, 1975).

McCarthy (1972) has reviewed the status of ultrasonic liver scanning before the introduction of grey-scale displays, and Wells (1971) has discussed the physical factors which controlled the diagnostic accuracy of the method. It was possible to see tube-like structures, including the portal vein, in the normal liver. There was a tendency for scans of patients with cirrhosis to contain "more" echoes than those of normals made under the same conditions: in this connexion, see Section 6.12.c. The detection of metastases was not very reliable, but solitary tumours usually revealed themselves as areas of increased echo density. Liquid-filled lesions, on the other hand, were well shown: an example is given in Fig. 6.74. The ability to detect liver abscess was of considerable clinical value. In relation to scintigraphy, ultrasound has the advantage of being able to confirm that a space-occupying lesion is liquid-filled, since it is relatively echo-free (McCarthy *et al.*, 1970; Monroe *et al.*, 1971; Matthews *et al.*, 1973); moreover, it may be used repeatedly to follow progress. The principal limitation with ultrasonic scanning is due to the inaccessibility due to lung and rib of the upper right lobe, and it is in this situation that scintigraphy may have the advantage (Leyton *et al.*, 1973). Once an abscess has been located using two-dimensional scanning, it can be aspirated by means of a needle inserted transcutaneously under ultrasonic control (Smith and Bartrum, 1975). The method is similar to that described in Section 6.16.b.vi; if the structures can be visualized, it may also be used to guide liver tumour biopsy (Rasmussen *et al.*, 1972) and porta hepatitis puncture for transhepatic portography (Burcharth and Rasmussen, 1974).

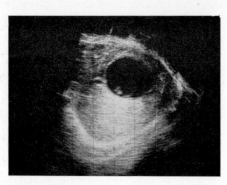
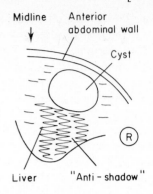

Fig. 6.74 Right subcostal oblique scan of liver, showing a cyst, anechoic save for a few reflexions near the posterior surface. Note "antishadow" beyond the cyst, due to overcompensating swept gain. (Courtesy F. G. M. Ross.)

A major breakthrough in the ultrasonic investigation of the liver came about with the introduction of grey-scale displays (Taylor *et al.*, 1973). A considerable amount of detail may be seen in normal liver, including vessels of only a few millimetres in diameter, as shown in Fig. 6.75. This degree of resolution is obtained using a non-compounded scanning technique. Even with perfect scanning geometry, it is doubtful whether this fineness of detail could be seen in a compounded scan, because of uncertainties in the position of the resolution cell (see Section 6.1.b) due not only to beam deviation and velocity changes but also to physiological movements during the scanning time. (In this connexion, it is interesting to note that a real-time grey-scale scanner* which has been available for

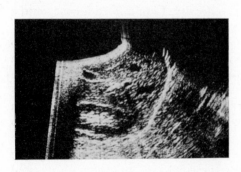
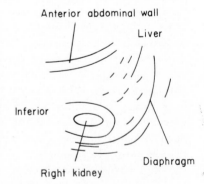

Fig. 6.75 Liver scan. Non-compounded, longitudinal, 50 mm right of midline. Note intrahepatic vessels (bile ducts, arteries and veins).

* "Vidoson" model 635ST: Siemens Aktiengesellschaft, Erlangen, West Germany.

many years is capable of producing excellent liver scans which lend themselves to quantitative analysis (see, for example, Rettenmaier, 1974). This machine seems to be in widespread use in West Germany, although it is rather seldom found elsewhere.) It is possible to see the portal vein, the middle and posterior divisions of the right hepatic vein, and the separate vein draining the caudate lobe into the inferior vena cava. Extrahepatic features which can be visualized include the right kidney, the aorta and the inferior vena cava. Against this background of normal anatomy, it is possible to detect abnormalities which are quite small in size, and this is of the greatest value in the care of the cancer patient. The management of the patient whose liver contains metastases is likely to be palliative, and the confirmation that this is the case may save him from a painful and unnecessary exploratory operation in the terminal stages of his life. Moreover, with the development of chemotherapy and immunology, the extent of liver involvement may become a decisive factor in clinical strategy.

Before the advent of grey-scaling, it was generally assumed that liver tumours appeared as areas of increased echo density. It is now clear, however, that this is seldom the case. For example, the hepatoma shown in Fig. 6.76(a) is apparent because it is delineated, and not because it has higher amplitude echoes than the liver. Moreover, Taylor (1974) has reported that liver metastases are almost always more anechoic than the surrounding normal liver, returning echoes which are typically 8 dB lower in amplitude (see Fig. 6.76(b)). It seems that most metastases which produce echoes of higher amplitude than normal liver are treated tumours.

Judging from the enthusiastic report of Taylor and Carpenter (1975a), ultrasonic scanning of the liver is beyond question more valuable than scintigraphy in the management of the cancer patient. Thus, in a series of 120 patients, the diagnosis was confirmed by ultrasonic scanning in 82%, but only in 4% by scintigraphy. Moreover, the scintigraphic findings were spurious in 27% of patients, but only in 8% of patients examined ultrasonically. Another situation in which ultrasound is more reliable than scintigraphy is in monitoring the results of chemotherapy of liver metastases. The chemotherapeutic agent may interfere with the distribution of the radiopharmaceutical (Gilby and Taylor, 1975).

In the case of jaundiced patients, it is important to distinguish between those requiring surgical treatment, and those who do not. Surgery may be necessary if the patient has pancreatic or biliary cancer, strictures or gallstones in the biliary system, or if there is compression of the biliary system by extrinsic tumour. Medical causes of jaundice include obstruction by metastatic disease, viral hepatitis, cholestasis, cholangitis and cirrhosis. Because of the limitations of radiological procedures in the jaundiced patient, ultrasonic scanning is the method of choice at least for initial studies. Using a single-sector longitudinal scan pattern, with the probe

12

positioned just below the costal margin, Taylor and Carpenter (1974) were able to distinguish obstructive jaundice caused by multiple intrahepatic space-occupying lesions, and by extrahepatic causes which generally require surgical relief. If the presence of liver metastases can be demonstrated in this painless way, the patient may be spared an exploratory operation in the terminal stages of his life.

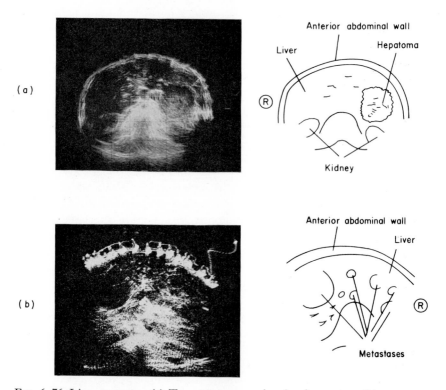

FIG. 6.76 Liver tumours. (a) Transverse scan, showing hepatoma; (b) transverse scan, showing multiple metastases giving rise to anechoic areas. ((a) Courtesy F. G. M. Ross; (b) courtesy C. F. McCarthy.)

It is difficult, even with a grey-scale display, to distinguish between a dilated portal vein and a dilated common bile duct. In the presence of biliary obstruction, Taylor and Carpenter (1975b) have reported that the dilatation of the biliary canaliculi can be detected. Moreover, an enlarged portal vein is shaped like a comma when scanned in longitudinal section: a dilated common bile duct is more uniform. Pulsed Doppler methods may be helpful here.

The diagnosis of diffuse liver disease by ultrasound is based, at the present time, on the change in the general level of amplitude of echoes originating from within the liver. The matter is reviewed in Section 6.12.c.

(iv) Gallbladder and bile duct

A long time ago, it was shown by Ludwig and Struthers (1950) that gall-stones could be detected in tissue by an ultrasonic pulse–echo method. Eleven years later this discovery was confirmed by Hill and McColl (1961), and subsequently applied to the problem of detecting gallstones at opera-tion (Knight and Newell, 1963). At cholecystectomy, the surgeon must decide whether or not to explore the common bile duct. The usual method of detecting gallstones at operation is cholangiography. This procedure is both dangerous and difficult. An alternative method is an ultrasonic search procedure which can ensure the examination of the entire length of the common bile duct, but not of the intrahepatic and common hepatic ducts. In Knight and Newell's (1963) series of eight patients, a 2·5 MHz probe of 3·5 mm diameter was used with an A-scope display; stones of greater diameter than 5 mm were found in three patients, the remaining five having no stones.

The A-scope has also been used to detect gallstones by means of a direct-contact probe applied to the anterior abdominal wall over the area of the gallbladder. There is no doubt that only those experienced in the method can hope to succeed: but after five years of practice, Hayashi et al. (1962) considered the ultrasonic method to be superior to cholecystography. Possibly more representative results are those of Tala et al. (1966). There were 33 patients in their series, of whom 28 were found at operation to have gallstones. Of these, 26 had previously been diagnosed by ultrasound, although stones had been demonstrated by cholecystography in only 22. The reliability of the method is placed in doubt by the fact that stones were not found at operation in five patients, in three of whom there were positive ultrasonic diagnoses.

A normal gallbladder can be seen in about 80% of individuals in both longitudinal and transverse two-dimensional scans and, according to Holm (1971), an enlarged gallbladder can always be visualized. In any event, the normal gallbladder is most likely to be seen in the fasting patient, and least likely, in the patient who has recently taken a fatty meal. It is not unusual for the gallbladder to remain non-visualized after double-dose oral cholecystography, and in this circumstance, and when the patient is unable to tolerate intravenous cholecystography, ultrasonic scanning may be extremely useful (Hublitz et al., 1972; Goldberg et al., 1974; Tabrisky et al., 1975). In view of the considerable success rate of the method—in one series (Doust and Maklad, 1974), the gallbladder was seen in 92% of patients, and in this group, there was 80% accuracy in the diagnosis of gallstones—it seems that ultrasonic scanning should be the first investigation to be used.

With grey-scale display, it would probably be possible to estimate the gallbladder volume from serial scans made in parallel planes, and to study some aspects of bile dynamics.

(v) Spleen

Ultrasonic scanning of the spleen is conveniently done with the patient lying in the right lateral position. The examination is generally begun by scanning along the tenth intercostal space: this permits the spleen size to be estimated by the length of its longitudinal axis. If the spleen is enlarged, particularly below the level of the costal margin, it can be visualized with the patient lying supine.

Little information apart from spleen volume—which can be estimated quite accurately by measurement from parallel scans (Kardel *et al.*, 1971)—can be obtained with low dynamic range displays (Lehmann *et al.*, 1966; Holm, 1971; Palo and Tähti, 1971). A grey-scale image may be more useful, however, and according to Taylor and Carpenter (1975b), splenomegaly resulting from portal hypertension is characterized by medium level echoes, greater in amplitude than those in neoplastic spleen, but lower than those in chronic inflammatory splenomegaly.

(vi) Pancreas

Investigation of the pancreas is a diagnostic challenge. A simple, safe and reliable method of examining the organ transcutaneously would be of great clinical value. At present, apart from ultrasound, there is no alternative to radiographic contrast study, X-ray tomography, or double-radiosotope scanning. Maybe computerized tomography will offer a solution, but it will never be cheap or radiologically safe.

Several attempts have been made to examine the pancreas by ultrasound. The first, such as that of Wagai *et al.* (1965), used the A-scope; but more recent results have been obtained with two-dimensional B-scopes, either of the direct contact or water-bath type. The frequencies have generally been in the range 2–3 MHz. The patient is examined in the supine position, and transverse scans are made close together to visualize the relationships of the dorsal surface of the liver, the shadow of the stomach, and the anterior surfaces of the aorta and vena cava. In the triangular space bounded by these three landmarks, the portal vein is normally the only echo-free structure, and the head and body of the pancreas occupy most of the remaining volume. The tail lies behind the gut. The full length of the pancreas can generally be displayed with the scan plane inclined at an angle of about 20° to the transverse, caudally to the right. The mesenteric artery may be visualized just below this scan plane.

Low dynamic range imaging of the pancreas seems only reliably to have been achieved in the presence of disease (Engelhart and Blauenstein, 1970; Filly and Freimanis, 1970; Holm, 1971; Kratochwil *et al.*, 1973). Since the normal pancreas is so difficult to identify on a two-dimensional *B*-scan, Rettenmeier and Gail (1972) pointed out that if the gland is visualized, it is likely to be enlarged due to disease. They used a real-time water-bath scanner (see Section 6.8) with a grey-scale display, which doubtless made the task of orientation easier, and they were able to distinguish between pseudocysts and neoplasms. They did not state, however, what degree of enlargement was necessary to make recognition of the organ reliable. Pseudocyst is probably the abnormality which is most reliably demonstrated.

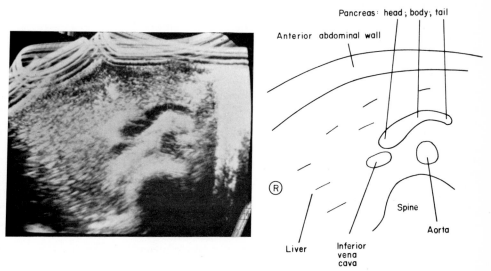

FIG. 6.77 Transverse oblique abdominal scan showing the normal pancreas. (Courtesy H. B. Meire.)

Stuber *et al.* (1972), using a 2·5 MHz direct contact two-dimensional scanner, have succeeded in obtaining quite good results in examinations of the pancreas. In a group of 18 patients in whom the diagnosis was subsequently confirmed by surgery, there was one false negative ultrasonic result. Moreover, they used a bistable display. Experience with grey-scale displays has been encouraging. A typical scan is shown in Fig. 6.77. For example, Lutz (1975) obtained correct diagnoses in 115 of 137 patients with disease of the pancreas; there were four false-negative results, and in the remaining patients the results were inadequate. There were six false-positives amongst 63 patients with apparently normal pancreases. When the nature of an enlarged pancreas is in doubt, ultrasonically guided fine needle biopsy may be helpful (Hancke *et al.*, 1975; Smith *et al.*, 1975). Although the false negative rate is around 10–20%, a positive biopsy confirming neoplasm may save the patient an unnecessary exploratory operation, since only 25% of pancreatic cancers are resectable, and the five-year survival rate is worse than 1%. Ultrasonically guided biopsy under these conditions is easily justified, even if there is a possibility of dissemination of metastases in the needle track.

Asher *et al.* (1975) have apparently been so successful in identifying the normal pancreas that they were able to cannulate the pancreatic duct in 23 out of 25 patients.

(*vii*) *Ascites*

The detection of ascites is quite suggestive of neoplasm, particularly in the peritoneal space, or of liver disease including cirrhosis. Clinical examination often leaves doubt (especially in the obese patient) as to whether or not there is any free abdominal liquid, and in order to resolve the question it may even be necessary, without the aid of ultrasound, to resort to four quadrant aspiration. Ascitic liquid, however, when favourably situated may be detected as an echo-free area immediately against the abdominal wall. Thus McCarthy *et al.* (1969) found that, by lying the patient on one side and ultrasonically scanning (*A*-scan or two-dimensional *B*-scan) the dependent part of the abdomen, they were able always to diagnose this condition provided that there was more than 500 ml of liquid: the smallest volume which they detected in their experiments was 300 ml. (Usually the most reliable results are obtained if the patient lies on the right side, so that the ascites collects between the liver and the abdominal wall.) Likewise Goldberg *et al.* (1970), using only an *A*-scope, were able to detect volumes as small as 100 ml. A more recent report of two-dimensional scanning has been presented by Hünig and Kinser (1973), who also pointed out the advantage of localizing the ascites before attempting aspiration for cytological examination.

6.16.e Neurology

(*i*) *Midline localization*

Although others may have previously and independently used the *A*-scope to study echoes received from within the intact living human skull, the first publication describing the method is that of Leksell (1956). His results were based on work apparently begun in 1953.

The basis of midline echoencephalography is that in the normal, the midline structures of the brain lie in a vertical *a–p* plane at the geometrical centre of the skull. This is at the time-centre of the corresponding *A*-scan produced by holding the ultrasonic probe in contact with the temporoparietal region just above the tip of the ear. This situation is disturbed by displacement of the midline. The criterion by which the midline echo is identified on the A-scan is that it is supposed normally to have the largest amplitude of all of the intracranial echoes.

Adequate swept gain compensation is provided, at frequencies of about 2 MHz and below, by arranging for the gain to increase to the maximum over a distance of about 50 mm (67 μs). If a substantially higher frequency is used, a two-stage swept gain may be necessary to compensate at the appropriate rates for the different attenuations in bone and brain.

Measurements made from a single A-scan are unreliable. It is much better—but far from foolproof—to examine the skull from each side in turn, and to display the two A-scans one above the other. Comparison is simplified if one of the two A-scans (usually the one obtained with the probe on the left side) is electrically inverted, so that the deflexions are in opposite directions from the two timebases, which lie close together near the centre of the display. A rather attractive possibility is to display the two A-scans simultaneously, by using two probes operating alternately, as suggested by Gordon (1959). This presents no electronic problems nowadays, but it is amusing to read in the literature of the trouble caused by an artifact at the time–centre of the A-scan due to poor isolation of the "inoperative" probe (Robinson and Kossoff, 1966; White and Blanchard, 1966).

Lithander (1960) developed the method, nowadays widely used, in which the time–centre of the skull is determined by transmission, and compared with the position of the midline as determined by reflexion. This technique is illustrated in Fig. 6.78. A displacement of 2–3 mm is generally considered to be within normal limits: to some extent, this reflects the inherent errors in the ultrasonic measurement, for so great an asymmetry would be unlikely in a normal patient.

There is quite a wide divergence between various authors in estimating the accuracy with which the midline can be localized. This is partly due to differing definitions of accuracy, but mainly to the surprisingly subjective nature of the test. Whether or not this is a valid criticism is a matter for personal opinion. There is no doubt that a skilled clinician can obtain high accuracy; thus, Brinker et al. (1965) claimed 97% in a series of 469 patients. On the other hand, White and Blanchard (1966) suggested that the objectivity of the test could be improved if the A-scan display is photographed with a time-exposure whilst small changes are made in the position and direction of the probe, since this seems to reduce the ambiguity in determining the position of the midline echo. Using this amplitude-averaging technique, White (1966) examined the results obtained in a series of 310 patients, and concluded that the echograms of nearly half of the patients with radiologically confirmed shifts could not be satisfactorily analysed, as compared with 10% of the whole group. This was presumed to be due to distortion of the midline structures which alters the characteristics of the midline echo so that it is no longer the intracranial echo of largest amplitude. As a screening method, the technique seems to be reliable: there were no errors when satisfactory echograms were obtained and no shift of the mid-

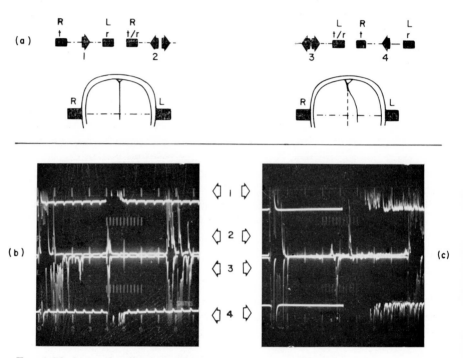

FIG. 6.78 A-scan localization of brain midline structures. (a) Diagrams indicating positions of probes in standardized examination. *t*, transmitting probe; *r*, receiving probe. Each of the positions 1 to 4 corresponds to the appropriate scans in the composite displays (b) and (c); (b) scans of an individual with central brain midline structures; (c) scans of a patient with brain midline structures displaced by 6 mm towards the left side by an intracerebral haemorrhage on the right side. The time markers on the scans of the normal patient correspond to 10 mm distances in soft tissues. (Courtesy F. G. M. Ross.)

line was diagnosed. In a further analysis, White (1967) reported no false-negative errors in 2500 examinations.

It is a waste of everyone's time—patient, operator and doctor, not to mention the waste of money—to leave conventional A-scope echoencephalographic investigations to non-clinical personnel. The reasons for this have been powerfully argued by White *et al.* (1969) and implicitly admitted by Schiefer *et al.* (1968). This restriction on the method effectively limits

its use to hospitals which already have alternative diagnostic capabilities, and even at these centres ultrasound may have fallen into disuse, or may not be available at all times.

Recognizing these deficiencies, Galicich and Williams (1971) have developed an instrument*, restricted solely to the location of the midline structures, which substitutes automatic pattern recognition criteria for operator decision. In this way, the operator can concentrate his attention on the positioning of the ultrasonic probe on the patient's head. Moreover, the acquisition and recording of sufficient data makes it possible to establish statistical confidence in the result.

The principles of the operation of the instrument (Williams, 1973) are as follows. A conventional ultrasonic probe is held on the patient's head in the usual way. A timing clock is triggered by a transmit search pulse. Echoes are amplified and gated into distal and middle memories. These memories are interrogated by a pattern recognition circuit, which either starts the computer or resets the whole system, depending on whether or not the received echoes were acceptable. The basis of acceptance of the distal echo pattern is the receipt of an echo doublet that exceeds a threshold level in amplitude and arises in a range gate opened approximately 100 mm beyond the probe. The round-trip time from the probe to the skin–air interface (the leading edge of the second echo in the doublet) is stored digitally as a number of timer counts. A successful measurement triggers a 250 Hz tone to alert the operator, and simultaneously institutes a search for echoes in the midhead region. Thus, every midline determination is normalized to the corresponding head width. The first single echo, or the first of two echoes which are separated by no more than 4 mm, that has an amplitude above a fixed threshold and which lies within the middle gate, is accepted as an echo from a midline structure. This gate is set automatically to occupy the distance $\pm 20\%$ from the true centreline of the head; and so, for example, it has a width of 30 mm if the temporoparietal diameter is 150 mm, and in this case no echo originating from a position more than 15 mm from the centreline would be accepted. If an echo group of characteristic midpattern is received, the difference between its distance from the probe, and that of the centreline, is computed and displayed as a shift to left or right, by a numerical indicator calibrated in millimetres. At the same time, a 500 s^{-1} tone is generated to inform the operator that the determination has been completed. On the other hand, if an acceptable midecho is not received within the same 2 ms period as the distal echo (the pulse repetition frequency is 500 s^{-1}), the whole memory is erased and the procedure is repeated. The brevity of this total search period ensures that

---

* Automatic Midline Computer: Diagnostic Electronics Corporation, Lexington, Massachusetts, USA. A similar instrument (Digiecho 1000) is manufactured by Radionics Ltd., Montreal, Canada.

every midline measurement is normalized to the corresponding head width.

As the location of each midecho is registered on the digital display, it is plotted manually to build up a histogram. The measuring process is then restarted, and so on until sufficient data points have been collected to allow the histogram to be interpreted.

Automatic echoencephalography has been evaluated by White and Hanna (1974) in 3333 consecutive patients. The great advantage of the technique seems to be the infrequency of false negative errors, although this depends on correct positioning of the probe. In patients with acute head injury, the diagnosis of an undisplaced midline can be accepted with a high degree of confidence, so that requests for many emergency angiograms can be avoided. The false-positive rate is around 15–20%.

Almost all are agreed that automatic techniques for ultrasonic midline localization have established an invaluable place in the care of the trauma patient. As White (1972) has pointed out, they make ultrasonic diagnosis available where the neurological need is greatest: this is in places without specialized equipment or personnel.

The increased reliability which became available with the advent of the automatic methods of midline localization led White and Curry (1974) to carry out experiments to determine the magnitudes of the various sources of error to which the method is subject. They investigated the following aspects:

(i) *Indentation of the scalp by the probe.* This does not introduce errors in conventional A-scope echoencephalography and other methods using two probes, one on each side of the head, simultaneously indenting the scalp by equal amounts. In techniques using only one probe, however, when measurements are compared with a centreline calculated to be at half the distance to the far-side scalp surface, the error is always decremental and approximates to 0·75 mm of soft tissue;

(ii) *Unequal thickness of the opposite sides of the skull.* This error may be incremental or decremental, and may be as much as the equivalent of 0·75 mm in soft tissue; and

(iii) *Refraction of the ultrasonic beam.* This may be due to rocking of the probe or inequalities in the skull thickness, or to the shape of the skull preventing a perpendicular orientation of the beam to the sagittal plane. Whatever the cause, the distance to the closest interfaces in the median sagittal plane is not measured. The error is always incremental, and typically is equal to 1–2 mm of soft tissue in magnitude.

One way of minimizing errors discussed under (i), whilst at the same time ensuring that sufficient couplant is trapped between the probe and the scalp, is to fit a "jelly bag" in front of the probe (Wealthall and Todd, 1972). The "bag" may consist of a latex membrane, held on to the probe by means of a collar. The difficulty with this gadget, however, is that multiple re-flexions occur within the jelly: but they are easy to recognize. Apparently, it is possible to incline a low megahertz frequency probe through an angle of 15° from the normal before these artifacts become troublesome.

(ii) A-scope studies of the brain

According to Kazner and Hopman (1973), ultrasonic investigations of the cerebral ventricles are more important clinically than measurements of the position of the midline structures. The widths of the third and lateral ventricles, and the distance from the lateral wall of the temporal horn to the inner skull table, can all be measured in suitable patients using the A-scope. In children, all three measurements are generally possible even in the absence of dilatation; but in adults, the width of the lateral ventricles can only be measured when they are substantially dilated.

The method has particular value in the investigation of hydrocephalus. Quite a sensitive measure is afforded by deriving a quantity—the cella-media index—equal to the ratio of the lateral ventricle width to the bi-parietal diameter. Values over 4·1 are normal; normal, slightly or moder-ately dilated ventricles have values in the range 4·1–3·8; values below 3·8 are always associated with abnormality. The diagnostic significance of the temporal horn echo is deduced from its position in relation to the midline and the end echo, expressed as the brain–mantle index. Values of 2·0–2·2 are normal. In posterior fossa lesions, values of 2·8–3·2 are common; higher values may occur in aqueduct stenosis or in infantile hydrocephalus.

It was reported by Kienast et al. (1971) that the amplitude of the midline echo decreases with the occurrence of brain death. This observation is relevant to the selection of organ donors for transplant, and to the ethics of continued life support.

A word of caution may be appropriate here. The identification of echoes arising from within the skull is, at best, difficult; great skill and clinical acumen are necessary if reliable results are to be obtained. With this in mind, it is interesting to read the Japanese accounts, such as that of Wagai et al. (1965), in which A-scans of the brain are interpreted as if the skull had no distorting influence. When the skull has been removed, it is possible to do this with much more confidence. Thus Müller (1972) has developed a method of exploring the brain following craniotomy whilst the patient is anaesthetized with the surface of the brain exposed for direct access. In this way gliomas, meningiomas, metastases and haematomas can be localized and distinguished, thus allowing the surgeon to plan the operation more logically.

Since ultrasonic scanning of the brain through the intact skull is so very liable to be spoilt by artifacts, the possibility that access to at least part of the brain might be gained by scanning through the superior orbital fissure deserved the careful investigation that it has received from Curry *et al.* (1973). Using this route, they hoped to visualize the structures in the posterior part of the cranium above the tentorium cerebelli. Experiments on skulls and fixed, post-mortem brains showed that to use this window it is essential that the beam should be accurately centred on both axes of the fissure. It was found that bones sufficiently thin to act as ultrasonic transparencies frequently occur in the margins of the orbit. When such a transparency is present in the greater wing of the sphenoidal bone, the acoustic window transmits more energy and has a larger aperture. Under these circumstances, and especially if the transparency is present only on one side, the images displayed from the two sides may be sufficiently dissimilar to cause errors in diagnosis.

(*iii*) Intracranial pulsations

The amplitude of the echo from the midline structure of the brain normally oscillates in sympathy with the cardiac cycle. Jeppsson (1964) demonstrated that the rise-time of the maximum excursion of the midline echo amplitude, normalized to the heart rate, is significantly decreased in patients with raised intracranial pressure. The ultrasonic information may be presented in the form of a time–amplitude recording of the signals fed from an electronic integrator. It was suggested by ter Braak and de Vlieger (1965) that this change in echo amplitude may be due to alterations in the curvature of the surface from which the midline echo originates, and that the extent of these alterations depends upon the magnitude of the intracranial pressure. This theory is supported by the apparent existence of horizontal echo pulsations along the time-base, associated with the variations in echo amplitude.

The character of intracerebral echo amplitude pulsations seems to be related to other clinical conditions in addition to the pressure of the cerebrospinal fluid (see, for example, de Vlieger, 1967). Richardson *et al.* (1972) have shown that these pulsations may result from the slow pressure waves which occur in patients with raised intracerebral pressure. In this connexion, it is relevant that Quaknine *et al.* (1973) included confirmation of the absence of intracerebral echo-pulsations as one of a battery of tests of brain death. Similar changes have been reported by Oka *et al.* (1974).

Despite the rather encouraging impression which may be given by this superficial review, it is as well to know that, on the basis of a careful study, White and Stevenson (1975) concluded that the recording of the amplitude and pulsation of the echoes from intracranial interfaces gives little information, and is very likely to mislead.

According to ter Braak and de Vlieger (1965), the amplitude of the pulsating shift in the position of an echo-producing interface in the brain is very small, being around 0·1 mm. On purely physical grounds, the measurement of so small a shift occurring synchronously with a variation in echo amplitude is subject to relatively large errors, due to the effect of the latter on the range resolution (see Section 6.1.b). Thus, although these pulsations may be related to clinical conditions (Avant, 1966; Jenkins *et al.*, 1971), it would be unrealistic to suggest that the method has yet been developed to a degree that is acceptable in clinical diagnosis.

(iv) Two-dimensional visualization of the brain

Possibly the first attempt to obtain pulse–echo two-dimensional ultrasonic scans of the brain through the intact skull was that of de Vlieger *et al.* (1963). Their initial experiments with a water-bath arrangement, in which the cranium was immersed, and a seal in the side of the tank achieved with an inflated pneumatic tyre, were disappointing because of the air which was trapped in the hair, the multiple reflexions in the water, and compression of the head by the sealing tyre. Therefore they developed a contact scanner, which produced some encouraging results, particularly in patients with hydrocephalus. As might be expected, attempts to scan the adult brain through the normal skull were, for all practical purposes, failures because of the distortion introduced by the skull. A similar approach was adopted by Brinker and Taveras (1966). It is not surprising that another water-immersion scanner, that of Makow and Real (1965), also failed to image the contents of the adult brain, with the exception of the midline structures.

Air bubbles trapped in hair, and multiple reflexions, are practical limitations which doubtless could be overcome if ultrasonic two-dimensional scanning through a water bath was capable of visualizing the brain through the intact skull. There is ample evidence (see, for example, White *et al.*, 1969), however, that the distortion of the ultrasonic beam which is caused by the skull is so great that it is simply impossible to obtain images of the brain using a conventionally narrow beam and ordinary scanning methods. Fortunately, in infants, and in patients with hydrocephalus, this limitation is not so serious. This explains the success of de Vlieger *et al.* (1963), and of Wealthall and Todd (1973). Similarly, Kossoff *et al.* (1974) and Garrett *et al.* (1975), using a grey-scale system, have reported the visualization of quite fine details of intracranial anatomy. It also is compatible with the excellent results which have been obtained by Freund (1974) and Kamphuisen (1974), using the electronically steered array of Somer (1968). This array is held motionless on the scalp, whilst a two-dimensional image is constructed in real time, as described in Section 6.10.c. Distortions due to the skull do not vary with time, and so the anatomical features can generally be identified.

It has been demonstrated by Fry (1968), using the rhesus monkey, that it is possible ultrasonically to visualize *in vivo* anatomic features of the ventricles, cisterns, sulci and major blood vessels, and the internal surface of the cranial vault, if access to the intracranial structures is provided via an opening in the skull. In these experiments, the animals underwent craniectomy to provide this access; the ultrasonic studies were carried out after the scalp had healed. Water-bath coupling was employed. The transmitting transducer had a diameter of 25 mm; the receiving transducer was mounted coaxially with the transmitter, at the minor focus of an ellipsoidal mirror with an aperture of 140 mm. The frequency was 2·5 MHz. The data were presented as two-dimensional sections at 1 mm intervals. Fry (1970) and Heimburger et al. (1973) were fortunate enough to have as a volunteer an individual who had several years earlier had a craniotomy for therapeutic purposes. Thus they were able to demonstrate intracranial anatomy in man with a resolution similar to that previously achieved in the monkey.

It is encouraging that Fry et al. (1974) found that the resolution of this wide-aperture system was not intolerably degraded by the presence of interposed skull, scalp simulator and hair. In their experiments, they measured a maximum shift in azimuth at the focus of 1·5 mm. The variation in echo amplitude was considerable, the difference between two skulls being 11 dB: but here, conditions of storage of the skulls might have differed, and the problem might be less in the intact living patient.

At the present time, when computerized tomography is de rigueur in brain visualization, it is natural that enthusiasm to develop two-dimensional ultrasonic imaging of the brain in the normal intact skull is somewhat dulled. Some even say—for example, White (1974)—that the advantage of real-time imaging is unlikely to warrant the expenditure of more time, effort and money. Those familiar with the practical inconveniences of computerized tomography—problems of immobilization, processing time, X-ray dosage and expense—may feel that ultrasound still has some potential for development.

6.16.f Obstetrics and Gynaecology

(i) Early diagnosis of pregnancy

During the first few weeks of pregnancy, the uterus is normally situated within the pelvis and so it is inaccessible to ultrasonic investigation. Donald (1963) demonstrated that it is possible to scan the uterus in very early pregnancy through the bladder, if the bladder is first allowed to become filled with urine. Pregnancy can thus be diagnosed within the first five to six weeks after the last menstrual period in a normal cycle, and occasionally even before the urine tests are positive. A scan obtained by this technique is shown in Fig. 6.79.

Donald (1974) thinks that a routine ultrasonic examination should be made of every pregnancy, between weeks 20 and 24, to establish maturity, to detect multiple pregnancy, and to locate the placenta. Ultrasonic scanning also has an important role in the diagnosis of pregnancy failure. This has been reviewed by Robinson (1975).

(ii) Diagnosis of multiple pregnancy

Multiple pregnancy can be reliably diagnosed by the demonstration of more than one foetal head, as shown in Fig. 6.80. Caution is necessary because it sometimes happens that a section through the foetal trunk is mistaken for a head. This error is less likely with a grey-scale scan, since structures apart from the foetal brain midline can be identified with certainty.

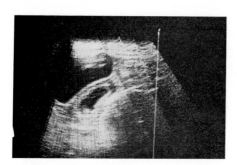
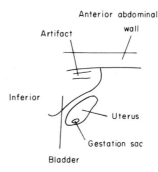

FIG. 6.79 Normal pregnancy, eight weeks gestation. Longitudinal section 10 mm right of midline. (Courtesy F. G. M. Ross.)

Campbell and Dewhurst (1970) have described how they used this method to diagnose a quintuplet pregnancy at nine weeks menstrual age, in a patient who had received hormone treatment for infertility.

(iii) Visualization of placenta

The first description in the literature of placental localization by two-dimensional ultrasonography seems to be that of Gottesfeld *et al.* (1966). They used an instrument with a bistable display—i.e. with zero dynamic range—but nevertheless noticed that the placenta gives rise to a characteristic pattern. This first report was followed by many others, such as those of Donald and Abdulla (1968), Campbell and Kohorn 1968), Morrison *et al.* (1972) and Kukard and Freeman (1973). The posterior placenta posed the major problem in detection, but accuracies were high for other placental sites, particularly when the internal os, or at least the vagina, could be visualized. Some papers appeared which compared the accuracy of ultrasonic localization with that of other methods, such as radioisotopes (Cohen *et al.*, 1972), radioisotopes, radiography and thermo-

graphy (Aanta, 1971), and radioisotopes, radiography and Doppler ultrasound (Brown and Young, 1972). Interesting though these comparisons
are, they are largely of historical value now that grey-scale echography has
eliminated many of the uncertainties of earlier methods (Kossoff and
Garrett, 1972a). Thus, in a series of 145 consecutively examined patients,
referred for general obstetrical reasons and not necessarily for placental
localization, the placenta was seen in 143 (nearly 99%); it was seen in all
20 patients for whom placental localization had been specifically requested.
Typical grey-scale scans are shown in Fig. 6.81.

Grey-scale scans reveal much detail in the placenta (Kossoff *et al.*, 1974).
Thus, the attachment of the cord may be seen, and infarcts and bleeding
are readily demonstrated. Calcification produces relatively strong echoes.

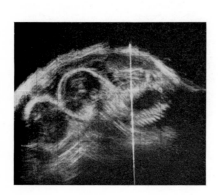
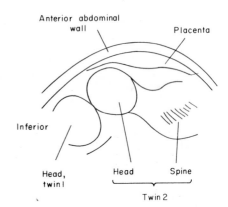

FIG. 6.80 Twin pregnancy, 29 weeks gestation. Longitudinal section 10 mm right
of midline. (Courtesy F. G. M. Ross.)

The scans may be helpful in patients with suspected rhesus iso-immuniza-
tion, but caution is needed because occasionally in the normal the placenta
may be remarkably thick. In this connexion, an attempt has been made to
estimate the volume of the placenta from scans made in longitudinal and
transverse planes (Hellman *et al.*, 1970), making the assumption that the
placenta is a convex–concave solid of resolution. The ultrasonically determined volume was consistently more than that measured by water displacement after delivery; this was presumably due to blood loss.

There are two circumstances in which ultrasonic placentography may be
especially helpful. The first is when placenta praevia is suspected, usually
as a result of vaginal bleeding. The second is as a preliminary to amniocentesis (Abramowski *et al.*, 1971; Bang and Northeved, 1972; Jonatha,
1974). In this application, in a series of 175 patients subjected to amniocentesis under ultrasonic guidance, Miskin *et al.* (1975) found that, in
comparison with results obtained with the aid of ultrasound, the number of

abortions dropped from 5 to 3%. The number of blood stained taps fell from 22 to 7%. The number of failed amniotic fluid cultures fell from 16 to 1·5%.

(iv) Assessment of foetal development

The measurement of foetal biparietal diameter is of established value in the assessment of maturity. The ultrasonic technique first suggested by Donald

(a)
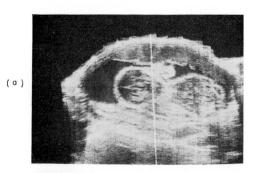
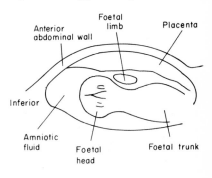

(b)
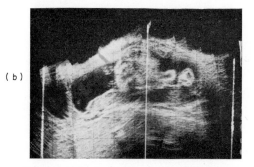
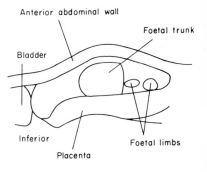

FIG. 6.81 Longitudinal scans illustrating placental sites. (a) Anterior placenta, 26 week pregnancy; (b) posterior placenta praevia, 28-week pregnancy. (Courtesy F. G. M. Ross.)

and Brown (1961) and introduced into clinical practice by Willocks et al. (1964), Thompson et al. (1965), and Durkan and Russo (1966), was placed on a firm scientific basis by Campbell (1968). Longitudinal scans are first made with a two-dimensional scanner, until the foetal head is identified. The angle between the vertical and the line of echoes from the midline structures is measured, and a transverse scan is made with the plane of the scan set to this angle with respect to the vertical. The plane of this scan is adjusted until the foetal head is seen as an ovoid with the midline echo bisecting its longest axis. This scheme can only be followed if the vertex

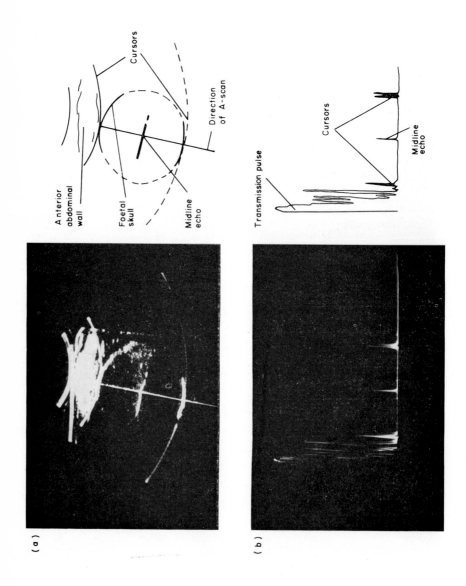

(a)

(b)

is in the occipito-transverse position; interpretive skill is otherwise required in adjusting the scan plane, and it is essential that the midline structures should be visualized if reliable results are to be obtained. Small adjustments are then made, until the maximum diameter has been found. Once the appropriate scan plane orientation has been achieved, there are various methods by which the diameter may be measured. The simplest is to measure directly from the B-scan: but this is not to be recommended. It is much better to align the ultrasonic beam so that its path may be seen on the B-scan to pass along the biparietal diameter, and to measure the diameter as the distance between electronically generated markers positioned on the skull echoes, either on the B-scan or on the A-scan (Hall et al., 1970). These markers appear as brightened dots on the displays. A typical result is shown in Fig. 6.82. The distance between them may be read off from a calibrated control, or a digital display (Bowley et al., 1972, 1973; Whittingham, 1973).

The measurement of the biparietal diameter by Campbell's (1968) method is liable to several errors (Davison et al., 1973; Watmough et al., 1974b). One of these errors is due to poor display of the midline structures, which may appear to be discontinuous. Christie (1974) has put these matters into perspective. To some extent, the difficulties are likely to disappear as grey-scale displays allow intracranial structures to be identified so that the exact sectional plane may be determined (Kossoff and Garrett, 1972b). In the meanwhile, measurements may be made in both longitudinal and transverse sections, with greater confidence being given to the result when these measurements agree. Moreover, the use of a third electronic marker, automatically generated midway between the markers positioned on the opposite sides of the skull, assists in identifying the midline echoes (Watmough et al., 1974a).

It may be possible to measure the biparietal diameter by means of a small, hand-held, real-time scanner. This proposal has been tested by Fleming (1974), who constructed a scanner based on a single transducer motor-driven repetitively through a 60° sector at 0·75 s per sweep. The technique seems to work, but there are a number of difficulties. Apparently the complete freedom which the operator has in positioning the scan plane makes orientation with the anatomy more difficult, because he has mentally to relate changes in the image on a stationary display, to changes in spatial position.

Fig. 6.82 Technique of biparietal cephalometry. The appropriate section through the foetal skull is first identified using the two-dimensional B-scope, as shown in (a). The cursors of the electronic caliper are set to coincide with the parietal bones. The display is simultaneously presented on an A-scope, and the cursors are adjusted more exactly, as shown in (b). The biparietal diameter is read off from the calibrated control. (Courtesy J. E. E. Fleming.)

No matter how accurately the ultrasonic beam may be aligned with the parietal bones, and the electronic markers may be positioned on the skull, the accuracy of measurement of the biparietal diameter depends on the choice of the value of the velocity. Indeed, it has even been suggested by Whittingham (1971) that it might be better not even to pretend to convert the time measurement into "distance". The sparse reference to this in the literature is worrying, since it is a potential source of systematic error. The velocity is generally assumed to be 1600 m s⁻¹, and this value is based on comparisons between antenatal ultrasonic time measurements and post-natal caliper distance measurements (Willocks *et al.*, 1964). Recent data of Wladimiroff *et al.* (1975) disagree with this value: at term, the velocity was found to be 1540 m s⁻¹, whilst it was 1517 m s⁻¹ at 18 weeks gestation. The situation is complicated since the markers are in practice positioned on the proximal surfaces of the foetal skull, so that the measured distance includes one two-way transit through the skull. The velocity in foetal skull is certainly higher than that in soft tissues. Therefore 1600 m s⁻¹ may be a reasonable estimate of effective velocity near term, but the possibility of a lower velocity in earlier pregnancy should not be forgotten.

There is reason to doubt, on purely physical grounds, that an accuracy of measurement of much better than 1 mm could be possible with present techniques of ultrasonic foetal cephalometry. Ultrasonic frequencies of 3 MHz and less seem to be used. At 3 MHz, a distance of 1 mm corresponds to two wavelengths. The measurement is based on the estimation of the time–position of two echoes: for an overall accuracy of 1 mm at 3 MHz, the position of each echo needs to be estimated to better than about one wavelength. It is explained in Section 6.1.b that such a resolution would require quite stringent conditions of dynamic range. The situation is proportionately worse at lower frequencies.

The measured value of foetal biparietal diameter may be used as an index of foetal maturity. The relationship between the biparietal diameter and the gestational age in normal pregnancy is shown in Fig. 6.83. The pre-diction is best made in early pregnancy (13–20 weeks), when the rate of growth is high, but predictions can be made up to 30 weeks: moreover, Lunt and Chard (1974) found that their results were most reproducible between weeks 23 and 31. Campbell (1969) made maturity predictions in 170 patients in whom the foetal maturity was in doubt; delivery occurred within nine days of the date predicted from the ultrasonic measurement in 84% of patients in whom labour began spontaneously and who were delivered of mature babies. There is thus an obvious advantage in screening all patients with suspect dates—amounting to about 40% of the population—by ultrasonic examination in early pregnancy.

Foetal growth may be followed by serial measurements of the biparietal diameter. A foetus with small biparietal diameter in relation to supposed age but which is growing normally is assumed to be a case of mistaken maturity, and the patient is allowed to proceed past the conventionally expected date of delivery. Thus, the method ensures proper management of clinically small-for-dates pregnancy, and it is preferable both to urinary oestrogen assay (Campbell and Kurjak, 1972), and to other biochemical tests (Robinson *et al.*, 1973).

The prediction of birth weight from a single biparietal diameter measurement in late pregnancy is not reliable (Ianniruberto and Gibbons, 1971;

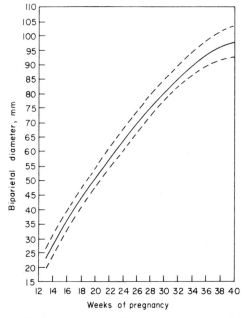

FIG. 6.83 Relationship between gestational age and biparietal diameter. The dotted lines represent the ±2 standard deviation limits. (Data of Campbell, 1969.)

Varma, 1974). A more promising method is based on the measurement of the dimensions of the foetal body (Hansmann and Voigt, 1973; Ylöstalo, 1974), and in this connexion it is the area of the cross-section of the abdomen which is probably most useful, as this is not constrained by the skeleton.

Although the systematic errors of different measuring methods may differ, the results are clinically useful provided that internal consistency is maintained. This is well illustrated by the data of Flamme (1972), whose distance measurements are some 5% less than those of Campbell (1969).

It is not possible to measure the biparietal diameter in very early pregnancy. Between weeks 6 and 14, however, the maturity of pregnancy may be predicted to within three days from measurement of the foetal crown–rump length (Robinson, 1973). During this period, this rate of growth has an average value of around 10 mm per week. The technique of measurement is not easy, however, and it is necessary to align the scan plane so that the long axis of the foetus lies within it. Compound scanning is not helpful; grey-scale display is.

(v) Foetal anatomy

A significant proportion of patients admitted to hospital with bleeding in early pregnancy are finally diagnosed as having blighted ova. The term "blighted ovum" is used to describe an impregnated ovum whose development has become arrested before the completion of the first trimester. Ultrasonically, according to Donald et al. (1972), the condition may be diagnosed with two-dimensional scans from the following features: loss of definition of the gestation sac within the first few weeks of pregnancy; absence of foetal echoes, which in a normal pregnancy may be seen from eight weeks amenorrhoea onwards; small-for-dates gestation sac; failure of growth; and low position of the sac, as a prelude to its expulsion. Using these criteria, Donald et al. (1972) examined 141 women with bleeding in the first trimester of pregnancy. In 66 patients who aborted, the ultrasonic appearances suggested blighted ova in 57. In 10 of the 75 patients whose pregnancy continued, the ultrasonic appearance was abnormal on at least one occasion. The use of modern techniques—for the detection of foetal heart motion (Sections 6.16.f.vi and 7.3.c), and grey-scale display—should enable more reliable diagnoses to be made.

When anencephaly occurs in a single pregnancy, the best management is early diagnosis and termination. The incidence of this complication of pregnancy is approximately 1–2 in 1000. Although the observation of anencephaly in two-dimensional scans was mentioned by Sundén (1964), apparently it was Campbell et al. (1972) who were the first to be sufficiently confident of their ultrasonic diagnosis to terminate an anencephalic pregnancy at 17 weeks after ovulation. Anencephaly in one of twins is very rare, but it has been confirmed by ultrasonic scanning at 32 weeks, in a patient described by Fisher et al. (1975).

Hydrocephaly is much less common than anencephaly, and the condition has not yet been diagnosed sufficiently early in pregnancy to allow therapeutic abortion to be performed. Campbell (1973) mentions three diagnostic criteria. These are: a biparietal diameter (see Section 6.16.f.iv) exceeding 110 mm; a foetal head being more spherical than the normal ovoid, with the midline structures frequently asymmetrically positioned; and the ratio of the cross-sectional areas of the head to the thorax being at least two to one. Likewise in microcephaly, diagnosis has not yet been achieved early enough to permit termination, but a ratio of less than one to two in the cross-sectional areas of the head to the thorax is very suspicious.

Particularly in grey-scale scans (Kossoff *et al.*, 1974), it is possible to see foetal structures such as heart, large thoracic vessels particularly aorta, spine, liver, gallbladder, stomach, spleen, genitalia and extremities. Thus, Garrett *et al.* (1970) have diagnosed polycystic kidneys in the foetus (even without grey-scale); and hydronephrosis, megaureter and urethal obstruction have been diagnosed by Garrett *et al.* (1975b), whilst Garrett *et al.* (1975a) have described the visualization of a foetal lung tumour and associated abnormalities. Duodenal atresia has been demonstrated antenatally by hydramnios and fluid-filled spaces (the duodenum and the stomach) in the foetus at 34 weeks; this was confirmed by neonatal radiography and corrected successfully by surgery (Loveday *et al.*, 1975). Even with a low dynamic range display, Campbell *et al.* (1975a) were sufficiently confident to diagnose spina bifida in one foetus out of three, two of which subsequently proved to have neural-tube defects. Although this excited some controversy (Gray, 1975; Kitau *et al.*, 1975; Goldie and Monk, 1975; Campbell *et al.*, 1975b), it seems reasonable to expect the method will become more reliable as the instrumentation is improved, and that prenatal ultrasonic diagnosis of spina bifida will be of major social importance.

(vi) Foetal heart rate

Detection of the pulsation of the foetal heart by means of a Doppler probe placed on the abdominal wall is unreliable before the twelfth week of pregnancy (see Section 7.3.c). A large proportion of threatened abortions present before this period. Robinson (1972) has developed a method using pulse–echo ultrasound, giving reliable detection by an abdominal approach from the forty-eighth day of pregnancy onwards (menstrual age). The uterus is visualized on a two-dimensional scan made in longitudinal section using the full-bladder technique. The foetus is located, and electronic markers are positioned so that, with the probe in contact with a chosen point on the abdomen, one marker lies on each side of the foetus. Small angular adjustments are made to the direction of the ultrasonic beam until echoes are seen between the markers on a simultaneous A-scan display, which pulsate in range and amplitude at the foetal heart rate. A time position recording system is then used to record these movements over a period of time, and hence it is an easy matter to measure the heart rate.

The detection of the foetal heart movement—or the confirmation of its absence—may be helpful in the management of recurrent and threatened abortion, and in the confirmation of pregnancy. Robinson and Shaw-Dunn (1973) found that in threatened abortion the foetal heart rate is not statistically different from that in normal pregnancy. The human embryonic heart probably starts to function approximately 21 days after conception.

The heart rate, as measured ultrasonically, rises from 123 min^{-1} at 45 days to a maximum of 177 min^{-1} at 64 days, and gradually falls to 147 min^{-1} at 100 days. These changes in heart rate correlate with the morphological and physiological changes which occur in the foetal heart during the period of gestation.

In studies of the foetal heart in late pregnancy, Murata *et al.* (1971) were able to distinguish between echoes from the mitral and tricuspid valves, and the interventricular system.

(vii) *Foetal breathing*

Dawes *et al.* (1972) have described how they recorded tracheal fluid flow in the foetal lamb, by means of an electromagnetic flowmeter transducer introduced *in utero*. The records show a remarkable episodic cyclical rhythm of breathing movements during each 24 h period, apparently correlated to changes in foetal blood gases. Changes in oxygen and carbon dioxide partial pressures do affect foetal breathing, but they do not normally vary much during the course of a day. The onset and cessation of rapid irregular foetal breathing movements are associated with changes in the state of sleep, breathing being present during rapid-eye-movement sleep and disappearing at the onset of quiet sleep. Rapid irregular breathing movements only occur during periods of rapid-eye-movement sleep: their incidence during these periods is decreased by foetal hypoxemia, and increased by hypercapnia.

The feasibility of detecting foetal breathing in pregnant women by means of pulse–echo ultrasound was first demonstrated by Boddy and Robinson (1971). They used an A-scope display, and an external probe held on the abdominal surface in a universal joint. The probe was orientated so that the rapid movements of the foetal heart could be seen on the display. The anterior foetal thoracic wall gives rise to an echo nearer in range than the heart, and the movements of this echo were obtained with a time-to-voltage analogue converter (see Section 6.9) and recorded on a polygraph. Using this technique, Boddy and Mantell (1972) succeeded in recording foetal breathing movements in all of a series of 34 pregnant women.

These observations confirm that the physiological systems of the foetus are exercised, though discontinuously. Dawes (1973) has discussed the relationship between foetal breathing and status. In general during the last 20 weeks of pregnancy, movements of the foetal chest occur at a frequency of 40–70 min^{-1} for 70% of the time (Dawes, 1974). This rhythmic movement is normally broken up by very short periods of apnoea. The normal breathing pattern is disturbed under adverse circumstances such as hypoxia or hypoglycaemia: extended periods of apnoea with episodes of gasping movements may then be seen. When the foetus is in great distress or even in imminent danger of death, the breathing movements cease except for occasional gasps. As Boddy and Dawes (1975) themselves were the first to point out, these results seem almost too good to be true, since high-risk foetuses can be identified whether from clinically high-risk or normal pregnancies. Thus it may become possible to identify, before the onset of labour, those foetuses to which the scarce facilities of continuous monitoring might be most advantageously directed.

It is certainly not easy to monitor foetal chest wall movements with an A-scan ultrasonic system. It is difficult to aim the ultrasonic beam and to adjust the swept gain and the analogue gate. The criteria by which the thoracic wall echo is recognized is that it moves rhythmically, asynchronously either with the maternal respiration and pulse, or the foetal pulse: the rate is 30–100 min^{-1} and the amplitude is up to 6 mm. The problems of satisfying these criteria have been discussed by Farman and Thomas (1975) and Farman et al. (1975): they recommended that a two-dimensional B-scanner is necessary to ensure an appropriate orientation of the monitoring beam, although this is clearly unnecessary if the operator is skilled in obstetrics and ultrasound. Likewise, Meire et al. (1975) found it helpful in achieving proper orientation to make a conventional two-dimensional B-scan, or at least to locate the foetal heart with a Doppler detector (see Section 7.3.c). Moreover, they used an unusually big probe, with a transducer diameter of 28 mm, operating at the rather low frequency of 1 MHz. (Reports are beginning to be published—see, for example, Hohler and Fox, 1975—of the visualization of foetal breathing movements by real-time ultrasonic two-dimensional scanning.) There is no doubt, however, that the present techniques cannot be used for routine monitoring, since it would be unreasonable to expect nurses to devote undivided attention to the procedure. The development of a simple-to-use system is very desirable. It may be that a pulsed Doppler (see Section 7.2.f) could be aimed at the foetal heart—and this is regularly done by nurses with continuous wave Dopplers—and that gates could be automatically adjusted to detect movements from the regions which must be occupied by the foetal thoracic wall when the beam is appropriately orientated. Furthermore, compensation could be made for movements such as those due to maternal respiration: in principle, these displace opposite walls of the foetal thorax in the same direction, whereas foetal breathing movements are in opposite directions.

(viii) Foetal urine-production rate

In middle to late pregnancy, urine in foetal bladder may be visualized as an echo-free area low in the abdominal cavity (Campbell et al., 1973). It is more easily seen if a grey-scale display is used. The volume of the bladder may be estimated by measuring three radii, mutually at right angles, from appropriately orientated scans, and by multiplying the product of these radii by $4\pi/3$. The greater the volume of urine, the more accurate the estimation. In a series of 33 patients with normal pregnancies of 32–41 weeks, the duration of the bladder cycle was found from serial measurements to lie between 50 and 155 min. Such measurements also allow the rate of urine production to be estimated. Wladimiroff and Campbell (1974) studied 92 patients with normal pregnancies, and found the mean hourly urine production rate to increase from 10 ml at 30 weeks to 27 ml at 40 weeks. No circadian variation was demonstrated. In about 50% of 62 patients with complicated pregnancies, the urine-production rate was less than that of all but 5% of the normal foetuses. There was a highly significant increase in the number of growth-retarded babies in this group, but no correlation was found between reduced urine-production rate and perinatal hypoxia.

(ix) Diagnosis of foetal death

Possibly the simplest test of foetal life is the detection of foetal heart movements by means of an ultrasonic Doppler instrument (see Section 7.3.c). Failure to detect movements by this method sometimes occurs even though the foetus may be alive. Certain changes occur within the tissue of the foetus after death, however, and these produce echo patterns which may be recognized on two-dimensional ultrasonic scans (Thompson, 1973). There is an increased density of interfaces within the thorax and the skull, the chest wall is thickened and irregular in shape. Moreover, growth ceases and this may be confirmed by serial measurements of biparietal diameter over a period of, say, 5 days.

(x) Hydatidiform mole

A hydatidiform mole can be identified as it appears on the scan as a mass of uniformly distributed echoes filling the uterus (Donald and Brown, 1961; MacVicar and Donald, 1963; Birnholz and Barnes, 1973). The echoes almost all disappear when the sensitivity of the system is reduced, although the mass remains transonic so that the posterior uterine wall can still be seen. A typical scan is shown in Fig. 6.84.

In a series of 115 patients in whom hydatidiform mole was suspected, and who were scanned by Kossoff et al. (1974) using a grey-scale system, 21 were diagnosed as having moles: of these, one was a missed abortion, and in another, the foetus was dead. The remaining 19 patients were correctly diagnosed.

(xi) Detection of intrauterine contraceptive devices

Janssens et al. (1973) considered that ultrasonic two-dimensional scanning was a good, but not perfect, method of detecting intrauterine contraceptive devices, except when pregnancy coincided. It was not good at distinguishing between Dalkon shield and Copper-7 IUCDs, but the Lippe's loop did

give a characteristic pattern. Similarly, in every one of 51 patients subsequently confirmed to have an intrauterine contraceptive device, the device
was seen by Zelnick *et al.* (1975) on ultrasonic scanning. It was not seen in
either of two patients who were pregnant, presumably because the echoes
from the device were indistinguishable from those from the gestation.

The main value of ultrasonic scanning in the management of patients
suspected of having lost IUCDs (maybe because the threads are missing)
is as a preliminary investigation. If the device can be seen in the uterus, all
is well. If it cannot, abdominal radiography or some other search procedure
must be instituted to test the possibility of translocation (MacKay and
Mowat, 1974; Vrijens *et al.*, 1974).

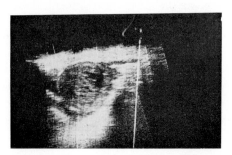
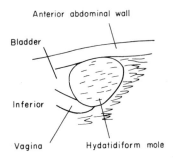

Anterior abdominal wall

Bladder

Inferior

Vagina

Hydatidiform mole

FIG. 6.84 Hydatidiform mole. Fourteen weeks amenorrhoea. Longitudinal section, 10 mm right of midline. (Courtesy F. G. M. Ross.)

(*xii*) *Abdominal tumours associated with pregnancy*

It occasionally happens that pregnancy may be complicated by the occurrence of an abdominal tumour such as an ovarian cyst, or fibroids. The
treatment of the patient is determined by the type of tumour: a cyst
requires surgery, whereas fibroids may be allowed to remain at least for
the duration of the pregnancy. Another consideration is that a tumour may
prevent the presenting part from engaging, and thus it may obstruct labour.
The differential diagnosis is not easy with a low dynamic range display,
since fibroids in pregnancy may be almost as anechoic as a cyst. They do
attenuate ultrasound more rapidly, however, and Donald (1972) has pointed
out that the distal wall of a fibroid may give rise to a weaker echo than
that of a cyst, particularly if a high frequency (5 MHz) is used. No doubt
the differential diagnosis would be easier with a grey-scale display.

(*xiii*) *Gynaecological tumours*

The common gynaecological tumours amenable to ultrasonic diagnosis are
carcinomas of the ovary, uterus and cervix, ovarian cysts, and fibroids.
The differentiation between ovarian cyst and fibroids is discussed in the

previous Sub-section. The partitions within multilocular cysts can be visualized. Malignant ovarian cysts appear in scans as more bizarre and disorganized tumours. Ultrasonic examination is particularly valuable in the very obese patient, where palpation is futile. Surgical strategy can be planned more effectively where the size of the tumour is accurately known, especially when it is desirable to remove the tumour intact in order to minimize the possibility of neoplastic spread.

6.16.g Oncology

(i) Ultrasonic scanning in radiotherapy and chemotherapy

Ultrasonic visualization of malignant lesions may be of great clinical value in planning radiotherapy, and in assessing the effects of treatment, both by radiotherapy and by chemotherapy.

The high degree of accuracy which is potentially available with computerized planning in radiotherapy is not matched by the usual methods for obtaining data on patient contours and tumour location. Often only guesswork is used. This is most unsatisfactory, since there is no doubt that effective radiotherapy depends on accurate planning. For example, Herring and Compton (1971) have predicted that the probability of a cure may fall from 80 to 26% if the radiation dose fraction is reduced by 10% in a standardized situation.

Brascho (1974) has developed a system which accepts information obtained from ultrasonic scanning, and enters it directly into the computerized radiation treatment planning routine. This information includes the surface geometry of the patient, and the locations of solid tumours and normal organs. Contact scanning is used. The ultrasonic scan, displayed on a storage oscilloscope, is inspected by the clinician who is able to delineate regions of interest using a light pen. These data are stored in the computer, and may be displayed for subsequent amendment if necessary. Once the clinician is satisfied that the information is accurate and complete, the computer is allowed to proceed with the preparation of the optimal treatment plan.

Similar methods have been described by Jentzsch et al. (1974) and by Slater et al. (1974). The latter report is particularly interesting because a sonic graph-pen digitizer is used to trace outlines on the ultrasonic scan.

The technique probably has its most important applications in planning radiotherapy of the retroperitoneal lymph nodes, the pancreas, the adrenals, the kidneys, the uterus, the ovaries, the bladder, and the prostate. Results in visualizing the lymph nodes have been presented by Asher and Freimanis (1969), Damascelli et al. (1969) and Holm (1971); the other organs are discussed elsewhere in this Section. The method is useful not only in the location of areas for treatment, but also in the delineation of intolerant structures. For example, Sanders *et al.* (1974) have pointed out the advantages of identifying unaffected parts of the genito-urinary tract so that their irradiation may be avoided.

It seems that a randomized controlled trial might be appropriate to test the contribution which ultrasonic scanning could make in improving the effectiveness of radiotherapy. Moreover, most contemporary radiotherapy planning procedures are essentially conducted in two dimensions. Three-dimensional ultrasonic scans (see Section 6.11) or, at least, three-dimensional ultrasonic data, might give more realism to the calculations.

Another, rather specialized, application of two-dimensional ultrasonic scanning is in the acquisition of data for the calculation of dose distributions resulting from radium (and similar) insertions in the treatment of gynaecological tumours (Mayer *et al.*, 1975).

In electron therapy of the chest wall, it is important to know the thickness of the wall so that the irradiation may be adjusted to spare the lungs. This thickness may be measured either by an A-scope (Whittingham, 1962; Jackson *et al.*, 1970), or by a B-scope with water-bath coupling.

Scanning is also useful in the assessment of the effect of irradiation: the lack of radiosensitivity of certain tumours can be discovered earlier than by other methods, and the radiotherapist can change the treatment schedule accordingly. The first reference to this seems to be in an article by Goldberg *et al.* (1968): using an A-scope, they followed the regression of brain tumours by measuring the return of the echoes from the midline structures towards the centre of the skull.

Direct observation by two-dimensional scanning of tumours treated by radiotherapy or by chemotherapy is helpful in evaluating regression (Brascho, 1972; Kobayashi *et al.*, 1972a, b, 1974). The method has been further developed by Eule *et al.* (1973), who enlarged their scans to life size, and drew aruond the features of interest on tracing paper. Likewise Tolbert *et al.* (1974) used tracings of serial ultrasonic scans to monitor spleen-tumour volume in chronic lymphocytic leukaemia, and liver-tumour volume in retroperitoneal rhabdomyosarcoma.

The growth rates of intracranial neoplasms have been studied by Heimburger *et al.* (1973) in three patients, using ultrasonic scanning through the healed scalp following surgical removal of a portion of the skull and the insertion of a stainless steel wire mesh prosthesis (see Section 6.16.e). Fissures, sulci, ventricles, cisterns, blood vessels, and some grey-matter interfaces were visualized. Fine details of tumour proliferation and regression were accurately delineated, thus making it possible to follow the effects of radiotherapy.

(ii) Investigations of the breast

The breast is amongst the most accessible of structures to ultrasonic examination. Therefore it is not surprising that first medical ultrasonic pulse–echo two-dimensional images, made in 1950, using a frequency of 2 MHz, were of this organ (Howry *et al.*, 1954). A-scan studies were first reported two years earlier (Wild and Reid, 1952), and the results demonstrated that, at 15 MHz, malignant and non-malignant tissues could be differentiated. The distinction was made on the basis of the so-called "area ratio"; this is the ratio between the area under the A-scan display of the suspect tissue, to that of the control (usually the other breast). The ratio was greater than unity if the lesion was malignant, and less than unity if it was benign. Further A-scan results have been reported by Laustela *et al.* (1966).

Most breast studies have been of the female. Disease of the male breast is rare, but similar considerations apply to its ultrasonic visualization (Jellins *et al.*, 1975a).

For two-dimensional scanning, a water-bath technique is most convenient. Contact scanning, whilst being possible (Damascelli *et al.*, 1969, 1970), is difficult because the pressure of the probe distorts the breast, and the transmission pulse makes it impossible to recover echoes from near the skin. (Real-time scanners may alter this situation: see, for example, Cole-Beuglet and Beique, 1975.) Three different arrangements of water bath have been constructed. In one, the patient lies supine, and the edge of an aperture in plastic sheet is fixed with adhesive to the skin; the outer edge of the sheet is supported above the patient so that a trough is formed within which the breasts tend to float upwards when immersed in water. The probe is mounted so that it is directed downwards into the tank. This arrangement has been used by Deland (1969), Jellins *et al.* (1971, 1975b) and Fry *et al.* (1972). Another approach is to scan the breasts through a plastic membrane at the base of a water tank, again with the patient supine. This method, used by Hayashi *et al.* (1962) and Wagai *et al.* (1965)—and their colleagues in subsequent studies—and by Evans *et al.* (1966), seems to be better suited to the Oriental than the Western breast. The third method of scanning, which seems to be the best (notwithstanding natural prejudice!) is that of Wells and Evans (1968): the patient lies prone, and her breasts dip into a water tank through an appropriately shaped aperture in the couch, whilst the ultrasound is directed upwards from an immersed probe or transducer array. This technique is convenient and fast, since it avoids the need to seal a membrane to the skin, and at the same time retains the advantages of direct immersion. A typical scan is shown in Fig. 6.85.

The normal breast is a complex structure which gives rise to numerous echoes, presumably from the interfaces between fatty, glandular and fibrous tissues, and the duct system and vascular trees. Cysts appear on echograms as anechoic areas surrounded by echoes from the normal breast. Solid lesions are less well delineated and defined. The identification of an abnormality is made easier if both breasts are shown on the same scan, so that any asymmetry is more obvious.

It is really only in Japan that a serious attempt has yet been made to distinguish between the histologies of different types of solid breast lesions. Wagai *et al.* (1967) classified two-dimensional linear or radial (i.e. non-compounded) B-scans of breast cancer into three categories. Type A is a strong irregular pattern characterized by localized, rather bright echoes arising from inside the breast tumour, with irregular boundary echoes. Type B is a relatively homogeneous pattern characterized by irregular boundary echoes with persistence of the distal limit of tumour echoes as sensitivity is reduced; this pattern is similar to that produced by benign fibrocystic lesions. Type C is similar to type B, but the distal echoes are relatively smaller in amplitude. Type C is most significantly related to the

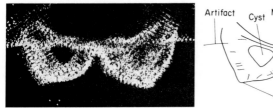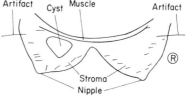

FIG. 6.85 Scan showing normal right breast, and cyst in left breast. Made using a water-immersion scanner, operating at 2 MHz. The artifacts, which appear on both sides of the scan, are due to reflexions at the water surface. (Courtesy K. T. Evans.)

presence of malignancy, as confirmed by Kobayashi *et al.* (1972c, d) and other investigators mentioned in the review of Kobayashi (1975).

Grey-scale breast scanning is better able to display the characteristics of the tissues and the nature of lesions, than is possible with a restricted dynamic range. Thus, using a water-bath scanner operating at 2 MHz, Jellins *et al.* (1975b) correctly interpreted 90% of the scans of 43 patients, with malignancy being correctly diagnosed in 85%.

There appear to be two chief factors which militate against satisfactory diagnostic information being presented as a compound breast scan, and which to some extent account for the relative success of non-compounded scans. Firstly, according to Jellins and Kossoff (1973) the average velocity of ultrasound in the breast varies from 1430 to 1560 m s^{-1} (see also Chapter 4). For example, there is a tendency for the velocity to be lower in older individuals. Therefore, registration of targets within the breast may be degraded in range, and refraction may occur at the surface of the breast where there may be a difference from the velocity in the coupling water. (Jellins and Kossoff (1973) have developed a method of compensating for both these effects, and doubtless this contributes to their excellent results.) Secondly, non-compounded linear scans, such as those used by the Japanese, are merely distorted by registration errors due to velocity uncertainties in the breast, and refraction is less of a problem in the East, where breasts tend to be smaller. Moreover, linear scans, and, to a lesser extent, radial scans, allow the shadows or "antishadows" behind lesions to be seen, so that the attenuation characteristics may reveal the presence of an abnormality and give a clue about its nature. This is much less likely with a compounded scan, in which the information is obscured by scan lines from other directions.

It has to be admitted that the present pulse–echo ultrasonic diagnostic techniques do not seem to be suitable for clinical use in relation to breast disease. In order to have any impact on the health of the population, ultrasound would need to give an earlier detection of breast lesions in the apparently healthy, so that treatment might be begun earlier. Whether this would merely increase survival time, which is the time between diagnosis and death, or actually postpone death, is a matter for conjecture. Some of the frightening logistic problems of mass screening have been discussed by Weiss (1974). Since breast cancer is the main cause of all deaths amongst women between ages 40–44 years (during which period about 1 in 200 Western women die of the disease each year), it seems to be important to try to improve ultrasonic screening methods. One way in which this might be done would be to exploit another characteristic apart from echo amplitude as the identifying feature of abnormality. The most promising characteristic for this purpose is attenuation, and it is possible that two-dimensional maps of attenuation distribution might be constructed by computer analysis of the echo amplitude decrements with range obtained by a conventional compound scanner (see also Section 6.12).

One area in which ultrasound might have an impact on patient care, which does not seem yet to have been explored, is in the search for positive nodes in women known to have breast cancer. Almost 40% may be missed by clinical examination. Their presence or absence is the most accurate indicator of the patient's prognosis: for example, when the nodes are negative, 80% of patients survive at least five years. There is much controversy concerning the surgical approach, and whether or not a radical mastectomy is only necessary if the nodes are involved. Sooner or later these questions will be resolved, and ultrasound may then have an important application in determining surgical strategy.

6.16.h Ophthalmology

(i) A-scan studies

Mundt and Hughes (1956) recognized the potential of pulse–echo ultrasonics in the diagnosis of tumours and retinal detachments, and in the localization of foreign bodies. The eye is a most suitable structure for ultrasonic investigation, since it is accessible without overlying bone or gas, and it is small and superficial.

Oksala (1968) has reviewed the applications of A-scan echography in the diagnosis of intraocular diseases. Frequencies in the range 6–12 MHz are generally used, with transducer diameters of between 2 and 8 mm. The probes are either round with a straight handle (and frequently fitted with a water delay, as illustrated in Fig. 6.86, thus allowing the anterior components of the eye to be examined without interference from the transmission pulse: see Leary, 1967), or L-shaped (Buschmann, 1965) with the ultrasonic beam at a right angle with the handle to examine the equatorial region. The interpretation of the echograms demands a good knowledge of normal anatomy. In idiopathic retinal detachment, the space behind the

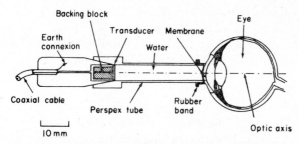

FIG. 6.86 Ultrasonic probe for measurement of the axial length of the eye, shown in relation to an adult human eye.

retina is echo-free; in secondary detachment of the retina, due, for example, to haemorrhage or tumour, weak echoes arise from behind the retina. Foreign bodies, even those which are radiotranslucent, may be located as isolated echo-producing targets (Bronson, 1965). Intraocular tumours can likewise be detected, and Ossoinig (1974) has described criteria by which different types of tumour may be identified according to their echo-producing characteristics.

The axial lengths of the various components of the eye can be measured with good precision using an A-scope. Generally, up to about 20 MHz, higher frequencies allow the echo arrival times to be measured with increasing accuracy. The method is more convenient and rapid than phacometry (Sorsby et al., 1963). Jansson (1963) compared radiographic and (4 MHz) ultrasonic measurements of the axial lengths of 36 normal eyes, and found that the ultrasonic method had the smaller error. Coleman and Carlin (1967) have developed an improved technique, in which the axis of the eye is optically aligned with that of the ultrasonic beam. Thus they claim a precision of 0·1 mm, using a 50 MHz clock as the timing reference. The conversion from the measurement of time to the estimation of distance involves the assumption of velocity. The following values may be assumed at 37°C: cornea, 1600 m s⁻¹; aqueous, 1532 m s⁻¹; lens, 1641 m s⁻¹; vitreous, 1532 m s⁻¹; retina, 1550 m s⁻¹; choroid, 1550 m s⁻¹; and sclera, 1650 m s⁻¹ (see Giglio *et al.*, 1968). Based on these values of velocity, a 20 MHz instrument is capable of measuring refractive length, and thickness and spacing of the optical interfaces, to an accuracy of better than ±0·03 mm.

One practical problem in investigations of the eye with a contact probe is that blinking and involuntary movements require that the eye should first be anaesthetized (for example, with a drop of Novesine: 0·4% oxy-buprocaine, 0·01% chlorhexidine acetate). This is a nuisance, particularly in axial length measurements of populations such as children. In order to overcome this difficulty, Giglio and Meyers (1969) have developed a system capable of horizontal forward movement of an ultrasonic probe into contact with the eye, with a maximum overtravel of 0·09 mm. The probe is retracted after a dwell of 10 ms, and the whole operation is accomplished in 100 ms, which is the average time of the blink reflex.

(ii) B-scan studies

The first paper describing ultrasonic two-dimensional visualization of the eye seems to be that of Baum and Greenwood (1958). They used a 15 MHz system, with the patient's eyes looking into the water bath, his face sealed by a rubber mask. The images produced by this instrument, and by some of those constructed later, reveal amazing detail of both the normal and abnormal anatomy of the eye and orbit. Whether such images are more helpful in patient care than the information which can be obtained with an A-scope by a skilled operator is open to question; but undoubtedly they are of enormous potential value because they are relatively easily interpreted.

Almost all two-dimensional ophthalmic scanners use water-bath coupling. Coleman (1972a, b) and Coleman and Jack (1973) have used a hand-operated water-bath scanner of the type described by Coleman *et al.* (1969), and have demonstrated that the method is reliable and that the results are clinically useful in the diagnosis of many kinds of ocular abnormalities. Orbital scans are more difficult to interpret, but the ability to map out the position and extent of a tumour can be decisive in planning treatment. More recently, Sutherland and Forrester (1974, 1975) and Sutherland *et al.* (1975) have reported encouraging results obtained with a conventional abdominal contact scanner modified to visualize the eye through a water bath. Scans obtained with the holographic system of Aldridge *et al.* (1974), operating as a B-scanner, are shown in Fig. 6.87. Although in some of these articles allusions are made to wide dynamic range displays, the potential of grey-scale imaging has been quite thoroughly investigated by Dadd *et al.* (1974, 1975). Using a frequency of 7·5 MHz, the method provides views of orbital contents which are otherwise unobtainable.

One exception to the water-bath type of scanner is the simple automatic contact instrument which has been described by Bronson (1972). It consists of a hand-held housing with a Mylar window, approximately 3×25 mm, behind which a 7·5 MHz probe (focal length 15 mm) oscillates through an arc of approximately 30°. The probe oscillation is provided by an electric motor, driven at a sufficient speed to give an acceptably flicker-free display; the ultrasonic pulse repetition rate is 4000 s^{-1}. This real-time system gives good visualization of posterior globe and orbit, and some of its clinical advantages have been reviewed by Bronson (1974).

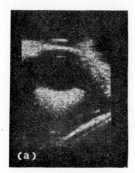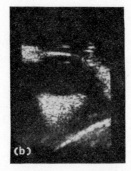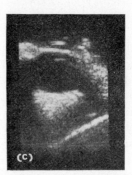

FIG. 6.87 Two-dimensional B-scans of normal eye. (a) Regular processing; (b) overcompensated swept gain, showing loss of resolution in orbital fat; (c) grey-scale display. (Courtesy R. C. Chivers.)

6.16.i Orthopaedics and Rheumatology

(i) Soft tissue thickness and oedema

The measurement of soft tissue thickness is chiefly important in two clinical situations. Firstly, in anthropometry, ultrasound A-scope methods have been used to estimate soft tissue thickness. Most investigators (for example, Whittingham, 1962; Bullen *et al.*, 1965; Booth *et al.*, 1966; Sloan, 1967; Jackson *et al.*, 1970) have used probes with the transducer in contact with the skin, although some (for example, Ramsden *et al.*, 1967) have used a perspex rod to space the transducer from the skin, thus avoiding confusion due to the transmission probe. In the measurement of subcutaneous fat, Bullen *et al.* (1965) found that the correlation between needle puncture and ultrasonic measurement at a site 20 mm below and to the right of the umbilicus was 0·98 in a series of 100 individuals. Booth *et al.* (1966) considered that the ultrasonic method was more accurate than measurements made with Harpenden calipers.

The second clinical application is in the measurement of chest wall thickness, either to plan electron radiotherapy to spare the lung (see Section 6.16.g), or to estimate by external detectors the activity of high-energy radionuclides inhaled as a result of an accident.

The soft-tissue structures of the limbs, and particularly of the leg, may be demonstrated by ultrasonic two-dimensional scanning (Holmes and Howry, 1958; Horn and Robinson, 1965; Howry, 1965). Generally, compound water-bath scanners operating at around 2 MHz have been used. The scans are capable of showing great detail, and they are helpful in the assessment of oedema. Contact scanners are certainly useful too, and have been used to distinguish between Baker's cyst and thrombophlebitis (McDonald and Leopold, 1972), and to diagnose and assess popliteal cysts (Meire et al., 1974).

(ii) Assessment of fracture healing

The results have been reported of some preliminary experiments designed to test the possibility of assessing fracture healing in limbs in terms of the attenuation of shear waves transmitted across the fracture (Horn and Robinson, 1965). The rationale of the method is that shear waves are rapidly attenuated in fluids, so that the transmission of a shear wave across the region of a fracture is controlled largely by the extent of bone fusion, since liquid fills the space where fusion has not occurred. Although the results were encouraging, the technique does not seem to have been introduced into clinical practice.

It has been reported by Abendschein and Hyatt (1972) that the propagation velocity through bone specimens is related to the degree of union of fractures. How it came about that the reduction in velocity was up to almost 50% in their experiments is hard to explain, and in the absence of more information about their apparatus it would not be wise to become too excited.

(iii) Assessment of osteoporosis

The absorption of monoenergetic photons has for many years been used as an index of skeletal status in terms of mineral content. This is not an adequate measurement in relation to the assessment of osteoporosis. It has been suggested by Rich et al. (1966) that bone mass could be estimated from ultrasonic velocity measurements, but this approach has not been used clinically. A sonic—as distinct from ultrasonic—method has been proposed by Jurist (1970a), in which the mechanical resonance frequency of a driver-arm combination is measured. This appears to be related to osteoporosis (Jurist, 1970b), but the method has not been widely introduced, nor is its physical basis fully understood (Davies and Wells, 1971; Jurist and Kianian, 1973).

6.16.j Otorhinolaryngology

Pulse–echo ultrasonics can be used to record the movements of the vocal tract without the use of transducers within the tract. This is potentially of importance in the study of both normal and pathological speech production.

In order to study movements of the pharyngeal wall, the ultrasonic probe is placed in contact with the skin at the side of the neck, about 10 mm below the angle of the mandible, and the ultrasonic beam is directed towards the lateral wall of the pharynx (Kelsey *et al.*, 1969b). The ultrasonic measurements, made at a frequency of 2·3 MHz and a repetition rate of 5000 s⁻¹, are most conveniently presented as time–position recordings (see Section 6.9), and in this form they correlate well with cinéradiographic studies (Kelsey *et al.*, 1969a). The ultrasonic recordings are obtained without exposing the patient to the hazards of X-rays, and may have some value in assessing cleft palate patients prior to therapy, and in the rehabilitation of patients following laryngectomy.

The vocal movements of the vocal folds can also be studied, if the probe is placed normal to the skin about 10 mm below, and lateral to, the thyroid prominence (Hertz *et al.*, 1970). Time–position recordings obtained in this way are relevant to speech research (see, for example, Hamlet, 1972).

During speech production, the velocities of the pharyngeal walls and the vocal folds may be very rapid. Pulse–echo measurements of these velocities depend on sequential sampling of the corresponding positions of the echo-producing surfaces, and the sampling rate needs to be as high as possible in order to achieve the best time resolution. In practice, 10 kHz might be the maximum pulse repetition frequency, and this might require an ultrasonic frequency of 10 MHz to be used to minimize reverberation problems. This difficulty does not arise with the continuous wave Doppler method of studying structure movement (see Section 7.3.e).

Brzezińska (1972) has described how the pulse–echo technique may be used, with a 3 MHz A-scope, to detect the presence of liquid in the maxillary sinus. The 10 mm diameter probe is held in contact with the skin on the face over the sinus. If the sinus contains liquid, an echo is received from its posterior wall; if it contains air, no posterior wall echo is received. Thus the ultrasonic technique should reduce the necessity to X-ray individuals—particularly children—suspected of having sinus problems. Moreover, using a smaller probe operating at 8 MHz, Brzezińska (1972) demonstrated experimentally that liquid could likewise be detected if present behind the tympanic membrane.

In one of the surgical procedures for the ultrasonic destruction of the labyrinth for the treatment of Ménière's disease (see Section 10.4), the aim is to leave a bone thickness of about 0·5 mm over the lateral semicircular canal. It has been suggested that this thickness could be measured by an ultrasonic pulse–echo technique, and Johnson *et al.* (1966) have reported encouraging results using a 4 MHz probe.

6.16.k Urology

(*i*) *Kidney*

A very early use of ultrasound in urology allowed the lower pole of the kidney to be detected transcutaneously by means of an A-scope as a preliminary to biopsy (Berlyne, 1961). In some centres, developments of this technique are in routine use. In this application, movement of the kidney with respiration may help in its identification.

The A-scope was used by Schlegal *et al.* (1961) to detect renal calculi at operation. Others have occasionally reported their results with the procedure (see, for example, Heap, 1968). It has not come into general use, principally because once the kidney has been subjected to surgery, air may enter the organ, giving rise to artifact echoes of large amplitude.

Since the publication of an article by Holmes (1966a), there has been an increasing interest in ultrasonic pulse–echo examination of the kidney. Several reviews of the pre-grey-scale era of ultrasonic kidney scanning have been published: see, for example, Barnett and Morley (1971, 1972); Mountford *et al.* (1971); and Kristensen *et al.* (1972).

Two-dimensional scanning is usually carried out with the patient prone. Both kidneys can normally be seen in either longitudinal or transverse sections, but the scans may be degraded by the necessity for the ultrasound to pass through the ribs. The right kidney can also be visualized with the patient supine, by scanning through the liver. No restriction of breathing is usually necessary. Contact scanners operating at 1·5–3 MHz have generally been used. Typical scans are shown in Fig. 6.88.

In essence, ultrasound may be of value when intravenous pyelography has failed to demonstrate a nephogram, as in uraemia, vascular occlusion and congenital absence of the kidney. It has a place in the differentiation between solid and cystic renal lesions. It may be used to determine the optimal site of cyst puncture or tumour biopsy. It is usable even when radiography is undesirable, as in pregnancy or long-term serial follow-up. Polycystic disease has characteristic appearances in the scan. In children, ultrasound is helpful when Wilms' tumour is suspected (Hünig and Kinser, 1973).

The considerable potential value of pulse–echo ultrasound in its ability to distinguish between cystic and solid masses in the kidney was pointed out by Goldberg *et al.* (1968). In general, cysts return no echoes from within, but have well-defined, smooth boundaries; in tumours, the opposite is true. Provided that the mass can be located with sufficient accuracy, and is large enough, the diagnosis can be made by inspection of the A-scan.

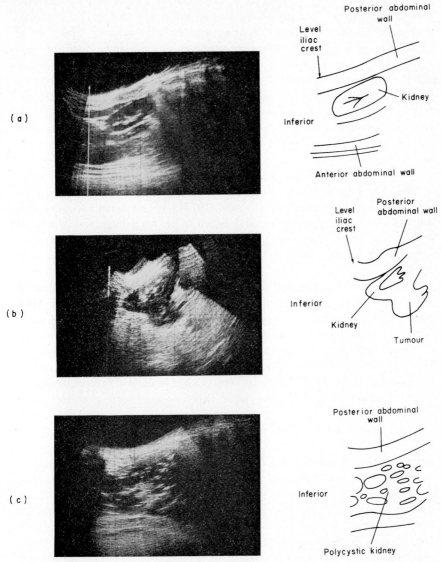

FIG. 6.88 Kidney scans, longitudinal sections. In these posterior scans, the patient's head is to the right, and the scan plane 60–70 mm from the midline. (a) Normal kidney; (b) kidney with anterior tumour; (c) polycystic kidney. (Courtesy F. G. M. Ross.)

Goldberg and Pollack (1971) have taken the process a step further: the instrument settings may be adjusted using the full bladder and the normal kidney as "echo-free" and "echo-producing" references. This use of "biological standards" may allow three groups of lesion to be distinguished. Cysts, hydronephrosis, and haematoma are relatively free of internal echoes. Renal cell carcinoma gives rise to quite large-amplitude echoes. Necrotic renal cell carcinoma, polycystic disease, renal vein thrombosis, Wilms' tumour and abscess are all associated with echoes of intermediate amplitude. It is questionable, of course, how much confidence should be placed in individual circumstances, involving such subtle distinctions.

Correlation of ultrasonic scans and intravenous pyelograms may confirm a diagnosis which would otherwise require retrograde pyelography or aortography. Thus Asher and Leopold (1972) recommended a step-by-step approach involving the minimum of insult to obtain a diagnosis. Moreover in the case of a radiographically non-visualized kidney, ultrasound may reveal agenesis, end-stage hydronephrosis, polycystic disease or vascular thrombosis.

Because of its considerable advantages, von Micsky *et al.* (1974) routinely scan with ultrasound all children who would otherwise certainly have intravenous pyelography. They use a 5 MHz contact scanner with a weakly focused beam. It is a nuisance that restless children need to be sedated for ultrasonic scanning in this way. This difficulty can generally be avoided, however, by using a water-bath coupling. In this situation, most children are happy to lie quietly or even to sleep. Lyons *et al.* (1972) have described a simple modification which makes this possible with a conventional contact scanner.

Renal cyst aspiration can be carried out by ultrasonically guided puncture with an A-scope display (Goldberg and Pollack, 1973), or, if the cyst is more difficult to locate, with a two-dimensional B-scope. If ultrasound is not used, X-ray screening is necessary, with the intravenous injection of contrast medium, to visualize the kidneys and to choose an appropriate site for the needle puncture; the depth of the cyst can only be determined by trial and error, and the needle may be inserted too far. As described in connexion with pericardiocentesis (see Section 6.16.b.vi), the tip of the needle generally produces an identifiable echo on the echogram. It is, however, sometimes rather difficult to see the tip echo if the needle is coated with teflon.

The improvements in diagnosis which result from grey-scale displays have yet to be assessed. No doubt the method will reduce errors such as confusion between highly vascular tumours and cysts. It will allow abnormalities of smaller size to be detected and studied; in this connexion also, close inspection of the scan sometimes reveals that multiple reflexion artifacts are falsely giving the impression that echoes arise from within a space which is in reality anechoic.

Two-dimensional ultrasonic scanning may be helpful in the management of patients who develop complications following renal transplant. According to Morley *et al.* (1975), it is often possible to diagnose and localize pelvic fluid collections, and it is a reliable method of excluding pelvic and perirenal abscess in pyrexia.

(*ii*) *Bladder*

The patient is usually examined in the supine position. It is generally easy to measure the distance between the anterior and posterior walls of the bladder by means of an A-scope (Holmes, 1966a, b), but this dimension is not closely correlated with the urinary volume. The volume may be estimated, however, from serial two-dimensional scans made in transverse parallel planes, using a planimeter to determine the area of each bladder cross-section. Thus Holmes (1966b) found an average difference of 25% in a comparison between ultrasonic and voided volume measurements in a series of 26 patients. Apparently results of similar accuracy can be achieved, however, in estimates based on a single transverse and a single horizontal scan. Using this method, Alftan and Mattson (1969) had a mean error of 28% in the urine volumes measured in 50 patients, provided that the volume was greater than 100 ml. With smaller volumes, the ultrasonic estimate was very inaccurate.

Although radiology and cystoscopy can be used to demonstrate most tumours of the bladder, they have several disadvantages, such as X-ray hazard, risk of infection, and discomfort. Moreover, radiology is ineffective in poor renal function, and cystoscopy is especially difficult in stricture. It was demonstrated by Damascelli *et al.* (1968) that tumours could often be visualized by two-dimensional ultrasonic scanning through the intact abdominal wall and the urine-filled bladder. The technique has been refined by Barnett and Morley (1971), and their results, obtained using a contact scanner which apparently had some grey-scale capability, are very encouraging. The size and exact location of a bladder neoplasm can be shown. The extent of the bladder base can be assessed, and infiltration of the bladder wall and extension into the pelvis may be recognized. The reliability with which these studies may be made is greatest when the bladder has a large capacity and the tumour is on the posterior wall. The lower part of the bladder behind the symphysis pubis is anatomically rather inaccessible, but the anterior wall should be more clearly seen if a water-bath scanner were to be used.

(*iii*) *Prostate*

The prostate is not readily accessible to diagnostic examination. It lies on the musculofascial diaphragm of the pelvis beneath the arch of the pubis, and, apart from the possibility that computerized tomography may prove to be useful, conventional diagnostic procedures involve exploration through the rectum or the urethra.

Transrectal ultrasonic scanning of the prostate, apparently first proposed by Takahashi and Ouchi (1963), has been developed into a routine clinical technique (King *et al.*, 1973). The instrumentation has been described by Watanabe *et al.* (1971). The probe consists of an outer, stationary tube containing inflow and outflow liquid ports, and an inner transducer assembly (with a radial ultrasonic beam axis) that can both rotate and move longitudinally. The tip of the probe is covered with a soft polyethylene tube to avoid damaging the rectal mucosa. The probe is encased in a thin rubber condom, which is filled with degassed water and further inflated to make contact with the rectal wall after the tip of the probe has been introduced for a distance of 80–90 mm above the anal verge. The transducer, which is weakly focused, has a diameter of 10 mm and operates at 3·5 MHz; transverse scans are made at 10 mm intervals beginning at the level of the bladder and seminal vesicles and moving down the rectum past the region of the prostate. The patient requires no special preparation, apart from taking a mild laxative during the evening prior to the examination, and being asked to allow his bladder to fill with urine. It is probably better for the patient to be in a sitting position rather than in lithotomy, since this reduces the possibility of interference with the scan by air bubbles.

The normal prostate appears in cross-section as a symmetrical, triangular space enclosed within the fibrous prostatic capsule, with more echoes arising from the posterior part of the gland, than from the anterior. The size of the gland, which is generally enlarged in disease, can be quite accurately estimated. Distortions of the shape of the prostate, resulting from advanced local malignancy, are also reliably detected; but without grey-scale display, tumours within the prostate are rather difficult to detect.

Barnett and Morley (1971) mentioned that they experienced no difficulty in visualizing, in two-dimensional scans made transcutaneously through the anterior abdominal wall, the enlarged prostate protruding into the urine-filled bladder. This approach is much less of a nuisance than transrectal scanning: the apparatus is widely available, and the patient is subjected neither to indignity nor discomfort. The method has been developed by Miller *et al.* (1973) and Whittingham and Bishop (1973) to estimate the volume of the prostate. With the bladder as distended with urine as is tolerable to the patient, both longitudinal and transverse scans are made over the lower abdomen. The outlines of the bladder and the prostate can be seen in appropriate longitudinal sections, but full visualization is impossible because of the intervention of the pubis: this is the reason why transverse scans are required. The estimation of the volume may be made by assuming an ellipsoidal shape, with the diameters being taken to be the largest measured dimensions in each set of scans. Allowance needs to be made for any obvious irregularities. It is simpler, but presumably less accurate despite the rather conflicting results of Miller *et al.* (1973) and Whittingham and Bishop (1973), to assume that the gland is spherical and to guess the diameter. In any event, the estimate is sufficient to enable a gland to be judged to be small, medium or large: this helps the surgeon to choose between open surgery and transurethral resection.

(*iv*) *Testis*

The testis is hardly a convenient organ for examination with a direct-contact scanner, but Miskin and Bain (1974) have succeeded in doing this through the intact scrotum using a 5 MHz instrument. The scans were indistinguishable from those in normal individuals, in oligospermic and azoospermic patients. On the other hand, hydrocele, testicular abscess and tumour produced abnormal scans. Better results might be obtained more conveniently with a specially designed water-bath instrument with a grey-scale display.

7. DOPPLER METHODS

7.1 TRANSMISSION METHODS

The Doppler effect is described in Section 1.15. The earliest use of the ultrasonic Doppler effect in medical diagnosis seems to have been in the measurement of blood flow velocity, particularly in intact vessels. The original flowmeters developed for this purpose were based on the measurement of the effective ultrasonic velocity between two transducers arranged at a fixed distance apart on the outside of the vessel. The difference between the apparent measured velocity, and the velocity in the absence of flow, is equal to the flow velocity. In biological systems, the flow velocities are much less than the ultrasonic propagation velocity, and so a balanced system is used which is sensitive to the small difference in the transit times of signals travelling up and down stream. The original instrument of Kalmus (1954) was not developed specifically for biomedical applications, but Baldes *et al.* (1957) described an experimental system for blood flow velocity measurement. The best transducer arrangement for this application seems to be that of Franklin *et al.* (1959), illustrated in Fig. 7.1. The assembly is constructed in two parts, which are clamped together to form a collar around the blood vessel. Neglecting the effect of the part of the ultrasonic path which does not lie in the moving liquid (the respiration monitor described by Blumenfeld *et al.* (1974) takes this into account; the catheter-tip arrangements for bloodflow monitoring described by, for example, Fricke *et al.* (1970) and Borgnis (1974) avoid this problem), and assuming "plug" flow at velocity v, the difference Δ_t between the up-stream and down-stream transit times is given by:

$$\Delta_t = d\{1/(c - v \cos \theta) - 1/(c + v \cos \theta)\} \qquad (7.1)$$

In practice, $c \gg v$, and Eqn. 7.1 can be simplified to:

$$v = \Delta_t c^2/(2d \cos \theta) \qquad (7.2)$$

In a typical arrangement, $d = 25$ mm and $\theta = 15°$. The ultrasonic velocity in blood is about 1570 m s^{-1} (see Fig. 4.6(b)). Substitution of these values in Eqn. 7.2 indicates that $\Delta_t = 0\cdot02$ ns (mm s^{-1})$^{-1}$. Thus, a flow velocity of 10 mm s^{-1} causes a difference of $0\cdot0013\%$ between the up-stream and down-stream transit times. In the system of Franklin *et al.* (1959), the up- and down-stream transit times of 3 MHz pulses are compared by in terms of the amplitudes of the output from a time-to-voltage analogue converter. The difficulty with this technique is to ensure that the triggering levels for pulses travelling in both directions are the same, since they determine the precision of the time measurements. Farral (1959) tried to solve this problem by using alternately one of two pairs of transducers, switched at a rate of 100 s^{-1} to provide up-stream and down-stream comparisons of the phases of 380 kHz ultrasonic pulses. Expressed in terms of phase difference, $0.003°$ corresponds to a flow velocity of 1 mm s^{-1} over a path length of 25 mm. Although it was a good idea to use the phase comparison method, drifts in zero calibration affect its accuracy in the same way as they affect the transit time method, and neither is really satisfactory at velocities of less than about 10 mm s^{-1}.

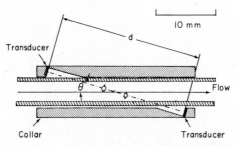

FIG. 7.1 Arrangement of transducers for measurement of flow velocity by transit time difference in up-stream and down-stream paths.

It has been pointed out by Franklin and Kemper (1974) that any transit-time instrument operating at a fixed ultrasonic frequency may suffer from multiple reflexion artifacts. They have described a method which avoids this problem. Each transducer serves simultaneously as a transmitter and as a receiver, and the signals applied to both transducers are frequency modulated through a frequency corresponding to a shift of 20 kHz for a single transit, about a resonance frequency of 10 MHz at a rate of 500 Hz. Therefore a signal undergoing two transits is shifted in frequency by 40 kHz, and so on. Low pass filters are used to eliminate multiple transit signals, so that the relatively small, true Doppler shift signals may be extracted without ambiguity.

7.2 REFLEXION METHODS

7.2.a Basic Principles

The Doppler shift in the frequency of reflected ultrasound may be used as a measure of the velocity of movement of the reflecting surface. The relationship between the Doppler shift frequency f_D (which is equal to $f_r - f$, where f_r is the received frequency), the transmitted ultrasonic frequency f, the vector component v_i of the interface velocity along the direction of the ultrasonic axis, and the ultrasonic propagation velocity c, is given by Eqn. 1.63. If $c \gg v_i$ (as is always the case in physiological systems), this equation can be simplified to:

$$v_i = -f_D c / 2f \tag{7.3}$$

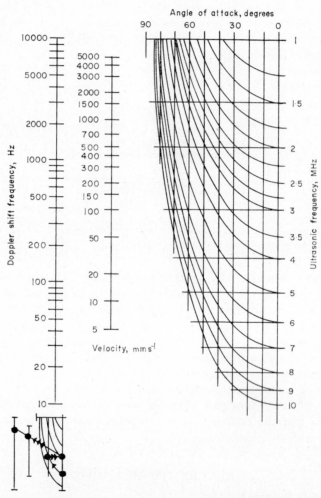

FIG. 7.2 Nomogram showing relationships between reflector velocity, Doppler shift frequency and ultrasonic frequency for various angles of attack. Values calculated for blood, velocity = 1570 m s^{-1}. (After Wells, 1969.)

Where the various velocities do not all act along the same direction, the appropriate velocity vectors must be used for the calculation of f_D. Thus, if γ is the angle of attack (defined as the angle between the direction of movement and the effective ultrasonic beam direction), Eqn. 7.3 can be modified to:

$$v = -f_D c/(2f \cos \gamma) \qquad (7.4)$$

where v = absolute velocity of the reflector along the direction of flow.

The algebraic sign of f_D is positive if flow is towards the transducer, and vice versa. The nomogram in Fig. 7.2 enables the relationships between v, f_D, f and γ to be found for the range of values which commonly occur in medical applications.

Ultrasonic Doppler systems are used in three main areas of clinical investigation. These are in blood-flow studies, in obstetrics, and in cardiology, as outlined in Section 7.3. For the study of blood flow, the choice of ultrasonic frequency is determined by a compromise between absorption and backscattered power, both of which increase with frequency. The optimal frequency f_{opt} (in MHz) has been shown by Reid and Baker (1971) for normal haematocrit to be given by:

$$f_{opt} \simeq 90/d \qquad (7.5)$$

where d is the soft-tissue distance (in mm) between the probe and the blood. Relatively higher frequencies are better, the lower the haematocrit, because the backscattered energy is reduced. As might be expected, however, the Doppler shift frequency in any particular flow situation is independent of the haematocrit (Michie and Cain, 1971). Most blood-flow studies are made at distances in the range 1–80 mm, and frequencies of 10–2 MHz are generally used. (The satisfactory performance at long range of frequencies rather higher than indicated in Eqn. 7.5 is due to the increase in backscattering volume which is associated with the increase in transducer size, and hence beamwidth, as the frequency is reduced: this point was overlooked by Reid and Baker (1971).) For the study of cardiac structure motion, including that of the foetal heart, frequencies of 2–3 MHz are usual; this choice is made to optimize the range of penetration, the directivity, and the detection, of both scattering and specular targets.

The backscattered Doppler method of blood-flow velocity measurement has two particularly important features, in comparison with other techniques. Firstly, there is no baseline drift, because when the flow velocity is zero, the Doppler shift frequency is also zero. Secondly, because of the similarity of the processing requirements for Doppler signals and for ordinary amplitude modulated radio signals, the circuitry is relatively simple and inexpensive. These advantages make the system attractive for use both in the clinical environment and for telemetry in man and other

animals. A typical arrangement is illustrated in Fig. 7.3. The principal
disadvantage of the Doppler method is that essentially it measures flow
velocity, and not flow volume, when used for blood-flow studies.

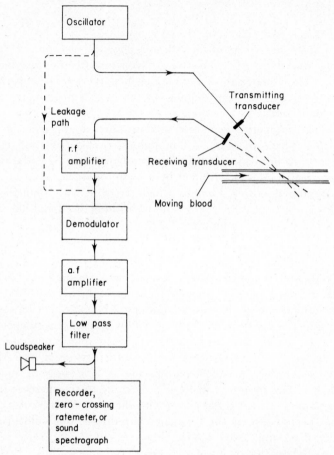

FIG. 7.3 Block diagram of a continuous wave Doppler motion detector.

7.2.b Transducer Arrangements and Beam Directivities

The construction of a typical ultrasonic probe is illustrated in Fig. 3.19.
This and other arrangements are shown in Fig. 7.4. In systems employing
a single transducer as both transmitter and receiver, the cross-talk is 0 dB
(because the output from the transmitter is connected directly to the input
to the receiver). This may lead to difficulty. In continuous wave operation,
the receiver may be saturated, and consequently be made insensitive to
Doppler shifted signals, and the noise of the transmitter may be trouble-

some. This is because the weakest signal of interest may be 120 dB below the transmitted signal. In the case of a common transducer acting both as transmitter and receiver, the amplitude modulation of the transmitter would have to be less than 1 part in 10^6 to be unobtrusive.

There are two ways around this difficulty. If it is desirable to use a single transducer, a bridge circuit can be used to balance out the direct signal from the transmitter at the input to the receiver (Reid *et al.*, 1974). The second solution, which is presently by far the more common, is to use separate

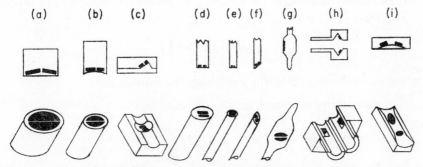

FIG. 7.4 Diagrams showing the transducer arrangements in typical ultrasonic Doppler probes (not to scale). (a) For obstetric use (Wells, 1970), transducer diameter = 25 mm, frequency = 2 MHz; (b) for blood flow studies (Baker, 1970), transducer diameter = 10 mm, frequency = 5 MHz, polystyrene lens focal length = 30 mm; (c) and (d) for blood flow studies*, each transducer element = 1.6×4.8 mm, frequency = 10 MHz; (e) for catheter-tip blood flow studies (Benchimol *et al.*, 1969), transducer diameter = 1 mm, frequency = 8 MHz; (f) for blood flow studies in arteries, scanning from veins (Duck *et al.*, 1972), transducer diameter = 2 mm, frequency = 8·5 MHz; (g) for blood flow studies in aorta, scanning from oesophagus (Side and Gosling, 1971), transducer diameter = 5 mm, frequency = 5 MHz; (h) for periarterial blood flow studies*, each transducer element = 1.6×4.8 mm, frequency = 10 MHz; (i) for blood flow studies from the walls of major vessels (Peronneau *et al.*, 1972), transducer diameter = 5 mm, frequency = 4 or 8 MHz. (After Wells, 1974.)

* Parks Electronics Laboratory, Beavertron, Oregon, USA.

transducers, acoustically and electrically isolated, one as the transmitter, and the other, as the receiver. Details of such an arrangement are shown in Fig. 3.19. Important features include: the use of an acoustic insulator, such as Corperne (Higgs and Erikson, 1969) or Nebar*, which decouples the transducers from the probe casing, and from each other; the inclination of the rear surface of the epoxy resin backing, which is cast at an oblique angle in order to reduce reverberations; the separately screened electrical

* Trade name of James Walker & Co. Ltd., Woking, UK.

connexions, which minimize cross-talk; and the acoustic load matching layer, which increases the gain-bandwidth product of the probe.

In probes in which separate transducers are used as transmitters and receivers, consideration needs to be given to the measurement of the effective direction of the ultrasonic beam in determining the angle of attack γ as defined for Eqn. 7.4. Two situations can be identified, as illustrated in Fig. 7.5. The actual directions of the beams may be determined more by the relative positions of the transducers and the moving target (or ensemble of targets), than by the orientation of the transducers, although the latter may be chosen to optimize the system performance. It is shown in Section 1.15. (Eqn. 1.63) that:

$$f_D = \left(\frac{c - v_r}{c - v_s} - 1 \right) f$$

where v_r = velocity of receiver away from the source; and

v_s = velocity of source in same direction as v_r.

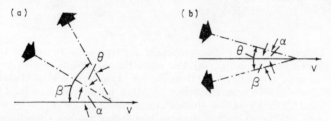

FIG. 7.5 Diagrams illustrating the calculation of the angle of attack in systems employing convergent transmitting and receiving ultrasonic beams.

When both the source and the receiver are stationary, a moving reflector may be considered to act as a moving receiver which itself re-radiates a frequency-shifted wave to behave as a virtual source moving with respect to the receiver. Substitution of the appropriate vector components of v for v_r and v_s gives:

$$f_D = \left(\frac{c - v \cos \alpha}{c + v \cos \beta} - 1 \right) f$$

and hence, if $c \gg v$,

$$f_D = -(fv/c)(\cos \alpha + \cos \beta)$$

This can be rearranged to give:

$$v = -(f_D c)/[2f \cos\{(\alpha + \beta)/2\} \cos\{(\alpha - \beta)/2\}] \tag{7.6}$$

Comparison of Eqns. 7.4 and 7.6 shows that:

$$\cos \gamma = \cos\{(\alpha + \beta)/2\} \cos\{(\alpha - \beta)/2\} \tag{7.7}$$

In Eqn. 7.7, the angle $\{(\alpha+\beta)/2\}$ is the angle between the direction of movement, and the line which bisects the angle between the transmitting and receiving beams. The angle $(\alpha-\beta)$ has a value which lies between the angle of convergence θ of the transmitting and receiving beams (Fig. 7.5(a)), and zero (Fig. 7.5(b)). The angle θ is typically about 10° in foetal blood-flow detectors, and about 30° in peripheral blood-flow Dopplers. The errors introduced by assuming that $\gamma=(\alpha+\beta)/2$ in calculating f_D from the nomogram in Fig. 7.2 for these two types of transducer arrangement have maximum values of about 0·5 and 3·5% respectively. These errors lead to underestimation in the calculated value of reflector velocity from any given Doppler shift frequency.

In foetal monitoring (see Section 7.3.d), it is desirable to have as broad a beam as possible, so that small changes in the position of the foetus do not vitiate the results. Commercial transducers for this purpose have convex, wide-angle transmitters surrounded by an array of similar receivers.

It has been suggested by Jethwa *et al.* (1975) that a small disc transmitting transducer, with a coaxial annular receiver, is particularly favourable from the point of view of achieving a narrow beamwidth. This arrangement is not new: indeed, it was used by Satomura (1957) in his pioneering work, and later by Lubé *et al.* (1967). Moreover, the beam shape has been quite thoroughly investigated by Wells (1970).

One of the important problems in backscattered Doppler measurements of velocity is that the angle of attack γ is frequently unknown. If γ is within 25° of true direction of motion, an error of only 10% is introduced even if cos γ is assumed to be unity. Unfortunately, however, the anatomical relationships may be such that a more oblique angle of incidence is inevitable. It was pointed out by Fahrbach (1970) and confirmed by Duck and Hodson (1973) that the Doppler shifts measured by two "beams" mutually at right angles and crossing in the moving target (probably blood) allow the target velocity to be calculated without additional information. Another method, due to P. L. Hansen, G. Cross and H. Light (quoted by Woodcock, 1975) uses two transmitting beams, mutually at right angles, bisected by a single receiving beam. The point of intersection lies at the position of the moving target. The transmitters are driven at slightly different frequencies, generating a moving fringe pattern. Provided that the target is moving within about 25° of normality with the receiving beam, the amplitude modulation frequency of the received signal by the fringe pattern is proportional to the flow velocity.

When separate transducers are used as transmitter and receiver in a conventional arrangement, the position of maximal sensitivity is closer to the probe than the cross-over point of the beams (Wells, 1970). The distribution of sensitivity for omnidirectional scattering targets is equal to the product of the transmitting and receiving beam shapes, modified by the ultrasonic attenuation. In principle, the situation could be analysed using the theory outlined in Chapter 2. In practice, however, it is generally more reliable to measure the effective sensitivity distribution, using one of the following methods:

(i) Echo amplitude measurements from stationary target

The method is similar to that used with pulse–echo transducers (see Section 3.7.1), but it is necessary to modulate the transmitter with long pulses so that the echo from the target may be identified (Wells, 1970). The duration of the pulse has to be sufficiently long for it to be permissible to assume steady-state conditions in the ultrasonic field. Typical beam distributions measured in this way are illustrated in Fig. 7.6. (Long pulses can also be used to measure the frequency response of the transducer.)

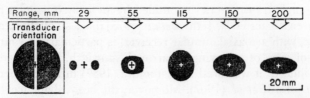

FIG. 7.6 Cross-sectional beam profiles for the ultrasonic Doppler probe illustrated in Figs. 3.19 and 7.4(a). The diagrams show those parts of the beam which return echoes of not more than 10 dB below the amplitude of the maximum (which occurs at a range of 110 mm on the central axis). The position of the central axis is marked + on each diagram. (After Wells, 1970.)

(ii) Moving targets

Three techniques have been devised in which indications of the field distributions of Doppler probes may be obtained by the use of moving targets. These methods can involve the complete Doppler system to convert the frequency-shifted echoes into audible signals, and the measurements may thus be influenced by the signal processing characteristics of the receiver, and in particular, by signal suppression and dynamic range compression.

In one method (due to D. Gordon), a steel sphere of about 3 mm diameter is set into vibration in water, parallel to the central axis of symmetry of the transducer array, at a frequency of 1–2 Hz. The Doppler shift signal is taken from the output of the r.f. section of the receiver. In another method (L. H. Light, unpublished), a rigid tube is terminated by a rubber membrane of about 4 mm diameter. Pressure changes are applied to the membrane through air driven by a pump at about 100 s^{-1}, and these cause the membrane to pulsate in the water in which the Doppler field is to be measured.

The third method (Baker and Yates, 1973) is particularly suited to the measurement of sample volume in range-finding Dopplers. The test probe emits an underwater jet seeded with silicone antifoam emulsion: this gives rise to Doppler-shifted signals as a result of scatterer motion. A collection tube can be arranged to collect the spent scatterers, so that water in the tank is not contaminated.

(iii) Schlieren visualization

The beam shape of the transmitting and receiving transducers of a Doppler probe can be visualized by schlieren optics (see Section 3.7.i), by connecting each transducer in turn to an appropriate oscillator. The Doppler field is the product of these two fields, and its position and extent may be estimated from the schlieren images.

7.2.c Analysis of Backscattered Doppler Signals

In considering the performance of a Doppler blood-flow velocity measurement system, the total backscattered power is spread over a frequency spectrum, the power density distribution of which is a convolution of the number of scatterers and the volume distribution of the velocity of the scatterers within the ultrasonic beam. Starting from these considerations, Flax *et al.* (1971) have analysed the statistics of the blood flowmeter for various conditions of geometry and fluid flow. The flow situations which they investigated were those of a parabolic profile, in which

$$v_r = v_m[1 - (r/H)^2] \qquad (7.8)$$

and a blunt profile, in which

$$v_r = v_m[1 - (r/H)^5] \qquad (7.9)$$

where v_r = velocity of blood in "cylinder" of radius r;

v_m = maximum velocity (at the vessel centre); and

H = vessel radius.

The theoretically predicted results are illustrated in Fig. 7.7. The maximum frequency f_m corresponds to the velocity of the most rapidly moving blood, and in the absence of noise the cut-off should be rapid. The shape of each frequency spectrum represents the corresponding volume–velocity distribution along the beam. Flax *et al.* (1971) demonstrated satisfactory agreement between the theoretical predictions and experimental results.

(i) The ear

In many kinds of clinical examinations, a diagnosis can be made by listening to the Doppler shift in frequency. This can often be made easier by electrically filtering out the components of frequency below about 100 Hz, which otherwise tend to mask the important frequencies in the range 200–1000 Hz. Aural analysis is generally not satisfactory in cardiological investigations, because the ear is not very good at detecting small differences in sound spectra which are not particularly musical. Thus although the trained investigator can obtain some information by listening to the Doppler signals, there are many situations in which quantitative analysis is helpful. The various methods which have been used to obtain such analyses are discussed in the following Sub-sections.

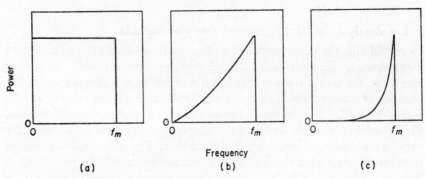

FIG. 7.7 Relative Doppler frequency spectra predicted for parabolic flow profile. (a) $W > H$; (b) $W = H$; (c) $W < H$; where W = width of beam, and H = diameter of vessel. (After Flax et al., 1971.)

(ii) Zero-crossing ratemeters

In classical papers on the statistical properties of random noise, Rice (1944, 1945) predicted the number of zero-crossings which occur with any given spectral distribution of input power, from the probability density of finding a zero-crossing in a given interval. This probability is described in terms of the autocorrelation function R and its second derivative R'', evaluated at time $t = 0$. The density ψ of zero-crossings is given by:

$$\psi = (1/\pi)\{-R''(0)/R(0)\}^{1/2} \tag{7.10}$$

and hence, if $\omega(f)$ is the power density spectrum,

$$\psi = \frac{\int_0^\infty f^2 \omega(f)\,df}{\int_0^\infty \omega(f)df} \tag{7.11}$$

Flax *et al.* (1971) developed equations for the signal power in the Doppler-shifted spectrum, and, regarding this as a "random noise" distribution, they substituted Eqn. 7.11 to show that:

$$\psi = 1\cdot29 f_m \qquad (7.12)$$

for all zero-crossings, both positive and negative, in the case of a parabolic flow profile producing the spectrum represented in Fig. 7.7(a). Since with parabolic flow the maximum velocity is twice the average velocity, the "velocity" indicated by a zero-crossing detector is nearly 30% greater than the average velocity (which should be used to compute flow volume). In a slightly different context, Reneman and Spencer (1974) refer to this as the "riding high" phenomenon! In physical terms, the high frequencies "ride" on the low frequencies, and this results in a reduction in the number of zero-crossings. It has been shown by Reneman *et al.* (1973) that this effect may be minimized if a high-pass filter (a "differentiator") is inserted in the circuit before the zero-crossing counter.

Another source of error with the zero-crossing ratemeter is due to the presence of noise. If *a priori* assumptions concerning the Doppler frequency spectrum can be made, the signal may be fed through a bandpass filter to "improve" the signal-to-noise ratio, as explained by Flax *et al.* (1971).

Equation 7.11 relates to a zero-crossing ratemeter responding to all transitions through zero, both positive-going and negative-going. Such an instrument would give an output (in counts per second) equal to twice the input frequency, in the case of a noise-free sine wave. Most practical zero-crossing ratemeters are arranged to respond only to transitions in one direction, and moreover a set–reset system is normally used (Lunt, 1975) to improve the noise rejection. The set–reset system operates in the following way. An output pulse is generated as the signal amplitude moves through a threshold level. The output is inhibited then until the input signal has passed through a second threshold, equal in magnitude but opposite in sign to the first. The threshold levels are chosen to be just large enough for the output to be zero when the input consists of noise alone. In the presence of a sine wave input the amplitude of which exceeds the threshold level, with or without noise, the output from the zero-crossing ratemeter is equal to the true frequency of the input signal.

(ii) Sound spectrographs

The principle of the sound spectrograph was proposed by R. K. Potter. The sound is analysed to produce a chart in which time and frequency are represented on the x and y axes respectively, and the corresponding amplitudes are represented by the degree of blackening of the recording.

Koenig *et al.* (1946) constructed the first practical sound spectrograph. The basic principles are as follows. The sound to be analysed is recorded in such a way that it can be replayed over and over again. The continuously replayed sound is then analysed by means of a modulator and variable frequency oscillator which shifts each part of the recorded spectrum in sequence to the passband of a fixed frequency filter. The output from the filter is arranged to control the degree of blackening of the recording. The recording paper and the replayed sound are synchronized so that the x-axis represents time. The position on the y-axis of the write out is arranged to correspond to the instantaneous value of the frequency being analysed. Electrically sensitive paper is used, and the dynamic range of the recording is about 12 dB.

Spectrographs based on these principles are available commercially*. In comparison with the zero-crossing counter, a sound spectrograph has several important advantages, which centre around the ability of an interpreter to use his experience in pattern recognition to identify artifacts, such as noise, and to interpolate across parts of the recording which have poor quality. Thus in many applications, spectrographs based on Koenig *et al.*'s (1946) design are entirely satisfactory. They do have two limitations, however, which may make them unsuitable for some purposes. Firstly, they can analyse only rather short samples of signals, typically of about 3 s duration. Secondly, the time necessary to analyse a 3 s sample is about 1 min, and this precludes the possibility of an interactive type of investigation in which the operator optimizes the recording during a clinical study.

Several methods of real-time spectral analysis have been developed, which are free from the limitations of the off-line instrument. Two of these methods are described in the following paragraphs.

Light (1970) has constructed a sound spectrograph in which the signal to be analysed is fed to a bank of 18 bandpass filters connected in parallel. The output from each filter is fed to one of an array of electrodes arranged on one side of a continuously moving strip of moist chemically treated paper which is blackened according to the current which passes through it to a stainless steel electrode on the opposite side. Thus the recording consists of 18 parallel lines, modulated to produce a spectrogram similar to that of an ordinary spectrograph, but with relatively poorer resolution.

Coghlan *et al.* (1974) have described a real-time sound spectrograph which uses time compression so that the frequency sweeping process (as employed in conventional spectrographs and described earlier in this Sub-section) is applied to high frequency signals with a consequent increase in sweep speed. The instrument has two main parts. Firstly, there is a digital memory which accepts the signals to be analysed in real time after analogue-to-digital conversion. The digital output from the memory is multiplied by a weighting function to compensate for the finite gathering

---

* For example, type 6061B: Kay Elemetrics Co., Pine Brook, New Jersey, USA.

time. The time compression factor is 256, and with an approximate input frequency range of 0–10 kHz, the memory output signal after digital-to-analogue conversion covers the approximate frequency range 0–2·3 MHz. The second part of the instrument is a conventional "swept filter" r.f. spectrum analyser, which consists of a swept frequency oscillator and a mixer, followed by a fixed frequency filter with a bandwidth of approximately 30 kHz. This bandwidth corresponds to a real-time bandwidth of just over 100 Hz. The output is presented on 80 parallel spectral lines on a fibre-optic recorder.

(iii) Other methods

The sound spectrograph is undoubtedly the instrument which is least likely to mislead in studying Doppler signals. Unfortunately it is expensive, and the interpretation of the recording requires training and skill. Therefore attempts have been made to develop processing techniques for blood-flow studies, which avoid both the limitations of the zero-crossing ratemeter and the expense and complexity of the sound spectrograph.

One of the expensive components in a sound spectrograph is the write-out system. It has been suggested by Flax *et al.* (1971) that an instrument could be designed which would track the high-frequency leading edge of the spectrum, which is shown in rather an idealistic way in Fig. 7.7. The frequency of the leading edge is proportional to the maximum flow velocity. The instrument could be based on a variable bandpass filter driven by a negative feedback loop designed to intersect a constant segment of the voltage spectrum. The loop would be driven towards lower frequencies when too little signal passed through the filter. Automatic gain control would be required to maintain the amplitude of the leading edge at a constant level despite changes in the frequency distribution of the scattered power. Whether or not the degradation due to noise in a practical system would be intolerable remains to be determined, but it is only fair to express pessimism.

Arts and Roevros (1972) have devised a system which determines the frequency of the mean of the scattered power spectrum. The instrument uses analogue circuits to determine $\Delta\omega_{av}$, the difference between the average angular frequency of the power density spectrum of the received signal and the angular frequency of the transmitted signal, from the equation:

$$\Delta\omega_{av} = \frac{1}{N} \sum_{i=1}^{N} \Delta\omega_i \qquad (7.13)$$

where N = number of particles in backscattering volume;

$\quad i \quad$ = number of any particular backscattering particle; and

ω_i = angular frequency shift associated with each corresponding particle.

Although the feasibility of this system has been tested experimentally, the idea does not seem to have been applied to the solution of clinical problems.

7.2.d Directional Detectors

Simple Doppler systems merely measure the magnitude of the frequency difference between the transmitted and received ultrasonic signals, and not the sign of the difference. As indicated in Eqn. 7.4, this sign carries the information about the direction of the movement of the target, either towards or away from the probe. This is another way of describing whether the Doppler shifted signal forms an upper or a lower sideband to the carrier signal. In many clinical problems, a knowledge of the flow direction is of crucial importance.

There are two situations which can be identified. In the first, the anatomy is such that the Doppler signal consists, at any instant in time, of flow in only one direction. Therefore, it is only necessary to determine whether the flow is forward or reverse. McLeod (1967) has developed a quadrature phase detector which produces two voltages, one of which leads the other by 90°. Which of the two leads the other depends on the sign of the Doppler shift. If only unidirectional, single-valued flow is present, the signals can be satisfactorily processed by logic circuits which allow the leading zero-crossing signals to pass into one of two channels, according to the sign of the Doppler shift.

The second kind of clinical situation arises when flow exists in both directions simultaneously. This may be due to a complex flow profile, or to the ultrasonic beam passing simultaneously through an artery and a vein. The application of this type of signal to a system such as that of McLeod (1967) results in the total number of zero-crossings allocated to each channel not being proportional to the corresponding flow, and only a signal proportional to the differential flow velocity can be produced. In order to obtain separate simultaneous measurements of velocities in opposite directions, the flow direction separation must be performed before the zero-crossing frequency conversions, and a circuit designed to do this has been described by Nippa (1975) and Nippa et al. (1975). A block diagram of the system is illustrated in Fig. 7.8. The two product detectors result in audible Doppler-shift signals at $\pi/2$ relative to each other. The two bandpass filters are identical: their low frequency cut-off is 50 Hz (the lowest frequency of interest), and they have a phase error of less than $\pm 0.5°$ from 90° for frequencies in the range 50–7500 Hz. The combined phase and amplitude errors result in a channel separation of 42 dB.

The use of this circuit with separate zero-crossing ratemeters to indicate forward and reverse flow leaves unsolved the problems associated with this type of indicator (see Section 7.2.c.i). One way around the difficulty is to mix the received signals with a second locally generated signal which differs in frequency from the transmitted frequency by an amount equal to the largest Doppler shift which is expected. The output from the mixing stage then contains signals all higher (or lower) in frequency than the lowest (or highest) signal of interest. The transmitted signal also appears, shifted in frequency and with high amplitude, at the position in the spectrum corresponding to zero velocity. Cross and Light (1971) have developed an instrument based on this superheterodyne system, using a bandstop filter with extremely sharp characteristics to attenuate the zero-

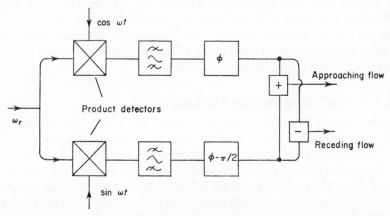

FIG. 7.8 Sideband separation method used by Nippa *et al.* (1975) in a direction-resolving Doppler system. The transmitted and received angular frequencies are respectively ω_t and ω_r.

flow signal. The success of the method depends principally on the performance of this filter. (A variant of this arrangement, for pulsed Doppler work, has been described by Haase *et al.* (1973): within the resolution cell, it may be assumed that flow is unidirectional.) In Cross and Light's (1971) instrument, the Doppler-shift frequency spectrum is displayed as a real-time sound spectrograph (see Section 7.2.c.ii). An alternative approach, due to Jong *et al.* (1975), is to derive the forward and reverse average velocities by the method developed by Arts and Roevros (1972), and described in Section 7.2.c.iii.

7.2.e Phase Detectors

Reid *et al.* (1967) have developed an instrument which derives a voltage proportional to the instantaneous position of a structure moving with respect to an ultrasonic Doppler probe, by phase detection of the reflected wave. The amplitude u of the reflected wave is given by

$$u = u_0 \cos(\omega t - \theta) \qquad (7.14)$$

where θ is the phase shift due to propagation delay over the distance x, and $\omega = 2\pi f$, the transmitted angular frequency, so that

$$\theta = 2\omega x/c$$

If the structure is moving at constant velocity v, then

$$x = vt$$

Even if x is an arbitrary function of time, measurement of the phase angle can directly yield the displacement distance over a limited range of amplitude. This limitation of range variation amplitude can be overcome by means of a phase lock loop, in which the frequency of the transmitted signal is varied to maintain a constant phase relationship with the signal received from the moving target (Baker *et al.*, 1967).

7.2.f Rangefinding Doppler Methods

Simple continuous wave Doppler systems are unable to measure the distance between the probe and the moving structure. Techniques were developed many years ago in radar by which the transmitted signal could be time-coded so that range information could be obtained by measuring time delays, whilst simultaneously velocity information could be extracted in the form of Doppler frequency shifts. Analogous techniques have recently been applied in medical ultrasonic diagnostics. They allow the movements of many targets to be studied virtually simultaneously, and blood flow profiles to be plotted. A detailed analysis of the performance of pulsed Dopplers, which is also of relevance to other rangefinding Doppler methods, has been made by Jorgensen *et al.* (1973).

A fundamental property of all methods designed to measure velocity and position simultaneously is that the velocity and range resolutions are inextricably linked. In physical terms, it is not possible to measure the velocity of a target the position of which is known precisely, because some movement is necessary to allow its velocity to be determined.

(i) Pulsed Dopplers

Apparently Baker and Watkins (1967) were the first to realize the possibility that range-selective Doppler information could be obtained by gating the output of a continuously running oscillator to transmit pulses, the phases of the echoes of which could be compared with that of the oscillator to give velocity information about targets lying within any chosen range interval.

Two years later it became apparent that other investigators had independently developed pulsed Doppler systems (Flaherty and Strauts, 1969; Peronneau and Leger, 1969; Wells, 1969).

A block diagram of a typical pulsed Doppler system is shown in Fig. 7.9. The pulse repetition rate is controlled by the clock, which triggers the monostable to open the gate to allow the transmitting transducer to be excited for a period corresponding to the width of the sample which it is desired to study. Echoes returning from the patient are amplified, and mixed in the demodulator with the signal from the oscillator (equal in

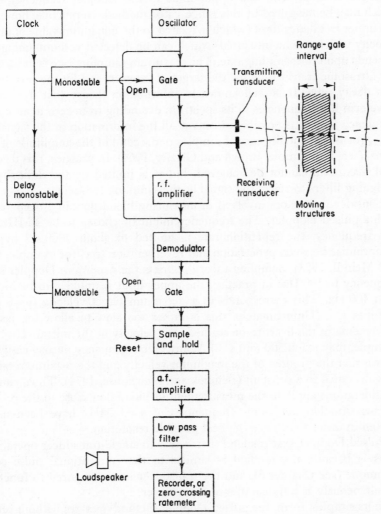

FIG. 7.9 Block diagram of typical pulsed Doppler system. (After Wells, 1969.)

frequency to that which was transmitted). The delay monostable triggers the monostable controlling the receiver gate, so that the gate opens to allow a voltage, which is in effect a sample corresponding to the instantaneous position of the target, to be stored in the sample and hold circuit. The sample and hold is reset immediately prior to being updated by a new sample corresponding to the following ultrasonic pulse. The output from the sample and hold is thus a square wave with a long mark, and a short space, the envelope of which is an audible signal representing the Doppler shifted information from the target under investigation.

There is in principle no upper limit to the Doppler frequency shift which may be measured by this range-gated method. In practice, however, the upper frequency limit (which is related to the maximum value of target velocity which can be measured) which can be detected without ambiguity depends upon the sampling rate. The maximum sampling rate is limited by the ultrasonic transit time for the target of interest, and by the reverberation decay time. It is well known in information theory that if a signal waveform has frequencies in its spectrum extending from zero to an upper frequency f_{max}, it is possible to convey all the information in the signal by $2f_{max}$ (or more) equally spaced samples per second of the amplitude of the signal (see, for example, Brown and Glazier, 1964). In practice, this theoretical maximum cannot be achieved, but it is limited by the difficulty of designing filters to reject the signal at the sampling frequency.

Consider the factors involved in measuring blood flow in a deep vessel with a pulsed Doppler. The frequency might be chosen to be 2 MHz. At this frequency, the repetition rate is limited to about 1000 s^{-1} by the compromise between penetration and reverberation (see, for example, Gill and Meindl, 1973). Sampling theory restricts the maximum Doppler shift frequency to 500 Hz; in practice, the upper limit is unlikely to be higher than 400 Hz. This corresponds to a maximum target velocity ($\gamma = 0°$) of 150 mm s^{-1}. (Unfortunately, this is rather too slow to allow the fastest movements in the heart to be studied: the velocity of the mitral valve, for example, may reach 500 mm s^{-1}.) At any given frequency, it may easily be shown that the product of the maximum velocity and the maximum target range is equal to a constant (Bendick and Newhouse, 1974). Thus, similar considerations apply to the measurement of blood flow close to the probe: in this situation, ultrasonic frequencies of 4–35 MHz have been used, chosen in order to achieve the best possible resolution.

Pulsed Doppler systems lend themselves to single-transducer operation. This is because the method is similar to the conventional pulse–echo technique (see Chapter 6), and the transducer is not required to function simultaneously as a transmitter and a receiver.

In its simplest form, the pulsed Doppler method operates without phase coherence between pulses. Baker's (1970) system is coherent in this respect:

the clock pulses are derived by dividing down from the master oscillator. The only advantage of this particular feature seems to be that every transmitted pulse is initiated at the same phase of the ultrasonic oscillator, thus avoiding "jitter" due to the restricted bandwidth of the transmitting transducer. Indeed, a fully incoherent system may be preferable in some circumstances. Thus, Atkinson (1974) has demonstrated that simple envelope detection of the long pulse reflected by a deep blood vessel and its walls, using the clutter signal as the reference, is better in separating the clutter and the blood Doppler frequency bands, than is any processing arrangement involving mixing with a coherent reference. In any event, spectral broadening inevitably occurs since the transmitted pulse, being of limited duration, contains energy spread over a finite range of frequency. This is in conflict with the concept of a phase-coherent reference, which strictly is relevant only in a continuous-wave system. The practical effect of this has general validity: improvement in range resolution is at the expense of velocity resolution. Some investigators (for example, Jethwa *et al.*, 1975) have suggested that it is possible that appropriately chosen signal processing arrangements may circumvent this limitation. There seems to be no theoretical justification for this. Expressed in physical terms, in the limit if the time spent in interrogating the target is infinitely short, perfect range resolution is achieved; but the target does not move in an infinitely short period of time, and so the echo carries no information concerning its velocity.

The clinical applications of pulsed Dopplers are reviwed in Section 7.3. Some of these applications involved the measurement of blood flow profiles. Instruments have been devised which display the data from multiplexed gates (see, for example, Peronneau *et al.*, 1970). Directional detection using the offset-frequency (superheterodyne) technique has been combined with multiplexed gating by Haase *et al.* (1973).

(ii) Time-coded Dopplers

An important limitation of the pulsed Doppler method is that the maximum velocity which may be measured at any particular range is restricted by ambiguity with the pulse repetition frequency. It was pointed out by Waag *et al.* (1972) that this limitation does not arise if the transmitted signal carries a random code. In their prototype instrument, continuous transmission of a carrier with phase modulation by pseudorandom binary sequence is used. The receiver correlates the received signal with delayed versions of the transmitted signal and then performs spectral analyses. The system can also operate in a coherent pulse mode by transmitting bursts of binary phase coded pulses.

As an alternative to pseudorandom pulse sequences, Bendick and Newhouse (1974) have used pulses of random noise. A block diagram of their system is illustrated in Fig. 7.10. The limiter protects the high gain amplifier from overload during transmission. The variable delay line determines the range corresponding to the target to be studied. As in a conventional pulsed Doppler, the duration of the transmitted pulse controls the length of the resolution cell. Both the echo and the delayed signals are clipped. This gives a slight reduction in the signal-to-noise ratio, but it allows the multiplication function necessary to correlate the two signals to be performed by simple "exclusive-or" circuit.

A similar system has been described by Jethwa *et al.* (1975), with the added refinement that directional information is retained by means of an offset-frequency (superheterodyne) detection arrangement.

Frequency modulation has been used for time coding by McCarty and Woodcock (1975). A block diagram of their system is shown in Fig. 7.11(a). The waveforms at the transmitting and receiving transducers with a

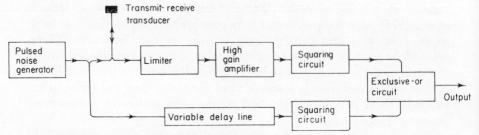

FIG. 7.10 Block diagram of pulsed random noise Doppler system. (After Bendick and Newhouse, 1974.)

stationary target at range R are illustrated in Fig. 7.11(b). The voltage ramp generator operates repetitively to sweep the frequency f_0 of the voltage controlled oscillator with a sawtooth waveform starting from frequency f_1. The echo at the receiving transducer is a version of the transmitted signal delayed by travelling through a distance of $2R$. This ultrasonic transit time is equal to $2R/c$, and so the difference between the transmitted and received signals is given by

$$f_r - f_0 = (2R/c)(df/dt) \qquad (7.15)$$

during the interval $t_1 < t < t_2$, where df/dt is the rate of change of frequency during sweeping. Typically $f_1 = 10$ MHz and $df/dt = 100$ MHz s^{-1}, so that the Doppler shift frequency $(f_r - f_0) = 6.7$ kHz for a target range $R = 50$ mm. Moreover, the shift frequency is proportional to the target range, and in a multiple-target situation the separate targets can be resolved as separate bands of frequency on the sound spectrograph. If the target is moving, a Doppler shift frequency which, to a first approximation, is proportional to the target velocity, is superimposed on the difference frequency. This shift frequency is either below or above the difference frequency, depending on whether the target is moving towards or away from the probe, if the sweep is increasing the transmitted frequency with time, and vice versa. Thus it is theoretically possible to derive flow direction, for example by using a trapezoidal waveform for frequency modulation. The method is still in the experimental stage. Whilst it is subject to the same fundamental limitations

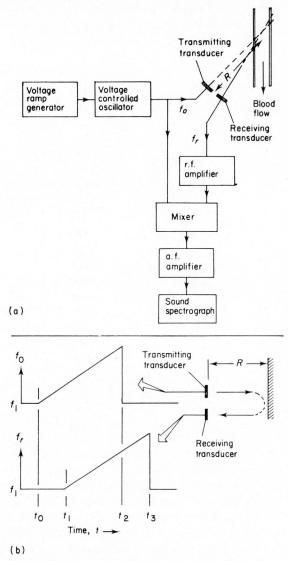

(a)

(b)

Fig. 7.11 Frequency modulated Doppler system. (a) Block diagram; (b) wave-forms with stationary target. (Based on McCarty and Woodcock, 1975.)

15

that apply to all range-finding Dopplers, the audible output might allow diagnostic information to be obtained with a simple instrument and without the expense of a sound spectrograph.

7.2.g Two-dimensional Doppler Imaging

In many clinical situations, adequate diagnostic information may be obtained with hand-held Doppler probes. The investigator needs to know the anatomy of the structures being studied, however, in order to interpret the results.

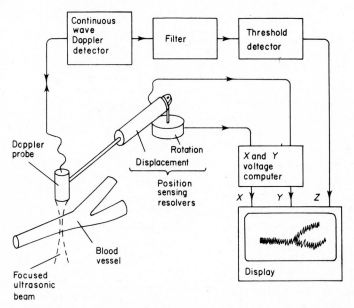

FIG. 7.12 Continuous wave Doppler system for two-dimensional visualization of blood vessels. (Based on Spencer *et al.*, 1974.)

   In blood flow studies, it is sometimes helpful to have a two-dimensional map showing the positions of blood vessels. An example of this type of image is the contrast angiogram familiar in radiology. The Doppler shift in the frequency of backscattered ultrasound is a special characteristic of flowing blood, and this was exploited by Reid and Spencer (1972) in constructing a simple instrument for non-invasive mapping of blood vessels. The basic principles, as subsequently developed by Spencer *et al.* (1974), are illustrated in Fig. 7.12. The probe is mounted on a two-dimensional coordinate measuring scanner, the resolvers of which provide data from which are computed x and y voltages to control the deflexion circuits of a direct view bistable electronic storage tube (see Section 6.6.b). The probe is arranged so that the ultrasonic beam is at least slightly inclined to the direction of flow in the vessels which it is required to visualize. When the beam passes through the moving blood, the Doppler detector generates an output which is filtered (to eliminate artifacts due to low velocity movements) and, provided that it exceeds a preset threshold level in amplitude, switches on the electron beam of the display. A two-dimensional map showing those regions in which flow is detected is constructed on the display by scanning the probe over the area of the patient's skin beyond which the blood vessel lies. Since arteries and veins are often close together, a directionally sensitive circuit is arranged to inhibit the display when flow is detected in the opposite direction to that in the vessel under study.

Continuous wave Dopplers lack range resolution. This may be a disadvantage in two-dimensional blood vessel visualization, if two vessels with flow in the same direction lie one above the other along the ultrasonic beam. Mozersky et al. (1971) and Fish (1972) have independently developed pulsed Doppler systems which, because of their range-finding capabilities, enable vessels in this situation to be separated. Both systems operate at 5 MHz. The essential difference between the continuous wave and pulsed Doppler instruments is that the former produces a plan of the blood vessels (a "Doppler C-scan") whereas the latter has three-dimensional data and so can produce a two-dimensional section (a "Doppler B-scan"). The natural development from single-element mechanical scanning to Doppler arrays has been begun by Hottinger and Meindl (1975).

All Doppler systems have the same inherent limitation in range resolution. At least two instruments have been constructed, which combine the velocity measuring capability of pulsed Doppler with the two-dimensional imaging capability of the pulse–echo method. In Barker et al.'s (1974) system, the same 5 MHz transducer acts alternately as a pulse–echo and as a pulsed Doppler probe. The transducer is rotated at 10 revolutions per second on the end of an arm within a circular water bath, and scanning takes place through a flexible rubber window. Only a small sector of rotation is used for imaging, amounting to 40° of a 75 mm diameter cylinder. The pulse repetition rate is 10 k s^{-1}, and the image has 111 lines. The system has adequate performance to produce a two-dimensional B-scan of superficial blood vessels such as the carotid arteries. The pulsed Doppler has 10 multiplexed gates, and the position of the Doppler beam can be selected to coincide with any chosen line on the B-scan.

A somewhat similar instrument has been described by Evans et al. (1974). Separate transducers are used for the pulse–echo system (10 MHz) and the pulsed Doppler (5 MHz). The image frame rate is 15 s^{-1}, and any selected blood-flow profile can be derived in real time from 20 multiplexed gates.

7.2.h Activity Monitors

Ultrasonic burglar alarms operate by detecting changes in the field distribution of low frequency ultrasound which pervades the sensitive volume. The same method has been used to monitor the activity of patients (see Section 7.3.f). A typical instrument has been described by Haines (1974). It is a replica of a conventional medical Doppler (see Section 7.2.a), except that it operates at a frequency of about 40 kHz. At this frequency, a small piezoelectric transducer is capable of insonating a volume large enough to enclose several individuals. Movement of any individual changes the signal detected by a second transducer acting as a receiver, and this change can be arranged to trigger a counter.

7.3 CLINICAL APPLICATIONS

7.3.a Angiology

(i) Arteries in the leg

The first application of the Doppler blood flow detector in the evaluation of arterial disease was simple in principle: the course of an artery was traced along the limb whilst the operator listened for sudden changes in the characteristics of the signal (Strandness et al., 1967). In the normal, the sound consists of two components superimposed on a continuous low-frequency signal. The first is high-pitched, and corresponds to systole, and the second is low-pitched, and occurs during diastole. It was soon found that compression of the limb produced changes in the distal flow pattern, and that these changes were different in normal and in occluded vessels (see, for example, Rittenhouse and Brockenbrough, 1969). The next step was the discovery that the blood pressure gradient along the limb could be measured using a Doppler detector on an artery in the ankle, with the sphygmomanometer cuff in turn placed around the upper and lower thighs, the calf, and the ankle (Allan and Terry, 1969). The gradient of blood pressure against distance down the limb is increased in patients with arterial disease of the leg. Another approach, developed by Lewis et al. (1972), is based on the observation that pressure changes in the leg seem to correlate with the level of disease. The blood pressures at the ankle (measured with an ankle cuff and a Doppler detector) does not alter greatly following exercise in the normal, but in disease it falls substantially (typically to 0–50% of the resting pressure) immediately after exercise, and the time which elapses whilst the pressure returns to the resting value may be up to 20 min. Moreover, these changes correlate with perfusion measurements of flow made using [133]Xe.

Johnston and Kakkar (1974) have described a non-invasive method of measuring the arterial pressure wave at the level of the ankle. An ultrasonic

Doppler detector was used to time the arrival of the pressure wave past a sphygmomenometer cuff, inflated in sequence to a series of increasing pressures, in relation to the R-wave of the e.c.g. Thus they were able to measure the mean systolic slope: this is reduced in stenosis or occlusion.

Woodcock (1970) was the first to describe the significance of changes in the velocity–time waveform, based on simultaneous observations of the arterial pulses at separate sites on the limb. Three quantities are determined. The first is the pulse *transit time* TT between any two measurement sites. The second is the *pulsatility index* PI at each site. This is defined as the sum of the maximum oscillatory energy of the Fourier harmonics of the Doppler frequency spectrum, divided by the mean energy over the cardiac cycle. The third is the *damping factor* DF between any two measurement sites, defined as the ratio of the PIs at the upstream and downstream sites.

An alternative and easier way of deriving the PI is to use a planimeter to obtain the integral, A, of the pulse waveform displayed on a sound spectrograph, corresponding to a complete pulse of duration T. Then:

$$PI' = |\hat{V}_{pk-pk}|/\bar{V} \qquad (7.16)$$

where $|\hat{V}_{pk-pk}|$ = peak forward velocity during the pulse, or difference between peak forward and peak reverse velocities if reverse flow occurs,

and $\bar{V} = \int_0^T V dt/T = A/T$

where V = velocity at time t.

Fitzgerald *et al.* (1971) described the use of these indices to grade arterial disease into four classes. Classification (a) is associated with short transit time and small damping factor; (b), with short transit time and large damping factor; (c), with long transit time and small damping factor; and (d), with long transit time and large damping factor. In physiological terms, these classifications correspond to (a) short, large diameter collateral; (b), short, small diameter collateral; (c), long, large diameter collateral; and (d), long, small diameter collateral. This scheme of classification has been subsequently refined. Thus, Fitzgerald and Carr (1975) have recently reviewed the status of arterial disease classification using this approach. Seven arterial pulse sites are examined, as indicated in Fig. 7.13. (Slightly different values of normal PIs and TTs are given by Gosling and King (1974).) Typical spectrographs and corresponding arteriograms are shown in Fig. 7.14. The aorta is monitored just above the level of bifurcation. The common femoral artery is located just below the inguinal ligament, the popliteal artery in the popliteal fossa, and the posterior tibial artery slightly above and behind the medial maleolus at the ankle. Finally, *blood pressure* BP is measured in the arm as a reference for systolic measurements taken in the limb. This is done using the Doppler probe on the ankle, to detect occlusions due to the sphygmomenometer cuff around the thigh, upper and lower calves in sequence.

The status of an artery may be classified into one of three broad groups. This is illustrated in Fig. 7.15. In Group I, there is no obstruction to arterial flow within the lumen, but there may be changes in the stiffness of the wall or the size of the lumen. In Group II, partial obstruction is present

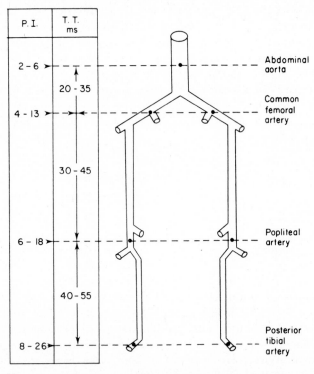

FIG. 7.13 Sites of measurement for the evaluation of lower limb arterial status, with normal values of PIs and TTs. (After Woodcock, 1970.)

in varying degrees of severity and distribution. In Group III, the artery is totally blocked, with collateral development in varying degrees. The letter N indicates normal values, as indicated in Fig. 7.13.

In Fitzgerald and Carr's (1975) series of 84 patients in whom the diagnoses were confirmed by arteriography, the ultrasonic diagnoses were correct in 83. The one error which was made with ultrasound was the diagnosis of a block in a popliteal–posterior tibial segment, which on arteriography was shown to be a severe stenosis which did not allow contrast medium to pass. These excellent results confirm that arteriography is certainly unnecessary except in patients in whom reconstructive surgery is a definite possibility. Moreover the ultrasonic method is economical: the cost of an ultrasonic examination is about one-third that of an arteriogram, and the capital investment in equipment is about one-tenth.

Measurement of the arterial function in terms of transit time and pulsatility index makes it possible to distinguish between poor arterial supply and

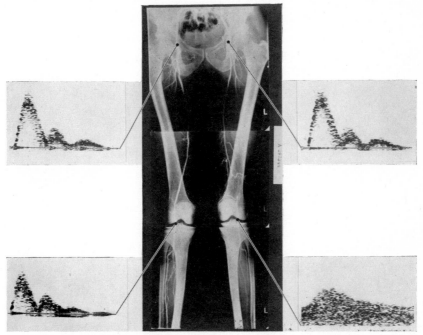

FIG. 7.14 Arteriogram and ultrasound Doppler frequency spectra of a patient with occlusive disease of the left (L) superficial femoral artery. Distal to the site of the occlusion, a large number of small vessels constitute the collateral circulation pathways; the right (R) limb appears to be normal. The Doppler frequency spectra do not distinguish between forward and reverse flow. (Courtesy J. P. Woodcock.)

poor venous drainage as the cause of ischaemic ulceration of the leg in those patients in whom this is not clinically obvious (Woodcock et al., 1974).

A new approach to the analysis of Doppler-shift arterial signals obtained from different sites on the leg has been described by Morris et al. (1975). The Doppler-shift signals at the input and at the output of an arterial segment are recorded simultaneously, and analysed by a sound spectrograph. In doing this, judgement is used to try to ensure that the signals are comparable: in principle, this requires that the angles of attack of the two ultrasonic beams are equal. The impulse response is derived by har-

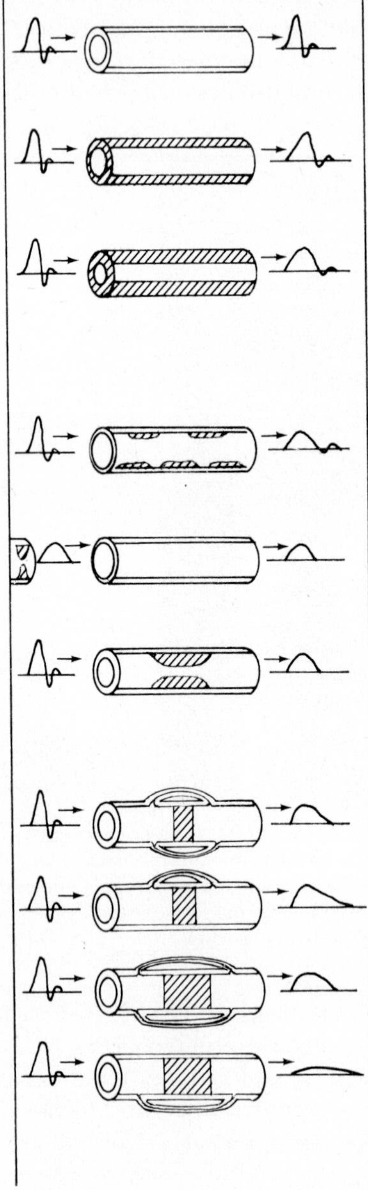

Group	Input	Output	P.I.$_i$	P.I.$_o$	D.F.	T.T.	B.P.
1A			N	N	<1,0	N	N
1B			N	≃N	<1,0	N	N
1C			≃N	≃N	<1,0	<N	≃N
2A			N	≤N	≤1,5	N	N
2B			<N	<N	<1,5	N	≤N
2C			N	<N	>1,5	≃N	≤N
3A			≃N	<N	<1,5	>N <70	<N
3B			≃N	<N	>1,5	>N <70	<N
3C			≃N	<N	<1,5	>70	<N
3D			≃N	<N	>1,5	>70	<N

FIG. 7.15 Classification of degenerative arterial disease of the lower limb. Group I, change in the vessel wall; Group II, partial occlusion; Group III, complete occlusion with collateral. (After Fitzgerald and Carr, 1975.)

monic analysis of the input and output maximum-blood-velocity/time waveforms. This is defined as the output of the system which would result from an input of infinitesimal duration and infinite amplitude. Alternatively, in certain circumstances the impulse response may be derived by correlation techniques, and in such cases the transfer function may be obtained directly from the input–output crosspower density spectrum. Woodcock *et al.* (1975) have used this approach to analyse the arterial status between femoral and popliteal detection sites in patients with disease of the superficial femoral artery. The time–position of the peak of the impulse response gives a measurement of the length of the vascular pathway; the occurrence of two peaks suggests two main pathways of different length. The shape of the impulse response is related to the impedance of the pathway: the "flatter" the peak, the worse is the collateral.

It has recently become clear that the impulse response approach has limitations, particularly in patients with normal circulation in whom the arterial segment has non-linear characteristics. Other analytical methods, however, including the calculation of Z-transfer function, have given encouraging results. It seems likely that it may become possible quantitatively to assess arterial status in terms of indices related to the mechanical properties of the blood vessels. This would have important applications in trials of the effects of lipid-removing drugs, and in the management of patients with atherosclerosis.

Two-dimensional visualization of arteries in the leg may also prove to be of value. Although the most relevant studies have been of vessels in the neck, it has been shown to be possible to examine vessels in the leg using two-dimensional scanning with pulsed Doppler (Fish, 1972; Fish *et al.*, 1972; Mozersky *et al.*, 1972).

Possibly the major limitation of simple Doppler blood-flow detectors is their inability to measure flow volume. Pulsed Doppler systems have been shown to be capable of doing this when the transducer is applied directly to the wall of the vessel, particularly in the case of the great vessels. Transcutaneous measurements in peripheral vessels would obviously be of substantial clinical value, and Histand *et al.* (1973) have shown in experiments on dogs that blood volume may be determined using transcutaneous Dopplers, with accuracy comparable to the electromagnetic flowmeter, which does require surgery. Moreover, according to Histand and Miller (1972), surgical exposure of an artery causes vasoconstriction which significantly changes flow characteristics.

(ii) Arteries in the head and neck

Methods of surveying the cerebral circulation by means of simple continuous-wave Doppler instruments have been described by several investigators. Despite the inherent difficulties associated with the zero-crossing counter and directional detection, it is possible to obtain clues concerning such disorders as carotid stenosis, arteriovenous aneurysm, subclavian steal syndrome, and innominate artery stenosis. For examples of relevant articles, see Mol and Rijcken (1974), Müller and Gonzalez (1974) and Planiol and Pourcelot (1974).

After the supraorbital artery has left the orbit, it passes over the smooth frontal bone of the forehead. Wyatt *et al.* (1973) have developed a method whereby the artery is compressed against this bone whilst the blood flowing through it is monitored by a Doppler detector. The pressure can be altered and measured, and the pressure at which blood flow is arrested is equal to the ophthalmic artery systolic pressure. In normals, this is about 50% of the brachial artery systolic pressure. Hypertensive patients generally have raised ophthalmic arterial pressures, whereas atherosclerotic patients have lowered pressures.

With anatomically accessible vessels, such as the carotid artery, it is possible simultaneously to visualize the diameter of the lumen, by means of a pulse–echo transducer and an A-scan display, and to measure the blood velocity, by means of a pair of Doppler transducers and a zero-crossing counter. This has been done by Olson (1974).

Although much useful diagnostic information can be obtained by a skilled observer using a hand-held Doppler probe, anatomical relationships can be more easily appreciated if it is possible to map the distribution of blood vessels by means of a two-dimensional Doppler scanner. There are three types of scanner, as described in Section 7.2.g: in increasing order of complexity, these are the continuous-wave, the pulsed-Doppler, and the combined pulse–echo and pulsed–Doppler instruments.

The continuous-wave two-dimensional instrument has been used chiefly for mapping the carotids (Spencer *et al.*, 1974; Thomas *et al.*, 1974). The operator is helped by listening to the Doppler signals whilst the scan is being formed on the display. A directional detector is arranged to separate arterial from venous flow, and to reject the latter so that it does not appear on the image. In the normal, the bifurcation is first imaged, and from this the internal carotid can be scanned as it moves posteriorly towards the mastoid process, and the external carotid, which is anterior and branches towards the mandible. A typical scan is shown in Fig. 7.16. In disease, there are four clues which can be gleaned, two from the scan, one whilst the scan is being made, and one from another observation. On the scan, occlusion of either the internal or external carotid artery is apparent by the failure to visualize the vessel. Calcification of atherosclerotic plaques results in high attenuation, and blood flow signals cannot be detected through such areas. During scanning, the Doppler shift signals may be audibly abnormal when detected from stenoses through which the velocity is increased together with turbulence. Finally, the direction of flow in the ophthalmic artery may be determined by placing the probe on the closed eyelid, with the beam directed posteriorly. Flow is normally towards the probe.

Two-dimensional mapping of blood vessels using the pulsed Doppler technique allows overlying blood vessels to be distinguished even if the flows are in the same direction. Mozersky *et al.* (1971) have made use of this in scanning the carotid arteries (in addition to the aortic arch, the abdominal aorta, iliac artery, and the femoral and popliteal vessels). The ultrasonic angiogram provides a simple, inexpensive, rapid and repeatable alternative to contrast radiology (arteriography). It may be better than

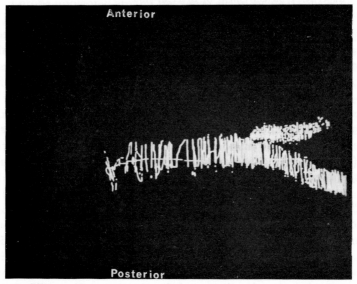

Fig. 7.16 Doppler flow map of the right carotid arteries of an asymptomatic volunteer. A, anterior, P; posterior. (Courtesy J. M. Reid.)

radiology in studying a localized lesion, because it simultaneously provides views in longitudinal, transverse and cross-sectional planes. Problems which remain to be solved are the rather large sample volume, which exaggerates the size of the vessel, and artifacts due to patient movement, which are particularly troublesome in neck scans, where swallowing or mumbling can spoil the image.

Combined pulse–echo and pulsed Doppler scanning of the carotids was first described by Barber *et al.* (1974). In their instrument, imaging is difficult in diseased patients, because pictures are only obtained when the beam is normal to the vessel. This is the most unfavourable orientation for Doppler detection. The rather disappointing results showed the great

Pulmonary embolism and death is an alarmingly common sequel to even minor surgical procedures. It is usually caused by thrombus detached from a clot in a deep vein of the leg. The matter has been reviewed by Evans (1971). One in seven hospital deaths is due to pulmonary embolism. Moreover, almost half of those who die from this cause in hospital have an otherwise normal life expectancy. Prevention by early diagnosis and treatment by anticoagulant therapy or vein ligation is obviously preferable to heroic surgery following collapse. Pulmonary embolectomy has a survival rate of only about one in four. Stimulated by these impressive data, Evans (1971) developed a simple method of screening for deep vein thrombosis. He used a 2 MHz continuous wave Doppler of the type intended for obstetrical use. The patient is examined in bed, sitting flexed at the hips to 45° or more, with ankles supported to allow good filling of calf veins. The sites studied are the superficial femoral vein 100 mm below the inguinal ligament, the common femoral vein, the external iliac vein, and the inferior vena cava. In the absence of a significant occlusion, compression of the calf—either by hand or with a cuff—produces a "swishing" sound in the Doppler shift signal.

In Evans' (1971) series of 60 legs in which there were proved thrombi in the popliteal or more proximal veins, the Doppler test was positive in 95%. (Most fatal emboli probably arise from popliteal or larger veins, rather than from smaller calf veins.) Likewise Moore et al. (1973) detected about 86% of thrombi in the deep veins, and most of their errors were failures to detect calf vein thrombi.

The method is speedy: thus McIrroy (1972) reported that only 30–40 min are required to examine the legs of 20 patients.

In connexion with the possibility of causing detachment of emboli by squeezing the calf, Bracey (1973) recommended squeezing the foot with an automatic cuff. It is also relevant here that distinctive "chirps" were heard with a 10 MHz Doppler placed on the femoral vein, in 21 out of 23 dogs following experimental fracture of the tibia and fibula (Kelly et al., 1972). These sounds were presumably due to fat emboli.

The relative values of transcutaneous Doppler, ^{125}I fibrinogen, and phlebography in the detection of deep-vein thrombosis have been compared by Negus (1972). Phlebography is a reliable method, since if the venous system is successfully visualized it is almost inconceivable that a significant clot could be overlooked. Doppler ultrasound is well suited to rapid examination of a patient, and twice-weekly tests of the femoral and iliac veins are advisable in postoperative patients during the period until the patient is fully ambulant. It is also helpful in deciding on the desirability of phlebography. In terms of diagnostic reliability, Doppler ultrasound and ^{125}I fibrinogen should be used together, since the former is better for investigating the upper part of the limb, and vice versa. Also the isotope test provides data on the production of thrombin, and so enables old and new thrombi to be distinguished. It cannot, however, be used repeatedly in the same patient, and in any case it is necessary to block the thyroid with oral inorganic iodide. Moreover, it is less useful than ultrasound since calf emboli are potentially less dangerous.

Entire limbs can be explored to discover incompetent perforating veins, using a Doppler blood velocity detector (Miller and Foote, 1974). The skin over the suspect area is marked with dots in a raster pattern, and the probe is placed normal to the skin over each dot in turn. At each position, the calf below the site, or the foot, is squeezed: if an incompetent perforator is present, the blood is heard to flow first in one direction, then in the other.

Patients with large tortuous varicose veins often have minimal symptoms of calf pump failure. Somerville et al. (1974) have determined the incidence of retrograde turbulent flow in superficial veins, and correlated this with assessments of the degree of varicosity and the severity of the symptoms. The presence or absence of turbulence in the long saphenous vein was determined by placing a Doppler probe at 45° to the vein in the region of the medial femoral condyle. With this lightly strapped in place, the patient was asked to stand up on her toes and relax down again: this produces reverse flow. The occurrence of turbulence can be detected by the presence of high-pitched signals when the sound spectrograph is examined. Three groups of patients can be identified. In Group I, there is laminar reverse flow, minimal varices and minimal symptoms; Group II has laminar reverse flow, minimal varices, severe symptoms and signs of calf pump dysfunction; and Group III has turbulent reverse flow, gross varices, negligible symptoms, and no evidence of calf pump dysfunction. The age distributions of the patients in this study suggested that Group I patients progress into Group II if left untreated, but not into Group III. Somerville et al. (1974) postulated that turbulence may damage the architecture of the vein wall or weaken the surrounding connective tissue, thus allowing dilation to occur.

Incompetence of the superficial and deep veins of the leg can be distinguished by testing the effect of occluding the superficial veins only by means of an ankle cuff (Lewis et al., 1973).

7.3.b Cardiology

(i) Cardiac function

The original suggestion that cardiac functional abnormalities might be reflected by changes in blood flow patterns in veins and arteries, which could be detected by Doppler shift signals, seems to have been made by Benchimol (1967). The present status of the method has been reviewed by Benchimol et al. (1973) and by Kalmanson et al. (1974). Right heart spectrum analysis; in his early experiments, an obstetric foetal heart detector was used, with off-line analysis by a sound spectrograph. Initially the probe was positioned in a left intercostal space, but in later work, the suprasternal position was adopted (Light and Cross, 1972). (This approach was also suggested, apparently independently, by Thompson and Mennel (1969).) The orientation of the aortic arch is such that the ultrasonic beam can, when directed from the suprasternal notch, intersect the direction of blood flow tangentially. Other angles of attack occur, due to the curvature of the vessel, but the highest Doppler shift frequency corresponds to the highest velocity vector within the beam. The use of a real-time sound spectrograph (see Section 7.2.c) to display directionally detected Doppler shift signals allows the operator to obtain optimal orientation, and to recognize flow signals from branch arteries which, since they serve the head and neck, are in the opposite direction to the flow in the aortic arch. The spectral display allows turbulence to be identified, and can be interpreted even if the signal-to-noise ratio is poor.

The clinical usefulness of transcutaneous aortovelography is still being assessed (Light, 1974; Light et al., 1974). The part of the aorta in which the flow velocity is monitored is close to the heart, so that information on left heart action is obtained. In any particular individual, instantaneous cardiac output is likely to be proportional to the measured velocity, provided that the systolic cross-sectional area of the aorta, the velocity flow profile, and the fraction of flow in the branches of the aortic arch, all remain constant. Preliminary observations bear out the validity of these assumptions, and therefore the method may be useful in critical care situations. The waveform of the envelope of the frequency spectrum also seems to reflect the cardiac performance in other respects. Thus, it is possible to estimate indices of early systolic acceleration, peak velocity, and durations of acceleration and deceleration phases of the systolic period. Because of the difficulty of absolute measurement, in clinical practice it is likely that changes in these indices will prove to be of more value than their actual values. In addition, the frequency spectrum may reflect functional abnormalities in the heart and aorta, such as aortic regurgitation, coarctation of the aorta, and so on.

Others who have developed transcutaneous aortovelographic instruments, and studied their performance, include Mackay and Hechtman (1975), who also used a frequency of 2 MHz, and Huntsman et al. (1975), who used 2·5 MHz, and a maximum frequency envelope detector.

(ii) Blood pressure

Indirect measurement of blood pressure depends on the equality of the external pressure applied to the arterial wall to that in a pneumatic cuff wrapped around the limb within which the artery lies. When the pressure in the cuff is greater than the systolic arterial pressure, no blood flows through the artery. As the pressure is decreased, blood begins to flow for a changing proportion of the cardiac cycle, until it flows without interruption when the cuff pressure is less than the diastolic arterial pressure.

There are various ways in which the arterial pulse distal to the cuff may be detected, in order to deduce the blood pressure from measurement of the cuff pressure. (This is usually measured by a mercury manometer in a sphygmomanometer, but other types of pressure gauge may be used. The traditional use of the mercury manometer has for years resulted in the measurement being expressed in units of "millimetres of mercury". Nowadays, the pressure should be measured in [kPa]; 1 kPa $\equiv 7\cdot5006$ mmHg.) The clinician usually detects the pulse either by palpation, or by auscultation, or simply by looking at the range of pressure over which the height of the mercury column in the manometer exhibits small pulsations whilst the cuff pressure is steadily reduced. R. W. Ware was apparently the first to suggest, in 1964, that the ultrasonic Doppler method might be used to detect these pulsations. The idea was soon taken up by many others (for example, Kardon et al., 1967; Kirby et al., 1969). It is certainly possible to detect the arterial pulsations and to measure the blood pressures in patients in whom other non-invasive methods would fail.

In unfavourable clinical circumstances, it is impossible to detect flow distal to the occluding cuff. The detection of arterial wall pulsations by Doppler ultrasound, however, is much easier. In a series of 495 comparisons between direct intra-arterial blood pressure measurements and indirect measurements using ultrasound, Dweck et al. (1974) found good agreements, particularly in the leg where experienced observers achieved correlation coefficients of 0·75 for systolic pressures, and 0·80 for diastolic pressures. (The same method had been used previously by Poppers (1973).) This technique seems to be more convenient than that described by Elseed et al. (1973), who apparently used the Doppler system to detect the flow of blood in the artery of the extremity, rather than the movement of the arterial wall.

Automatic blood pressure recorders using Doppler ultrasound to detect the presence or absence of the pulse have been developed (see, for example, Hochberg et al., 1973). Whilst these instruments are better than many others—particularly those using microphones—reservations about their performances have been expressed (Labarthe et al., 1973).

The Doppler method is usable in unfavourable environments, such as in high noise and vibration levels (Kopczynski, 1974), and during rapid accelerations (Forlini, 1974), and in such situations an automatic Doppler instrument may be the only alternative to an indwelling arterial line.

It has been pointed out by Harken and Smith (1973) that peripheral arterial flow is affected by vasoconstriction, so that, in the very ill patient, the peripheral blood pressure as measured by the Doppler detector may be substantially lower than the aortic pressure.

(iii) Respiration

Respiration rate may be monitored remotely by an airborne ultrasound Doppler system in which the patient's chest wall acts as a reflector (Stegall, 1967). The frequency is 25 kHz. The phase change of the received signal is directly proportional to the displacement of the thorax. A similar method, using a frequency of 40 kHz, has been described by Stegall et al. (1973) in connexion with infant apnoea monitoring.

The measurement of respiratory flow by transit-time Doppler instruments (see Section 7.1) has not achieved widespread acceptance. This is because the instrument at present commercially available is reported to have shortcomings which make its use impracticable (Blumenfeld et al., 1975). These problems include sensitivity to condensation, baseline drift, and mechanical weakness. In principle, it is possible to overcome these difficulties by mounting the transducers so that the ultrasonic beams are coaxial with the gas flow, and by improvements in circuitry.

7.3.c Gastroenterology

Side-to-side portacaval shunt is a surgical procedure sometimes carried out to relieve portal pressure. There is no general agreement concerning the haemodynamic changes which result from this procedure. Loisance et al. (1973) have used periarterial transducers operating with pulsed Dopplers to study flow in the hepatic artery and the portal vein in dogs, before and after the decompressive procedure.

Another interesting possibility is that of the transcutaneous measurement of flow in the portal vein. This vessel can be visualized by a two-dimensional scanner, and thus it is possible to interrogate it with a pulsed Doppler system. Atkinson (1974) has attempted to do this, using an ultrasonic frequency of 2 MHz, and has achieved some success, particularly with an incoherent reference (see Section 7.2.f.i). (The same method has also been used to study flow in the vena cava.)

7.3.d Obstetrics

(i) Studies of the foetal heart

The use of the ultrasonic Doppler frequency shift method for the detection of the movement of the foetal heart seems to have been first reported by Callagan et al. (1964). Johnson et al. (1965), using a 5 MHz ultrasonic instrument designed for blood flow studies, noticed two types of foetal sound. One of these is biphasic, and is assumed to arise from within the foetal heart. The other is monophasic and is probably due to blood flow:

foetal and maternal blood flow signals can be distinguished by their different cardiac rates.

Nowadays, 2 MHz systems, some with specially designed transducers, are almost always used in obstetrics. The movements of the foetal heart can often be detected at 9–10 weeks gestation, and almost always after 12 weeks (Bishop, 1966). The method is valuable in the diagnosis of intrauterine foetal death throughout the last six months of pregnancy, particularly in obese patients and in those with hydramnios where the foetal stethoscope is often unsatisfactory. It is also useful in the detection of multiple pregnancies, but care must be taken to avoid counting the same foetus twice.

In the perinatal period, the normal foetal heart rate is in the range 120–160 min^{-1}, there is no change in rate during uterine contractions, and there is a beat-to-beat variability $\geqslant 5$ min^{-1}. Unfavourable patterns include bradycardia without beat-to-beat variations, or with decelerations during contractions (this is usually due to foetal asphyxia), and tachycardia with decelerations during contractions. On the other hand, accelerations at the beginning of contractions are a good sign. Loss of beat-to-beat variations alone is not worrying (it may be due to maternal drugs). Further details of the relationships between foetal status and foetal heart rate have been discussed amongst others by Hon (1962), Baskett and Ko (1974), Tushuizen et al. (1974), Thomas and Blackwell (1975), and Liu et al. (1975). Beard et al. (1971) have correlated foetal heart rate with foetal pH.

The method is so simple to use that many obstetricians routinely monitor all deliveries for unsuspected foetal distress. Fully engineered instruments* are commercially available for the purpose, and comprehensive monitoring systems have been described in the literature (see, for example, Thomas et al., 1973).

Organ et al. (1973a) have shown that a signal corresponding to the opening of the foetal aortic valve (or pulmonary valve, which moves synchronously) can be identified in the filtered Doppler signals in more than three out of four patients examined during labour. In these individuals, it is possible to measure the pre-ejection period as the interval between the beginning of the QRS complex of the foetal e.c.g. (obtained using a scalp electrode), and the occurrence of the Doppler aortic valve signal. Studies on the foetal lamb have shown the pre-ejection period decreases with increasing myocardial contractility and hypoxaemic stress (Organ et al., 1973b), and assuming this also to be the case in the human foetus, the measurement might give a useful index of foetal status. Murata and Martin (1974) have extended these studies to measure the foetal ventricular ejection time, which is the interval between aortic valve opening and closing: the latter can be identified by a Doppler signal, and by the P wave of the

---

* For example, type FM3: Sonicaid Ltd., Bognor Regis, Sussex, UK.

e.c.g. The ventricular ejection time is related to the stroke volume, and varies inversely with heart rate and aortic blood pressure. More recently, Cousin *et al.* (1974) have developed an instrument automatically to obtain a continuous recording of the foetal pre-ejection period. No doubt this method of foetal monitoring will be further improved and achieve wider acceptance.

The umbilical vein can often be seen in two-dimensional scans of the foetal abdomen. It might be possible to obtain an index of foetal cardiac output by a pulsed Doppler system sampling the corresponding flow velocity. Another possibility of interest to obstetricians is that of monitoring flow in the uterine artery, by means of a Doppler probe positioned in the fornix.

(ii) Blood flow in the placenta

With experience and self-confidence, it may be possible to identify Doppler signals arising from blood flow in the placenta, using a transcutaneous approach. These signals are a mixture due to movements at the foetal heart rate, modulated by movements at the maternal heart rate. Naturally, some investigators have tried to map out the position of the placenta by examining the abdomen with a Doppler probe. During the last few weeks of pregnancy, an accuracy of about 75% was claimed in an early series (Bishop, 1966). Others have claimed higher accuracies. Thus, Hunt (1969) made one error in localizing the uterine segment containing the placenta in a series of 56 patients with "definite" confirmation of placental site; Cooper *et al.* (1969) achieved an accuracy of more than 90%, and Nelson and Parkes (1974) were correct in nearly 80% of their predictions. These results should be considered in the context of the practical clinical situation, however, and when this is done the conclusion must be reached that the test is not useful.

(iii) Foetal breathing

The potential value of foetal breathing monitoring in patient care is discussed in Section 6.16.f.vii. Progress in exploiting this index of foetal wellbeing is held back by the lack of convenient instrumentation. The Doppler method is basically better suited than pulse–echo techniques for detecting target movement. It may prove to be possible to devise a Doppler system which could separate the signals from the foetal thoracic walls (the breathing signals) from those originating in the foetal heart and as a result of maternal pulse and respiration. Hopefully such an instrument, which might use pulsed Doppler or phase-lock-loop techniques, would be both reliable and simple to use.

7.3.e Otorhinolaryngology

A continuous-wave 6 MHz Doppler system has been used by Minifie *et al.* (1968) to measure vocal fold motion during voice production. The probe is placed on the side of the neck immediately anterior to the oblique line of the thyroid cartilage at the level of the vocal cords. This non-intrusive method gives results which are in good agreement with those obtained by high-speed ciné films.

7.3.f Psychiatry

The level of activity of an individual may reflect his psychiatric status. Hyperactivity is certainly considered to be abnormal, but methods of quantitating this aspect of behaviour lack precision, both in definition and mensuration. Various techniques, reviewed by Johnson (1972), have been proposed and used. The use of ultrasound in this application, first suggested by Peacock and Williams (1962), depends upon the disturbance of a steady-state ultrasonic field by the movement of some structure within the field. This disturbance may be detected by the amplitude modulation of the signal received by a second transducer somewhere in the monitored room. A counter is arranged to record the number of such movements which occur over a chosen interval of time, and which exceed some threshold either in amplitude or in frequency, or both.

A description of an instrument designed to operate at a frequency of 40 kHz has been given by Haines (1974).

7.3.g Urology

The continuous wave Doppler method provides a rapid and reliable indication of the patency of the vascular supply to a transplanted kidney (Marchioro *et al.*, 1969; Sampson, 1969). The ultrasonic probe is positioned on the posterior abdominal wall, directly over the kidney. Doppler-shifted signals may be detected by aiming the probe medially so that the ultrasonic beam passes through the renal artery. Diminished flow velocity in an individual patient may warn that rejection is imminent. Experiments with dogs (Sampson *et al.*, 1972) have confirmed that transplantation is followed initially by an increased flow, but the flow progressively falls until the animal dies of rejection.

A combination of milk and sodium bicarbonate tablets taken orally several hours prior to voiding increases the urine pH and produces phosphate crystals in low, but adequate, density to provide scattered signals. The crystal diameter is around 10 μm. This useful effect, described by Albright *et al.* (1969), has been exploited by Albright and Harris (1975) in the measurement of average urine velocity, and the detection of turbulence and strictures, in the urethra in man. Since the urine flow volume can be measured directly, it is possible to calculate the urethral diameter.

Pedersen *et al.* (1975) have described the detection of torsion of the testis by means of a continuous-wave Doppler instrument designed for blood-flow studies. In this condition, the blood supply to the testis is impaired, and an abnormal sound spectrum is obtained with the probe positioned on the scrotum.

8. OTHER DIAGNOSTIC METHODS

8.1 TRANSMISSION METHODS

8.1.a Attenuation Methods

(i) Early work

The first attempts to use ultrasound for medical diagnosis were based on the expectation that it would be possible to demonstrate tissue masses by differential attenuation. Thus, the method is analogous to that used in conventional radiology. In radiology, the whole of the transmitted beam can be recorded by the exposure of a photographic plate. No comparable detector exists for ultrasound (with the possible exception of the enzyme system mentioned in Section 3.7.j). Therefore scanning is usually necessary with ultrasound to visualize the transmission characteristics of many separate tissue elements in order to produce a two-dimensional image.

The early investigators hoped in particular that the method might be used to visualize abnormalities of the brain. Before the development of scintigraphy and computerized tomography, the demonstration of such abnormalities by radiology was usually only possible by deductions based on procedures involving the injection of contrast media.

Dussik *et al.* (1947) constructed an ultrasonic scanner, based on an original suggestion of K. T. Dussik, in which a beam of ultrasound was directed through the patient's head, and detected by a receiver placed in line with the transmitter. This instrument produced a recording in the form of a plan in which the degree of blackening was related to the corresponding received intensity. The patterns thus recorded seemed to represent intracerebral structures, particularly the ventricles. Encouraged by these results, Ballantine *et al.* (1950) constructed a similar scanner, which was subsequently described in detail by Hueter and Bolt (1951). It operated at a frequency of 2·5 MHz, with a transmitted intensity of about 1 W cm^{-2}. In head scanning, the attenuation amounts to about 70 dB in the thicker parts of the skull, and to 40 dB in the brain. The receiver bandwidth was quite narrow, so that the equivalent input noise was only about 2 μV. Hueter and Bolt (1951) concluded that "a preliminary evaluation indicates that the echo-reflection method is considerably less promising" (than the transmission method) "for general ventriculography, mainly because of the small amount of reflection at the interface between the tissue and the ventricular fluid". It was not long before this rash statement was refuted! Thus, Güttner *et al.* (1952) pointed out that the attenuation due to the ventricles is small compared with that of the brain and the skull, and that the skull distorts the ultrasonic scan. Variation in the characteristics of skull and brain mask the changes due to the ventricles, and it is merely fortuitous that the skull happens to have a transmission pattern which resembles the shape and position of the ventricles. Ballantine *et al.* (1954) reached a similar conclusion, and the method was never developed for clinical application.

This early disappointment has held back progress in transmission methods of ultrasonic diagnosis. Less ambitious projects, not involving scanning, have produced interesting results. Thus, Crawford *et al.* (1959) reported a correlation between the attenuation of continuous wave 1 MHz ultrasound through the thorax in man, and the movement of intrathoracic structures. Horn and Robinson (1965) have proposed a method for the assessment of fracture union in bone, in which both longitudinal and transverse waves were transmitted simultaneously. Using a brass bar, they demonstrated that the shear waves are attenuated if a fracture is present, whereas the longitudinal waves are substantially unaffected. (According to Kossoff (1975) the method fails in clinical practice because of multiple path propagation in the soft tissues surrounding the bone.) Kossoff and Sharpe (1966) have detected the presence of gas within the pulp chamber of the tooth in degenerative pulpitis by an increase in the attenuation of 14–18 MHz ultrasound; the technique is simpler to use than the pulse–echo method, particularly as it is not affected by the inclined surfaces which occur in the pulp chamber. Again, Hamlet and Reid (1972) have reported how the transmission of 3·2 MHz through the larynx is modified by glottal closure, vocal-fold thickness, vocal-fold vibratory pattern, and thyroid cartilage ossification.

(ii) Frequency spectral modification

The measurement of attenuation over a range of frequencies, from observations of the changing amplitude of a pulse propagated through tissue, is discussed in Section 4.3.a. Holasek *et al.* (1973) have suggested that tissues might be identified by unique attenuation/frequency characteristics, and that these could be obtained quickly and automatically from pulse transmission data.

(iii) Image converters

The ultrasonic image converter (see Section 3.7.k) can be used either as a detector of backscattered ultrasound, or to form a two-dimensional attenuation map by detecting transmitted ultrasound. (This latter method is analogous to the use of the fluoroscopic image converter in radiology.)

A large source-to-specimen distance is necessary to avoid the inhomogeneity of the ultrasonic field in the near zone. The specimen is placed as close as possible to the image converter to obtain the best resolution and the least degradation from scattering, refraction, and diffraction. Alternatively, a lens can be used to focus the image on the transducer (Smyth *et al.*, 1963). Jacobs (1967) has pointed out, however, that a lens system involves oblique incidence on the transducer, and that optimal resolution is only obtained at normal incidence. In this connexion, according to Jacobs (1965), the smallest resolvable detail with normal incidence is a cylindrical volume whose length and diameter are both equal to the thickness of the transducer.

Although the ultrasonic image converter was originally expected to have a number of applications in biomedicine, none has yet achieved widespread acceptance. Multiple reflexions and standing waves occur both in the

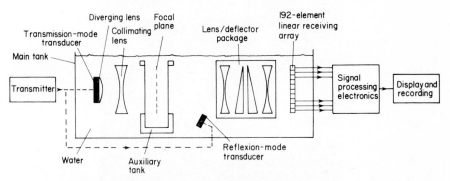

FIG. 8.1 Simplified block diagram of real-time ultrasonic camera using mechanically scanned linear array. (After Suarez *et al.*, 1975.)

specimen and in the water used for coupling, and these give rise to artifacts which spoil the image. To some extent these difficulties are reduced in real-time studies of moving structures; but this cannot be illustrated in a book.

(iv) Scanned arrays

In order to obtain real-time through-transmission images in two dimensions, Green *et al.* (1974) have developed an ultrasonic scanner in which a linear array of 192 elements is scanned mechanically in a direction normal to the long axis of the array. The basic principles of the instrument are illustrated in Fig. 8.1. (The instrument can also operate in the reflexion mode.) An ultrasonic pulse of 6 μs duration, centred at a frequency of 2 MHz, is propagated through the water and scattered and attenuated by the object to be visualized in the focal plane. The transmitted ultrasound is collected and focused by a pair of polystyrene lenses on to the piezoelectric receiving array. Each pulse results in one line of the image. Two-dimensional imaging is achieved by counter-rotation of the two polystyrene prisms in the lens deflector package, thus sweeping the ultrasonic field across the array. The resultant image consists of approximately 400 interlaced lines, each containing 192 picture elements. The frame rate is 15 s^{-1}, and the object size is 150 mm square. Synchronization of all the pulse, gating and deflexion waveforms is based on signals sent from prism position sensors. The detection sensitivity is about 10^{-11} W cm^{-2}. A typical scan is shown in Fig. 8.2.

The use of a pulsed system eliminates problems due to multiple reflexions in the water tank, but those within the specimen (or patient) may remain. Moreover, in common with other transmission methods, the

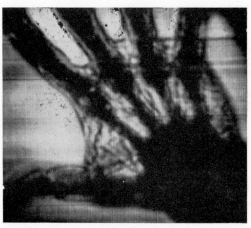

FIG. 8.2 Transmission image of living human hand, made using the ultrasonic camera illustrated in Fig. 8.1. (Courtesy P. S. Green.)

information may be degraded by gas or bone in the propagation path. Experimental results *in vitro* (Marich *et al.*, 1975) have been encouraging, however, and detailed images of excised organs such as liver, kidney, spleen and uterus reveal good detail. Image degradation due to diffraction and refraction effects are less troublesome with real-time display, than appears to be the case from still photographs. Preliminary *in vivo* results have been described by Zatz *et al.* (1975), using an immersion technique. The prototype clinical instrument (Zatz, 1975) is designed to examine the abdomen, to which ultrasonic coupling is made anteriorly and posteriorly through flexible membranes. Different planes within the patient can be imaged by changing the position of the focal plane. Perhaps the fairest way to summarize the conclusions of this work is to quote from one of these articles: "Degradation of information content due to complex surrounding tissues continues to be a problem. While *in vitro* studies have provided potentially useful images, this potential has not been achieved *in vivo* because of diffraction and refraction effects which degrade the images and produce spurious shadows in areas which should be clear. It is essential that further research be done on this problem if real-time transmission ultrasonic instruments are to find their way into clinical practice."

Two-dimensional arrays with fully electronic scanning are likely to have no inherent advantages in relation to the mechanically scanned one-dimensional linear array. (Nor, for that matter, are image converters, which are in principle two dimensional arrays with electronic scanning and the additional disadvantage of lateral coupling particularly with oblique incidence.) The arrays described in Section 6.10.c. for pulse–echo applications may generally be operated as receivers in transmission imaging ar-

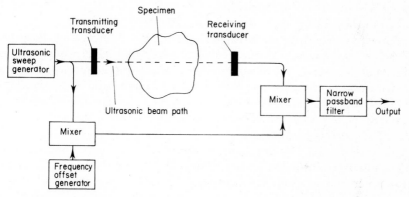

FIG. 8.3 Block diagram of time delay spectrometer. (Based on Heyser and le Croissette, 1974.)

rangements. One system which seems to have been developed specifically for use as an ultrasonic image converter is that of Harrold (1969).

(v) *Time delay spectrometry*

This technique, developed by Heyser and le Croissette (1974), involves the transmission of an ultrasonic beam, modulated with a linear frequency sweep, through the specimen under investigation. The elements of the system are illustrated in Fig. 8.3. The received signal is reduced in amplitude and delayed in time by transmission through the specimen. The first signal to be received is normally that which has travelled along the direct path (line-of-sight) from the transmitting to the receiving transducer. Since the transmitted frequency is a linear function of time, the difference between the transmitted and received frequencies is constant for a given transit time. The output of the frequency offset generator is mixed with the transmitted signal to give a sweep shifted by an amount corresponding to this transit time, and when this signal is itself mixed with the output of the receiving transducer, a constant frequency signal results which corresponds to the ultrasound which travelled along the direct path. This signal is separated from other signals by means of the narrow passband filter.

The transmitted signal has a frequency spectrum in which each frequency component is time-coded. Upon emergence from the specimen, the frequency components with a given time delay are reassembled to yield the frequency spectrum. This is the time delayed spectrum by which the process is named.

Some of the difficulties experienced with other continuous-wave transmission imaging systems arise because they have no means to reject late-arriving signals (see Section 8.1.a.i). In principle, time delay spectrometry offers a method to overcome this difficulty, and by incorporation in a suitable scanner it gives a shadowgraph picture which can be related to losses in the direct path, without ambiguity.

An experimental system has been used to make transmission images of biological specimens. A linear frequency sweep of 1 MHz was used, over the range 2–3 MHz. Two distinct types of image can be formed. The first is a conventional shadowgraph in which the brightness of the display is related to the corresponding transmission loss through the specimen. A second type of image, showing transmission time through the specimen, is described in Section 8.1.b.ii.

Time delay spectrometry, being a transmission technique, requires only a low ultrasonic intensity. Unfortunately, however, the range of anatomical sites potentially available for this type of investigation is very restricted.

(vi) Computed tomography

Since Bracewell and Roberts (1954) obtained three-dimensional information in radioastronomy from two-dimensional projections, the technique of algebraic reconstruction has been used to solve several imaging problems. In medicine, the technique forms the basis of computerized axial tomography (Hounsfield, 1973), which has revolutionized neuroradiology, and which is being extended to the investigation of other parts of the body.

The theory of image reconstruction in computed tomography has been reviewed by Brooks and DiChiro (1975). The algebraic reconstruction technique was used in the first successful X-ray CT-scanner.* The basis of this method is illustrated in Fig. 8.4. Better reconstruction methods have since been developed, and the filtered back-projection technique is presently *de rigueur*.

---

* EMI Medical Ltd., Hayes, Middlesex, UK. CT-scanners presently manufactured by this company use more advanced reconstruction algorithms.

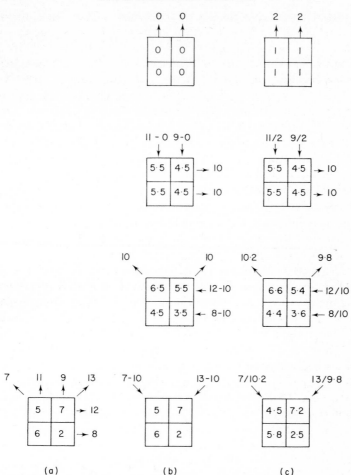

(a)   (b)   (c)

FIG. 8.4 Numerical example of algebraic reconstruction technique (ART). (a) Original object consisting of four elements of differing attenuation: the total attenuations measured along six separate ray-paths are indicated; (b) reconstruction by additive iterative correction. The upper box shows the starting values (0). A correction is first applied for the two vertical rays by subtracting the calculated values (0 and 0) from the measured values (11 and 9) and distributing the difference between the two cells that make up each ray (second box). This process is repeated for the two horizontal rays (third box) and diagonal rays (fourth box), thus completing one iteration. In this simple example, the reconstruction is perfect after one iteration; (c) reconstruction by multiplicative iterative correction. The starting values (1) shown in the upper box are multiplied by the ratio of the measured vertical ray sums (11 and 9) to the calculated values (2 and 2). This procedure is repeated for the horizontal and diagonal rays. In this example, errors persist and further iterations are required. (After Brooks and DiChiro, 1975.)

In principle, analogous images should be obtainable using ultrasound. Greenleaf *et al.* (1974) have described an experiment designed to test this possibility. They scanned a phantom, and an excised dog heart, by means of two transducers, separated by a distance of 150 mm, operating with pulses at a frequency of about 5 MHz, and bandwidth 2 MHz. At each angular position of the transducers, 200 equispaced lines were interrogated over a distance of 150 mm. The amplitude of each received pulse was digitized and stored, together with positional data, in a CDC 3500 computer. The specimen was thus scanned in 35 discrete steps of angle through a total of approximately 180°. This procedure resulted in 7000 data values, from which simultaneous equations were set up and solved by the computer to generate a matrix of 64×64 picture elements representing the attenuation distribution within the specimen. The solution of these equations was accomplished by an algebraic reconstruction technique developed by Herman and Rowland (1971). The algorithm required 2·5–3·5 min to reconstruct an image plane.

The images thus obtained were interesting, but not excellent. It appeared that degradation by refraction was significant. Greenleaf *et al.* (1975) have pointed out that this invalidates the assumption that the line integrals through the three-dimensional functions, which represent the points on the two-dimensional function, or shadow, are on straight lines. They are not. It may be that the difficulty could be reduced by using more highly focused beams, or possibly swept focusing (see Section 6.10.c.iii), and by reducing the spacing between the transducers. Alternative reconstruction algorithms might also result in improvements. Meanwhile, however, Greenleaf *et al.* (1975) seem to be concentrating on time-of-flight profiles (see Section 8.1.b.iii).

(vii) Transmission oscillator ultrasonic spectrometry

Although both gaseous and solid microemboli may be detected by pulse–echo (see Section 6.16.a.iii) and Doppler (Section 7.3.a.vi) methods, these and other techniques have failed to quantify the number and size of the particles. Clark *et al.* (1974) have developed an on-line, continuous, non-invasive method which does do this, by the use of a transmission oscillator ultrasonic spectrometer. The blood is arranged to flow between two 10 MHz transducers, positioned face-to-face in a resonant chamber. A standing wave is established in the blood. The presence of any inhomogeneity in this field produces a small increase in attenuation, the effect of which is multiplied by a sensitivity enhancement factor due to resonance. The analogue electronics portion of the monitor consists of a gain-stabilized amplifier that is made to oscillate by providing it with a feedback path through the ultrasonic resonator. Extremely high sensitivity to small changes in attenuation is achieved by operating the system on the verge of dropping out of oscillation. According to Dietz *et al.* (1974), the output from this circuit consists of pulses of which the amplitudes are proportional to the cross-sectional areas of the microemboli, and the durations, to the transit times through the resonator.

The instrument has been used to manage prolonged cardiopulmonary bypass surgery, by providing an indication of the development of microemboli, and of their reduction by the administration of anticoagulants. It also makes it possible to compare the performances of oxygenators, pumps, and filters.

(viii) Noise modulation

Multiple reflexion artifacts are likely to degrade transmission images. Such signals are troublesome because of their inherent ambiguity. It has been suggested by Fry and Jethwa (1975) that this particular problem could be avoided by the use of incoherent Gaussian noise modulation.

8.1.b Transit Time Measurements

(i) Dimensional measurements

Rushmer *et al.* (1956) used an early version of their transit time flowmeter (see Section 7.1) to measure the left ventricular size of the heart. Two transducers, one for transmitting and the other for receiving, are sutured one on each side of the ventricle in an experimental animal. The transit time is measured by a time-to-voltage analogue converter somewhat similar to that described in Section 6.9. The pulse repetition rate is between 1000–2500 s^{-1}, so that the time-resolution is very good. Horwitz *et al.* (1968) refined the method by implanting the transducers on the inside of the ventricle, thus making it possible to measure the ventricular cavity diameter. In this connexion, the implantation of transducers in the ventricular endocardium by a simple and relatively atraumatic approach through the left atrium has been described by Stinson *et al.* (1974).

The method is chiefly useful in experimental studies of cardiac physiology in animals. Thus, for example, Suga and Sagawa (1974) have found, in excised dog heart, that the left-ventricular volume V is given by

$$V \simeq 1 \cdot 2 D^3 \qquad (8.1)$$

where D is the ultrasonically measured ventricular diameter, and that the standard deviation of the method is around 8%. Another useful measurement of cardiac function is given by the rate-of-change of chamber diameter, which is related to the myocardial contractility.

Continuous measurement of left ventricular wall thickness has been achieved by Guntheroth (1974), using transducers attached on the endocardium and the epicardium in dogs. This dimension was found to increase by 9% during ejection, and to decrease by 2% during isovolumic systole.

The velocity of the changing separation of the transit-time-measuring transducers may be obtained by differentiating the instantaneous value of the displacement signal. (In principle, it might be better to obtain this information in terms of the Doppler shift signal: see Section 7.1.)

An ingenious method which in principle makes it possible to measure left ventricular diameter in man by the transit-time technique has been described by Kardon *et al.* (1971). They have constructed a catheter with one transducer at the tip, and another, approximately 80 mm behind the tip. This is introduced via the mitral valve, the aorta and the femoral artery, so that it curves around the apex of the left ventricle. In this way, the two transducers come to face each other across the ventricular cavity. Another method, potentially applicable in man, is the use of a pair of transducers mounted on wires which spring apart to bring them into contact with the opposite walls of a blood vessel into which they have been introduced at the tip of a catheter (Stegall, 1974).

Using three transducers positioned on relatively stationary parts of the maternal abdomen, and operated in sequence as pulse transmitters, and one transducer attached to the foetal presenting part, acting as receiver, Wolfson and Neuman (1973) have measured the rate of foetal descent during labour, by triangulation calculation.

Another application of transit time measurements in obstetrics has been described by Zador *et al.* (1974). They have devised small ($1 \times 1 \times 5$ mm) transducers which may be clipped to diametrically opposite parts of the cervical lips during labour. The degree of dilation of the cervix may thus be measured, provided that the direct path between the transducers remains occupied by foetal parts. Apparently the transducers neither interfere with clinical management, nor do they change the mechanical properties of the cervix.

Mullins and Guntheroth (1966) have developed a method for measuring changes in mesenteric blood volume. A small sample of intact mesentery is inserted between two transducers held by a rigid frame so that their axes are in line, the ultrasonic beam passing through the sample. Mesentery consists mainly of fat, blood vessels and blood; the fat is forced in and out of the frame by changes in the blood volume. The ultrasonic velocity in blood is about 8% greater than that in fat (see Fig. 4.6(b)), and so changes in the proportion of blood in the sample can be estimated from changes in the transit time between the two transducers. The resolution using pulses of 3 MHz nominal frequency across a transducer spacing distance of 15 mm allows changes of 0·2% in blood volume to be detected.

A transmission technique which involves scanning has been described by Rich *et al.* (1966). Differences in transit time are assumed to be related to bone mass, when scanning across a limb. The transit times of 3 MHz pulses are measured by means of a time-to-voltage analogue converter. The transmitting and receiving transducers are mounted in line so that they can be scanned together across the specimen. A recorder is coupled to the position of the transducer assembly, so that the results are presented in the form of a graph showing the variation in transit time with position. The results of preliminary experiments on samples of cortical bone and rabbit humerus (either in an intact limb or stripped of soft tissues) showed good agreement between the predicted mass of calcium and that subsequently determined chemically.

The method of deriving the trigger pulse for the "stop" logic of the time-to-voltage analogue converter is usually to amplify the output of the receiving transducer, and to feed this through a threshold detector. In poor signal-to-noise conditions this is not satisfactory, however, since there may be a danger of triggering from noise if the sensitivity is sufficiently high to respond to the weakest signals. Thus, according to Häusler and Klauck (1970), there may be a variation of 80 dB in the signal level received across the ventricular cavity in a cardiac cycle, due primarily to variation in angulation of the transducers, even when small transducers are used. Although convex plastic lenses do reduce this problem by increasing the beamwidth, it has been shown by McGough *et al.* (1973) that a better solution may be to use an extremely short exciting pulse for the transmitter. Another solution is to use a tracking gate, which is relatively insensitive to amplitude variations (Stinson *et al.*, 1974). A block diagram of the arrangement is illustrated in Fig. 8.5. The Colpitts oscillator is pulsed by the astable multivibrator to excite the transmitting transducer to emit 1 μs bursts of 8 MHz ultrasound at a repetition rate of 5600 s^{-1}. The signal fed to the preamplifier contains a capacitively coupled component which occurs simultaneously with the pulsed output of the oscillator (this does not affect the operation of the circuit), and an acoustically coupled component delayed by the propagation transit time between the two transducers. The tracking gate is a second order closed loop system which locks on to the arithmetic mean of the acoustically coupled component of the received signal. Because of the memory characteristics of the low pass filter and integrator in the feedback loop, the tracking gate tends to follow the signal even in low signal-to-noise situations, such as occur periodically during the cardiac cycle. When the gate generator is triggered, it produces two 2 μs gate pulses, one immediately following the other. The time position of this event is determined by comparison of the output of the integrator and the sawtooth output of the ramp generator which is reset each time that a pulse is transmitted. During the first of the two gate pulses, the received ultrasonic signal is rectified and amplified by the tracker in the negative direction; during the second, the signal is amplified in the positive direction.

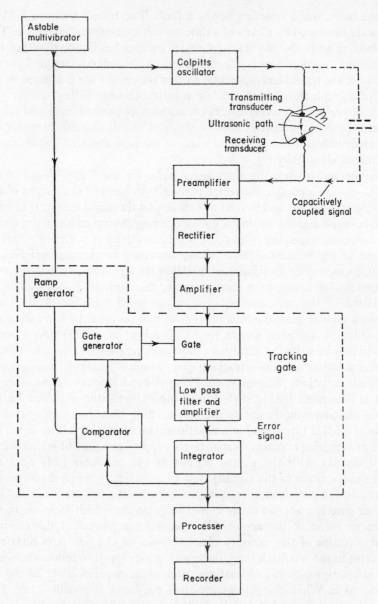

FIG. 8.5 Transit time measurement by means of a tracking gate. (Based on Stinson *et al.*, 1974.)

At all other times the input is grounded. Therefore, if the gates are centred on the acoustically coupled signal, the positive and negative components cancel each other, and the error signal is zero for any constant separation of the transmitting and receiving signals. Similarly, there is a constant error signal for constant velocity of transducer separation.

An alternative to time–domain displacement measurement is frequency–domain measurement using frequency modulation to code the transmitted signal. This method is discussed in Section 7.2.f.ii.

(ii) Time delay spectrometry

This technique is discussed in relation to attenuation measurements in Section 8.1.a.v. It has been shown by Heyser and le Croissette (1974) that images may also be formed by a phase comparison technique in which successive dark bands on the display correspond to phase changes of 180° over the complete frequency sweep. This type of display has no analogue in contemporary medical imaging methods using either ionising or ultrasonic radiation.

(iii) Computed tomography

The rather disappointing results which have so far been obtained in attempts to use the algebraic reconstruction technique to image the ultrasonic attenuation distributions of biological structures are discussed in Section 8.1.a.vi. At the present time, it seems that computed tomographic images of velocity distributions are more promising. Thus, Greenleaf et al. (1975) have described the production of pictures with a matrix of 64 × 64 elements, from transit time measurements of 10 MHz pulses, basically using the system previously described for attenuation mapping. Whether this approach will prove to have any diagnostic application in clinical practice remains to be seen, but its potential advantages are that it eliminates the requirement for swept gain, its inherently better signal-to-noise performance in relation to pulse–echo methods, and the absolute nature of the measured quantity. Practical disadvantages will doubtless be due to problems with transmission through gas and bone, and the consequently rather limited range of anatomically suitable structures, and to difficulties in acoustic coupling.

8.1.c Microscopy

The idea of an acoustic microscope is not new: according to Kessler (1974), in his review of the subject, it was first proposed in 1936 by S. Y. Sokolov. Sokolov's suggestion (Devey, 1953) was that an ultrasonic image converter might operate at such a high frequency that its resolution would be high enough to reveal microscopical detail. Thus, Jacobs (1967) has discussed the factors which would affect the performance of an image converter (see Section 3.7.k) operating at a frequency of 3 GHz. New transducers would be required, and formidable problems would need to be solved, before such a converter could be constructed. A resolution of around 50 mm^{-1} was predicted for a system in which the specimen was in contact with the transducer. Such a system has not yet been realized, and the first practical ultrasonic microscope for biomedical applications seems to have been constructed by Dunn and Fry (1959). In this instrument, the differential attenuation of a complex specimen is scanned by a small thermocouple. A structure with a diameter of 25 μm can thus be recorded using 0·1 s duration pulses at a frequency of 12 MHz, with a thermocouple of about 13 μm diameter. It was concluded from these results that it should be possible to detect a structure with a diameter of less than 1 μm (i.e. resolution > 1000 mm^{-1}) by the use of 1 μs pulses of 1 GHz ultrasound at an intensity of 1 kW cm^{-2}, with a thermocouple of 0·1 μm diameter and a pulse repetition rate of 1000 s^{-1}. Like the piezoelectric image converter, however, this approach has not been pursued.

At present, two different methods of acoustic microscopy seem to be receiving most attention. The first of these is somewhat similar to the original idea of using a piezoelectric image converter, but the image is detected by optical scanning of a reflecting surface distorted by the ultrasonic field to be visualized (Korpel *et al.*, 1971). The optical scanning is at a frame rate of 30 s^{-1}, and an ultrasonic frequency of 100 MHz allows details of 25 μm in size to be resolved. (More recent work, at 220 MHz, has apparently improved this performance to 10 μm: see Kessler (1964).) The instrument with which most of the published results have been obtained is illustrated in Fig. 8.6. At 100 MHz, the attenuation in tissue structures of around 25 μm size is insufficient to cause observable contrast, and it is primarily structures which differ significantly from their neighbours in characteristic impedance which are visualized.

At gigahertz frequencies, the contrast due to attenuation differences in microscopic structures is greatly enhanced in relation to that which exists at a few hundred megahertz. Moreover, the contribution of viscosity as an absorption mechanism becomes relatively important in relation to relaxation (see Sections 4.5 and 4.6). It is difficult to design an imaging system which could operate at these high frequencies, in which the specimen is uniformly irradiated whilst the scanning process is essentially one of sampling the transmitted (or scattered) ultrasonic field. The problem has been solved by Lemons and Quate (1974), by the ingenious expedient of scanning the specimen with a highly focused ultrasonic beam. Their first instrument operated with reflected ultrasound at a frequency of 600 MHz, and the diameter of the minimum resolvable element was 2 μm. The transducer was a zinc oxide film, and the lens, made from sapphire, had a diameter of 0·2 mm and an aperture of *f*0·75. More recently, Lemons and Quate (1975a) have constructed a transmission microscope operating at frequencies of up to around 1 GHz; this is illustrated in Fig. 8.7. Typical images of biological specimens have been presented by Lemons and Quate (1975b) and Kompfner (1975). These images confirm that unstained biological specimens can be visualized with good contrast. Materials such as

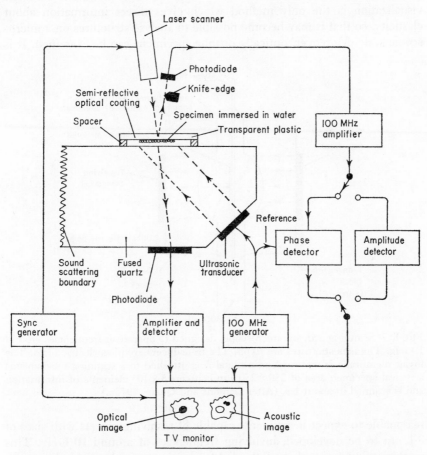

FIG. 8.6 Acoustic microscope based on optical detection of surface deformation. The instrument simultaneously produces acoustic and optical images of the specimen, which can be displayed separately (as shown here), or superimposed. The probing laser beam focused upon the semireflective coating of the plastic mirror becomes spatially modulated by the localized surface distortion produced by ultrasound transmitted through the specimen. A fraction of the light is transmitted through the mirror and the specimen to produce the optical image. In this diagram, the effects of refraction on the ray paths have been neglected. (Based on Korpel *et al.*, 1971; Kessler *et al.*, 1972.)

collagen and connective tissue have particularly marked attenuations. Consequently information can be obtained that otherwise is available with light microscopy only after time-consuming staining procedures. Moreover, the method is compatible with frozen sectioning techniques.

As acoustic microscopy develops to provide greater resolution and new kinds of display, new aspects of the structural organization of biological materials will become available for analysis for the first time. Acoustic visualization is the only method which gives direct information about elasticity, so that it may become possible to analyse structures on a microscopic scale. Moreover, optically opaque specimens can be examined. It is

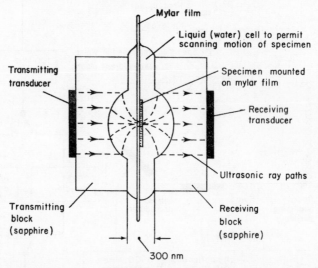

FIG. 8.7 Scanning acoustic microscope, designed to operate at frequencies around 1 GHz. The lens apertures are $f0.65$. The transducers are piezoelectric films. The mylar membrane is mounted on a metal ring attached to a scanning mechanism: a typical specimen area of 250×250 μm contains 5×10^4 elements of information and is scanned in about 1 s. (After Lemons and Quate, 1975a.)

reasonable to expect instruments capable of resolving objects with sizes of 0·1 μm to be developed, involving frequencies of around 10 GHz. This resolution surpasses that of the light microscope, and would allow very basic biological phenomena, such as cell differentiation and development, to be studied *in vivo*. The potential importance of all these possibilities cannot be overemphasized.

8.1.d Thermo-acoustic Sensing Technique

Sachs *et al.* (1972) have developed a technique for studying biological tissues which depends on the disturbance of the ultrasonic propagation characteristics of the tissues which occurs as a result of heating by a focused ultrasonic beam. The disturbance is sensed by a "thermometer beam" of pulsed ultrasound directed through the focal volume of the "heating beam", the two beams being effectively at right angles. The whole of the path of the thermometer beam is interrogated by a sampling process in which the heating beam is tracked across the tissues. One thermometer beam pulse precedes the heating pulses, another follows it. The difference in transit times between the two sense beam pulses is related to the vascular perfusion and the attenuation coefficient of the target tissue. Some aspects of these relationships have been discussed by Sachs (1973). The technique may have applications in tissue identification.

8.2 HOLOGRAPHY

Ultrasonic holography is a two-stage process in which the diffraction pattern of an object irradiated by ultrasound is biased by a coherent reference wave and recorded to generate an ultrasonic hologram. A three-dimensional image of the object is created when the ultrasonic hologram is illuminated by a coherent light source. Thus, the principles are the same as those of optical holography.

There are many different arrangements by which ultrasonic holograms may be obtained. Some are illustrated in Fig. 8.8. These various arrangements may be classified according to the type of detector which they employ. Detailed information may be obtained by consulting the following representative articles:

(i) *Liquid surface levitation* (see Section 3.7.e.v): Weiss and Holyoke (1969); Anderson and Curtin (1973); Holbrooke *et al.* (1973, 1974); Brendon (1974).

(ii) *Optical interferometry* (see Section 3.7.i.ii): Korpel and Desmares (1969); Gabor (1974); Metherell (1974); Metherell *et al.* (1974); Erikson *et al.* (1975a, b).

(iii) *Scanned hydrophone* (see Section 3.7.a.ii): Aldridge *et al.* (1971, 1974); Chivers (1974).

(iv) *Pohlman cell* (see Section 3.7.e.iv): Lafferty and Stephens (1971).

The occurrence of standing waves and multiple reflexions may make ultrasonic holography impossible with continuous waves (Halstead, 1968). It is for this reason that most systems use a pulsed transmitter and gated receiver. The ultrasonic pulse duration, and the timing and duration of the receiver gate, need to be chosen carefully so that the received signal contains complete information with respect to both phase and amplitude of the entire scattered field.

In optical holography, it is generally necessary for the addition of the scattered and reference signals to take place before the hologram is recorded.

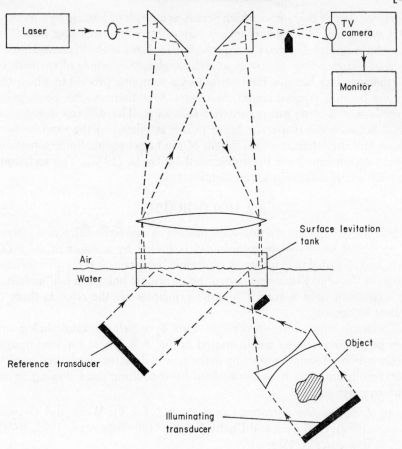

(a)

FIG. 8.8 Typical arrangements for ultrasonic holography. (a) Surface levitation detection arrangement. The reference field and the field carrying the diffraction pattern of the object are combined at the detector, which is illuminated by a parallel light beam, the reflected light being viewed through closed circuit television. The system may operate with ultrasonic pulses of 30–120 μs duration, repetition rate 60 s^{-1}, and maximum average intensity 20 mW cm^{-2}. (b) Linearized subfringe interferometric arrangement, sensitive to subfringe phase and amplitude changes. The reference signal is added optically. Acoustic hologram movies may be recorded at a frame rate of 16 s^{-1}, each frame being derived in 6 μs from a 100 μs burst of 1 MHz ultrasound, with an average intensity of around 10 mW cm^{-2}. (c) Scanned hydrophone arranged to generate a hologram by sampling. The reference signal is added electronically. One transmitted pulse is required for each position of the hydrophone; at a pulse repetition rate of 1000 s^{-1}, the scanning time would be 1000 s for 10^6 sampling points, with an average intensity of around 10 mW cm^{-2}. (Based on data given in papers listed in the text of Section 8.2, with modifications in the interests of intelligibility and simplicity.)

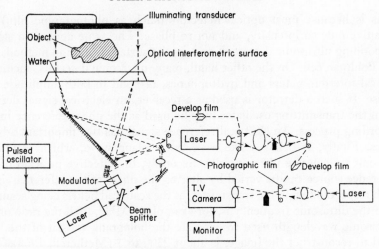

(b)

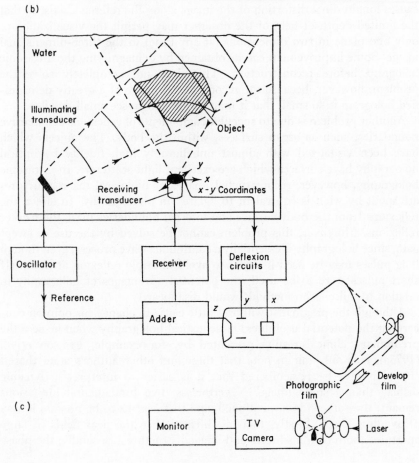

(c)

This is because most optical detectors (such as photographic film) are sensitive only to intensity, and not to phase. The same applies to slowly responding ultrasonic detectors, such as the surface levitation method, and the Pohlman cell. On the other hand, many ultrasonic detectors, including optical interferometers and hydrophones, respond to both amplitude and phase. If such a detector is used as a receiver, an electrical signal derived from the transmitting oscillator may be used as the phase reference in the recording process. An electrical reference signal has two important advantages. Firstly, it behaves like a perfectly plane wave, which would be difficult to generate ultrasonically. Secondly, the effective position of the reference source can be varied by altering the phase of the reference signal with respect to that of the transmitter, as the scattered field is being scanned.

If the ultrasonic frequency is, for example, 1 MHz, then the ratio of the ultrasonic wavelength used to generate the hologram, to that of the light used to reconstruct the image, is about 2300 to 1 (Metherell, 1968). This causes longitudinal distortion of the image along the reference axis, so that the limited depth-of-field of the observer may permit the visualization of only one plane in two dimensions (at any time) in the three-dimensional image. Some improvement can be obtained by demagnifying the ultrasonic hologram before reconstruction. This does not completely solve the problem, however, because the reconstructed image of a greatly demagnified hologram is so small that it may be difficult to see small details.

Another problem is due to specular components of reflexions at extensive boundaries, such as organ surfaces, within the body. The objects which have been visualized with almost unbelievably high fidelity by optical holography have surfaces which are excellent light scatterers. In ultrasonic holography, however, reconstructed images of biological macrostructures are spoilt by what is equivalent to "glare" in photography. In effect, the reflexions from the body surface and internal boundaries mask the weaker reflexions. Moreover, this problem cannot be solved by the use of swept gain, since holography is essentially a continuous wave process, even though long pulses may be used in order to avoid multiple reflexion artifacts. (If short pulses were to be used, the potential advantages of holography in relation to pulse–echo methods would disappear.)

Although the pragmatist will find little cause to change his opinion concerning the potential usefulness of acoustical holography when he sees the preliminary clinical results presented by, for example, Erikson *et al.* (1975a), it is only fair to note that these and other authors state that it should always be remembered that it is easier to interpret a dynamic display than a static image. Nevertheless, two fundamental limitations remain; they are seldom mentioned, and there seems to be no simple way of avoiding them. Firstly, there is diffraction in the near fields of large apertures, both of transducers and imaged structures. Secondly, the phase coherence is destroyed by variations in the velocities in different biological tissues. Therefore, new fundamental discoveries must be made if ultrasonic holography is to have a useful future in medical diagnostics: technology alone is not enough.

8.3 BRAGG IMAGING

Light interacts with the refractive index variations due to an ultrasonic wave travelling in a transparent medium, in a manner analogous to the interaction of X-rays with the lattice of a crystal in X-ray crystallography.

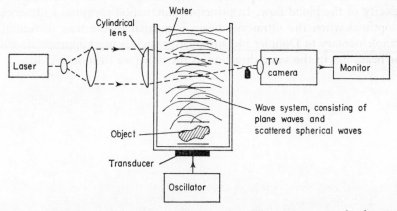

FIG. 8.9 Typical arrangement for Bragg imaging. The wave system in the water beyond the object acts as a three-dimensional diffraction grating. The illuminating light has a cylindrical wavefront, and the scattered light from each region of the ultrasonic field in which the Bragg condition is satisfied appears to emerge from a virtual line source displaced from the actual source, which is occluded. (Based on Landry et al., 1969.)

The phenomenon may be used as the basis of an imaging method. A typical arrangement is illustrated in Fig. 8.9. The method was proposed by Korpel (1966). It has real-time capability and is most suitable for imaging with ultrasound the wavelength of which is within one or two orders of magnitude of the interacting light. This is because this relationship corresponds to a convenient Bragg angle of a few degrees, for maximal light reflexion. Potentially the technique could be used to image biological materials (see, for example, Keyani et al., 1974), but it seems to offer no practical advantage in relation to more conventional methods. Moreover, the necessity to immerse the specimen and to operate at rather high frequencies are positive disadvantages.

8.4 FLUCTUATION MEASUREMENTS

Atkinson (1975) has described a method of measuring the flow velocity of liquid containing many scatterers, which does not depend on the Doppler effect. The flow velocity is related to the rate at which different distributions of scatterers move through the resolution cell. The size of the resolution cell is determined by the duration of the transmitted pulse, and the cross-section of the ultrasonic beam (which is arranged to be normal to the flow direction). The position of the resolution cell is determined by a time-gating circuit in the receiver. As the distributions of the scatterers in the resolution cell change, the reflected amplitude fluctuates. The rate at which these fluctuations occur depends, for a given size of resolution cell, on the velocity of the blood flow. In principle, fluctuation measurement, since it is optimal when the ultrasonic beam is normal to the flow direction, is complementary to Doppler measurement, which is most appropriate when the beam lies in the same direction as the flow (see Section 7.2.a).

9. BIOLOGICAL EFFECTS

9.1 EARLY INVESTIGATIONS

In 1927, Wood and Loomis described how filaments of *Spirogyra* were torn to pieces, and small fish and frogs were killed, during exposures of a few minutes to ultrasound at a frequency of 300 kHz, at an intensity which was probably about 10 W cm^{-2}. The following year, Harvey and Loomis (1928) reported how they had irradiated small organisms with ultrasound. Using a frequency of 406 kHz, they observed the effects by means of a microscope. They saw streaming within cells, and their eventual destruction, and they noticed a rise in temperature.

Schmitt *et al.* (1928) irradiated protozoa at a frequency of 750 kHz. Large specimens were killed, but small ones survived. It was suggested that the effect was due to denaturation of proteins, possibly by high pressure. Streaming of cell suspensions around a vibrating fine glass point was also observed, and protoplasmic changes took place when the point was inserted into a single cell. Schmitt (1929) extended this work, and observed protoplasmic rotation when a vibrating quartz needle was inserted into a cell in suspension in a liquid.

Johnson (1929) described the irradiation of protozoa and red blood cells, at frequencies between 0·75 and 1 MHz. He attached great importance to the formation during irradiation of minute bubbles of gas within the liquid, and he associated this with cell destruction. When this *cavitation* was eliminated, either by increasing the externally applied pressure, or by the use of a gas-free liquid, no destruction was observed (see Section 9.4).

In a review article, Harvey (1930) distinguished between two thermal effects. These are the heating of the medium due to the absorption of ultrasound, which may be eliminated by cooling, and local heating at interfaces in vibration, when thermal conduction is poor. Small crystals of ethyl stearate (melting point 30–31°C) did not show signs of surface melting when suspended in water and irradiated. Therefore he was quite certain that the biological effects which he observed with cells were not connected with local heating, if proper precautions were taken to reduce the average temperature of the liquid. (This conclusion is not incontrovertible, since the temperature reached by the ethyl stearate crystals may not be comparable with that reached by other systems irradiated under the same conditions, because of differences in characteristic impedance, absorption coefficient, and heat conduction.) He concluded that the mechanism of cell destruction by cavitation was due to the "rapid striking of cells by minute cavitated air bubbles, and violent commotion accompanying cavitation, rather than to the expansive bursting of the cell by gases cavitated within". He was unable to find any difference between irradiation at frequencies of 340 and 600 kHz.

The following year, Harvey and Loomis (1931) described a technique for the high-speed photomicrography of living cells subjected to ultrasonic irradiation. They demonstrated that the destruction of irradiated eggs of *Arbacia* took place in less than about 1 ms. During irradiation, the egg was drawn out into a spindle, which suggested that rapid tearing movements of the fluid might have been responsible for the destruction. No air bubbles could be seen in the photographs, but it was believed that the rapid movements of the fluid were the result of submicroscopic cavitation.

9.2 THERMAL EFFECTS

Ultrasound is attenuated as it passes through tissues. The absorption mechanisms are discussed in Chapter 4. The rate of absorption increases with frequency. At medium and high frequencies, it is often difficult to demonstrate non-thermal effects, since they may be masked by thermal effects, and for this reason a number of investigators believe that ultrasonic effects are due to heat alone. The matter has been summarized by Lele and Pierce (1972). Thus, Herrick (1953) irradiated various biological structures with ultrasound at a frequency of 800 kHz, and at powers of up to 5 W from a 5 cm^2 radiator. She demonstrated the selective heating of nerve and bone, and described the interruption of nervous conduction. Differential study of various fibres in frog sciatic nerve indicated that an analgesic application was unlikely to be successful, and she concluded that heat was responsible for the observed effects. A similar conclusion was reached by Lehmann (1953), but he also suggested that a decrease in the thickness of the diffusion layer at an interface resulting from mechanical stirring might be a possible mechanism for an increase in metabolite exchange rate.

Madsden and Gersten (1961) were unable to demonstrate any significant effect on the conduction velocity of the ulnar nerve in man after irradiation at 1 MHz, at intensities of up to about 2 W cm^{-2}, but their system was inaccurate, and measurements were made before and after, but not during, irradiation. Young and Henneman (1961) used a 2·7 MHz focusing equipment at an intensity of about 1·2 kW cm^{-2} to irradiate frog sciatic nerve. They were able to block the smaller fibres without affecting the larger fibres. Reversible and irreversible blocking of any fibre was possible by careful choice of irradiation conditions. A criticism of these experiments is that the irradiated nerve lay in a block of rubber, a situation shown by Lele (1963) to be accompanied by a considerable rise in temperature. Likewise Shealy and Henneman (1962) were able to produce reversible depression of the spinal reflexes in cat by irradiation with focused ultrasound, using the equipment of Young and Henneman (1961). In these experiments, however, the irradiated section of the nerve was in mineral oil, and so thermal effects must have been significant.

The irradiation system of Lele (1963) was designed to minimize the effects of heat and of standing waves. Using focused ultrasound at frequencies of 0·6, 0·9 and 2·7 MHz, he demonstrated enhancement, reversible and differential depression, followed by irreversible depression, of the action potential, during 450 experiments on peripheral nerves of cat, monkey and man, and the giant fibre of earthworm. He also recorded an increase in the conduction velocity of the action potential in irradiated nerve. These effects and the subsequently observed histological changes were considered to be thermal in origin, despite the precautions taken to minimize heat production during irradiation.

Hodgkin and Katz (1949) suggested that the disappearance of the nervous action potential at high temperatures is due to the rising phase of the impulse being overtaken by the permeability changes that lead to recovery. Wells (1966a) described an experiment in which the thermal origin of ultrasonically induced nerve block (at a frequency of 3 MHz) was demonstrated in the isolated giant axon of squid. Other experiments on the squid giant axon (Wells 1966b) have shown that, at 3 MHz, both the metabolic sodium pump and the conduction velocity are accelerated during irradiation, and that heat is an important, but not necessarily exclusive, factor which causes these effects.

Hughes et al. (1963) measured changes in frog muscle permeability after exposure to 1 MHz ultrasound at about 1 kW cm^{-2}. Immediately after irradiation, loss of potassium and gain of sodium were accelerated. Respiration was not significantly affected by irradiation, but other experiments indicated that the muscle might have become freely permeable to glucose. In intact muscle, there is a barrier to free glucose entry. No significant histological changes could be found in the treated muscle (which is rather remarkable). Temperature changes were not measured, but there is no doubt that thermal effects must have been important under the conditions of the experiment.

Using much lower intensities, of up to 34 W cm^{-2} at 3 MHz for 30 s, Carney et al. (1972) reported inhibitions in phosphate and sulphate uptakes, cell respiration and dehydrogenase activity, in guinea-pig ear skin. These effects were consistent with thermal damage to the skin cells, and this was supported by their histological appearances. More recently, Chapman (1974) showed that the effect of ultrasonic irradiation (1·8 MHz, up to 1·2 W cm^{-2}, up to 180 min exposure) on the potassium content of rat thymocytes *in vitro* was temperature-dependent.

Brain *et al.* (1960) irradiated the cat inner ear at a frequency of 1 MHz. They noticed a rise in temperature during irradiation, and, subsequently, various histological changes. McLay *et al.* (1961) irradiated the superior semicircular canal of guinea-pig, using a frequency of 1 MHz, at an intensity of about 1 W cm^{-2}, for period of between 15 and 30 min. Histological changes were seen after about four days, and the evidence of damage was more extensive in animals which were allowed to survive for longer times. They pointed out that one biological effect of ultrasound might have been a preliminary stimulation of endolymph production, followed by an atrophic change in the secretory epithelium and a consequently reduced amount of endolymph in the membranous labyrinth.

James *et al.* (1964) found an increase in endolymphatic sodium, and a decrease in endolymphatic potassium, in guinea-pig, following irradiation of the lateral semicircular canal for about 10 min at 3 MHz and at about 20 W cm^{-2}. In contrast, the sodium concentration falls and the potassium concentration rises in the perilymph after death. The rapid changes which were observed following irradiation could have been due to a failure of some secretory mechanism, or to a breakdown in the permeability barrier between endolymph and perilymph. In published discussion, Hughes (1965) considered that it is unlikely that a violent stirring of the solution would affect the permeability of cells, and suggested that the effect of ultrasound in causing a leakage of nucleotides may be similar to the effect of adding detergents which become bound to the membrane and appear to make it leaky. Another, more probable explanation, however, which might also account for the histological changes described by McLay *et al.* (1961) and Lundquist *et al.* (1971) in guinea-pig, and by James (1963) in sheep, is that the membranous canal which lies beneath the bone at the area of application of the ultrasound may be heated to a temperature of more than 50°C. This is because of the rapid attenuation of ultrasound in bone, which causes an increase in temperature which cannot be completely controlled by surface cooling: the matter is discussed in Section 10.4. It is probable that this temperature would irreversibly damage the membrane, whilst the neighbouring structures might remain unharmed. The resultant change in the ionic balance of the endolymph, due to the leakage through the membrane, might lead to the degeneration of the various structures which has been observed histologically. This possibility is compatible with the similarity between the effects of heat and ultrasonic irradiation on the semicircular canal of pigeon (Sjöberg *et al.*, 1963). In addition, Arslan and Sala (1965) and Drettner *et al.* (1967) were able to explain the ocular nystagmus observed during ultrasonic irradiation of the vestibular system on the basis of caloric response. Moreover, a thermal mechanism is not incompatible with the results of the experiments of Crysdale and Stahle (1972) on the guinea-pig cochlea: it seems reasonable to suppose that the preferential damage of the outer hair cells, in comparison with the inner hair cells, might be due to a greater sensitivity to an unfavourable environment. Likewise, the results of experiments on the irradiation of the vestibule of sheep using the round window approach (Barnett *et al.*, 1973) could have been due to heat.

As a substitute for lobotomy, Lindstrom (1954) employed prefrontal ultrasonic irradiation at a frequency of 1 MHz. A bone button was removed from over each prefrontal area, and ultrasound from a quartz disc (diameter 32 mm) was transmitted into the brain through a cone filled with circulating saline. In animals, intensities below 2 W cm^{-2} produced no damage, but 5–7 W cm^{-2} produced microscopic damage after 3–5 min of irradiation. The dura and the surface of the brain were not affected, but a volume of about 10 mm in diameter and 20 mm in length was damaged at a depth of about 10 mm. Such a distribution of damage might occur as the result of heat generated by the absorption of ultrasound in the brain, but with the brain surface kept cool.

Fry *et al.* (1957) concluded from histological examination of a series of irradiated cat brains that larger doses were needed to change irreversibly the grey matter than the white matter. Under specified conditions, the ratio was 2:1. It may be significant that grey matter has the lower absorption coefficient, and so would be heated less than white matter irradiated under the same conditions. They also concluded that ultrasonic irradiation is not followed by long-delayed effects similar to those which can be produced by ionizing radiation (see Section 9.11.e).

Basauri and Lele (1962) used focused ultrasound at a frequency of 2·7 MHz, and at an intensity of between 250 and 840 W cm^{-2}, to produce trackless lesions in the cat brain. In a series of experiments involving 654 animals, they found great reproducibility in the results. Lesions developed within 30 min after large doses, and the linear dimensions of the lesion were shown to be proportional to the logarithm of the irradiation time at any given intensity (see Section 9.11.a). The effects of multiple pulses were shown to sum in a manner inversely proportional to the interval between the pulses. The probability of producing a lesion was increased when the cranial circulation was temporarily arrested, presumably as a result of the absence of cooling by blood.

Using apparatus which was simpler and in some respects superior to those of Fry *et al.* (1957) and Basauri and Lele (1962), Warwick and Pond (1968) obtained results which were similar except for certain detailed histological differences. Their apparatus operated at a frequency of 3 MHz, which gives a satisfactory compromise between absorption and focal size in the brain of a small animal, and produced focal intensities of up to about

2·5 kW cm^{-2}. Self-focusing curved transducers were used, mainly operating at harmonics, with angles of convergence of about 50° (see Section 3.6.b.iv). Lesions of 0·5–3 mm in extent were induced reproducibly with exposure times of 0·2–2·5 s (see Section 9.11.a). The rate of change of temperature in the focal region during irradiation reached 180 degK s^{-1}, and heat leakage from the focus made the relationship between intensity and exposure non-reciprocal. The results indicate that the diameter of the lesion is linearly related to the logarithm of the irradiation time, for lesions of less than 2·5 mm diameter, and for intensities within the range 0·2–2·5 kW cm^{-2}. The relationship for an intensity of 1·5 kW cm^{-2} is shown in Fig. 9.1. Typically, the lesion becomes visible 4–9 min after irradiation,

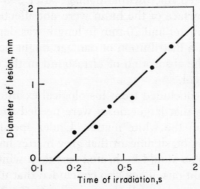

FIG. 9.1 The relationship between lesion diameter and irradiation time in ultrasonic neurosurgery, for an intensity of 1·5 kW cm^{-2} at a frequency of 3 MHz. (Based on data of Warwick and Pond, 1968.)

increases in size until 15 min after irradiation, and remains constant in size for 18 days; it then diminishes as part of a recovery process. Warwick and Pond (1968) considered that cavitation was eliminated as a factor leading to the results which they analysed, and they believed that thermal effects were predominant.

The results of experiments on two further types of tissue also appear to be compatible with thermal effects. Firstly, Smith *et al.* (1966) studied the effect of ultrasound on the gastric mucosa and its secretion of acid. Secondly, both Baum (1956) and Torchia *et al.* (1967) have studied the relationship between intensity and exposure time in damaging the eye, for continuous waves and pulsed irradiation respectively. In this connexion, it is relevant that the eye is considered to be a critical organ in microwave (electromagnetic) exposure, since it lacks a cooling circulation and it is sensitive to heat.

9.3 EVIDENCE OF NON-THERMAL EFFECTS

It was experimentally established by Freundlich and Gillings (1938) that ultrasonic waves can reduce the viscosity of colloidal solutions, and that such changes are not fundamentally of thermal origin. It was natural to assume that some biological effects might also be of non-thermal origin. Thus, Fry *et al.* (1950) attempted to identify non-thermal mechanisms in ultrasonically induced changes in living systems. Their ultrasonic source was a quartz crystal of 25 mm diameter, which operated at a frequency of about 1 MHz. The maximum intensity was between 30 and 40 W cm^{-2}. Irradiation of the commissure and two adjacent ganglia of the ventral abdominal nerve of crayfish was accompanied by an initial increase in the frequency of the periodically occurring action potentials, followed by a decrease in frequency to zero. After irradiation, the frequency gradually increased almost to the original rate. Temperature measurements made with a thermocouple in a similar preparation indicated a maximum rise of 1 degK during irradiation. (So small a temperature rise is rather surprising, since very large temperature gradients are known to occur under certain conditions involving the use of similar intensities.) Experiments were also described which showed that such a temperature rise (1 degK) might have produced an increase in discharge frequency by 4–5 s^{-1}. Thus, the ultimate effect of ultrasound in depressing the frequency of the discharge was in a direction opposite to the effect of the measured temperature change.

In a second group of experiments, prolonged exposure to ultrasound of excised frog sciatic nerve produced no detectable change in the waveform or the magnitude of the action potential, or in excitability. A rise in temperature of about 2 degK was recorded. In a third series of experiments, however, intact frogs were partially immersed in water at 21–25°C, and irradiated at the centre of the back over the lumbar enlargement. Complete paralysis of the hind legs occurred with exposures of 4·3 s duration. When the animals were first cooled to between 1–2°C, exposures of 7·3 s produced the same effects. Histological changes were evident in the tissues of para-lysed animals, fixed 20 min after treatment. Temperature measurements showed a rise of between 40 and 50 degK from room temperature, and to between 25 and 30°C from 1 to 2°C. It was found that frogs cooled to between 1 and 2°C, and irradiated for 4·3 s, did not suffer paralysis; but a second exposure of 4·3 s, 4 min after the first, did result in paralysis. This may be interpreted as being evidence of non-thermal damage. Control experiments were carried out where the animals were partially immersed in hot water: 6 min immersion at 40°C produced temporary partial paralysis.

It should be noted that the results of these experiments are not entirely satisfactory in demonstrating non-thermal effects. In particular, it may be significant that *in vitro* frog sciatic nerve was unaffected by prolonged irradiation, where as *in vivo* nerve could be blocked. In a later paper, however, Fry *et al.* (1951) showed that whatever mechanism was involved, it was unlikely to be cavitational, since considerable increase in applied pressure had little effect.

Takagi *et al.* (1960) used 1 MHz focused ultrasound at intensities of up to 120 W cm^{-2}, and 3 MHz unfocused ultrasound, to irradiate myelinated nerve, spinal cord and brain. The effects on the action potential, reflex discharge and electroencephalogram were reported to be dissimilar to those which were produced by heat. These results, however, are not in agreement with those of other investigators mentioned in Section 9.2.

Curtis (1965) irradiated the livers of intact mice with ultrasound at a frequency of 1 MHz. He thought that heat could have caused the histological damage which was found, at intensities below 60 W cm^{-2}, and this is in accord with the earlier findings of Bell (1957). At higher intensities, some other mechanism seemed to assume importance.

The existence of a threshold level of ultrasonic intensity, below which biological damage of any particular type, if it occurs at all, is thermal in origin, and above which a mechanical effect contributes to damage, has been demonstrated by experiments in which *Daphnia* was irradiated at a frequency of 3 MHz (Wells, 1968). The threshold intensity was between about 23 and 29 W cm^{-2} for an immediate effect on survival, and about 15 W cm^{-2} for a long-term survival effect. It is important, however, to realize that these threshold levels were probably most dependent upon the irradiation configuration, because the specimen was restrained within a small cylinder filled with water. The biological effects of the irradiation of smaller structures, such as biopolymers, are likely to be less dependent on the experimental arrangement.

Talbert (1975) has demonstrated an apparently non-thermal effect on the spontaneous activity of mammalian smooth muscle as a result of irradiation at an intensity of 1 W cm^{-2} at a frequency of 280 kHz. Similar effects produced by 2 MHz ultrasound seem to be due to heating. The suggested mechanism of the effect at the lower frequency is that the outer cell membrane may be depolarized (see Section 9.11.g).

More evidence of non-thermal effects of ultrasound is given in Section 9.11. In this connexion, it may be mentioned here that the visco-elastic properties of the protoplasm of *Helodea densa* are profoundly affected by exposure to 1 MHz ultrasound at 40 mW cm^{-2} for 3 min (Johnsson and Lindvall, 1969). It seems unlikely that this could be a thermal effect. Likewise, the morphological changes reported by Ravitz and Schnitzler (1970) to occur in muscle subjected to 85 kHz ultrasound were not due to heat.

Another extremely interesting phenomenon is referred to in Section 3.7.j.vi in connexion with the detection of ultrasonic waves. It appears that ultrasound at very low intensity can accelerate enzyme turn-over.

9.4 CAVITATION: PHYSICAL CONSIDERATIONS

The term *cavitation* is used here to describe the behaviour of gas bubbles in ultrasonic fields. Two situations may be distinguished: these are *transient* and *stable* cavitation.

Acoustic cavitation is an effective mechanism for concentrating energy (Flynn, 1964). It transforms the relatively low-energy density of an ultrasonic field into the high-energy density characteristic of the neighbourhood and interior of a collapsing or vibrating bubble. Because it concentrates energy into very small volumes, cavitation is able to produce drastic effects, of which the ultrasonic field propagating in a continuous medium would be incapable.

9.4.a Transient Cavitation

Transient cavitation is the phenomenon in which voids suddenly grow from nuclei in the supporting liquid, and then collapse, under the influence of the changing pressure in an ultrasonic field. The whole process occupies an interval of less than the wave period. The collapse of the cavity causes strong pressure pulses, or shock waves, in the supporting liquid. Cavitation may be suppressed by degassing the liquid, or by increasing the external pressure applied to the system (Harvey *et al.*, 1947). The pressure pulses which occur under conditions of increased external pressure are of larger amplitude than those associated with transient cavitation under similar ultrasonic conditions, but at lower external pressure.

Nottingk and Neppiras (1950) have developed a theory to describe the motion of bubbles in transient cavitation. It predicts that cavitation phenomena diminish and finally disappear as the frequency is increased. This has been demonstrated experimentally by Esche (1952) and by Gaertner (1954). During the adiabetic collapse phase, temperatures approaching 10^4 °K seem likely to occur within the bubble. According to Griffing (1950, 1952), such high temperatures can cause thermal decomposition of water, resulting in the formation of free hydroxyl radicals which are chemically very active. Similarly, Él'piner (1964) discussed the formation by ultrasonic cavitation of chemical free radicals and their biological effects.

The nature of the various types of nuclei from which cavitation bubbles may arise has been discussed by Sirotyuk (1963). It has been suggested that such nuclei may be due to thermal fluctuations within the liquid which give rise to tiny gas bubbles. Another possibility is that discontinuities in the tensile strength of the liquid may exist at interfaces with solid particles (Harvey *et al.*, 1944). Alternatively, the liquid may contain tiny gas bubbles, perhaps protected by unimolecular layers of fatty acids adsorbed on the bubble surface. Thus, evidence has been obtained by

Blake (1949) which indicates that bubbles of around $0·1$ μm radius are stabilized in ordinary liquids. Finally, it may be that microcavities so small that they could not function as cavitation nuclei are expanded by the vapour which forms due to the change in temperature which occurs during the passage of high-energy ionizing particles (Sette and Wanderlingh, 1962).

9.4.b Stable Cavitation

The behaviour of a gas-filled bubble existing in an ultrasonic field of intensity below that necessary to cause transient cavitation is known as stable cavitation. The matter was first investigated by Minnaert (1933), who showed that a resonant system is formed in which the surrounding liquid is the inert mass which is set into vibration, the elasticity being due to the gas in the bubble. The resonance frequency f_r of a gas bubble in a liquid is given by

$$f_r = (1/2\pi r_b)\{3\gamma(P_0 + 2\sigma/r_b)/\rho\}^{1/2} \tag{9.1}$$

where r_b is the bubble radius, γ is the ratio of the specific heats of the gas, P_0 is the hydrostatic pressure, σ is the surface tension, and ρ is the density of the surrounding medium. For an air-filled bubble in water at atmospheric pressure, Eqn. 9.1 simplifies to give $f_r r_b = 0·33$ m s^{-1}. At frequencies above about 10 MHz, the bubble becomes so small that surface tension effects become important.

9.4.c Cavitation Thresholds

The concept of *cavitation threshold* is a simple one. It defines the intensity below which, for a given irradiation situation, cavitation does not occur, and above which it does. The numerical values of cavitation thresholds for a given liquid depend on many variables.

Esche (1952) characterized the "cavitation threshold" as the onset of detectable wide-band noise occurring outside the frequency band of the applied sound field. The generation of such noise results from shock waves associated only with transient cavitation. Stable cavitation can occur at intensities much below this "threshold".

According to Flynn (1964), the most important factor which determines the cavitation threshold is probably the size distribution of nuclei, and this is often the most difficult parameter to specify except as it may be inferred from the history of a particular sample of liquid. The gas content of the liquid (Blake, 1949) and its history (Apfel, 1970) are crucial. Lauterborn (1969) has compared theoretical values of cavitation threshold in water with experimental measurements, and obtained fairly good agreement in the frequency range 1 kHz–10 MHz.

Other parameters on which thresholds may depend are equilibrium pressure (Blake, 1949), temperature, vapour pressure, surface tension, and the duration of the ultrasonic irradiation. Furthermore, Iernetti (1971) has investigated the increase in the cavitation threshold as the volume of the irradiated specimen is decreased.

Hill (1972) defined cavitation as the condition in which the following three experimental criteria are simultaneously satisfied:

(i) DNA in aqueous solution is degraded, on the evidence of viscometry, by at least 50% of its initial molecular weight (approximately 3×10^6). This criterion was chosen on the grounds that degradation, if it occurs to any detectable extent, is found to proceed readily at least to the 50% point (see Section 9.7);

(ii) Free iodine is released at a rate of at least 10^{-6} mol s^{-1} ml^{-1} (the minimum rate that is readily detectable) from a solution of potassium iodide in the presence of carbon tetrachloride (Weissler et al., 1950); and

(iii) The first half-order subharmonic of the driving frequency is detectable, by means of a hydrophone focused on the region of the irradiated specimen (de Santis et al., 1967; Eller and Flynn, 1969; Neppiras, 1969).

The absence of positive indications of cavitation on these criteria, however, cannot be taken as ruling out the possibility of its occurrence.

The frequency dependence of cavitation with intensity in air-equilibrated water is given in Fig. 9.2. Whilst at first sight these results may seem to be anomalous, they are consistent with differences in the criteria used by the various investigators. The phenomenon of the single transient cavitation event, studied by Coakley (1971), seems to exist in two different forms: one results in a bubble emitting a strong subharmonic signal, and shooting off tiny air bubbles when strongly excited, but without producing strong shock waves; the other radiates shock waves which may last (at 1 MHz) for several milliseconds.

Hill et al. (1969) made the important discovery that stable cavitation may be established in a liquid subjected to an ultrasonic beam of megahertz frequency, if the sample is rotated in relation to the ultrasonic axis. In the absence of rotation, cavitation bubbles are apparently driven by radiation pressure to the wall of the container, before they have time to produce effects in the medium. Furthermore, Hill (1972) reported the effects of various pulsing conditions (Fig. 9.3) and various applied pressures (Fig. 9.4) on the cavitation threshold. Cavitation is inhibited by the use of short pulses, low duty factors, and high ambient pressures. It is clear enough why cavitation—both transient and stable—should be inhibited by increasing external pressure: in this situation, the absolute value of the negative-going pressure excursion in the wave may never become negative at all. In connexion with the observation that cavitation is suppressed by the use of shorter pulses, it appears that stable cavitation may require at least about 1000 cycles to become established at 1 MHz. The explanation of this may be that a bubble is most effective from the point of view of cavitation if it is of resonant size (see Eqn. 9.1). It is likely that the bubble nuclei within the unirradiated liquid are smaller than this. During irradiation, these nuclei may grow by a process known as *rectified diffusion* (Eller, 1972). Over a relatively few cycles of oscillation, the ratio of the surface area to the volume of the bubble oscillates about a mean value. During negative-going pressure excursions, the area is greater than during positive-going

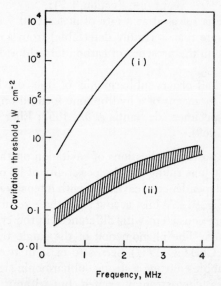

FIG. 9.2 Frequency dependence of cavitation threshold in water, for continuous waves. (i) Transient cavitation (data of Esche, 1952); (ii) stable cavitation in air-equilibrated water; the shaded area is the region between positive and negative indications of cavitation (data of Hill, 1972).

pressure excursions. The humidity within the bubble oscillates with the changing volume. The result is that more gas diffuses into the bubble during the negative-going pressure excursions, than diffuses out during positive-going pressure excursions. Therefore, the bubble grows, and, if the pulse duration is sufficiently long, it passes through resonance size. By this time, however, its dimensions may have become fairly stable.

Cavitation is also inhibited by increasing the viscosity of the supporting liquid, and by reducing the time duration of the irradiation (Briggs *et al.*, 1947). Thus, the transient cavitation threshold at 500 kHz and atmospheric pressure is between 130 and 260 W cm^{-2} in blood, and lies somewhere

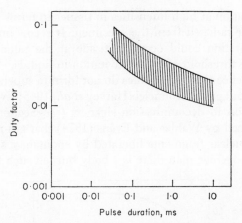

FIG. 9.3 Dependence of stable cavitation on pulsing parameters in air-equilibrated water. Frequency$=2$ MHz; intensity$=4\cdot7$ W cm^{-2}. The shaded area is the region between positive and negative indications of cavitation. (Data of Hill, 1972.)

above 400 W cm^{-2} in soft tissues (Esche, 1952). Hill (1972) has studied the occurrence of stable cavitation at megahertz frequencies in various media, including gels and biological tissues. His results are reproduced in Fig. 9.5. Although a considerable range of values of subharmonic signal occurs among normal liquids, mammalian tissues are very greatly separated from all of these and exhibit behaviour similar to that of gels, their subharmonic signals being in most cases below the limit of detection. Despite this difficulty, Lele *et al.* (1974) have apparently succeeded in quantifying

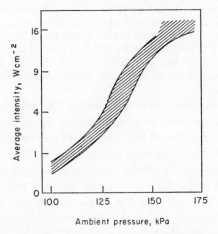

FIG. 9.4 Dependence of stable cavitation on applied pressure in air-equilibrated water, for continuous waves. Frequency$=1$ MHz. The shaded area is the region between positive and negative indications of cavitation. (Data of Hill, 1972.)

ultrasonic cavitation at high intensities in tissues in terms of the total sub-harmonic power radiated from the specimen. It seems unlikely, however, that stable cavitation could occur in tissue at the same intensities that characterize the threshold of stable cavitation in liquids.

There is evidence that gas bubbles do not form in supersaturated liquids or animals without gas micronuclei (Harvey *et al.*, 1945; Evans and Walder, 1969). In relation to decompression sickness (see Section 6.16.a.iii), it has been proposed by Walder and Evans (1974) that gas micronuclei may be caused by nuclear fragments liberated by spontaneous fission of ^{238}U, of which in the average man there is a body burden such that there is one

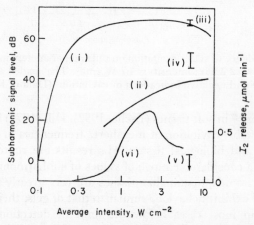

FIG. 9.5 Evidence from subharmonic measurements on cavitation activity in some liquids and tissues at 1 MHz. (i) Non-degassed water; (ii) degassed water; (iii) distilled water, tap water, liquid paraffin; (iv) transformer oil, glycerol, acetone, methyl alcohol, ethyl alcohol; (v) agar gel (1·5%), gelatine gel (5%), ox liver (fixed, mounted in 5% gelatine), ox liver (fresh, mounted in 5% gelatine), ox muscle (fresh, mounted in 5% gelatine), ox fat (fresh, mounted in 5% gelatine), rat liver (fresh, mounted in 5% gelatine), rat kidney (fresh, mounted in 5% gelatine); (vi) iodine release from non-degassed potassium iodide solution. (Data of Hill, 1972.)

disintegration about once every three weeks. The lifetime of microbubbles formed by this mechanism is not known, but it seems to be significantly long because the incidence of the bends depends on the time of exposure to high pressure which precedes decompression. Whether such bubbles contribute to ultrasonic bioeffects remains to be determined. It may be relevant that most of the body burden of uranium resides in bone: whilst this fact supports the correlation with decompression sickness (since the commonest symptom is bone pain), it does lessen the possibility of associa-tion with ultrasonic bioeffects.

If bubbles are present in a tissue or gel, at low frequencies it appears that they oscillate quite freely; they execute surface oscillations, generate microbubbles, and radiate spectra including subharmonics (Storm, 1974). There seem to be no data concerning direct observation of bubble activity under these conditions at megahertz frequencies.

9.5 ACOUSTIC STREAMING: PHYSICAL CONSIDERATIONS

It has been shown (e.g. by Nyborg, 1968) that the localized vibration of a small area of a membrane, such as a cell wall, results in an increase P^+ in static pressure at a given point by an amount

$$P^+ = C + \langle p^2 \rangle / 2\rho c^2 + \langle v^2 \rangle \rho / 2 \qquad (9.2)$$

where C is a constant; the second and third terms on the right-hand side of the equation are respectively the time-arranged volume densities of potential and kinetic energy. Close to a small source, such as the tip of a vibrating needle (see Section 3.5), the kinetic energy term predominates. Consequently, a particle suspended in the field is acted upon by unequal forces on its opposite sides such that there is a tendency for the particle to migrate towards the source if its density is greater than that of the medium, and vice versa.

Equation 9.2 fails when absorption mechanisms or boundary effects convert vibratory energy into heat. In the case of a membrane vibrating at low ultrasonic frequencies, the principal mechanism of energy loss is viscous drag in the boundary layer close to the surface. In this situation, streaming movements occur in which particles suspended in the medium may be set into rotation, or may tend to move in circulating paths. The subject of acoustic streaming has been reviewed by Nyborg (1965). The streaming which occurs in fluids near a vibrating membrane (Nyborg, 1958) is a special case of the streaming which tends to occur in any non-linear acoustic field. It is similar to the so-called "sonic wind" which is associated with vibrating plates in air and which was first noticed many years ago, and is a manifestation of radiation pressure (see Section 1.13).

The earliest investigations of acoustic microstreaming were made using vibrating needles, of the type described in Section 3.6.b.iii. Small-scale acoustic streaming, similar to that which occurs near the tip of a vibrating needle, may also be set up by bubble-scattered sound waves. The problem was first investigated by Elder (1959), who demonstrated and analysed four régimes of streaming, the transitions between which occur with changing amplitude. The various patterns are illustrated in Fig. 9.6. In this kind of situation, the calculation of the velocity gradient involves the consideration of several factors. It is based on an equation for a representative streaming velocity V_L near a pulsating hemispherical bubble on a solid boundary

(Nyborg, 1965), given by

$$V_L = v_b / 2\pi f r_b \tag{9.3}$$

where v_b is the radial velocity of the bubble surface.

In experiments on the biological effects of acoustic streaming, the transversely oscillating wire (Williams *et al.*, 1970; Section 3.6.b.vi) allows the physical parameters to be quite closely controlled. It can be

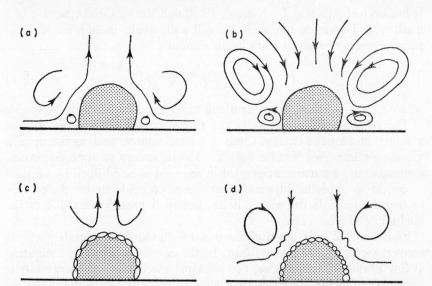

FIG. 9.6 Four régimes of streaming. The bubble (which is shown stippled) is excited by the vibration of the surface to which it is attached. (a) A surface-contaminated bubble in a liquid of low viscosity, oscillating at low amplitude; (b) a pattern observed over a wide range of amplitudes and viscosities; (c) a pattern which occurs at low amplitudes in low viscosities, and at high amplitudes in high viscosities; its appearance coincides with the onset of the first surface mode and the dissolution of régime (b) at higher amplitude; (d) a pattern which occurs only at low viscosities, and which seems to represent a return to régime (b) as the amplitude becomes too large to permit the existence of a single stable surface mode. (From Elder, 1959.)

shown (see, for example, Nyborg, 1965) that the magnitude G of the maximum velocity gradient associated with a transversely vibrating cylinder is given by

$$G = 2\pi f u_0 / a\delta \tag{9.4}$$

where δ is equal to $(\eta/\pi f \rho)^{1/2}$; η is the shear viscosity coefficient of the liquid, and the other symbols have their usual meanings. It turns out in practice, however, that the maximum velocity gradient produced by a transversely oscillating wire is critically dependent upon the geometry of the wire tip (Williams, 1972; Sanders and Coakley, 1972). Therefore, in order to obtain reproducible results it may be necessary to measure the pressure amplitude, and the so-called "bubblephone" of Nyborg and Rooney (1969) may be suitable for this purpose. This instrument consists of a long thin tube connected to a gas reservoir, and at the lower end of which a gas bubble is trapped. The application of an acoustic field to the bubble causes a related change in the gas pressure at which the bubble becomes untrapped.

9.6 BIOLOGICAL EFFECTS OF TRANSIENT CAVITATION

Ackerman (1952) used ultrasound to determine cell fragilities and resonances. He subsequently improved his apparatus, and in 1954 he showed that the maximum breakdown rate of red blood cells of *Amphiuma* occurred in a cavitating field at a frequency of 16·5 kHz. In 1960, he published a theoretical analysis based on a simple cell model which seemed to agree with experimental data obtained for a number of different types of cell. It may be significant, however, that (transient) cavitation was required, and in any event the published photographs bear a suspicious resemblance to the appearance of crenated cells.

Despite the controversial nature of the biophysical mechanisms involved, Ackerman's (1952) results showed that:

$$\ln (N/N_0) = - K v_0 t \tag{9.5}$$

where N_0 is the original cell concentration, N is the cell concentration after irradiation for time t, v_0 is the peak velocity of the source (space-averaged), and K is a breakdown constant. This result seems to be of quite wide validity, and similar equations have been verified by several investigators (for example, Neppiras and Hughes, 1964).

Goldman and Lepeschkin (1952) irradiated various botanical materials in standing wave fields, at frequencies of 0·4, 0·7 and 1·0 MHz. The specimens were usually held between thin glass plates, but were sometimes retained by hairs on single glass sheets. There was a cooling circulation, but the ultrasonic intensities were not measured. Marked variations in damage were found according to the position of the specimen in the standing wave field. Injury was slow without cavitation, but with transient cavitation it was widespread and rapid, being most marked at the pressure antinodes. The damage appeared to be dissimilar to that which would have been produced by heat.

The pressure pulses generated by transient cavitation may be of sufficient amplitude to disrupt cells (Hughes and Cunningham, 1963) and biological macromolecules (Tomlinson *et al.*, 1965). In this connexion, Howkins and Weinstock (1970) have shown that the ultrasonic intensity may be chosen so that irradiated blood is haemolysed if gas bubbles are introduced, but not in the absence of gas.

Freifelder and Davison (1962) reported partial degradation of DNA in a 10 kHz cavitating field. The degradation was shown to be by preferential halving of the DNA molecule, which is also the mechanism suggested by Doty *et al.* (1958), and shown to occur in shearing fields. This type of degradation is a non-random process, unlike the degradation induced both by ionizing radiation and by the enzyme DNAase, which act at random.

Figure 9.7 shows the results of some experiments of Neppiras and Hughes (1964), in which yeast cells were irradiated at 20 kHz under varying conditions of applied pressure and ultrasonic intensity. At any

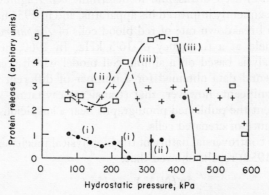

Fig. 9.7 Disintegration of yeast cells by 20 kHz ultrasound, under conditions of varying hydrostatic pressure and ultrasonic power. The cell disintegration was estimated from measurements of the quantity of protein released into the solution. Treatment time = 5 min. For each ultrasonic power, the corresponding curve and theoretical cavitation threshold pressure are marked by the same letter. (i) 5 W; (ii) 10 W; (iii) 15 W. (From Neppiras and Hughes, 1964.)

fixed intensity, the rate of disintegration (i.e. the disintegration which occurs during a fixed interval of time) increases to a maximum value as the ambient pressure is increased, and thereafter decreases rapidly. The maximum rate of disintegration occurs at higher ambient pressures with increasing intensity. The threshold pressures agree fairly well with those predicted by Neppiras and Nottingk (1951). The rather erratic behaviour observed at hydrostatic pressures greater than those needed to suppress cavitation has not been explained. Similar results in experiments in which *Chlorella* cells were increasingly destroyed under excess pressure conditions have been reported by Bronskaya *et al.* (1968).

Thacker (1973) has demonstrated a progressive shift towards smaller sizes in the distribution of suspensions of yeast cells subjected to cavitating ultrasonic fields, both at 20 kHz and at 1 MHz. The shift occurs more rapidly with diploid than with haploid cells; diploid cells are about 50% larger than haploid cells, and so are subjected to larger strains in a given velocity gradient. Moreover, cell killing does not occur in the absence of cavitation, nor when cells are placed in recently irradiated media: although this does not rule out an effect due to very short-lived cavitation-generated free radicals, it does eliminate H_2O_2 as a toxic agent.

At a frequency of 1 MHz, Coakley et al. (1971) have shown that destruction of an amoeba, Hartmannella, is correlated with the actual number of discrete cavitation events occurring during irradiation. Similarly, Coakley and Dunn (1971) found that degradation of DNA in solution depended upon transient cavitation at an intensity of 500 W cm^{-2}, but that at lower intensities (200–288 W cm^{-2}), DNA degradation was observed which did not depend on transient cavitation.

Hamrick and Cleary (1969) reported the breakage of particles of tobacco mosaic virus by acoustic transients generated by thermal gradients resulting from the rapid absorption of high-energy pulses of light from a Q-switched laser. The duration of the stress transient was about 10^{-7} s. No evidence of cavitation could be found—and this seems reasonable on account of the brevity of the disturbance—and it was calculated from the experimental results that a velocity gradient of 4×10^7 s^{-1} was sufficient to break a virus particle into halves. As in the earlier work of Pritchard et al. (1966) on DNA (see Section 9.7), this stress is an order of magnitude less than the theoretical bond-strength critical stress, and so non-mechanical factors (such as the solvent permeability of the particle) are probably important.

It is natural to enquire, in view of the very short duration of the stress transient known to damage the tobacco mosaic virus particle, whether the oscillating component of velocity gradient in a wave may be a factor contributing to damage in other situations. It is easy to show, from Eqn. 1.32, that the maximum value of this velocity gradient is equal to $(u_0\omega^2/c)$, and that, at a frequency of 1 MHz and an intensity of 1 W cm^{-2} in water, this corresponds to a maximum velocity gradient of 480 s^{-1}. This is a factor of about 10^5 less than that shown by Hamrick and Cleary (1969) to be necessary to break a tobacco mosaic virus particle.

Biological effects induced by cavitation occur only at intensities above a threshold value equal to the cavitation threshold.

9.7 BIOLOGICAL EFFECTS OF ACOUSTIC STREAMING

Migration of protoplasm towards a vibrating needle (at 25 kHz) was demonstrated in intact cells of Elodea by Nyborg and Dyer (1960). Selman and Jurand (1964) described the disorganization and subsequent recovery of the arrangement of the endoplasmic reticulum following irradiation for 5 min with 1 MHz ultrasound at intensities of between 8 and 15 W cm^{-2}.

Detailed observations of intracellular motion were made by Wilson *et al.* (1966), who studied certain marine eggs vibrated with needles at a frequency of 85 kHz and at peak-to-peak amplitudes of up to 5 μm. It was also shown by Hughes and Nyborg (1962) that the streaming of red blood cells in solution around a needle vibrating longitudinally with a tip excursion amplitude in the order of 10 μm at a frequency of 25 kHz resulted in shearing forces which haemolysed the cells.

It has been possible to apply acoustic streaming theory to certain aspects of streaming motion, particularly those observed experimentally in cell models (Jackson and Nyborg, 1958); but a complete description of the circulation which occurs in biological cells would need to be very elaborate, and has not yet been attempted. As far as plant cells are concerned, the situation has been reviewed by Gershoy and Nyborg (1973). With displacement amplitudes of around 0·1 μm at 85 kHz, distortions of the vacuolar membrane occur. These take the form of evaginations into the vacuole: it is supposed that they result from the flow of fluid along the parietal channel. Vibration at an amplitude of 0·2 μm causes rupture of the vacuolar membrane and fragmentation of the cytoplasm; plastid-containing fragments are then released into the vacuole. Motions in the vacuole include streaming, as well as particle migrations and spinning. There is considerable variation in post-irradiation response. (Studies made by Child *et al.* (1975) of the growth of pea roots after exposure to pulsed ultrasound, 2·3 MHz 10 W cm^{-2} peak, support the concept of a cavitational mechanism. It seems that air spaces exist in the root tissue, and that they act as cavitation nuclei. Moreover, the effect of irradiation becomes less marked as the pulse duration is decreased.) Some cells, in which there are no visible changes, die; others show a surprising ability to recover from apparently severe damage.

Quite steep local gradients in the acoustic field generated by a source much larger than the tip of a vibrating needle can occur in the presence of gas-filled bubbles. The behaviour of this form of stable cavitation is quite distinct from that of transient cavitation (see Section 9.4.b). Nyborg (1965) pointed out that the sound field used by Hughes and Nyborg (1962) in their experiments with a vibrating needle (amplitude 10 μm at 25 kHz) in which haemolysis occurred was similar in scale to that near a bubble resonating at 20 kHz (i.e. with a radius of about 160 μm) with a vibration amplitude of about 16 μm.

Whilst much of the work on acoustic streaming has been at the cellular or subcellular level, in this connexion it may be noted that streaming can separate biological aggregates, apparently without affecting the cells. Thus, Williams *et al.* (1970b) reported the break up of sludge flocs, and Williams and Slade (1971) described how aggregates of *Sarcina lutea* were dispersed: both these effects were observed with the 20 kHz field of a transversely oscillating wire.

Irradiation under conditions of stable cavitation has given much useful information about certain aspects of the biological effects of ultrasound. The subject has been reviewed by Nyborg (1974). Hughes and Nyborg (1962) devised a method for causing bubbles of suitable size to appear at low amplitudes of vibration, so that quite large volumes of sample could be treated quickly. The face of a metal plate, 20 mm in diameter, was drilled with a series of about 50 holes, each of 200 μm diameter and 200 μm in depth: thus each hole was somewhat larger than the dimensions of a bubble resonant at 20 kHz. At low vibration amplitudes (about 3 μm), bright and shining bubbles appeared to grow from the surface of the probe into the liquid, but did not leave the holes. It has been shown by Howkins (1965) that the resonance frequency of a bubble of given size is slightly lower when in contact with a solid boundary than in a free field. Degradation of certain biological structures was accelerated when the drilled probe was used in place of a polished probe, the two probes being driven at equal amplitudes below the threshold of transient cavitation.

Pritchard *et al.* (1966) and Peacocke and Pritchard (1968) investigated the ultrasonic degradation of DNA under conditions of stable cavitation, using an apparatus slightly larger but otherwise similar to the drilled probe arrangement of Hughes and Nyborg (1962). An important advantage of this technique in comparison with the transient cavitation method previously used by Freifelder and Davison (1962) is that it was possible to calculate the maximum velocity gradient within the sound field, and to relate this quantity to the biological effect. Figure 9.8 shows how the initial rate of degradation increased with increasing velocity gradient; there was a limiting degree of degradation at each value of velocity gradient. It was possible to demonstrate a linear relationship between the number of breaks per original average molecule and the velocity gradient, a single break being produced by a velocity gradient of about 12×10^4 s^{-1}.

It seems certain that the effect of ultrasound in this situation is due to hydrodynamic shearing of long molecules subjected to a velocity gradient. There is apparently good agreement between the value of the mechanical shear calculated to produce a given degradation (Levinthal and Davison, 1961), and that believed to exist in the ultrasonic field which produces the same degradation. The mechanical situation, however, was analysed from considerations based on the behaviour of a simple model which is not entirely satisfactory. It should be possible to calculate the breaking strain (and consequently the velocity gradient to produce breakage) by considering the molecular shape, the molecular bond strengths and the viscosity of the medium. In a velocity gradient, the force distribution over a rigid rod is parabolic with the maximum at the centre; the maximum tensile force varies with the square of the length of the rod. However, the calculated values (Harrington and Zimm, 1965) are greater by a factor of about 30 than those believed to exist in the ultrasonic field which produces comparable degradation. It has been suggested that this discrepancy may be due to solute–solvent interaction.

Williams *et al.* (1970a) reported that the haemolysis of red cells in suspension was associated with a well-defined threshold of acoustic streaming generated by a wire oscillating transversely at 20 kHz. Similar results were obtained by Rooney (1972), who used a bubble-generated streaming field. Here again, shearing forces seem certain to be responsible for the observed effects. In this connexion, it is interesting that the threshold shear stress for haemolysis decreases by a factor of two from that necessary

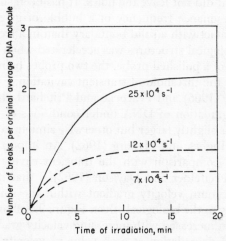

FIG. 9.8 The relationship between the degradation of DNA and the time of irradiation under conditions of stable cavitation at 20 kHz, for various maximum values of velocity gradient. Approximate initial molecular weight $= 6 \times 10^6$. (Based on data of Pritchard *et al.*, 1966.)

in the temperature range 20–40°C, when the temperature is increased to 45°C.

Hawley *et al.* (1963) demonstrated the degradation of DNA by ultrasound, allegedly in the absence of cavitation. At a frequency of 1 MHz, and at intensities of up to about 30 W cm^{-2}, the molecular weight of DNA was reduced; the temperature increased by less than 5 degK. It was suggested that the mechanism of destruction was the relative motion of the molecules and the medium. (This mechanism is the same as that shown by Pritchard *et al.* (1966) to be responsible for DNA degradation at much lower frequencies, in the presence of stable cavitation.) No delayed effects were observed, and it was concluded that "ultrasound acts at a level of structure closely associated with cell function, and not at a level which results in physiological changes after a time delay." In the light of the results of Hill *et al.* (1969), however, the claim that DNA was degraded at megahertz frequencies in the absence of cavitation must be treated with some reservation. As mentioned in Section 9.4.b, it is certainly possible for the cavitation field to be stabilized at quite low intensities at high frequencies, and Hill *et al.* (1969) were unable to degrade DNA in the absence of cavitation.

In somewhat similar experiments on certain enzymes, irradiated at frequencies in the range 1–27 MHz, Dunn and Macleod (1968) were unable to detect degradation unless transient cavitation occurred in the ultrasonic field. Thus enzyme molecules are not subjected to shearing forces large enough to cause breakage, unless cavitation is present. Completely negative results have been reported by Robinson *et al.* (1972) in experiments on placental enzymes following 8 h of irradiation with either 6·3 W cm^{-2} continuous waves, or pulsed waves with peak intensity 80 W cm^{-2}, average 24 mW cm^{-2}. Likewise, the results of the experiments of Woodcock and Connolly (1969) in which the hydrolysis of sucrose solution was accelerated, may have been dependent on the existence of stable cavitation.

The circumstances under which stable cavitation can occur in liquids at megahertz frequencies are discussed in Section 9.4.c. The relevance of this to the cumulative effects of pulsed ultrasound is discussed in Section 9.10. In this connexion, no distinction is made between the biological effects of streaming whether resulting from stable cavitation or not.

The possibility that stable cavitation might occur in tissues at megahertz frequencies is discussed in Sections 9.4 and 9.11.a. It seems unlikely that stable cavitation could occur at low intensities, and if biological effects are due to streaming in this region, the mechanisms must be very sensitive.

9.8 DOSIMETRY

In considering the biological effects of ultrasound, it is necessary to know the following physical parameters (Wells, 1973):

  (i) The frequency (or the frequency spectrum) of the energy;
 (ii) The total energy flux across the region of interest;
(iii) The spatial distribution of the energy (i.e. the beam profile: this includes, in particular, the value of the spatial peak intensity); and
(iv) The time distribution of the energy (i.e. the pulse shape and repetition rate).

In the light of these requirements, many of the data on the biological effects of ultrasound which are recorded in the literature are unsatisfactory, and the precise conditions of irradiation are left to speculation. In particular, it may be important to distinguish between exposure (i.e. the ultrasonic field parameters to which the tissue in question is exposed) and dose (in the sense of the quantity of energy absorbed by a tissue element as a consequence of an exposure). Thus, an exposure parameter, such as peak particle displacement amplitude, might be of relevance if some biological change were related to the degree of mechanical stress experienced by a tissue element during the passage of an ultrasonic wave. On the other hand, the absorbed dose would be the quantity of interest in a situation where temperature rise was the biologically significant consequence of ultrasonic irradiation. This distinction bears an analogy to current practice in ionizing radiation dosimetry, but entails a shift from the existing, rather vague practice in ultrasound work, where the term "dose" is often used interchangeably to cover the different concepts of exposure and absorbed dose.

For clarity in this book, the following terms are used to describe exposure conditions:

> On-intensity: the intensity of the ultrasound when the beam is switched on (equal to the intensity during the pulse, in the case of a repetitively pulsed beam);
> Pulse-duration: the duration of the ultrasonic pulse (i.e. each single pulse in the case of a repetitively pulsed beam);
> Duty cycle: the product of the pulse duration and the pulse repetition frequency (equal to unity, in the case of a single pulse); and
> On-time: the product of the total time of exposure and the duty cycle (equal to the pulse duration, in the case of a single pulse).

9.9 FREQUENCY DEPENDENCE OF BIOLOGICAL EFFECTS

It is convenient to make a broad distinction between the mechanisms of the biological effects induced by low-kilohertz ultrasound, where cavitation and associated phenomena are of major and obvious importance (see Section 9.4.a), and those responsible for the effects of low-megahertz ultrasound, where the interactions are at present only rather poorly understood.

Some of the published data concerned with the frequency dependence of ultrasonically induced biological effects are summarized in Table 9.1. At very high intensities (the value quoted is 620 W cm^{-2}), an equal on-time is required to damage brain with a single pulse, in the frequency range 1–6 MHz (Fry *et al.*, 1970). At the much lower on-intensity of 10 W cm^{-2}, however, ultrasound pulsed at a duty cycle of 0·09, with pulse durations of 10 ms or 20 μs, is more damaging at low frequency (0·5 MHz) than at high frequency (4·9 MHz), when the damaging ability is taken as the reciprocal of the on-time required to damage spinal cord (Taylor and Pond, 1972). On the other hand, low frequencies (0·5 MHz) are less damaging than high frequencies (3·2 MHz) when the index of damage is taken to be the reduction in cell electrophoretic mobility (Taylor and Newman, 1972); and here

TABLE 9.1

Data for frequency dependence of biological effects, low megahertz range

Frequency (MHz)	Minimum on-time(s) for damage		Equilibrium reduction % in cell electrophoretic mobility (note iii)	Cavitation threshold (W cm⁻²) (note iv)
	Brain (note i)	Spinal cord (note ii)		
0·5	—	18	6	0·08
1	0·45	24	11	0·2
2	0·45	27	16	0·7
2·7	0·45	—	—	1
3	0·45	—	—	2
3·2	—	—	22	3
3·5	—	30	—	4
4·2	—	45	—	6
4·9	—	>120	—	—
6	0·45	—	—	—

(i) Single-pulse, on-intensity 620 W cm⁻² (collected data quoted by Fry et al., 1970).
(ii) Pulse duration 10 ms, interval between pulses 100 ms, 50 W cm⁻² on-intensity; similar effect produced with pulse duration 20 μs, duty cycle 0·09 (Taylor and Pond, 1972).
(iii) On-intensity 10 W cm⁻², duty cycle 0·09; similar effects may occur with pulse durations 10 ms, 1 ms, or 20 μs (Taylor and Newman, 1972), although Joshi et al. (1973) disagree with the short-pulse data.
(iv) Values for continuous waves in air-equilibrated water (Hill, 1972).

again the effect is independent of the pulse duration (10 ms, 1 ms, or 20 μs) at a duty cycle of 0·09; although this finding for short-duration pulses has been questioned by Joshi *et al.* (1973). The heating effect, expressed in terms of the distance rate of energy deposition, increases with frequency at a fixed intensity, because absorption increases with frequency. Conversely, cavitation becomes less likely with increasing frequency, and it is also inhibited by pulsing (see Section 9.4.c).

9.10 CUMULATIVE EFFECTS

Biological effects which are apparently similar may be produced by ultrasound delivered under differing conditions of pulsing. Some of the published data are summarised in Table 9.2. At fixed on-intensity, the on-time required to produce nerve block increases rapidly as the pulse duration is decreased from about 7 s to about 3 s, if there is a long interval between the pulses (Fry *et al.*, 1950). A reduction in this interval, from about 250 s to 400 ms, allows quite short pulses, of about 100 ms, to become effective. With a pulse duration of 10 ms, the threshold for damage to spinal cord is associated with a constant on-time at a fixed on-intensity, for intervals between pulses in the range 100–400 ms (Taylor, 1970). Likewise, a constant on-time produces a constant reduction in cell electrophoretic mobility, whether the pulse duration is 10 ms or 20 μs (Taylor and Newman, 1972); although this finding has been questioned by Joshi *et al.* (1973), who failed to reproduce the result with mouse lymphoma cells. Similarly there is a cumulative effect, although not one of simple addition, in cell mortality resulting from irradiation with pulses of 10 ms duration, and duty cycle 0·09, and in which stable cavitation is the main damaging factor (Clarke and Hill, 1970). But shorter pulses, of 1 ms duration, are ineffective in this situation, even with much longer on-times, at least when the interval between the pulses exceeds 1 ms. Also, very short pulses of 0·5 μs duration, with a low duty cycle (0·0005), are without effect even at quite high on-intensity; but this has been tested only with a rather short on-time. For a given on-time and a duty cycle of 0·09, however, pulses of 20 μs duration are more damaging to liver than those of 10 ms duration, whereas those of 150 μs are less damaging (Taylor and Connolly, 1969). This may be due to stresses being established at membranes immediately upon the arrival of each pulse. Such stresses have visco-elastic relaxation times of around 400 μs, so that pulses arriving every 200 μs cause additive strains; but the stresses decay during intervals of 1500 μs. With an on-time of 10 ms, the strains reach a maximum value during the pulse. In contrast, a pulse duration in excess of 1 ms at 1 MHz (i.e. more than 1000 cycles) is necessary for non-collapse cavitation to cause degradation of DNA in solution (see Section 9.7). In this situation, 30 ms is the most effective pulse length for

TABLE 9.2

Data relating biological effects to pulsed irradiation conditions

Degree of damage	Pulse duration	Interval between pulses	On-time s	On-intensity W cm⁻²	Frequency MHz	Effect studied	Reference
+	7.3 s	—	7.3	35	1	Sciatic nerve paralysis, frog	Fry et al. (1950)
+	4.3 s		8.6				
+	3.3 s	240 s	9.9				
+	2.8 s		1400				
+	80 ms	420 ms	29				
−	10 ms	40 ms	>120				
+	10 ms	100 ms	27	25	3.5	Spinal cord damage, rat	Taylor (1970)
+	10 ms	200 ms	29				
+	10 ms	300 ms	29				
+	10 ms	400 ms	29				
−	10 ms	100 ms	16				
−	10 ms	200 ms	23				
−	10 ms	300 ms	23				
−	10 ms	400 ms	23				
+	30 s	—	30	1	1	Mortality, mouse lymphoma cells	Clarke and Hill (1970)
+	10 ms	10 ms	30	5.75			
		100 ms					
−	1 ms	1 ms	1640	5	2		
		10 ms					
−	0.5 μs	2200 μs	>1.6	98			
+	10 ms	90 ms	27	10	3.2	Cell electrophoretic mobility*	Taylor and Newman (1972)
+	20 μs	180 μs					
*+	10 ms	100 ms	27	105	6	Liver damage, rat	Taylor and Connolly (1969)
*++	150 μs	1500 μs					
*+++	20 μs	200 μs					

+ Shortest on-time for positive results.
− Longest on-time for negative results.
*+ Suprathreshold damage.
*++ Greater suprathreshold damage.
*+++ Greatest suprathreshold damage.
** The validity of the short-pulse data has been questioned by Joshi et al. (1973).

the establishment of cavitation and the optimum interval between pulses is 100 ms. Under these conditions, bubbles may recycle continuously through resonant size.

In summary, for a fixed on-intensity, pulses of around 10 ms duration, separated by intervals of not more than about 400 ms, may summate so that the cumulative effect increases with the on-time. Irradiation may become less damaging as the interval between the pulses is increased, even when the pulse duration is also increased. At 1 MHz, effects due to stable cavitation are most important when the pulse interval is around 100 ms, but they are suppressed by shortening the pulse duration to 1 ms or less, even when the on-intensity is increased. With a duty cycle of around 0·1, other effects, possibly due to mechanical stress, may remain cumulatively related to the on-time even when the pulse duration is reduced to 20 μs, and such short pulses may be more damaging than pulses of 150 μs duration. In this situation, an interval of around 200 μs between pulses may be most damaging, but here there are at present insufficient data concerning the effects of very short pulses.

9.11 OTHER INVESTIGATIONS OF BIOLOGICAL EFFECTS

9.11.a Production of Focal Lesions in Brain

Data are available principally from three laboratories, in Illinois, London and Massachusetts, concerning the relationship between intensity and single-pulse time duration necessary to produce threshold lesions in white matter of mammalian brain. Fry *et al.* (1970), of the Illinois group, have collected the data of J. B. Pond (London) and P. P. Lele (Massachusetts) and combined it with their own, to compile the graph reproduced in Fig. 9.9. There is remarkably good agreement between the results obtained in the different laboratories. Although no marked discontinuities exist in the intensity–time relationship, there are two (or possibly three) distinct mechanisms involved, one (or two) of which only become significant at intensities above particular levels.

Pond (1970) developed a method to calculate the temperature cycles at the centre of the focal volume of a pulsed ultrasonic beam irradiating brain tissue. He compared the lesions produced by ultrasound with those produced by thermal cycles generated by applying pulses of electric current to embedded resistance wires. At an intensity of 320 W cm^{-2} and a frequency of 3 MHz, with 3 s pulse durations, the temperature cycle was adequate to explain the lesion formation. Another model, due to Robinson and Lele (1972), has yielded similar results. Precooling the brain inhibits the production of lesions by ultrasound. Pond (1970) has pointed out, however, that under similar conditions, but with intensities of 720 W cm^{-2}

and beyond, the thermally induced lesions were significantly less marked than those due to ultrasound.

In the intensity range from 700 to approximately 1500 W cm^{-2}, the ultrasound is supposed to disrupt biological structure partly by mechanical means (e.g. stable cavitation), and the histological response to the ultrasonic irradiation has been described in great detail (Fry, 1958). Briefly, white matter exhibits the lowest threshold and the lesion results in demyelination of the axis cylinders. Grey matter is more resistant, and the dose must be increased by about 30% in order to produce lesions of the same volume. Glial structures and the vascular system are even more resistant, and, for threshold lesions, there is no interruption of the blood supply. In this

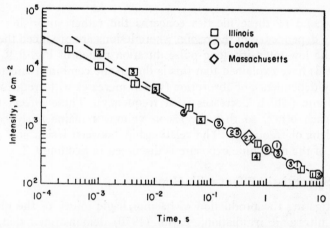

FIG. 9.9 The relationship between intensity and single-pulse time duration, for threshold lesion production in white matter of the mammalian brain, at various frequencies, as indicated in MHz. (From Fry et al., 1970.)

connexion, the effect of focused ultrasound on arteries has been studied by Fallon et al. (1972), who found that arterial tissue suffers severe damage at intensities comparable with threshold intensities for nervous tissue. They suggested that, in certain circumstances, nerve damage by ultrasound may well be a secondary phenomenon due to small vessel damage followed by ischaemic changes in the locality.

At intensities above about 2 kW cm^{-2}, and with pulse durations of less than 40 ms, the threshold lesion is probably partly due to transient cavitation. In this connexion, it has been suggested by Lele et al. (1974) that cavitation and heat due to ultrasonic irradiation might be synergistic. From Fig. 9.9, it can be seen that the dosage to produce a lesion in this region is greater at higher frequency, and this is in accord with cavitation phenomena (see Section 9.4.c). (The role of frequency has recently been studied in greater detail by Dunn *et al.* (1975).) These transient cavitation lesions differ significantly from those induced at lower intensities. Thus, they appear immediately (at lower intensities, about 10 min typically elapses between irradiation and the appearance of histological evidence of the lesion); they may not be found at the focus of the ultrasonic beam, but rather at interfaces between neural tissue and fluid-filled spaces; and they do not exhibit tissue selectivity.

There are two theoretical niceties which may be mentioned here in connexion with focal lesion formation. Firstly, it has been pointed out by Pierce (1973) that, for a given ultrasonic power at the transducer, the intensity at the focus may tend to decrease with time because the velocity in tissue increases with temperature. Typically, this intensity reduction might be 25%.

The second of these niceties concerns the rather surprising lack of frequency dependence in the region where lesions are produced thermally. This is the low-intensity, long-pulse duration region of Fig. 9.9. Lerner *et al.* (1973) have explained that this is due to the combined effects of the frequency dependence of absorption (which increases with frequency) and focal volume (which decreases with frequency). These effects tend to balance each other, so that the lesion volume remains fairly constant, independent of frequency. The relationship between lesion size and the duration of the ultrasonic exposure is discussed in Section 9.2.

9.11.b Synergistic Effect with Hypoxia

In investigating the production of haemorrhagic injury of the rat spinal cord by ultrasonic irradiation, Taylor (1970) demonstrated that, at 3·5 MHz, the presence of hypoxia decreased the exposure time required for injury by 40%. In subsequent experiments, Taylor and Pond (1972) studied the effect of changing the ultrasonic frequency. They used an on-intensity of 25 W cm^{-2}, with a pulse duration of 10 ms and a duty cycle of 0·09. The damaging ability (the reciprocal of the on-time required to cause damage) was greater in the presence of hypoxia by a factor of about 40% at frequencies in the range 0·5–3·5 MHz, but this enhancement rapidly became less with increasing frequency, and approached zero at 4·9 MHz.

9.11.c Synergistic Effect with Sterilizing Chemicals

The microorganism *Bacillus subtilis* is used to test the sporicidal activity of sterilizing systems. Glutaraldehyde (pentanedial) is commonly used in aqueous solution as a sterilising agent for surgical instruments. A 1% solution of glutaraldehyde is effective against a wet suspension of *B. subtilis* spores (10^7 ml^{-1}), in 60 min at pH 8 and 55°C, and in 10 min at pH 3·3 and 65°C. These times are reduced to 5 min and 4 min respectively in a cavitating 20 kHz ultrasonic field (Last and Boucher, 1973).

9.11.d Effect on Blood Flow

Dyson *et al.* (1971) described how the flow of blood through the vessels of a chick embryo at the 3·5 day stage of incubation may be arrested by the application of an ultrasonic field of 3 MHz frequency. The irradiation chamber used in this experiment has been described by Pond *et al.* (1971). It consisted of a trough with internal dimensions $160 \times 50 \times 6$ mm depth, containing saline. The transducer was a rectangular element of lead zirconate titanate, 30×5 mm in size; it was fixed at one end of the trough, the other end of which reflected the ultrasound to establish a standing wave field. The particulate matter—mainly red cells—within the arrested blood aggregated into clumps arranged into vertical planes at right angles to the direction of propagation of the ultrasound. These aggregates were spaced at half wavelength intervals throughout the field. The cause of the effect has not fully been explained, although Dyson *et al.* (1974) have discussed several possibilities, and it has been pointed out by Nyborg and Gershoy (1974) that acoustic streaming, which gives rise to inter-particle forces of attraction, may contribute to the tendency of the cells to form aggregates. A detailed analysis has been made by Gould and Coakley (1974). Wladimiroff and Talbert (1973) have pointed out an interesting aspect of the phenomenon: the velocity in the erythrocytes aggregated into the bands is greater than that in the fluid in which they are suspended, and the resultant refraction may account for the small instabilities which have been observed in the striations.

The intensity required to produce stasis may be less than $0·5$ W cm^{-2}, depending on the diameter of the blood vessel and the undisturbed flow velocity. The intensity threshold at any given site is proportional to the heart rate (Dyson and Pond, 1973). The stability of the arrested blood depends on the orientation of the ultrasonic field: it has been demonstrated by Baker (1972) that, if the wave is horizontal, the cells tend to fall downwards along the bands in which they are trapped. In general, the phenomenon is reversible, although some small vessels do remain blocked with immobile blood cells. Moreover, the endothelial lining of some blood vessels is damaged by the irradiation, the most usual form of damage being to the cell membrane on the luminal aspect of the endothelial cell.

The phenomenon may have at least two serious consequences. Firstly, there is the possible hazard of a reduction in the oxygenation of surrounding tissues. In the chick, for example, it is even possible to arrest the flow in the embryonic ventricles during diastole (Taylor and Dyson, 1972). Secondly, there is the possibility that Doppler blood flow detectors used in diagnostics may emit ultrasound of sufficient intensity to interfere with the flow which they are being used to measure.

9.11.e Effects on Malignant Tissues

In concluding their paper on the effects of ultrasonic irradiation at megahertz frequencies on normal and neoplastic tissues in the intact mouse, Southam *et al.* (1953) wrote "These studies give no reason to believe that ultrasonic energy might be useful in the treatment of inoperable neoplastic disease of man". Likewise, Cerino *et al.* (1966) demonstrated that the effects of heat and ultrasound (frequency 0·5–0·75 MHz) on a particular type of bone tumour are similar. They also showed that, under their experimental conditions, the effect of a rise in temperature of 13 degK for 10 min was far greater than the effect of an ultrasonic field with intense cavitation in the relative absence of heat.

It has been suggested that simultaneous irradiation with ultrasound increases the efficacy of ionizing radiation in the treatment of cancer. Thus, Lehmann and Krusen (1955) found a substantial reduction in the X-ray dosage required to produce regression of a given type of experimental tumour, when simultaneously irradiated with ultrasound at a frequency of 1 MHz and at an intensity of 8·4 W cm^{-2}. They concluded that the effect was due to heat produced within the tumour by the absorption of the ultrasound.

Woeber (1965) reported a striking increase in the regression of experimental tumours simultaneously treated by X-rays and ultrasound, in comparison with those treated by X-rays alone. The X-ray dose to produce a given regression was reduced by a factor of up to 1·7. He also described the improvement in the therapy of superficial cancer in man, which resulted from simultaneous ultrasonic and X-irradiation. He considered that 80% of this improvement was due to heat, and 20%, to some unspecified mechanical effect.

The synergism between ultrasound and X-rays in tumour therapy has been further investigated by Clarke *et al.* (1970). They carried out experiments both *in vitro*, using mouse lymphoma cells irradiated in gelled suspension culture, and *in vivo* using implanted tumours in rats: 1 MHz ultrasound was used at intensities of 5 and 1 W cm^{-2} respectively in the two experiments, and care was taken to minimize changes in temperature. In the gel experiments, treatments of 5 min were given, concurrently with X-ray doses of 1·0, 1·5, 2·0, 3·0 and 4·0 Gy; in the rats, the treatments were of 35 min duration, with 20 Gy of X-rays. In addition, various combinations of irradiation modalities were investigated. Under these conditions, no significant evidence for synergism could be found; the upper limits for dose modification factors in the two experiments were 1·2 and 1·3 respectively.

There is evidence that there is a useful therapeutic ratio between at least some forms of cancer and normal tissue when exposed to heat treatment (Muckle 1974). Whilst ultrasound, either alone or in combination with ionizing radiation, may have little to contribute to cancer therapy through its non-thermal effects, it may be that some tumours could be more easily heated by ultrasound, with its directional and focusing properties, than by other means. This possibility is of great potential importance, and it deserves investigation.

In connexion with the treatment of malignant brain tumours, Heimburger et al. (1975) have suggested that ultrasound may act synergistically to improve the effectiveness of chemotherapy. This suggestion was based on the results of the treatment of four patients, who were irradiated with ultrasound (3 W cm^{-2}, 1 MHz, through a bone flap port) simultaneously with the administration of chemotherapy. These authors admit, however, only a longer series with considerable improvement in survival could confirm that the method has any significant advantage.

A rather surprising phenomenon has been reported by Gavrilov et al. (1975). Tests on mice with transplanted sarcoma 37 malignant tumours indicated that preliminary irradiation of the tumour with 1 MHz ultrasound in the intensity range 0·5–2·5 W cm^{-2} for periods of 1–5 min enhanced the sensitivity of its cells to the subsequent action of γ-radiation. For example, in comparison with matched controls, there was nearly a threefold increase in the proportion of resolved tumours, the growth rate of the remaining tumours was reduced by 30%, and the 25 day mortality fell from 42 to 10%, in mice treated first with ultrasound for 3 min at 0·5 W cm^{-2}, followed after 7 min by 3·5 Gy delivered in 4·8 min. (Although discovered in another context, it may be relevant that water previously irradiated at 800 kHz for 1 min at 1 W cm^{-2} reduces the viscosity of synovial fluid more than the addition of an equal quantity of untreated water: see Pospíšilová (1968).) Whatever the biophysical basis of these encouraging results, it is clear that this approach to cancer treatment should be thoroughly investigated.

9.11.f Effect on Tissue Regeneration

The stimulation of tissue regeneration by ultrasound has been reported by Dyson et al. (1968). They measured the rate of repair of experimental wounds consisting of 10 mm square holes made in the ears of rabbits. This technique allowed the progress of regeneration to be studied quantitatively without additional trauma, and the external nature of the wound simplified the irradiation procedure. In each animal, the healing process in the wound of the untreated ear was compared with that in the ear which was irradiated by ultrasound. The equipment which was used has been described by Pond and Dyson (1967). The frequency was 3·6 MHz. Each treatment lasted 5 min, and three treatments were given each week. The intensity was either 0·1 W cm^{-2} continuously applied, or lay within the range 0·25–8 W cm^{-2} pulsed at various duty cycles. The regeneration rates of the irradiated wounds were significantly more rapid than those of the controls. The maximum mean growth increase, which was about 1·3 times that of the control, was found 21 days after treatment at 0·5 W cm^{-2}, pulsed 2 ms on, 8 ms off. It was shown that the corresponding temperature rise was about 1·5 degK, and this was presumably too small an increase to account for the observed effects. It was suggested that streaming may play an important part in the process.

9.11.g Effect on Cell Surface Charge

A reduction in the electrophoretic mobility of Ehrlich cells, after irradiation with ultrasound, was reported by Repacholi et al. (1971). Suspended cells were exposed to 1 MHz ultrasound, on-intensity 10 W cm^{-2}, pulse duration 10 ms, duty cycle 0·1, for periods of 5 min. This resulted in a 15% reduction in mobility. 10 Gy of 220 kV X-rays gave the same reduction; combined treatment gave a reduction of 30%. Taylor and Newman (1972) extended these experiments, varying the ultrasonic frequency, the irradiation time, the pulsing parameters, and the hydrostatic pressure: the detailed results are recorded in Sections 9.9 and 9.10. It was suggested that the mechanism of this effect did not involve cavitation, particularly as it was uninhibited by an increase of 70% in the applied pressure, and occurred with pulses even as short as 20 μs. In a series of similar experiments with mouse lymphoma cells, however, Joshi et al. (1973) were unable to reproduce the results of the earlier investigators. Using a frequency of 2 MHz, they found that there was no effect on cell electrophoretic mobility either when the applied pressure was doubled, or when pulse durations of 20 μs were used. Only under conditions conducive to cavitation was the electrophoretic mobility reduced. Furthermore, reduction in the mobility of an irradiated cell population was found to be accompanied by an approximately proportional degree of cell disintegration, but the surviving population was unaffected in its ability to proliferate, and its mobility was found to return to normal within 48 h of irradiation. The finding that cavitation is required for this effect implies that it is most unlikely to occur in vivo under normal therapeutic or diagnostic conditions of exposure (see Section 9.4.c).

9.11.h Effect on Recalcification Time

It has been shown by Williams (1974) that ultrasonic irradiation of platelet-rich plasma, by means of a transversely oscillating wire at a frequency of 20 kHz, results in an increase in the rate of release of serotonin. There appears to be no intensity threshold for this effect, the response being proportional to the square of the wire-displacement amplitude. This relationship indicates that hydrodynamic shear stress due to velocity gradient is the mechanism, and suggests that it might occur at megahertz frequencies. In this connexion, the following is the published abstract of a paper on the subject presented by A. R. Williams and W. D. O'Brien at a Colloquium on Ultrasound Bioeffects and Dosimetry, held in July 1974 at Imperial College, London:

The recalcification time of platelet rich plasma, PRP, was decreased following ultrasonic irradiation. Fresh human blood, anticoagulated with citrate, was spun gently for 10 min to obtain PRP which was then incubated at room temperature for an hour to oversensitize the clotting system. The PRP was irradiated in a siliconized, cylindrical pyrex chamber (inside diameter 11 mm, volume 1·5 ml), with its ends covered with Saran Wrap. The chamber was immersed in a water bath and positioned on axis with the Saran Wrap window closest to the transducer 25 mm from the transducer. The 38 mm diameter, 1 MHz, PZT4 transducer was operated at its fundamental frequency. The intensities reported are spatially averaged over the area which the Saran Wrap occupies but determined in the absence of the chamber. Four exposure conditions have been examined, viz., 65 mW cm^{-2}, 330 mW cm^{-2}, 770 mW cm^{-2} and 1·5 W cm^{-2}, each for 5 min. Following ultrasonic irradiation, the recalcification time irreversibly decreased from the control value to an asymptotic level which was 8–20% lower. This asymptote was reached within 30 min following irradiation. It is believed that the ultrasound affects the initiation of the clotting process by stimulating the release of platelet factor 3, a heterogeneous population of phospholipids found within the secretory granules and non-vesicular membranes of intact platelets, which is a potent clot initiating and promoting factor.

In a personal communication, A. R. Williams and W. D. O'Brien were unable to make a positive statement as to the presence or absence of a dose–effect relationship in their observations. A complication in these preliminary results was due to the intake, by some of the female blood donors, of oral contraceptives: this has the effect of reducing the recalcification time by a factor of about two. Moreover, Williams (1974) has pointed out that there is no unambiguous information available on the *in vivo* clinical hazard of thrombi due to the release of small quantities of human platelet pro-coagulation factors. It is probable that for the healthy individual the risk of thrombus formation due to diagnostic ultrasonic irradiation (see Section 9.12) is no greater than that following moderate exercise where the increased hydrodynamic trauma within the circulation undoubtedly disrupts the most fragile platelets.

Williams (1975) has successfully tested his suggestion that thrombi may be formed in blood vessels by the direct application of localized, low frequency (25–80 kHz) vibrations to the outer surface of the surgically exposed vessel. Quite low amplitudes ($\sim 10 \ \mu$m) cause thrombi within about 5 min, as a result of local turbulence. This may provide a useful model in experimental measurements of the efficacy of anticoagulant therapy.

9.11.i Evidence of Genetic Effects

(i) DNA degradation

Ultrasonic irradiation of DNA in solution can result in a reduction in molecular weight by a non-random process of mechanical shearing. The matter is discussed in Section 9.7. Incorporated within the cell, however, it seems unlikely that shearing would preferentially act on DNA, but rather that the whole of the cell contents would be disorganized. Also, the viscosity of cytoplasm is substantially greater than that of water, and so it is certain that a greater intensity would be required to establish a given velocity gradient.

(ii) Chromosome damage

Thacker (1973) has reviewed many of the papers, published up to 1972, concerning the effect of ultrasound on chromosomes. Amongst the data not considered in that review, mention should be made of the reports of Šlotova et al. (1967) that an increase in chromosome aberrations was observed in the cells of the meristem of *Vicia faba* following ultrasonic irradiation at 800 kHz, and that this increase was independent of intensity in the range $0 \cdot 2$–3 W cm^{-2}, and of irradiation time in the range 1–20 min. The frequencies of the aberrations in the large and small chromosomes were proportional to the corresponding total metaphase lengths. On the other hand, Hill et al. (1972) found no significant increase in the chromosome aberration rate in Chinese hamster cells, following exposure for 1 or 2 h to 1 MHz ultrasound at an on-intensity of 150 W cm^{-2}, 50 μs pulse duration, duty cycle $0 \cdot 05$. Also Galperin-Lemaitre et al. (1973) found that $0 \cdot 87$ MHz ultrasound at 1–$1 \cdot 5$ W cm^{-2}, with an exposure of 2–5 min, did not damage bone-marrow chromosomes. In contrast, Serr et al. (1971) concluded that there was some suggestion (not statistically significant) that chromosome damage may occur in foetal cells obtained by amniocentesis following irradiation for 10 h at 22 mW cm^{-2} (at the transducer) at a frequency of 6 MHz. On the other hand, Ikeuchi et al. (1973) found no evidence of embryonic chromosome damage in foetuses irradiated at 40 mW cm^{-2}, 2 MHz, for 5 min, before therapeutic abortion.

In addition to these reports, there has been much interest in the effect of ultrasonic irradiation on human lymphocyte chromosomes. Macintosh and Davey (1970) reported that 22–50 aberrations per 100 cells occurred in human blood cultures exposed to ultrasound for 1 or 2 h at a frequency of $2 \cdot 25$ MHz, and at intensities of 8–17 mW cm^{-2}. The corresponding incidence in unirradiated cells was 5 aberrations per 100. More detailed data (Macintosh and Davey, 1972) seemed to indicate a threshold intensity of 8·2 mW cm^{-2} for zero increase in chromosome damage, with a linear increase in aberration frequency with the logarithm of the intensity, at greater intensities. The aberrations were predominantly in the chromatids. This is inexplicable, since the lymphocytes in the peripheral blood are in the G_1 stage of the mitotic cycle, and if the chromosomes are broken by a mutagen they should react as if they are single-stranded (Wolff, 1968). When the chromosomes are seen at the next mitosis, the aberrations are seen in the chromosome rather than the chromatid.

These reports led to the publication or rediscovery of many papers reporting failures to reproduce these results (Fischer et al., 1967; Abdulla et al., 1971; Bobrow et al., 1971; Boyd et al., 1971; Coakley et al., 1971; Buckton and Baker, 1972; Coakley et al., 1972; Rott et al., 1972; Watts et al., 1972; Watts and Stewart, 1972; Brock et al., 1973; Mermut et al., 1973; Braeman et al., 1974): many of these experiments were carried out at much higher intensities and with longer irradiation times than were used by Macintosh and Davey (1970, 1972). Inconclusive data were reported by Bugnon et al. (1972). Apparently the only other positive results are those of Kunze-Mühl and Golob (1972) and Fischman (1973). Kunze-Mühl and Golob (1972) reported an increase in the number of chromosome aberrations in cells irradiated at 2 MHz for 1 h at an intensity of 20 mW cm^{-2}, but this could be ascribed to experimental technique. Fischman (1973) reported a significant increase in chromosome aberrations irradiated at 1·3 MHz for 2 min, at intensities of 22 and 40 W cm^{-2}, in an asynchronous population of human lymphocytes.

Controversy raged for four years from 1970: in retrospect, the matter was probably given undue importance, for, as Thacker (1973) pointed out, it seems likely that most chromosome lesions due to ultrasound are lethal, and that genetic damage does not occur. In any event, however, the matter was resolved, possibly as far as it ever could be, in a lecture given by I. J. C. Macintosh at Colloquium on Ultrasound Bioeffects and Dosimetry, held in July 1974 at Imperial College London. His lecture was entitled "Failure to reproduce chromosome aberration attributed to ultrasound". The abstract, published in the programme, reads as follows:

Experiments performed in Cape Town have been repeated using the original apparatus and conditions. Published experiments using a modified Doptone apparatus operating at 2·25 MHz, as well as unpublished experiments at 1 MHz, under conditions which included cavitation, were repeated. No evidence of chromosome damage was found.

Details of these experiments have subsequently been published (Macintosh et al., 1975).

(iii) Cell proliferation

An aqueous suspension of mouse leukaemia cells exposed to 1 MHz ultrasound, at 15 W cm^{-2} spatial peak, for 10 s, has been shown to be most susceptible to damage in the M-phase of the cell cycle (Clarke and Hill, 1969). This phase is the period of mitosis. There seem to be two possible explanations. Either the cells surviving the ultrasonic irradiation have been modified in a manner affecting their progress through the cell cycle, or there may be some variation in cell fragility around the cell cycle. That the latter is the case has been established by the observation that cell death occurs immediately after irradiation, rather than being a delayed effect. The increased fragility may be a result of the changes which take place in the cell wall and the internal organization of the cell during mitosis. Likewise Loch *et al.* (1971) found that proliferation of cultured human cells *in vitro* was inhibited by 10 min exposure to 870 kHz ultrasound at intensities above 0·1 W cm^{-2}, whereas exposure to pulsed ultrasound from a diagnostic instrument (2·5 MHz, 0·01 W cm^{-2} mean intensity) for up to 45 min was without effect. Here is a clearly defined threshold: whether the supra-threshold biological effects are thermal or non-thermal has not yet been established. An example of sub-threshold irradiation has been described by Brown and Coakley (1975), who exposed gelled suspensions of *Acanth-amoeba* to 1 MHz ultrasound at continuous and pulsed intensity-time régimes which would result in lesions in solid tissues. Samples from logarithmically growing and from synchronous cultures were treated both in free field and standing waves. No difference was observed in the growth of treated and control samples.

There were early fears that ultrasonic examination might affect the growth of amniotic-fluid cells in culture. Mahoney and Hobbins (1973), however, found no effect following irradiation with a conventional pulse–echo machine, and Robinson (1973) considers that this possibility may be discounted.

Bleaney *et al.* (1972) irradiated suspensions of Chinese hamster lung cells with 1·5 MHz ultrasound. On-intensities of up to 15 W cm^{-2} were used, and the exposure conditions ranged from continuous waves for up to 1 h, to pulses of 1 ms duration with duty cycles of down to 0·14. There was no evidence of stable cavitation occurring in the samples. When the temperature remained below 45°C, there was no reduction in cell survival. Any reduction in survival was always associated with a lethal temperature, resulting from absorption of the ultrasonic energy in the polyethylene containers used to hold the cells during irradiation. It was considered that ultrasound has no direct effect on cell reproductive integrity.

Further evidence of the inhibiting effect of ultrasound on mitotic activity has been published by Serr *et al.* (1971). They found a great reduction in mitosis in human foetal fibroblasts *in vitro*, as a result of irradiation for 10 h at 2·2 MHz, either at 1 or 2 W cm⁻². Brock *et al.* (1973) reported similar results with human blood cultures. Using 1·9 MHz ultrasound at an intensity of 0·06 W cm⁻² to irradiate the liver in rat for 5 min, Kremkau and Witcofski (1974) found a reduction of 20–80% in mitotic index.

Root growth in seedlings of the broad bean, *Vicia faba*, results from division of cells in the meristem, which remains approximately constant in size, producing cells for differentiation and elongation. This normal growth pattern may be modified by ionizing radiation (Hall, 1963): the dividing cells are damaged so that the growth, which typically remains unchanged for the first day following irradiation, falls to a minimum at about five days, and then increases gradually back to the same rate as unirradiated

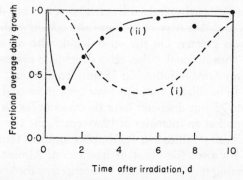

FIG. 9.10 Variation of average daily growth of *Vicia faba* roots (expressed as the fraction of the corresponding average growth for control roots of the same age) following irradiation. (i) X-rays, 1·25 Gy; (ii) ultrasound, 1·5 MHz, 3 W cm⁻², 15 min. (From Bleaney and Oliver, 1972.)

roots after about 10 days. In this context, "growth" is defined as the ratio of the increase in root length in the irradiated group to that in the control group of the same age.

The results of a comparison between the effects on growth of an exposure to ionizing radiation and ultrasound are shown in Fig. 9.10. In contrast to the effects of ionizing radiation, following ultrasonic irradiation the growth rate falls to a minimum in the first day after exposure, and recovers gradually to the control value over eight days. Bleaney and Oliver (1972) investigated the effects of several ultrasonic exposures, and concluded that the interference with growth increased with both exposure time and ultrasonic intensity. These results indicate that cells sterilized by ultrasound are not able to undergo any division, and the radiation damage becomes immediately apparent in relation to growth. Furthermore, the response was shown to be unchanged if the exposure was split into two fractions, separated by 24 h. This indicates that sublethal damage is not repaired during this interval.

The results of Bleaney and Oliver (1972) have been substantially reproduced in a more extensive series of experiments by Gregory *et al.* (1974). They used a frequency of 2 MHz, and a rather complicated time–dose distribution, but they did not test the inability to repair sublethal damage. They did notice, however, that ultrasonic irradiation was followed by a reduction in lateral root formation and mitotic index. Likewise Hering and Shepstone (1972) reported similar modification of the growth of roots of *Zea mays*: their experiments, at 1 MHz, included observations with both continuous wave irradiation, and with pulses of 2 ms duration, duty cycle 0·2. They found that similar responses resulted from 30 min exposures to continuous waves of 0·62 W cm^{-2}, and to pulses of 0·21 W cm^{-2} average intensity. This indicates that pulsed irradiation was more damaging under these conditions, and this may be because the corresponding on-intensity (1·05 W cm^{-2}) was greater. On the other hand, with an even higher on-intensity from a conventional pulse–echo diagnostic system, Hering *et al.* (1974) observed no damage following 15 min irradiation.

Temperatures in irradiated root tips have been measured by Eames *et al.* (1975), with 50 or 75 μm diameter bare thermocouples. When exposed to 2·3 MHz ultrasound at an intensity of 10 W cm^{-2}, the temperatures of the root tips rose to limiting values 3–6 degK above ambient temperature (about 23°C) within 2–4 s after the onset of irradiation. Almost the same time course of root heating may be obtained by immersing the root tip in a warm bath. Whilst the growth rate was modified by ultrasonic irradiation for 1 min under these conditions, heating for the same time even to 12 degK above the same ambient temperature did not affect the growth rate.

The initial rate of change of temperature in response to an ultrasonic wave depends only on the acoustic absorption coefficient. The measurements of Eames *et al.* (1975) indicate that $\alpha = 10$ dB cm^{-1} at 2·3 MHz in the root tip; this is five times greater than the absorption in typical mammalian soft tissues (see Section 4.4). Plant tissues may have a high acoustic absorption because of intercellular air spaces and cellulose walls. Moreover, the presence of these air spaces may enhance streaming (see Section 9.7), and this might be the mechanism by which the growth rate is reduced in botanical preparations. This conclusion is supported by the observations of Leeman *et al.* (1975) that growth-rate inhibition is more marked at 1·5 MHz than at 3 MHz; this is the opposite to the trend which would be expected with a thermal mechanism.

(iv) Mutagenesis and teratogenesis

Wallace *et al.* (1948) irradiated various botanical materials and young adult *Drosophila*. The frequency which was used was 400 kHz, and the power, determined calorimetrically, was 150 W. Various growth abnormalities were observed in the treated specimens. Unfortunately, these data are not very useful because the physical conditions of the experiment are not clearly stated in the article. The physical conditions in the experiments of Fritz-Niggli and Böni (1950) are better defined. Using a frequency of 800 kHz and intensities between 0·4–4 W cm^{-2}, they irradiated specimens of *Drosophila* in a water-filled tube. The damage produced depended on the stage of development of the animal at irradiation, and evidence was presented which was alleged to show that the effects on survival were closer to those of ionizing radiation than to those of heat. They were unable to demonstrate that ultrasound could increase the mutation rate. Selman and Counce (1953), on the other hand, demonstrated developmental abnormalities in *Drosophila* following the irradiation of eggs on agar discs in a water medium, using a frequency of 1 MHz and an exposure of 30 s, with intensities between 0·3 and 0·5 W cm^{-2}.

The article by Kato (1966), in which mutations of *Drosophila* were reported, unfortunately contains inadequate data concerning the irradiation conditions. Apparently adult flies were irradiated: it is not clear how this could have been done at a frequency of 560 kHz, since the animals cannot be immersed for long periods.

Using exposure conditions far greater than those experienced in contemporary diagnostic procedures, Thacker (1974) concluded that abnormal genetic effects generally did not occur in irradiated yeast cells, even when the cells were killed to 0·1% of the survival of the controls. This seems to be a consequence of the all-or-none response of cells to ultrasound. Because of the difficulties inherent in extrapolation, however, he considered that tests should be carried out on genetically well-defined multicellular organisms in order to assess the risk in man. Likewise Combes (1975) found no increase in the back-mutation of an auxotrophic strain of *Bacillus subtilis* following irradiation for 5 min with 2 MHz ultrasound at up to 60 W cm^{-2} on-intensity, pulse duration 20 μs, duty cycle 0·004. Moreover he was unable to detect mutagenic lesions after *in vitro* irradiation of transforming DNA. Like Thacker (1974), he also suggested that tests using genetic systems of higher organisms are necessary to assess possible effects in man.

Taylor and Dyson (1974) have examined chick embryos for abnormalities following ultrasonic irradiation. Great care was taken to ensure that the control and irradiated groups were identical in all respects except for irradiation. Scoring was blind. These precautions are of crucial importance —and so they are in many other experiments. At 1 MHz, the ultrasound was pulsed: the pulse duration was 20 μs, and the duty cycle was 0·1. Early embryos, corresponding to about three weeks development in man, were affected by exposures of 5 min to on-intensities of 25 W cm^{-2}, but not of 10 W cm^{-2}. Slightly older embryos, corresponding in development to about six weeks human gestation, were unaffected even at an on-intensity of 100 W cm^{-2}. Likewise, irradiation at a frequency of 2·2 MHz for 24 h from a Doppler diagnostic instrument (electrical input power 100 mW cm^{-2}) was without effect on developing embryos.

Smyth (1966) found no congenital abnormalities in 348 offspring of mice irradiated at 2·3 MHz, 10 mW cm^{-2}, over extended periods of time. Likewise Warwick et al. (1970) found no change in gestation time, foetal weight, litter size, incidence of resorptions, or abnormalities, in the foetuses of 223 mice irradiated at megahertz frequencies at on-intensities of up to 490 W cm^{-2}, and average intensities of up to 27 W cm^{-2}, in comparison with 132 unirradiated controls. Somewhat similar results were obtained by Bang (1971). Negative results have also been reported by McClain et al. (1972), who searched for changes in litter size, foetal weight, resorptions, and foetal soft tissue and skeletal abnormalities, following the irradiation of pregnant rats during the period day 8–13 of gestation, with 2·5 MHz ultrasound at 10 mW cm^{-2} with exposures of 30 min or 2 h. The results of Shoji et al. (1971), however, are less reassuring. They irradiated the foetuses of anaesthetized mice for 5 h with 2·25 MHz ultrasound at an intensity of 40 mW cm^{-2}, on the ninth day of gestation. These animals, together with unirradiated controls, were sacrificed on day 18 of gestation. All living foetuses were examined for the occurrence of gross external malformations. The resorption sites and placental remnants were considered to correspond to dead foetuses. Although an increase in foetal abnormality was found in the irradiated group when compared with control groups, the difference was not significant; the increase in foetal mortality was significant. Measurements of body weight did not reveal any growth-inhibiting effect. One foetus with exencephaly did occur in the irradiated group. This abnormality was not found in 1797 living foetuses derived from 272 untreated mice, although it has been demonstrated in many experiments with X-rays and other teratogenic treatments. It is a worrying result: the only comfort is that it has not been repeated in independent experiments. Earlier negative results have already been mentioned. Since the publication by Shoji et al. (1971, 1972)—which first received attention in the Western world in the summer of 1973—Mannor et al. (1972) have reported that they found no differences between the abnormality rates in the foetuses, or in subsequent brother–sister crossmatings, in unirradiated mice and in mice irradiated at 2·28 MHz, at up to 1·05 W cm^{-2} for up to 60 min per day for up to five days, between day 8–20 of gestation. Likewise, mice between the ages of one to seven days were ultrasonically irradiated at a frequency of 1 MHz by Kirsten et al. (1963). Whole body irradiation was administered, either continuously or in pulses, at on-intensities ranging from 0·14 to 10 W cm^{-2}, for periods of 5 min. Burning and paralysis occurred in some animals. The unaffected mice were bred brother–cross–sister for six litters, and the average litter size was comparable with that of the control group.

Garrison *et al.* (1973) reported that normal development occurred in rats in which the ovaries were exposed to ultrasound for 10 min each on day 8 of pregnancy. There was no effect on resorption rate. In three experiments, the effects of two dose régimes were tested: 10 W cm^{-2} on-intensity, 10 ms pulse duration, 0·1 duty cycle; and 100 W cm^{-2} on-intensity, 0·6 ms pulse duration, 0·006 duty cycle. Since the ovaries are essential for the maintenance of pregnancy in the rat, it may be concluded that the function of the ovaries was unaffected by the particular conditions of irradiation to which they were exposed.

Tests for genetic damage in mice have been made by Lyon and Simpson (1974). The gonads of anaesthetized, submersed animals were exposed to 1·5 MHz ultrasound for 15 min. The exposures used were 1·6 W cm^{-2} continuous wave; 6·4 W cm^{-2} on-intensity, pulse duration 1 ms, duty cycle 0·25; and 45 W cm^{-2} on-intensity, pulse duration 30 μs, duty cycle 0·02. The results were compared with those from similarly anaesthetized and submersed animals, both unirradiated controls and exposed to 1·0 Gy of X-rays in air. In comparison with the control group, the males in the ultrasonic group showed no evidence of induction of dominant lethal mutations or sterility, no change in testis weight or sperm count, and no induction of translocations or chromosome fragments in spermatocytes, for up to at least eight weeks after treatment. Similarly in the females there was no evidence of dominant lethal induction in the period from several days before mating to the day of mating. On the other hand, genetic damage was observed in the animals treated with X-rays. Sterile matings among females —as distinct from genetic damage—were significantly increased in animals treated both with pulsed ultrasound at 45 W cm^{-2} on-intensity, one to several days prior to mating, and with continuous waves on the day of mating. Thus, the irradiations were near the maximum that could be used without sterilizing the animals. These results indicate that it is unlikely that antenatal ultrasonic diagnosis presents any genetic hazards to mother or foetus.

(v) *Other evidence*

Several investigators have sought to discover biological changes following the irradiation of various living systems with ultrasonic energy from instruments designed for diagnostic purposes. Entirely negative results were obtained by French *et al.* (1951), Donald *et al.* (1958), Garg and Taylor (1967), and Kohorn *et al.* (1967), in experiments on brain tissues. Similarly, Andrew (1964) irradiated samples of frog and perch spawn for periods of up to 24 h, apparently without effect.

Smyth (1966) was unable to demonstrate any change in behaviour, brain tissue, liver, gonads or heart of rats and mice exposed for periods of up to 2 h to pulsed ultrasound with a mean power of 10 mW cm^{-2} at 2·3 MHz. Likewise, using an instrument designed for ultrasonic diagnosis (2 MHz, 5 mW cm^{-2}: presumably the average intensity of a pulsed beam), Baethman *et al.* (1974) irradiated the brains of 10 craniotomized rats for 2 h each. These brains were examined following sacrifice 24 h after irradiation. In a second experimental group, the blood–brain barrier was assessed 24 h after irradiation. No significant changes were found in the electrolyte and water balances, nor in the blood–brain permeability to proteins. In an extension of this kind of investigation to man, Ford (1974) has reported the results of pathological investigations of the brains of 24 neurological and neurosurgical patients who had had multiple ultrasonic pulse–echo examinations of the brain at up to 120 days before death. He concluded that if diagnostic ultrasound does cause changes in brain tissue, then these changes must at worst only be slight.

There have been several attempts to detect harmful effects of ultrasonic irradiation by means of epidemiological studies of populations exposed to diagnostic procedures. Thus, Bernstine (1969) found no effects due to ultrasonic irradiation, either in various tissue cultures exposed for up to 18 h to 6 MHz ultrasound at 20–30 mW cm^{-2}, or in abnormality rate in 720 babies who had been exposed to ultrasound *in utero* for Doppler detection of the foetal heart. Similarly, clinical follow-up of 150 babies subjected to short duration ultrasonic irradiation for Doppler detection of the foetal heart *in utero* did not reveal any change in the expected rate of abnormality (Serr *et al.*, 1971). In what seems to be the most extensive study of this kind, Hellman *et al.* (1970) pooled the data from the diagnostic investigation of 1114 apparently normal pregnancies, in Glasgow, Lund and New York. The incidence of foetal abnormalities in the irradiated group was 2·7%; in a separate and unmatched survey of women who had not had ultrasonic diagnosis, the corresponding figure was 4·8%. These results principally serve not so much to inspire confidence in the safety of ultrasonic diagnosis —although they give no cause for alarm—but rather to highlight two perplexingly difficult problems in this kind of epidemological survey. Firstly, where ultrasonic diagnosis is available, both pregnant women and their doctors demand its use: interpreted at the extreme, this means that matched groups, irradiated and non-irradiated, cannot ethically be separated, thus making a randomized controlled trial impossible. Secondly, the use of ultrasonic diagnosis is one aspect of a high standard of medical care, and it may be that this is associated with a lowering in the foetal abnormality rate: therefore comparison with an unmatched group, with a generally lower standard of care, is not helpful.

(vi) Conclusions

The data in this Sub-section may be summarized as follows:

(i) It seems unlikely that ultrasound can cause genetic damage;

(ii) Chromosome damage, if it does occur as a result of ultrasonic irradiation, is likely to be lethal;

(iii) Ultrasonic damage to DNA is unlikely selectively to occur in cells;

(iv) Where mutations due to ultrasound do occur, they are likely to be caused by thermal shock;

(v) There is some evidence of ultrasonically induced teratogenesis (abnormal development induced by direct action on the embryo, rather than being mediated by hereditary change), and this requires further investigation; and

(vi) Ultrasonic irradiation inhibits growth by an all-or-none effect on the cell, which seems to be more susceptible during mitosis; there is no recovery process, such as occurs following damage by ionizing radiation.

9.11.j Effects on Plants

The literature is replete with generally hazy accounts of the "effects" of ultrasound on plant material. The subject has been reviewed by Gordon (1971). Evidently in this mass of data there are seldom enough concerned either with the physical conditions of the irradiations or with the physiological conditions of the tissues.

About three-quarters of the reports deal with the effect of ultrasound on the germination of seeds. One of the mechanisms involved seems to be acceleration of the entry of water into the seed. There is a tendency for the postharvest dormancy period to be reduced, provided that ultrasonic cavitation does not occur, and it seems that the rate of germination (i.e. the proportion of seeds which germinate) may be increased. The growth rate has also been alleged to be increased but this seems strange in relation to the effects on cell proliferation discussed in Section 9.11.i.iii. There are some claims that there may be an increase in marketable products, and that plants may mature or flower earlier. Mutations may also occur—see Section 9.11.i.iv.

It should be clear enough, from the vagueness of the evidence, that this subject requires—and probably deserves—a thorough investigation.

9.12 POSSIBILITY OF HAZARD IN DIAGNOSTICS

It is possible to define pairs of zones on charts of intensity and time, such that in one zone the conditions have been shown to produce biological effects, and in the other, they have not. It should be noted that not all biological effects are damaging. Three such pairs of zones are illustrated in Fig. 9.11. The lines separating these zones are based on interpretations of literature surveys. Many of the data used in this connexion are discussed earlier in this Chapter, but some additional results have been incorporated. (The possibility that ultrasound may disrupt platelets and so cause thrombus formation (see Section 9.11.h) has been neglected, and so has the report of David *et al.* (1975) that foetal activity, as judged by the movement count, increased by more than 90% during routine monitoring with a

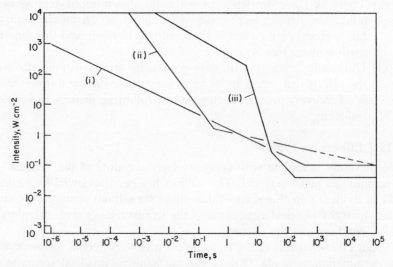

FIG. 9.11 Three pairs of exposure zones, showing "safe" and potentially hazardous conditions. Each line separates one pair of zones, the zone below the line being "safe". (i) Data of Ulrich (1971, 1974): the intensity is the average intensity (equal to the product of the on-intensity and the duty cycle), and the time is the total time of the exposure, including intervals between pulses if appropriate; (ii) data of Edmonds (1972), based on the envelope threshold of his Figs. 1–6; intensity and time generally defined as in (i); (iii) data of Wells (1974): the intensity is the on-intensity, and the time is the on-time.

continuous wave Doppler system. In view of the notorious sensitivity of the foetus to external stimuli (see, for example, Grimwade *et al.*, 1971), scepticism concerning the relevance of the ultrasound to the latter observation is understandable, and it seems reasonable not to give it too much attention.) In general, there are two schemes for classifying the exposure conditions: either the average intensity and the total time may be used, or the on-intensity and the on-time. In view of the evidence that ultrasonic damage may be cumulative (see Section 9.10), the latter scheme may be the better one; it is also more sensibly compatible with the concept of a "threshold" level of intensity, below which irradiation is incapable of affecting biological systems, no matter how long the on-time may be.

Since there is no general rule relating biological effectiveness to ultrasonic frequency (see Section 9.9), no attempt has been made here to separate data according to frequency in the range 1–15 MHz, so the conditions illustrated in Fig. 9.11 may be taken to apply in the usual diagnostic range. Moreover, there are no data to suggest whether long intervals of rest between exposures may be accompanied by the recovery of latent damage. Ulrich (1971) considered that his "safe" zone would be satisfactory in the case of an individual, for up to 10 exposures per month, and up to 30 exposures per year, provided that irradiation of the eye was excluded. On the other hand, Wells (1974) recommended no such exclusions, and considered that, for example, a Doppler detector operating at an intensity of less than 40 mW cm^{-2} could be used without time restriction, whereas a pulse–echo system operating with pulses of 0·7 μs duration and 30 W cm^{-2} on-intensity with a pulse repetition frequency of 1000 s^{-1} should not be used to examine any individual patient for a total time exceeding 5·5 h. Typical values of the output of various diagnostic systems are discussed in Section 6.14.

Once it has been recognized that a particular irradiation condition is potentially hazardous, the anatomical site of the irradiation becomes important. For example, it is more dangerous to irradiate a foetus *in utero*, than a blood vessel in an adult limb. Also, in scanning procedures, a particular tissue site may only be irradiated for a relatively small fraction of the total examination time.

In conclusion, it should be accepted that there is no simple answer to the question "is ultrasonic diagnosis safe?". Ultrasonic diagnostics depend upon the interactions between ultrasound and living tissues, and in certain circumstances these interactions may be destructive. Therefore there are only three situations in which the use of ultrasonic radiation to obtain information about function or structure in man could be justifiable. These are: firstly, in the ill or potentially ill patient, when the benefit which may accrue from the diagnostic data outweighs any forseeable risk; secondly, in situations where the risk is considered to be small, and it is ethically acceptable provided that it has been explained to, and accepted by, the patient; and thirdly—an alternative which present knowledge does not allow—when it is quite certain that the conditions of ultrasonic exposure are such that there is no risk.

9.13 EFFECTS OF AIRBORNE SOUND AND ULTRASOUND ON MAMMALS

A detailed discussion of this subject is beyond the scope of this book, but this short summary is included for completeness. For additional information, reference may be made to the articles by Knight (1967) and Acton (1974), which include quite extensive bibliographies.

It is convenient to express airborne sound and ultrasound intensities in decibels relative to a reference level. Intensities are then measured in dB SPL, the abbreviation SPL denoting the reference sound pressure level which is normally taken to be equal to 2×10^{-5} Pa. The principal hazard of airborne sound on man is that the intensity may be sufficient to produce either a temporary or a permanent shift to higher levels in the threshold of hearing. The damaging ability of a sound depends on its frequency, in roughly inverse proportion to the response of the ear. For this reason, a measure of intensity weighted according to this response may give an indication of hazard irrespective of the frequency. Such a weighted measurement is afforded by the dBA scale used in acoustics: Hill (1970) has discussed the matter, and set a level of 92 dBA as a practical damage risk criterion for occupational exposure to broad band noise. Where a monitor calibrated in dBA is not available, alternative maximum exposure levels have been proposed by Acton (1968): these are 74 dB SPL at frequencies below 16 kHz, increasing to 110 dB SPL at frequencies in the range 21–32 kHz. These conditions should prevent both auditory and subjective effects in the greater part of the population exposed over a working day. At higher intensities in the ultrasonic range, exposed individuals may suffer from fatigue, headache, nausea and vomiting. It does not seem to have been established, however, that these effects are actually due to ultrasound, and not to the audible noise which is usually generated in addition to the ultrasound, particularly in machines such as jet engines, or as a result of cavitation in a working liquid, or even to the cleaning liquids themselves!

The effects on small mammals cannot be extrapolated directly to man. The absorption of airborne ultrasound at 20 kHz is greater by a factor of about 200 if the body is covered with fur; the temperature control mechanism may be less effective in a small animal; and the lower ultrasonic frequencies may be audible to some small animals. Thus, whilst mouse, rat and guinea-pig are killed by exposures to 145–155 dB SPL, and rabbits, by 160–165 dB SPL, in man the lethal level is likely to be about 180 dB SPL.

9.14 BIOLOGICAL EFFECTS OF LOW-FREQUENCY VIBRATIONS

Low-frequency vibrations, in the frequency range 0·1–100 Hz, are strictly outside the scope of this book, and so only a brief note on their biological effects is included. Generally, man responds maximally to vibrations in the range 1–10 Hz, the response ranging from perception at an acceleration of around 0·002 gravity, through annoyance at 0·005 gravity, complaint at

0·01 gravity, tolerance limitation at 0·1 gravity, to pain at 3 gravity. Motion sickness occurs with vibration of around 0·5 Hz at an acceleration of 0·5 gravity. Vibration-induced disease is a syndrome of vasospasm and associated depression of the anticoagulation system, abnormal cardiac function, cochleovestibular disturbance, bone damage, and psychiatric disorder. Much of the literature on the subject is in the Russian or Eastern European languages: a collection of English abstracts appears in volume 8, number 1, pages 65–8, of *Acoustics Abstracts*, March–April 1974. A more accessible reference is to volume 4, page 367, of *The British Medical Journal*, 15 November 1975, which ends with a list of papers written in English.

10. FUNCTIONAL MODIFICATION: CLINICAL APPLICATIONS

10.1 PHYSIOTHERAPY

Physiotherapy is a branch of medicine which has been largely neglected by scientific investigators. It is important, however, not only because it forms part of the treatment of a great number of patients, but also because, by the very large scale of its application, it is a significant factor in the economics of health services.

There are five variables in ultrasonic physiotherapy. These are the frequency, the intensity, the duration of the treatment, the duty cycle of the irradiation, and the method of application. The frequency is usually within the range 1–3 MHz, and intensities of between 0·25 and 3 W cm^{-2}, averaged over a total transducer surface of about 5 cm^2, are generally used. The construction of a typical applicator is illustrated in Fig. 10.1. Each application may last for between 3 and 50 min, and this may be repeated perhaps 10 times during a course of treatment. Irradiation is either continuous, or pulsed with a duty cycle of about 0·2. Pulsing the ultrasound allows higher on-intensities to be used without increasing the temperature if the average intensity is kept constant; but Lehmann and Krusen (1958) were unable to detect any difference between the clinical effects of pulsed and continuous wave application when the average intensity was kept constant. According to Lehmann and Guy (1972), the temperature range which is effective in physiotherapy is around 40–45°C.

The various methods of application have been discussed by Summer and Patrick (1964). Coupling to the treated surface may be achieved in one of three ways:

(i) The ultrasonic source may be placed in a water bath, facing and in close proximity to the area of tissue which it is desired to treat;

(ii) The ultrasonic source may be held in contact with the surface of the skin, and air is excluded by a film of mineral oil, glycerine, or proprietary jelly; or

(iii) The ultrasound may be applied through a water-filled rubber or plastic balloon containing water.

Mineral oil or aqueous gel are both suitable coupling agents. In order to avoid losses due to gas bubbles trapped in the pores of the skin, it is sometimes helpful to clean the surface to be treated with a detergent (Pätzold *et al.*, 1951). This must be washed off thoroughly with water before the ultrasound is applied, in order to avoid skin irritation.

The machine should have a meter which accurately indicates the output —for convenience this may be expressed in units of [W cm⁻²] averaged over the surface of the transducer. Usually, the meter measures the voltage

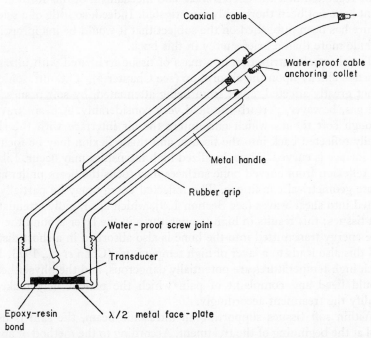

Coaxial cable

Water-proof cable anchoring collet

Metal handle

Rubber grip

Water-proof screw joint

Transducer

Epoxy-resin bond

λ/2 metal face-plate

FIG. 10.1 Construction of a typical ultrasonic applicator for physiotherapy. The transducer has a diameter of about 25 mm.

applied to the transducer, and so its accuracy depends on the proper tuning and calibration of the system. There should be some means of calibration: the radiation pressure balance is probably most convenient (see Section 3.7.e.i). It is important that the transducer mounting should be efficient, so that the applicator does not heat up excessively. If pulsed equipment is used, it is desirable that the pulses should be square (since, for a given average intensity, the corresponding on-intensity is constant and less than the peak in a "pulse" resulting from a lack of rectification and filtering in the power supply).

The poor performance of much of the equipment in clinical use is disconcerting. Thus, reporting on the status and use of ultrasonic therapy machines in a typical population, Stewart *et al.* (1973) stated that the majority of instruments in clinical use were incapable of delivering a prescribed amount of ultrasonic energy to the patient. The maximum indicated output error for 85% of the machines exceeded $\pm 20\%$. One third of the timers were in error by more than 10%.

Ultrasonic phsyiotherapy forms a part of many procedures thought to be helpful in relieving the symptoms of several unpleasant ailments, and it is to be regretted that the effectiveness and mechanism of this form of treatment have not been thoroughly investigated. Indeed, so little of a scientific nature has been published on the subject that it would be inappropriate to include more than a brief survey in this book.

The thermal distribution in a mass of tissue irradiated with ultrasound depends chiefly upon the absorption (see Chapter 4). The ultrasonic field is not greatly affected, apart from being attenuated, by soft tissues. Bone and gas, however, perturb the field very considerably. A beam travelling through soft tissues which encounters the air interface with the skin is totally reflected back into the tissues, and this reflexion may be focused if the surface is curved. Thus, localized high intensities may occur. Likewise the reflexion from curved bone surfaces may focus the beam under appropriate geometrical conditions. The reflected energy may be partially converted into shear waves (see Section 1.9), which are rapidly attenuated in soft tissues: this results in high temperatures in the layer around the bone. The energy transmitted into the bone is also absorbed in a short distance, and this also leads to a layer of high temperature (Chan *et al.*, 1973, 1974). Such high temperatures are potentially dangerous, and the physiotherapist should heed any complaint of pain which the patient may make, and modify the treatment accordingly.

Within soft tissues supporting an ultrasonic beam, the skin is usually cool at the beginning of the treatment. According to the method of application, the heat distribution during irradiation may be such that the surface is hottest, with a decrease in temperature along the beam as it is attenuated, or the surface may remain cool if the treatment is carried out under water or through a water bag. Locally within the irradiated tissue, flowing blood may carry away heat and so lower the temperature. An additional complication is due to the inhomogeneity of the near field of the ultrasonic beam (see Section 2.2), which in a stationary situation results in a non-uniform temperature distribution. For this reason, some physiotherapists recommend that the position of the treatment head should be continuously changed, using a kind of massaging technique.

For general guidance, some physiotherapists consider relatively high temperatures are helpful in the treatment of chronic disease processes— such as joint contracture, a result of scarring and shortening of the periarticular tissues. On the other hand, vigorous heating is undesirable in acute processes.

It is interesting to compare the heating due to ultrasonic physiotherapy with the intrinsic heating due to metabolism. Heart muscle has the highest continuous metabolic rate of all the tissues in the body, at about 30 W kg^{-1}. Kidney is next, at 20 W kg^{-1}. A simple calculation shows that 1 MHz ultrasound at an intensity of 1 W cm^{-2} deposits power at a rate of about 200 W kg^{-1} in a small volume of tissue if the attenuation coefficient is 1 dB cm^{-1}.

The biological mechanisms of ultrasonic physiotherapy have not been systematically investigated. It seems likely that the method is valuable chiefly because of the unique distribution of heat to which it gives rise; such distribution generally cannot be obtained by other means. There is now no doubt, however, that even low-intensity ultrasound can cause non-thermal biological effects (see Section 9.3), and such effects may be important in certain physiotherapeutic applications such as in the breakdown of fibrous adhesions at the site of an operative incision.

Lehmann (1965) reviewed the data which had been published up to the early 1960s. He concluded that ultrasonic physiotherapy increases blood perfusion of the limbs by up to about 25%, that this effect is due to heat, and that the frequency used to produce the heat is irrelevant. In this connexion, see Bickford and Duff (1953), Abramson et al. (1960) and Buchan (1970) for experimental evidence. Contradictory data also exists, however, and so it is difficult to know where the truth lies. Thus, the influence of ultrasound at physiotherapeutic levels (0·25–1·5 W cm^{-2}, 2–3 min, probably 1 MHz) on blood flow in cutaneous, subcutaneous and muscular tissues in normal individuals has been investigated by Paaske et al. (1973). The blood flow was measured by the ^{133}Xe washout technique. In cutaneous tissue the ultrasound did not change blood flow significantly. There was no correlation between ultrasonic intensity and either blood flow or change in skin temperature. In subcutaneous and muscular tissues, inconsistent and insignificant blood flow changes were recorded. In these tissues, too, there was no correlation between the measured physiological quantities. These particular results indicate that the eventual benefits of ultrasonic physiotherapy cannot be ascribed to augmentation of blood flow.

Lehmann (1965) has also reported that there is some suggestion that irradiation of main nerves has an analgesic effect on the areas which they supply. Muscle spasm is also reduced. Ultrasonically induced heat increases the extensibility of tendons by a factor of 5–10 times. There seems to be no difference between continuous wave ultrasonic irradiation, and pulsed irradiation of the same average intensity, save that the latter, having a correspondingly greater on-intensity, may be more dangerous since cavitation is more likely to occur. Apart from thermal effects, Lehmann (1965) concluded that the only ultrasonically induced process of beneficial effect in physiotherapy might be "the acceleration of the diffusion process across biologic membranes". In another context, data on this effect have been presented by Howkins (1969). That the acceleration of active transport is largely due to heat has been demonstrated by Wells (1966) (see Section 9.2).

The damaging effects of ultrasound on the eye have been discussed by Sokollu (1972). Ultrasound should not be applied to the eye in physiotherapeutic procedures (for fear of causing cataract), and great care is necessary when an area of the spinal cord is treated after laminectomy, when any anaesthetic area is involved.

Attention is also drawn to the effects of ultrasonic irradiation on haemodynamics, and their possible consequences, as mentioned in Section 9.11.d. It is reassuring that Dyson and Pond (1973) found that damage only occurred in vessels exposed to a standing wave field for more than 15 min without variation in the direction of the ultrasound, and even then the effects were only rarely seen.

The cautionary recommendation not to irradiate neoplastic tissue with ultrasound, lest metastases may be caused, is found from time to time in the literature. It seems to be a sensible precaution, but one which has not been scientifically tested. In this connexion, see Section 9.11.e.

In general terms, the indications and contraindications for ultrasonic physiotherapy are essentially the same as those for other deep-heating techniques.

Patrick (1971) has explained that she prefers a 1 MHz instrument to one operating at 3 MHz, on account of the greater penetration of the former. She also prefers a pulsed system—2 ms on-time, 0·2 duty cycle—but the reasons given for this are not entirely convincing. She has much experience in the use of ultrasound for physiotherapy, however, having been involved in the treatment of 12000 patients. Acute back pain, tenosynovitis, scar tissue, and acute shoulder pain, all respond to ultrasonic therapy; the sooner that the treatment is begun, the better is the result. Really chronic conditions seldom respond to ultrasound. Therefore, according to Patrick (1973), it is worth having ultrasonic physiotherapy machines in departments serving accident units, but not in departments which deal only with chronic medical conditions or acute surgery. This is because ultrasonic treatment is most effective following trauma causing soft-tissue lesions. The sooner after the injury that ultrasonic treatment and exercise therapy are begun, the better is the result.

Lanfear and Clarke (1972) reported that relief of the symptoms of tenosynovitis was generally obtained within a week of the injury, if treated daily with ultrasound at up to 3 W cm^{-2} at 1 MHz, for about 10 s cm^{-2}. It must be realized, however, that it is notoriously difficult to assess the effects, beneficial or otherwise, of physiotherapeutic procedures. Roman

(1960) attempted to do this with ultrasonic therapy for low back pain, bursitis of the shoulder, and myalgia. In each of these groups, which were also divided into subgroups, patients were either treated in the usual way with ultrasound, or they were subjected to an apparently conventional treatment whilst, unknown to them, the ultrasound was not switched on. A total of 100 patients were involved in the trial. Of the patients who received ultrasound, the results in 60% were classified as either good or normal; and in the sham group, 72% were in these categories! It would be foolish to rush to hasty conclusions on the basis of this one experiment, which is open to several technical criticisms: but it does highlight the difficulty of assessing the value of particular physiotherapeutic procedures, and lends support to the opinion that patients derive a great deal of benefit merely from receiving the care and attention of people in whom they have some confidence.

10.2 NEUROSURGERY

The first report of the use of focused ultrasound to produce lesions in living tissues seems to be that of Lynn and Putnam (1944). They used a spherical segment of quartz, resonant at a frequency of 835 kHz, with a diameter at the rim of 51 mm and ground to produce a focus at a distance of 55 mm from the concave crystal surface. They gave no information about intensity, and the transducer could not have been entirely satisfactory due to the unfocused nature of its polarization (see Section 3.6.b). Three dogs, 30 cats and four monkeys were used in the experiments. For the animals, the results were generally pretty catastrophic. Unfortunately, the importance of bone as an attenuator was not realized by these investigators: thus, they wrote "in contrast to the cats and dogs, the monkeys were especially satisfactory experimental animals because of the almost complete lack of radiation-absorbing muscle tissue over the skull areas . . ." Therefore, although Lynn and Putnam (1944) have historical precedence in the use of focused ultrasound, they do not have scientific pre-eminence in relation to the pioneering groups in Urbana, Boston and London.

The use of unfocused ultrasound in neurosurgery has been described by Lindstrom (1954). Twenty patients were treated, ultrasonic irradiation being used as a substitute for lobotomy. Sixteen of the patients were suffering from intractable pain due to metastatic tumours. The intensity used was 7 W cm^{-2}, applied for 4–14 min through a suitable hole in the skull, and the postoperative course in every case was reported to be satisfactory and without complication. Lindstrom and Beck (1963) used similar equipment to suppress movements in epilepsy experimentally induced in cats. They then treated three humans: an ultrasonic beam of

20 mm diameter was used, at an intensity of 8 W cm^{-2}, applied for 1 min. Satisfactory reductions were produced in the frequencies of the attacks.

The most important potential value of ultrasonic neurosurgery arises because it affords the only method by which damage can be induced in a deep part of the nervous system, without injury to the overlying tissues. This can be achieved most strikingly by the use of a focused beam of ultrasound, in which the focal volume is the only part of the field where the intensity is sufficient to cause damage. A typical arrangement is illustrated in Fig. 10.2. The relationships between the lesion size and the exposure conditions are discussed in Section 9.11.a. The chief disadvantages of the method are its complexity, the necessity to remove bone—a portion of skull or vertebra—which would otherwise absorb a large fraction of the ultra-

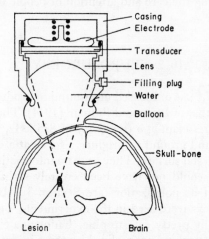

FIG. 10.2 A typical arrangement for ultrasonic neurosurgery. (Based on Lele, 1962.)

sonic energy, and the difficulty of providing a sterile liquid coupling with the tissue surface.

A graphic description of the histological appearances of ultrasonic focal brain lesions has been given by Warwick and Pond (1968). Lesions are sharply demarcated. Peripheral tissue in a lesion appears to have lost its affinity for most stains, leading to a startlingly punched-out appearance. Closer examination shows, however, that the effects on nerve cells and neuroglia extend a little beyond this region of decolourization: and many nuclei of surrounding cells are shrunken and intensely stained. The nuclei of affected cells show little or no internal structure, and nucleoli cannot be discerned within them. Specific myelin stains reveal some damage in this peripheral zone, but this is less severe than in the neighbouring pale zone of the lesion.

All except the smallest lesions display lamination. There is a central core, and outside this there is the region of damage previously mentioned. The pallor of this region is the most striking feature of a lesion. This appearance gives rise to a descriptive simile, the "island and moat". In the moat, cells and fibres are much altered, and all the surviving nuclei are deformed, shrunken and darkly stained. In the island, damage is less severe, and is to some degree selective: thus, neuroglial nuclei appear for the most part to be unaffected. Blood vessels are even less affected, and even capillaries may remain throughout the lesion, although they may become non-functional.

Perhaps the moat of the lesion is of the greatest interest in relation to its clinical usefulness, since it may safely be assumed that all neuronal elements within this border are either killed at the time of making the lesion, or are at least irreversibly damaged.

The following aspects, *inter alia*, of focal neurosurgery, summarized by Meyers *et al.* (1960), are relevant to the therapy of certain neurological disorders:

(i) Permanent lesions of any size, shape and orientation can be produced at any site in the brain; no disruption of intervening tissue occurs;

(ii) Changes in function of the tissues can be achieved, either temporarily or permanently;

(iii) The vascular system can be left intact and functional in cerebral regions in which all neuronal elements are destroyed;

(iv) White matter can be selectively damaged without involving grey matter; and

(v) Mortality and morbidity incidences are low.

The development of ultrasonic neurosurgery in the 1950s was carried on in an environment of depressingly hazardous "conventional" techniques. Neurosurgeons were familiar with their patients experiencing paraparesis and bladder dysfunction following arterolateral chordotomy, vegetation following prefrontal lobotomy, and hemiplegia following surgical treatment of basal ganglion disorders. Patients often died from haemorrhage resulting from electrocoagulative lesions. Set against this background, the possibility that ultrasonic focal neurosurgery might overcome these problems must have been enormously exciting (Fry *et al.*, 1954). People then could not know that advances in pharmaceuticals and direct surgical skills and techniques, and changing medical fashions, would make ultrasonic methods of treatment of brain disorders in man largely obsolete even before they became widely available.

The availability of such a powerful method—albeit costly—highlights the limited state of knowledge concerning anatomical schema relating to, for example, hyperkinesia, akinesia, and hypertonus (i.e. signs), and pain, dysesthesias, and paresthesias (i.e. symptoms), or parkinsonism and thalamic pain (i.e. syndromes). Meyers *et al.* (1960) wrote that "planful trial-and-error experimentation and prompt exploitation of newly acquired knowledge, both 'positive' and 'negative', appear essential to making rapid progress in this area of study". Alas, progress has not been rapid.

10.2.a Treatment of Parkinson's Disease

Surgical and related methods—such as proton radiotherapy—used for the treatment of parkinsonism are all aimed at interrupting, in some appropriate region of the brain, a neural pathway, possibly forming a portion of a reverberating circuit, the integrity of which is supposed to be a necessary condition for the appearance of hyperkinesia, or hypertonus. Since the discovery of the therapeutic value of levodopa (Cotzias *et al.*, 1967), procedures of this kind have generally gone out of fashion. The ultrasonic technique which was developed in the 1950s for the treatment of Parkinson's disease, however, is both of historical interest and of relevance to neuroanatomy, and so some details of the work described by Meyers *et al.* (1959) are recorded here. The principles of Horsley–Clarke stereotaxy, establishing certain cranial landmarks as "zero" planes and using craniocerebral coordinates based on these planes, were used to place ultrasonic focal lesions of the desired sizes, shapes and orientations at preselected sites within animal brains. These principles, however, were found to be inadequate to provide the accuracy necessary for optimal ultrasonic neurosurgery. Consequently, for irradiation in man, the skull was fixed by four pinions seated in small superficial cranial burr holes in the frontal and occipitoparietal bones. The intercommissural line and the mid-saggital plane of the third ventricle were used as references, and they were visualized by contrast radiography. The ultrasonic source, consisting of four separately focused transducers, was equipped with a retractable pointer, the tip of which was at the position of the common focus of the system. Thus it was possible precisely to position the transducers in relation to the head of an individual patient, by superimposing radiographs, in order to place lesions exactly where desired within the brain. It was also possible to decide the extent of the necessary craniotomy.

Meyers *et al.* (1959) carried out 15 operations on 12 patients, with the ansa lenticularis and the substantia nigra as targets. The total lesion volumes were built up from many juxtaposed single focal volumes. Eleven of these patients were suffering from parkinsonism, with or without rigidity. The time spent by each patient in the operating theatre was about 12–14 h, divided into two sessions: during the first session, occupying about 3–3·5 h, the craniotomy and landmarking procedures were carried out. For the irradiation, coupling between the transducers and the surface of the exposed dura was provided by means of saline filling a hopper, clamped and sealed to the skull. The patient was observed, as the irradiation progressed and being under local anaesthesia, in order to notice any modifications of tremor or rigidity. The irradiation was continued until a satisfactory result had been obtained, as judged from the behaviour of the patient. It appeared that the most economical treatment for hyperkinesia and hypertonus was the irradiation of the caudal half of the substantia nigra and its superior medial neighbourhood. The region of the ansa lenticularis in the control of rigidity was less consistent.

10.2.b Hypophysectomy

Hypophysectomy affects the hormonal activity of target organs. The withdrawal of the pituitary stimuli to the adrenals and ovaries is especially relevant to the control of breast cancer, particularly with bone metastases. To some extent, the effects of withdrawal can be brought about by the removal of these endocrine glands, but in many patients adrenalectomy with or without oophorectomy is unsuccessful: these patients may respond to hypophysectomy. The procedure may also be helpful in patients with advanced cancer of the prostate with bone metastases, and in those with diabetic retinitis, with malignant exopthalmus, with Cushing's syndrome, or with acromegaly.

Interruption of pituitary function may be achieved by surgical excision (see, for example, James, 1969), by implanted radiation sources (Rand et al., 1962), by external radiation, particularly by heavy particles (Lawrence et al., 1963), or by stereotactic cryosurgery (Rand et al., 1964, 1969). None of these methods is completely satisfactory either technically, since all are associated with the possibility of postoperative complications, such as cranial nerve involvement—and, in general, James' (1969) technique of trans-ethmoidal–sphenoidal excision seems to be the method of choice—or strategically, since complete functional suppression of the pituitary, which necessitates hormone substitution therapy, may be undesirable—for example, only the anterior part of the gland is involved in diabetic retinitis.

The possibility that ultrasonic energy might be used to inhibit pituitary function is an attractive one, since it might eliminate at least some of the difficulties associated with the other techniques. Two distinct ultrasonic methods have been investigated, and these are described in the following Sub-sections.

(i) Transcranial irradiation with focused ultrasound

Krumins et al. (1965) reported how they made ultrasonic lesions of a variety of shapes and sizes in different positions in the anterior pituitary of cats, and the resultant cellular changes were studied following sacrifice after periods of from 1 h to three months. The lesions were produced by a 5 MHz focused beam irradiating through the brain exposed by craniotomy.

An intensity of 2.7 kW cm^{-2} was used, and the lesions were built up by a series of exposures, each of about 0.5 s, separated in space by 0.2–0.3 mm. Two groups of pituitary cells were studied—the acidophils and basophils. Damage was observed which resulted either from a direct transfer of heat from bone (in which absorption is very rapid: see Section 4.7), or from interaction between ultrasound and the tissue of the pituitary. At sacrifice within three days, in thermal lesions the nuclei are destroyed, whilst the cytoplasm remains intact; in ultrasound lesions, the nuclei are relatively unaffected, whilst a large proportion of the secretion granules are depleted. After a longer period before sacrifice—21 days—there is a general absence of acidophil cells in the lesion, and those basophils which are present are regenerated cells. This distinction becomes more marked as time progresses. Preliminary results indicated that hormonal changes were associated with the histological damage.

If ultrasonic energy could be applied selectively to depress the acidophil population, this would be of great medical significance since the acidophils are associated with the production of growth hormone. It is relevant to note that Yoshioka and Oka (1965) reported a reduction in the number of β-cells following irradiation of the pituitary with focused ultrasound, so there is at least an element of uncertainty here.

There are only scanty data concerning the clinical application of the method in man. In retrospect, it may seem that this work was premature. But it is often easy to be critical of clinicians faced with appallingly difficult problems in patient care: and, given the state of knowledge which then existed, it is clear that the doctors acted in the best interests of their patients.

In a series of five female patients with advanced breast cancer, beyond any expectation of cure, Hickey *et al.* (1961) irradiated the pituitary with focused ultrasound, using techniques similar to those described for the irradiation of brain structure (see Section 9.11.a). No unequivocally favourable alterations in the growth patterns occurred, and one patient, who was not benefited by ultrasonic treatment, enjoyed a marked improvement following subsequent adreno-oophorectomy. Every patient developed diabetes insipidus following ultrasonic irradiation, and three suffered from cranial nerve palsies. In every case, there was a postoperative increase in the urinary 17-ketosteroids. These results were not at all encouraging. The complications—polyuria, paralysis of extraocular muscles, visual interference, and hemiplegia—were considered by Hickey *et al.* (1963) to be sufficiently serious to prevent the treatment of further patients.

(ii) Direct transdural ultrasonic irradiation

Arslan (1964) was the first to describe a technique for hypophysectomy by direct irradiation by means of a probe introduced along the trans-ethmoidal

–sphenoidal route. Apparently the first operation of this kind in man was carried out in 1957. The irradiation was performed using a probe similar to that designed for the treatment of Menière's disease (see Section 10.4), but with an appropriate extension of the cylindrical end of the velocity transformer. The frequency was 3 MHz, the intensity, 2·5 W cm^{-2}, and the irradiation time, 20–40 min. The ultrasound was applied to the dura anterior to the pituitary, exposed by the trans-ethmoidal–sphenoidal route. The potential advantages of the method are that the dura remains intact, so that the possibility of cerebrospinal fluid rhinorrhea is eliminated, and that, by an appropriate choice of ultrasonic frequency and intensity, it might be possible to destroy only a selected region of the gland.

Arslan (1964) reported his results with a series of 15 patients with advanced cancer of breast or prostate, and four with Cushing's syndrome. In every case, there was some degree of postoperative improvement, although in only 11 of the cancer patients were the 17-ketosteroid and 17-hydroxicorticoid levels reduced, and in two of these patients, second applications of ultrasound were necessary in order to achieve this objective. At least one of the cancer patients developed diabetes insipidus, but apart from this the procedure was free from postoperative complications. In a later report, Arslan (1967) reported satisfactory results following direct ultrasonic irradiation of the pituitary in 14 patients with Cushing's syndrome: postoperative recovery was apparently very good in all cases, and in some, normal regular menstruation reappeared. Three patients with acromegaly benefited from the procedure, and one patient with diabetic retinopathy was improved, requiring only half the insulin dosage which was necessary before irradiation. The clinical impression was that pituitary function was "normalized", rather than eliminated, by the treatment.

Although the trans-ethmoidal–sphenoidal approach has the advantage of being relatively comfortable for the patient, the alternative trans-septal–trans-sphenoidal approach has the advantage of allowing the route to be in the midline, which allows easy orientation, and consequent safety. This operative procedure has been described in detail by Giancarlo and Mattucci (1971). Having exposed the dura over the gland, they applied ultrasound at 2–3 W cm^{-2} for 20–25 min in their early patients, but for 40 min in more recently treated individuals. The only other data about the ultrasonic probe were that it employed a velocity transformer, and had a tip diameter of 5 mm. All 15 of their patients were suffering from diabetic retinopathy, but no information was presented concerning their postoperative progress, except that hormone replacement was minimal, and varying degrees of insulin sensitivity were demonstrated; there were no renewed retinal haemorrhages and but one patient noted immediate improvement in visual acuity. The only problem was a technical one: the difficulty of approaching the pituitary in patients with the conchal type of sphenoid was considered to be sufficient to contraindicate the operation in this group. The authors concluded that "it remains to be seen whether the modality of ultrasound will offer a temporary or permanent beneficial response".

Arslan et al. (1973) have summarized the results of an eight-year follow-up of 167 patients. Unfortunately, the endocrinologist will be disappointed by the lack of data. Ultrasonic hypophysectomy seems almost invariably to be followed by the onset of diabetes insipidus. This is a distressing complication for the patient; but the literature contains no useful discussion of its severity and management.

There is no clinical evidence whatsoever that ultrasound can be used selectively to destroy cells of a specific type in the whole gland.

10.2.c Ultrasonic Focal Lesions in Neuroanatomical Studies

Focused ultrasonic techniques allow the effects of damage to a selected portion of the brain to be assessed, for example in the study of nervous pathways within the brain, and in the treatment of experimentally induced abnormalities. Thus, Lele (1962) described the single transducer focusing system illustrated in Fig. 10.2, which operates at a frequency of 2·7 MHz. Some results using this equipment have been reported by Basauri and Lele (1962), Manlapaz et al. (1964) and Young and Lele (1964). In this application, the relationship between lesion size and the duration of the exposure is discussed in Section 9.2, whilst the threshold conditions relating intensity and the duration of the exposure are considered in Section 9.11.a.

Young and Lele (1964) have produced focal ultrasonic lesions within the brains of foetal and of growing rabbits. Production of such lesions in foetuses in utero by irradiation through intact scalp and skull, in particular, opens up many possibilities in neuroembryology. The major difficulty is that of foetal movement during alignment and irradiation.

The present status of this area of investigation has been summarized by Fry (1972). Ultrasonically generated lesions provide the necessary precision in terms of lesion size, shape and placement, to permit resolution of problems of neuronal organization in brain stem nuclei which could not previously be solved. It is anticipated that this technique will make it possible to relate many aspects of function and behaviour to defined structures.

10.2.d Commissurotomy

In the spinal cord, the beta sensory fibres ascend ipsilaterally in the posterior columns. Impulses arising from stimulation of gamma, delta and C fibres have been detected contralaterally, and have been shown to cross in the posterior commissure in cats (Shaffron and Collins, 1964). It is not known whether they cross in the anterior commissure. Although they also transmit other impulses, gamma, delta and C fibres are known to transmit pain in man, whereas beta fibres do not (Collins *et al.*, 1960).

Direct surgical spinal commissurotomy enjoyed a brief vogue in the late 1920s and early '30s, as an unique method for the relief of pain. It soon fell into disfavour, however, because of the paralysis which frequently resulted from surgical disruption of the posterior spinal artery. Focused ultrasound offers the possibility of disrupting the centre of the spinal cord, whilst sparing the surrounding structures.

Richards *et al.* (1966) performed ultrasonic commissurotomies in a series of 35 cats, and made observations of the effects on nervous pathways. The operation involved laminectomy followed by the making of 40 focal ultrasonic lesions, 0·6 mm apart in the caudal–rostral plane. A frequency of 2·7 MHz was used, and the dose was such that each lesion was vertically elliptical, and measured about $1 \times 0·5 \times 1$ mm in size. In acute experiments, the transmission of electrically stimulated impulses through various fibres of the cord past the irradiated region was observed. Evoked potentials were blocked in more than 50% of gamma, delta and C fibres, by a commissurotomy of two spinal segments. Thus, it appears that the majority of fibres crossing to the contralateral cord do so shortly after their entrance into the cord. In chronic experiments, there was no weakness, sensory loss of pinch or pin prick, or loss of bladder control.

The results of these experiments indicated that ultrasonic spinal commissurotomy was a technically feasible procedure for the relief of pain, and that motor and sphincter control would not be sacrificed.

In the spinal cord, grey matter is spared selectively, and when the midline branches of the anterior spinal artery are involved in the ultrasonic lesion an obliterative arteritis results (Griffith *et al.*, 1973). Even in the presence of this vascular change, the motor neurons of the anterior horns—which are especially liable to ischaemic or mechanical damage—may not show pathological changes.

10.2.e Reversible Ultrasonic Lesions

In certain applications, an additional advantage of ultrasonic neurosurgery is that it seems to be possible to adjust the dosage so that induced functional damage is temporary (Lele, 1967). This may make it possible to test the effect of a treatment before permanent damage is induced. Moreover, pulse–echo techniques (see Chapter 6) using the surgical transducer can give information about the adequacy of the extent of the craniectomy, of the acoustic coupling to the brain, and of the general physiological condition as reflected in the cardiovascular and respiratory pulsations. It can also be used to locate structures within the brain, to act as references in the positioning of lesions (Lele, 1966). Results of an analytical and experimental study of the acoustical scattering properties of ultrasonic focal lesions in terms of their effects on plane waves have been presented by Matison and Lele (1974). These results indicate that direct echoes from reversible lesions within the brain are beyond the limits of detection by so many orders of magnitude that their existence must be considered to be theoretical only. The same may be true for permanent lesions. Indirect echoes—i.e. the modulation of the echo from some structure lying beyond the lesion—do not seem to be reliable for several reasons: brain is inhomogeneous and contains interfaces which generate interfering echoes; brain does not possess an uniform surface for reflecting indirect echoes; and the acoustic properties of brain do not change very rapidly with temperature. The only remaining possibility is detection of change in the energy scattered forward from the lesion: but this would require two craniotomies.

10.3 NON-INVASIVE STIMULATION OF NEURAL ELEMENTS

A method of electrically stimulating neural elements deep in the brain has been proposed by Fry (1968). Whilst this is not basically a surgical technique, alternative methods of stimulation do involve surgery. The scheme is based on the partial rectification in the focal region of an ultrasonic field of an alternating current flowing through a large portion of the brain in response to an externally applied electric field. Since the magnitude of the electrical conductivity decreases with increasing temperature, the adiabatic changes in temperature produced by the ultrasonic pressure wave cause a periodic variation in conductivity that results in a direct current electrical flow when the two frequencies are equal and appropriately adjusted in phase. Calculations indicate that an order-of-magnitude safety factor between the conditions for stimulation and for brain damage may be achieved using 1 ms pulses of 4 MHz ultrasound, focal intensity 10 W cm^{-2}, with a current density of about 10 A cm^{-2}. The total non-oscillatory temperature rise would be about 4 degK.

10.4 VESTIBULAR SURGERY

Menière's disease is due to a disorder of the vestibular end organ, possibly of psychological origin, which results in the spasmodic occurrence of attacks of vertigo of varying duration and severity. The disease presents no threat to life, except from consequential accident, but its effects are most damaging psychologically and may interfere so much with locomotion as to render the patient's life almost intolerable. These patients are ready to submit to almost any treatment, even to the infliction of total deafness, to rid themselves of their attacks.

The process that triggers off an acute attack is still a matter of conjecture.

It may be due to a rupture of the saccus, mixing perilymph with endolymph. The deformation of the cupula by the bulging of the saccule may supply the initial stimulus. The capillary circulation may be interrupted by the raised labyrinthine pressure. Whatever the cause, however, fortunately the symptoms of most (more than 80%) patients can be controlled by medication and appropriate diet. The remainder require some form of surgical treatment, however, as do a proportion of patients suffering from various other related disorders of the inner ear.

None of the conventional surgical alternatives reviewed by James *et al.* (1960) is entirely satisfactory. Either the hearing is lost in addition to the balance function in the diseased ear, or the operation is associated with a significant risk to the patient. Thus, unilateral total destruction of the whole inner-ear function provides dramatic relief for these patients. Such radical treatment may be afforded by labyrinthotomy and avulsion of the endolymphatic canal, by alcohol injection through the oval window, by alcohol injection of the lateral canal after labyrinthotomy, or by electro-coagulation. In general, however, it is undesirable to sacrifice any hearing which the patient may still possess despite the disease. Procedures which retain the hearing whilst relieving the symptoms of the disease are operative division of the vestibular branch of the eighth nerve, and the induction of vestibular neuronitis by streptomycin. The former is dangerous (although it may be safer than some of its opponents suggest), and the latter affects both ears. A possibly satisfactory method of treatment is cryosurgery (Cutt *et al.*, 1965; House, 1966).

Ultrasonic treatment was first proposed by Krejci (1952), who, following some experimental work on animals, irradiated the vestibular end organ of a patient suffering from Menière's disease. The patient lost the balance function in the irradiated ear, and so was cured of the symptoms of the disease. Equally important, he retained his hearing.

It was M. Arslan who pioneered the introduction of the ultrasonic technique. In his original description of the method, Arslan (1955) advised that the ultrasonic source—in his apparatus, a solid metal rod of 5 mm diameter driven at 1 MHz—should be applied direct to the prominence of the bone over the external semicircular canal, and that the field should be kept completely dry. The fact that this method largely prevents the transmission of ultrasound into the labyrinth caused scepticism amongst those who naturally assumed ultrasonic energy to be the agent responsible for the beneficial effects of the treatment. In retrospect, however, it does not seem so dubious (see Section 9.2) and, although the techniques which were later developed may give more favourable heat distributions—and certainly do, from the point of view of the risk of damage to the facial nerve—Arslan's (1955, 1958) reports of satisfactory results support the hypothesis that the mechanism is one of thermal damage to the membranous labyrinth.

For reasons which are clear now, but which may not have been apparent then, Arslan (1958) developed the technique in which the lateral semi-circular canal is exposed by surgery, so that direct application of the ultrasound is possible.

A typical procedure employed in irradiation of the lateral semicircular canal has been described by James (1963). The operation is performed under local anaesthesia with sedation, so that the progress of the treatment may be assessed by observing the eye movements resulting first from the irritation, and later from the destruction of the vestibular end organ, and so that watch may be kept for any sign of facial nerve involvement. A drill is used for the bone work, as patients seem to tolerate it very much better

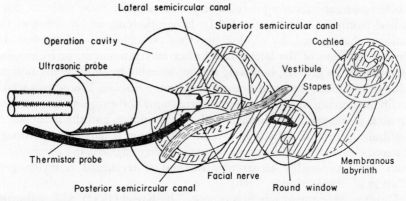

FIG. 10.3 Diagram showing the right labyrinth, with the lateral semicircular canal exposed by surgery. The ultrasonic probe of James *et al.* (1963) is in position for irradiating the lateral semicircular canal, and the thermistor probe is arranged to measure the temperature of the irrigating fluid flowing through the ultrasonic probe into the operation cavity.

than the mallet and gouge; they do not object to forceps being used to nibble bone at certain stages in the approach to the lateral canal. The bone of the mastoid is taken down well forward towards the attic to expose the short process of the incus, and to allow plenty of room to watch the application of the probe to the bone over the canal. Using an operating microscope, a clear blue line (the semicircular canal seen through the bone, which is at this final stage about 0·5 mm in thickness) is exposed for a distance of about 5 mm. Using the probe illustrated in Fig. 3.11(b), the tip is placed in contact with the bone immediately over the canal, as shown in Fig. 10.3, and the saline is allowed to flow continuously. Its temperature, monitored by a thermistor in a probe within the cavity, is maintained at 37°C. The ultrasound is first switched on at a fairly low intensity— 10 W cm⁻²—and within a few moments the patient may develop vertigo and irritative nystagmus to the operated side, or deviation to the opposite side. As soon as the vertigo becomes more tolerable, the intensity is increased progressively in steps of a few watts per square centimetre, until it has reached 22 W cm^{-2}. It is explained later in this Section that this intensity is the maximum which can be used without risk of damage to the facial nerve. At this intensity the irritation normally ceases after a few minutes, and after a further 2 min the irradiation is interrupted for 15 s. If irritation is not observed following this intermission, the application is continued for a further 5 min. If irritation returns, however, the procedure is as before, and when 2 min free from irritation have passed, the labyrinth is allowed to recover for 15 s. The irradiation is terminated only when a 15 s interval has been followed by 5 min without any sign of irritation. The wound is then closed completely without drainage.

At the end of the operation, the patient is generally very giddy with paralytic nystagmus (i.e. with nystagmus away from the operated side). This condition gradually diminishes, disappearing usually within a week. Facial nerve paralysis, which is a rare complication, if it occurs at all is generally seen during the first six postoperative days. Patients are warned that they must not be alarmed if they have some vertiginous attacks: following a successful operation, these attacks decrease to an insignificant frequency over a period of a few months. It is wise for the patients to restrict fluid intake, and to continue a vitamin B supplement.

A procedure similar in principle but differing in detail from that described by James (1963) has been adopted by Kossoff and Khan (1966). They used an electronystagmograph to monitor nystagmus: but this would not be appropriate in the absence of nystagmus, if, for example, it was suppressed by drugs.

The uncomplicated cases of Menière's disease respond best to ultrasonic treatment. The earlier that surgery is undertaken, the better is the chance of a happy result. The method has proved very useful, however, where previous labyrinth surgery, including labyrinthotomy and alcohol injection, have been unsuccessful.

As far as clinical results are concerned (James, 1963), the most important is that vertigo is abolished in all but about 15% of patients. It is reduced in about 10%, and worse in fewer than 2%.

Roughly a quarter of all patients given ultrasonic surgery for Menière's disease lose their tinnitus, and in a similar fraction, the hearing is improved. In about one half, tinnitus is reduced; it is unchanged in the majority of the remainder, but worse in about 5%. Hearing is unchanged in about one half, but worse in about a quarter.

The clinical results reported by Kossoff and Khan (1966) for a series of 55 patients were as follows. The hearing improved in 15%, was unchanged in 55%, decreased by between 10–20 dB in 20%, and was lost in 10% of patients. Vertigo was abolished in 75%, and a further 5% were helped by second irradiations. Six patients with positional vertigo and normal hearing were treated, with excellent results.

The method is now in routine clinical use. Several instruments designed for the purpose have been described (see, for example, Gordon, 1962; James *et al.*, 1963; Kossoff, 1964; Johnson, 1967). All these instruments are capable of delivering up to at least 0·7 W of ultrasound from an area of between 2 and 5 mm in diameter, at frequencies of from 1 to 3 MHz. The designs of Gordon (1962) and James *et al.* (1963) both have the advantage that a continual flow of saline issues from the tip of the probe: this serves to couple the ultrasonic energy from the transducer to the patient, and to cool both the transducer and the irradiated surface. Of these two probes,

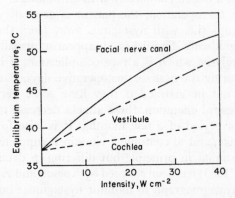

FIG. 10.4 Equilibrium temperatures at various sites measured in human post-mortem temporal bone, during irradiation with the 3 MHz ultrasonic probe of James *et al.* (1963). The bone was prepared as for an operation. Equilibrium temperature is reached within about 30 s of the commencement of irradiation. Temperatures normalized to 37°C at zero intensity. (Data of James, 1963.)

that of James *et al.* (1963) is small enough to fit inside the operative cavity in the mastoid bone, as shown in Fig. 10.3. In J. A. James' last (unpublished) series of 310 patients, the average duration of irradiation was 21 min, with an average dose of 800 J.

The chief hazard of the operation is that of damage to the facial nerve, which lies close to the exposed part of the lateral semicircular canal. The risk arises because the nerve, although not itself irradiated, may be heated by thermal conduction from irradiated areas to such an extent that it subsequently becomes oedematous and fails to conduct. Some of the results of temperature measurements made by means of small thermocouples inserted into post-mortem temporal bones, prepared as for an operation, are shown in Fig. 10.4. By restricting the maximum intensity (total power divided by radiating area) to 22 W cm^{-2}, the temperature of the facial nerve canal does not exceed 48°C. Exposing the nerve to this temperature for at least up to about an hour does not have any untoward effect. At this intensity, the temperatures within the vestibule and the cochlea are about 44 and 39°C respectively: but the temperature within the lateral semi-circular canal immediately beyond the site of application of the ultrasound is probably about 54°C (Wells, 1962).

The operative approach to the lateral semicircular canal requires much surgical skill. If by accident the bone left over the canal is cracked, the hearing function of the patient is lost as a result of ultrasonic irradiation (James, 1963). It may be that this is due to the entry of gas bubbles which amplify the mechanical effects of the ultrasound (see Section 9.7). Even when this hazard was avoided, however, in one series the hearing of 28% of patients was made worse by the operation (James, 1963). Kossoff *et al.* (1967) suggested that the loss of hearing in these patients may have been due to the arrival in the cochlea of too high a proportion of the ultrasound applied to the lateral canal. In order to avoid this complication, they con-structed a probe small enough to be applied directly to the round window. The rationale is that the ultrasonic dose to the cochlea is thus reduced, whilst that to the vestibular end organ is increased. The probe consists of a cylinder of 2 mm diameter, 2 mm long, containing a 3·5 MHz transducer of 1·5 mm diameter. Using an ultrasonic power of about 50 mW, the clinical results in a series of seven patients were encouraging, although the vestibular function was not destroyed. This latter observation suggests that the technique may eliminate damage to the end organ hair cells, whilst relieving the excessive endolymphatic pressure—hydrops—which is believed to cause the symptoms of the disease. The theory of Kossoff *et al.* (1967) concerning the distribution of ultrasonic energy in the labyrinth cannot be accepted, however, without some experimental confirmation. Nevertheless, there are several potential advantages in the round window approach. Firstly, a smaller degree of surgical skill is required; secondly, a lower ultrasonic power is necessary; thirdly, the round window is so far from the facial nerve that the risk of facial paralysis is reduced. On the other hand, the probe is very difficult to construct and it is rather fragile.

Measurements made by means of tiny thermocouples in post-mortem temporal bones irradiated through the round window indicate that, at the power which would be used during an operation, the temperature of the membranous lining of the labyrinth in the region of the probe may exceed 53°C (James and Halliwell, 1970). Kossoff (1972a) measured a temperature rise of 8 degK at 50 mW (but found no effect on the cochlear microphonics) in cats. Such a high temperature would probably cause a permanent inter-ruption of the permeability barrier between the endolymphatic and peri-lymphatic systems (see Section 9.2).

According to Kossoff (1972b), in the semicircular canal approach the ultrasound enters the labyrinth and travels along the lumen of the canal—which is about 0·8 mm in diameter—and enters the vestibule. He states that "the method by which ultrasound effects the treatment is not clearly understood". It is explained in Section 9.2, however, that the mechanism may be that the ultrasound interferes with the permeability of the membranous labyrinth as a direct result of heat immediately under the area of application of the ultrasound, and that this results in a disturbance of the composition of the endolymph. The abnormal physiological environment of the vestibular receptors may thus cause the relief of symptoms and the histological changes which have been observed in experimental animals. Also the endolymphatic pressure may fall due to the leakage of the membrane. Although the round window technique offers surgical advantages, the hypothetical mechanism of the therapeutic effect—thermal damage of the membrane—seems equally plausible. Amongst the surgical advantages are that it is necessary only to deflect the tympanic membrane in order to gain access to the round window, and that the low ultrasonic power—0·1 W—applied some distance from the facial nerve is associated with a reduction in the likelihood of facial paralysis, so that this complication did not occur in a series of 75 patients. In both techniques, intensities at 3 MHz of around 10 W cm^{-2} are used, with irradiation times of around 20 min. The lower intensity used with the Australian equipment, in comparison with the British equipment of James et al. (1963), may be due to the efficient surface cooling provided by the latter instrument.

With the round window approach, in a series of 75 patients the postoperative hearing loss was greater than 20 dB in only four patients. Seventy-five per cent of patients were helped by the first irradiation; 10% benefited from a repeat irradiation.

Originally some trouble was experienced with the reliability of the round window applicator, but this difficulty has now been overcome.

Arslan (1968) has tried the effects of irradiation through both the round and the oval windows, using the same endaural approach which is adopted in stapes surgery. In the case of the oval window, the tip of the probe—having a diameter of 1·5 mm—can be easily inserted between the crura, going on to the inferior part of the stapes. The ossicles thus remain in the normal positions. The probe used by Arslan (1968) was a modified version of the original metallic velocity transformer, but with a decreased flare and a greater length (120 mm). For round window irradiation, the power was 0·025–0·060 W; and, for the oval window approach, it was 0·08–0·10 W, the higher intensity being necessary to penetrate the bone of the platina. The rationale of the oval window irradiation is that ultrasound thereby enters the vestibule, and does not impinge directly on the tympanic scale and the cochlear duct. Whether or not this represents a real advantage depends on the biophysical mechanism of the interaction of ultrasound with the end organ, and on the optimum placement of the lesion in securing the therapeutic effect. If, as seems likely, the basic mechanism is one of interruption in the permeability barrier between endolymph and perilymph by thermal damage of the membranous labyrinth, then the site of the lesion would be related to the distribution of abnormal physiological environment with the ear. Presumably, in Menière's disease, this should preferentially involve the vestibular end organ, rather than the cochlea. The cause of associated tinnitus may also be relevant, however, and if tinnitus is particularly troublesome, the round window approach may be better.

10.5 OTHER APPLICATIONS OF HIGH-FREQUENCY ULTRASOUND

10.5.a Treatment of Warts

From time to time, euphoric papers have been published in the literature, purporting to demonstrate that ultrasound cures plantar warts.

One of the first reports seems to be that of Rowe and Gray (1960), who by 1965 had built up a series of 100 patients. For their treatment, they used mineral oil as a coupling fluid and applied 870 kHz ultrasound at 0·6 W cm^{-2} (from an ordinary physiotherapy instrument) for 15 min, at weekly intervals, for a maximum of 15 weeks. The warts disappeared in 84 patients; there was no control group for comparison. Cherup *et al.* (1963) mentioned the use of five patients as controls; these patients did not respond to simulated treatment, and it was concluded that this "eliminated the possibility of improvement by psychic effect"! Kent (1969), quoting his results with a series of 1000 patients, went so far as to state that he "felt that controls could serve no useful purpose under the limitations imposed by this type of study".

Fortunately Braatz *et al.* (1974) have conducted a double blind study of the method. They restricted their material to warts of age less than six months. The treatment consisted of preparation by soaking in tepid water, swabbing with hydrogen peroxide followed and the removal of the callus by shaving. Ultrasound (1 MHz, 0·8 W cm^{-2}, 12 min) was then applied through a coupling gel. The process was repeated weekly for a maximum of 17 treatments. Of the 32 patients in the study, 17 were given ultrasound therapy with 82·3% effectiveness; 15 were given placebo treatments, with 86·6% cure. It may be concluded that ultrasound applied under these conditions is of no value in the treatment of plantar warts. Moreover, it is worth pointing out that higher intensities cause pain which the patient finds it hard to tolerate.

10.5.b Treatment of Laryngeal Papillomatosis

Of the benign epithelial tumours of the larynx the common type is the single papilloma. Multiple papillomata are unusual: they are even less common in adults than in infants and young children. There is no really satisfactory method of dealing with the problem, either surgical, medical or physical. Being a rare complaint, and liable to spontaneous remission, it is hard to assess the efficacy of any kind of treatment.

The use of ultrasound for the treatment of laryngeal papillomatosis was first reported by Birk and Manhart (1963). They applied the ultrasound by direct contact between the source and the skin over the larynx, and used intensities of 1–2 W cm^{-2}, for times of 2–10 min, once or twice a day, for up to 10 days. Rudimentary measurements of temperature suggested that this did not increase by more than about 2 degK. All five patients treated in this way apparently did very well.

Jenkins (1967) has reported the results of ultrasonic treatment of juvenile laryngeal papillomatosis, in a series of six patients. He used a 3 MHz ultrasonic source, applied with continuous irrigation to the skin over the thyroid cartilage, initially for 5 min, twice daily for 10 days. If the treatment was repeated, it was extended to 10 min (5 min each side) daily for six treatments. The intensity which was used is not clear, but the article states that "care must be taken not to turn the sound up too high as a prickling sensation ensues and makes the child restless". Later it is recorded that "the dose was increased to 3–5 W". The results were not consistent: four patients were improved to varying degrees; one seemed to be no better; and one was still receiving his first treatment. Jenkins (1967) ascribed this variability to faulty technique, and expressed the opinion that direct application of ultrasound to the papillomata would be preferable to irradiation through the neck.

According to Fairman (1972), both H. G. Birk and J. C. Jenkins have given up applying ultrasound externally to the larynx, and now use some form of intralyngeal probe. Either method may be preceded by surgical removal of the papillomata. White *et al.* (1974), in their series of 12 patients, used ultrasonic transducers of 5 mm diameter operating at 9 MHz, applied directly to the tissues to be treated. The ultrasonic power was 0·15 W, corresponding to an "average" intensity of 9 W cm^{-2}. The time of irradiation is not stated in the article, but it may be deduced from Fairman (1972) that the duration of a single treatment was 5 min. Furthermore, the rise in temperature was around 25 degK, and this could account for the therapeutic effort if the disease is due to a virus, as has been suggested. Clinically, the use of ultrasound seems to decelerate the rate of growth of laryngeal papillomata; but treatments need to be given at frequent intervals, not more than three months in children, until control has been established.

10.5.c Termination of Pregnancy

Sikov (1973) has proposed that pregnancy might be terminated by the delivery of ultrasound, either through the cervical canal, or focused transabdominally.

10.6 SURGICAL PROCEDURES DEPENDENT UPON THE DIRECT MECHANICAL EFFECTS OF ULTRASONIC VIBRATIONS

The use of ultrasonic cutting and drilling machines is widespread in industry (see, for example, Ensminger 1973). A slurry consisting of abrasive particles in a low-viscosity liquid is washed over the end of a tool shaped to conform to the desired geometry of the impression to be made. The tool is mounted at the tip of an ultrasonic source (usually a resonant velocity transformer: see Section 3.5) by which it is vibrated normally to the surface of the work, at a frequency of a few tens of kilohertz. The peak displacement of the tool is typically a few microns: the zone through which the tool vibrates is practically impenetrable. The cutting slurry is driven by the tool into the work for only a very small fraction of each cycle of oscillation, so that the cutting action is analogous to that of a pneumatic road-drill, but on a miniature scale.

The method is especially suitable for machining hard and brittle materials, where conventional rotary machines suffer from rapid wear and the danger of shattering the work.

10.6.a Dental Applications

In the early 1960s, ultrasonic techniques seemed to have a bright future in dentistry. At the time when they were being developed, however, the high speed rotary drill was introduced. This instrument is capable of operating at speeds of up to about 300000 rev min^{-1}; it can cut tooth structure faster than the ultrasonic drill, but, like the ultrasonic drill, it requires only very light pressure. Dentists familiar with the conventional rotary drill quickly learned to use the new high-speed drill. Thus ultrasonic cutting techniques never really gained acceptance in dentistry. The remaining potential applications of the ultrasonic instrument have been reviewed by Balamuth (1967); they include cleaning and calculus removal, gingivectomy, root canal reaming, orthodontic filing, and amalgam packing and gold foil manipulation. Although the dentist has fairly satisfactory conventional techniques for all these tasks, there is no doubt that the silence and ease of the ultrasonic method relieves the patient of much of the stress associated with dental treatment. It was estimated by Lees (1972) that at that time there were 50000 ultrasonic instruments in dental offices in the USA. Perhaps two factors are responsible for the obvious rarity of ultrasonic dental instruments in most other parts of the world: these are the cost of the equipment, and the general lack of knowledge and training concerning its use.

10.6.b Disintegration of Calculi

The objective of any method of ureteral lithotresis is harmlessly to break up the stone into fragments so small that they can be flushed out of the ureter immediately, or pass naturally without excessive pain, damage, or likelihood of later forming nuclei for more stones. Apart from the possibility that this objective might be achieved by ultrasonic energy, no realistic proposals have been made. Lamport and Newman (1956) described how they devised a method of making plaster-of-paris stones in the ureters of cadavers, to simulate ureteral calculi. Such stones were used as models in the design and development of ultrasonic lithotresor. There seemed to be no difficulty in transmitting 25 kHz ultrasound along four metal ribbons within a No. 11 catheter, to vibrate a hollow tool with an amplitude of 0·02–0·05 mm. The difficulties arose in maintaining contact by suction between the calculus and the tool: the tendency was for the tool to slip to one side of the calculus, and to cut a groove on its surface whilst also partially in contact with the wall of the ureter. This is not totally unsatisfactory, since the ureter suffers little damage, on account of its compliance, and it might allow conventional extraction instruments to be used where otherwise they would fail. Despite these rather encouraging experimental results, Lamport and Newman (1956) did not feel justified in using the method in man, since they feared the possibility of some unknown hazard resulting from the use of ultrasound. In this connexion, Howard *et al.* (1972) and Davies *et al.* (1974) studied the damage to the epithelial lining of the ureter and bladder in dogs resulting from the procedures which would be involved in the ultrasonic disintegration and subsequent removal of calculi. Generally, it appears that damage would be no worse than that caused by other methods of removing calculi, and that healing would be complete with about one month.

Unfortunately, Goodfriend (1973) gave no information concerning the ultrasonic parameters which he used to disintegrate calculi introduced in the ureters of dogs. Apparently the stones were broken up without gross injury to the wall of the ureter provided that the duration of the ultrasonic exposure was less than 10 s. He used the same method to disintegrate a calculus in the ureter of a patient who had had repeated attacks of renal colic. It seems that the procedure was ultrasonically to vibrate a long wire manipulated into position on the calculus by means of a cystoscope, within which the wire probe was introduced. Following the disintegration of the stone, the patient happily passed the fragments, and made an uneventful recovery.

It seems fairly clear that the major problem which remains to be solved in the development of a practical method of dealing with ureteric calculi with ultrasound, is the maintenance of contact between the stone and the vibrating tip of the ultrasonic tool. Davies *et al.* (1974) have constructed an expanding cage consisting of six wires which are contained within the lumen of the catheter. Once trapped in this cage, the stone is appropriately positioned for ultrasonic disintegration. The difficulty is to manoeuvre the cage around the stone in the first place.

In order to complete this review, mention must be made of the description of the breakdown within 5–15 min of calculi irradiated *in vitro* at intensities of 1·5–3·5 W cm^{-2}, at a frequency of 800 kHz (Velea *et al.*, 1972). Oxalate calculi differed from others, in that they did not break down so readily. Whether this effect could be used clinically remains to be tested, but it would be wrong to be optimistic.

10.6.c Emulsification and Aspiration of Cataracts

Congenital cataracts may be aspirated through an incision of only 2–3 mm in length; but this is not possible with senile cataracts, due to their consistency, and conventional removal requires an incision of 10–15 mm, encompassing 180° of the capsule.

Kelman (1967) has described the use of an ultrasonic instrument to emulsify the senile cataract *in situ*, thereby making aspiration possible. The system is illustrated in Fig. 10.5. The working tip, which is driven by a transducer and velocity transformer similar to that used in dentistry, consists of a hollow titanium needle with an outside diameter of about 1 mm, and a very slightly tapered point, with a loosely fitting protective sleeve made from teflon (PTFE). Irrigating solution is introduced through the space between the sleeve and the needle, at a pressure which is less than 3·3 kPa. Suction is applied to the hole in the centre of the needle: a roller type suction pump is used to provide a constant, controllable rate of fluid withdrawal. A bypass valve allows fluid to run off even if the suction pump is not operating. A thermocouple embedded in the protective sleeve is arranged to cut off both the ultrasound and the suction, if the temperature of the tip should become dangerously high as a result of a failure of the irrigation flow.

The surgical technique, described in detail by Kelman (1967), was developed in experiments with cadaver and animal eyes. A well-dilated pupil is essential: this is obtained by injection and instillation of adrenalin. An operating microscope is necessary. In brief, the procedure is as follows. An incision of 2–3 mm is made at the limbus, and aqueous is allowed to escape. Air is injected into the anterior chamber to expose the anterior surface of the lens. The anterior part of the capsule is cut with a cystotome, and removed through the incision, and the lens is manoeuvred out of the remaining part of the capsule. The ultrasonic probe is introduced through the incision into the anterior chamber, and chilled irrigation fluid (Baxter solution, or artificial aqueous) is allowed to flow slowly into the eye, until the temperature is 10°C or less. The suction pump is then started, by means of a foot switch; and the ultrasound is switched on for brief periods, using a second foot switch, and the resultant emulsion of nucleus and

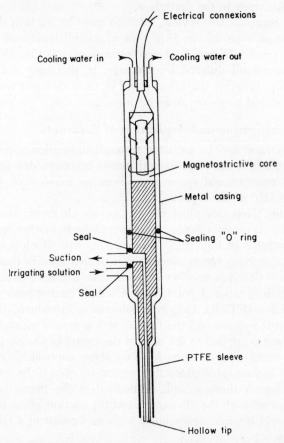

Electrical connexions

Cooling water in   Cooling water out

Magnetostrictive core

Metal casing

Seal   Sealing "O" ring

Suction
Irrigating solution

Seal

PTFE sleeve

Hollow tip

FIG. 10.5 Probe for phaco-emulsification. The diameter of the casing is about 15 mm, and that of the tip, about 1 mm. (Based on Kelman, 1969.)

cortical material is aspirated from the eye immediately after it has been formed. After several minutes, the lens material anterior to the capsule is completely removed. Material trapped between the anterior capsule is freed by a blunt aspirator, and subsequently emulsified and removed by the ultrasonic probe. The remainder of the procedure is concerned with mechanical removal of the remnants of the capsule.

The usefulness of the method has been assessed by Kelman (1969) in the clinical results achieved in a series of 12 patients. Eight of these patients had retinal disease or degeneration which precluded the possibility of achieving any useful vision no matter what the method of surgery: they hoped that the removal of their cataracts would improve their peripheral vision. In the other four eyes, there was a chance that vision might be regained. In every case, the visual result was as would have been expected with conventional surgery. Because of the small size of the incision, the postoperative progress was more rapid, and none of the operative or post-operative complications could be attributed to the use of ultrasonic energy. Mechanical difficulties, particularly in the balancing of input and output of fluid during aspiration, were largely overcome towards the end of the clinical series.

Further details of the operative procedure have been given by Arnott (1973). The advantages are the short convalescence—patients may be discharged after two days—the safety of the procedure, and the freedom from astigmatism. That the method has achieved considerable popularity, particularly in the USA, is clear from a series of articles in the *Transactions of the American Academy of Ophthalmology and Otolaryngology*, vol. 78, 1974, pp. 3–40.

Phillips and Williams (1972) have described a refinement of the procedure, using two Mason horns, each with a central hole, the two holes being connected to a pair of push–pull syringes. The tips of the two horns are introduced through opposite sides of the corneo-scleral junction, and the driving frequency is such that these junctions lie at nodal points, thus minimizing undesirable trauma.

10.6.d Other Applications in Eye Surgery

According to Youdin (1969), rabbit blood clots *in vitro*, and blood clots in the anterior chamber of cat and rabbit eyes, have been liquified by means of 60 kHz ultrasound applied through a hollow probe (1·3 mm outside diameter, 0·6 mm inside diameter) driven at peak-to-peak displacement amplitude of 0·05 mm. The hollow probe allows the removal of the liquified clot by suction, whilst the vitreous cavity is refilled with saline. Also Youdin (1969) has shown that, in the rabbit eye, a detached retina may be driven back by radiation pressure, using an ultrasonic frequency of 200 kHz, if air or silicone oil bubbles are introduced into the vitreous to act as a temporary tamponade against the retinal tissue. This method may prove to be a valuable adjunct in the treatment of giant retinal tears and the destruction of retinal adhesions without the necessity to subject the eye to the hazards of intravitreal surgery. Unfortunately, however, it has been found by Sokollu (1972) that the production of chorio-retinal lesions by ultrasound—using a trans-globe approach and frequencies in the range

3–15 MHz—is inferior to methods employing lasers and photocoagulation, so that a potentially elegant single-modality procedure is non-viable. This is because the ultrasonic technique has the disadvantages that injury may occur at the point of application of the probe, and at sites remote from the desired position of the lesion as a result of reflexion. Likewise ultrasonic cyclodiathermy—irradiation of the ciliary body to reduce intraocular pressure—has no advantage over the present conventional methods.

10.6.e Cleaning and Decalcifying Blood Vessels and Cardiac Valves

Arteriosclerosis is a common disease in developed countries. Its cause is not understood, but it may be associated with the stress of modern living. As the disease progresses, fatty material lines the walls of affected blood vessels. Initially this material has a consistency like that of soft cheese, but as time passes it hardens and becomes impregnated first with fibres and then with calcium. The effect is to restrict the blood flow, to change the shape of the pressure pulse, and sometimes, to embolize.

Mechanical scraping has been tried in order to clean blood vessels, but the wall of the artery may suffer damage, and detached deposits may travel downstream and block smaller vessels. Yeas and Barnes (1970) have experimented to determine whether it might be possible ultrasonically to remove these atheromatous deposits without damaging the blood vessel, forming particles so small in size that the dangers of occlusion would be eliminated. *In vitro* irradiation for 158 s of a segment of diseased artery with 72 kHz cavitating ultrasound resulted in substantial erosion of the fatty tissue without significant damage to the vessel. Most of the eroded material was of 1–7 μm in size, with a few pieces up to 25 μm. Particles of this size would not be troublesome, if the artery *in vivo* could be isolated during treatment. Subsequent experiments both *in vitro* and in dogs *in vivo* (Davies *et al.*, 1974) have confirmed that the softer elements of plaques can be pulverized and dispersed without difficulty, but calcified or rubbery areas are largely unaffected. This is rather discouraging, but it may be that a rotary cutting action could be used to detach this type of plaque.

The destruction and removal of thrombus from within blood vessels has been achieved by means of a specially designed ultrasonic probe (Stumpff *et al.*, 1975). The active part of the probe is the tip of a hollow waveguide. The waveguide is mounted coaxially within a sleeve, through which irrigating liquid (saline) is introduced to wash the liquidized thrombus into the waveguide and so out of the system. Two probes have been tested. One has an outside diameter of 3·4 mm, with a waveguide of 2·0 mm outside diameter and 1·4 mm inside diameter, and a length of 290 mm. The corresponding dimensions of the other are 3·0, 1·2, 0·8 and 210 mm. Both operate at 26·5 kHz. The dissolution and removal of thrombus are influenced by the shape of the tip of the waveguide. Best results are obtained, in terms of maximal dissolution rate, freedom from blockage, and minimal damage to the vessel wall, if the tip is rounded and the diameter of the hole at the end of the tip is rather less than the internal diameter of the remaining length of the waveguide. The suggested biophysical mechanism is that of cavitation. Experiments with thrombi induced in the iliac veins of dogs confirmed that clots of up to nine days old could be removed in 2·5–10 min. Older thrombi are organized by fibrous tissue, and cannot be removed in this way.

In clinical practice, the removal of thrombi by this method might be a dangerous procedure, since any small clots which become detached without being sucked out would be likely to cause occlusions in small arteries elsewhere in the body.

If the annulus of a cardiac valve is heavily calcified, the incidence of complications following its replacement by a prosthesis is increased. The common complications are heart block, separation of the aorta or the atrium from the ventricle, late aneurysm formation, paravalvular leak, and haemolysis. Brown and Davies (1972) have described the disintegration of calcific masses by means of an instrument designed for ultrasonic dental surgery (see Section 10.6.a). Preliminary experiments were made using valves excised during the course of prosthetic replacement surgery. Solid, ripe condensations of predominately mineral calcification were easily and quickly removed, but institial cartilaginous deposits were more difficult. In clinical prosthetic valve replacements, the method allowed good clearances of the annuli to be performed in six out of seven patients, in one of whom an earlier operation had been unsuccessful because of calcification. In comparison with conventional techniques, ultrasonic decalcification leaves the adjacent tissues relatively undamaged, and with good suture-holding properties. Furthermore, two elderly patients with pure calcific aortic stenosis were successfully treated by debridement of the aortic valve with ultrasound.

10.6.f Cutting and Welding Procedures

Some surgical techniques using low frequency ultrasonic probes, although little known in the English-speaking world, have been enthusiastically described by Goliamina (1974). More detailed information may be gleaned from Nikolaev (1973), who stated that more than 1000 operations using ultrasonic surgery had been carried out in the USSR up to 1972. Recently a review article has been published in English (Volkov and Shepeleva, 1974).

There are two distinct procedures. These are cutting and welding. In cutting procedures, the tool—a saw or a scalpel—is mounted at the end of a velocity transformer (see Section 3.5), and driven with an amplitude of

50–80 μm at 20–50 kHz. The cutting speed may be 50 or more times faster than with conventional methods. Generally the force which needs to be applied is only 10–20% of that required without ultrasound: this greatly reduces surgical trauma. Another advantage is that the tendency to bleed is greatly reduced. In cutting bone, the ultrasonic saw is 10 times faster than an ordinary saw. It is easy to control the cutting geometry, and the procedure is both relatively bloodless and free from pain.

In bone welding, a monomer of ethyl-alphacyantacrilate (cyacrine) is polymerised by ultrasound (20–50 kHz) within a few tens of seconds. The application of pulsed ultrasound (vibration amplitude 40–60 μm) to the bone tissue by means of a metallic velocity transformer causes deep penetration of the cyacrine, and thus ensures that a rugged, strong joint is made. The bone collagen enters into reaction with the cyacrine, and forms a single unit with it. Thus the action of the ultrasound is to bring about physicochemical processes, and to raise the temperature to 50–70°C.

The joint is generally formed from auto- or hetero-bone chips mixed with cyacrine. Bone ends may be butt-jointed or angled seams may be made to weld bone plates. The bone chip filler may be used to restore a cavity left by the removal of a tumour.

Bone welding is a temporary expedient which holds the various pieces together while natural regeneration occurs. Live cells eventually cover or penetrate the seams, and the filler material becomes perfused by blood. The method is apparently useful in orthopaedic surgery, and in the treatment of complicated fractures of the skull.

10.6.g Stapes Surgery

In stapes surgery for the treatment of otosclerosis, the most difficult part of the procedure is generally the removal of the footplate. The inner ear may be damaged by conventional techniques, whether a cuvette, a hook, or a microdrill is used. The drill is most dangerous, since it produces heat, and may cause microfractures in the petrous bone.

Apparently an ultrasonic drill has been developed which eliminates these risks (Anon., 1967). The ultrasonic frequency is 40 kHz—well above the audible range—and a velocity transformer is used to drive the cutting tip. No other technical details have been reported. In experimental tests on unspecified animals, histological studies made 15 days to three months after the surgery showed that the procedure produced no injury when used on the edges of the oval window, but damage to the inner ear was observed if the probe had been applied to the promontory or apical turns of the labyrinth. In clinical use, the probe is applied to the bone for not more than 4 s at a time, with 5 s intervals to allow the heat to be dissipated.

Those who try to reproduce this work may experience some difficulties. At least one attempt to construct a probe, using a length-expanding ceramic tube transducer, has been largely unsuccessful (J. A. James and P. N. T. Wells, unpublished).

10.7 CELL DISINTEGRATION AS A MANUFACTURING PROCESS

Low frequency cavitating ultrasound is used in many biological laboratories and in some manufacturing plants to disrupt cells or tissues and thus to release intracellular materials (see Section 9.6 and Hughes, 1961).

Using yeast as an experimental organism, Hughes (1961) showed that cell disruption is independent of ultrasonically generated free radicals, but enzyme (alcohol dehydrogenase) inactivation is accelerated by free radicals. Thus a compromise is necessary in order to obtain the most economic yield of active enzyme. Coakley and James (1971) extended this work with yeast, and studied the activities of both alcohol dehydrogenase and p-nitropheno-lase. They found that the rate constants for enzyme denaturation are both very much less than the rate contents for enzyme release, but that the former are functions of the protein concentration. They concluded that, for optimum results, the cell concentration should be high. Brown $et\ al.$ (1974) have developed a model, based on the assumption that the material is released intact and subsequently damaged, to enable the conditions to be optimized. The fraction x of protein released from cells after a treatment time t is given by:

$$x = 1 - e^{-k_1 t} \qquad (10.1)$$

where k_1 is the protein release rate constant. Once released the proteins are liable to sonochemical inactivation: the inactivation rate constant k_2 is proportional to the total protein concentration, and has a minimum value $k_{2\ min}$ when all the cells are disrupted. The inactivation rate at time t is given by:

$$k_2 = k_{2\ min}/[1 - \exp(-k_1 t)] \qquad (10.2)$$

The ratio $k_{2\ min}/k_1$ is a constant for the release of a given product from a given type of cell suspension, and may be determined experimentally. If D is the fraction of the total pool of product in solution at time t, then the equation

$$\Delta D/\Delta(k_1 t) = \exp(-k_1 t) - k_{2\ min} D/\{k_1[1 - \exp(-k_1 t)]\} \qquad (10.3)$$

may be integrated to obtained D as a function of $k_1 t$ for different values of $k_{2\ min}/k_1$.

10.8 PREPARATION OF TISSUE SPECIMENS FOR HISTOLOGICAL EXAMINATION

The conventional methods used to decalcify bone and to prepare soft tissue specimens for microscopy are slow. This may have an adverse effect on patient care, quite apart from being a nuisance in the laboratory.

Gagnon and Katyk (1960) have demonstrated that these processes may be greatly accelerated by the use of ultrasound, and that specimens prepared in this way are of good microscopic quality. They used an ultrasonic cleaner, operating at 37 kHz. Tissue fragments were successively fixed, dehydrated, clarified and included in paraffin wax under the action of ultrasound in liquid media: a specimen of 2 mm thickness may be processed in about 1 h. Compact bone fragments of the same thickness were decalcified within 4 h, either in 5% hydrochloric acid, or in successive baths of phloroglucinol-nitric acid and hydrochloric acid. Spongy bones required only half this time. The histological images showed only a minimum of artifacts. Conventional stains were used.

These exciting results have been confirmed by Thorpe *et al.* (1963) and Poston (1967). Since the method is inexpensive and simple, it is remarkable that it has apparently not been widely used.

10.9 AEROSOL THERAPY

When a beam of ultrasound of sufficient intensity is passed through a liquid and directed at an air interface, "atomization" of the liquid may occur. Liquid particles are ejected from the surface into the surrounding air, following the disintegration of capillary waves. Under suitable conditions, very fine dense fogs may be produced.

The production of ultrasonic aerosols has been investigated by Long (1962). He has shown that, at low production rates (less than about 0·01 ml s^{-1} of liquid atomization per square centimetre of surface area),

$$d_m = 0·34(8\pi\sigma/\rho f^2)^{1/3} \qquad (10.4)$$

where d_m is the median particle diameter, σ is the surface tension of the liquid, and the other symbols have their usual meanings. Thus, the particle size may be controlled for a given liquid by variation of the exciting frequency. For example, the median particle diameter of a water aerosol generated at 1 MHz is about 4 μm.

High rates of production can be achieved, the amount of liquid which can be suspended in the air being limited only by the rate at which it falls out. At higher rates, however, larger particles tend to be formed by the coalition of smaller ones.

Ultrasonic nebulizers designed for medical purposes are available commercially. Instruments of several types have been described by Boucher and Kreuter (1968).

It has been shown by Goddard et al. (1968) that the droplet size generated by commercially available nebulizers is in good agreement with theory, provided that there is a continuous and rapid flow of air through the nebulization chamber. A typical machine operates at 1·4 MHz, and converts 5 ml of liquid to aerosol per minute. The median particle diameter is around 6 μm. Ultrasonic nebulization under these conditions is not detrimental to pharmaceuticals such as penicillin. Ultrasonic nebulization can be used directly into a tent or canopy, as an aerosol treatment alone, or by incorporation into intermittent positive pressure breathing therapy.

Ultrasonically generated aerosols are of considerable potential value in medical treatment. For example, Miller et al. (1968) have described the maintenance of a humid atmosphere in a ventilating assistor using an ultrasonic nebulizer. Pneumatic atomization is less satisfactory in this application because of the large gas volume required to generate fine particles.

A collection of papers on this subject appears in Volume 5, number 4, of the *Journal of Asthma Research*, June 1968.

The control of particle size which can be achieved by an appropriate choice of ultrasonic frequency does not yet seem to have been exploited clinically. The depth of penetration into the respiratory tract increases as the particle size decreases. Thus, for treating the larynx and the trachea, particles of 6 μm diameter might be suitable; whereas to reach the bronchioles, particles of less than 1 μm might be necessary. This potential specificity might have significant clinical importance. Moreover, it has been pointed out by Cheney and Butler (1968) that the ultrasonic nebulizer may provide a method of quantifying the reactivity of the airways of patients with obstructive airway disease.

Finally, it is as well to point out that ultrasonic nebulizers require careful maintenance and regular cleaning. There are many reports in the literature (see, for example, Ringrose et al., 1968) of the transmission of infections by contaminated nebulizers.

10.10 ELIMINATION OF OXYGEN BUBBLES FROM THE CIRCULATION

In some surgical bypass procedures, small oxygen bubbles, with an average radius of less than about 100 μm, may be introduced during artificial oxygenation of the blood. Such bubbles are dangerous, since they may block small blood vessels and so cause thrombi to develop.

A practical solution to the problem would be to trap and possibly to extract the bubbles, before the blood is returned to the patient. Preliminary experiments have been carried out by Macedo and Young (1973) in order to test their theory that gas bubbles may be brought to a standstill on the wall of a tube through which liquid is flowing, by an ultrasonic field. They investigated the effect of irradiation in the frequency range 18–22 kHz, for flow velocities of up to 85 mm s^{-1}, through a tube of 15 mm diameter. The behaviour of air bubbles of 50–200 μm radius was studied, both in distilled water and in polymer solutions, one of which had rheological properties similar to those of blood.

The trajectory of the bubble motion depends on all the parameters investigated. By increasing the acoustic pressure amplitude (up to a maximum of 20 kPa), or by decreasing the flow velocity or liquid velocity, all the bubbles could be brought to a standstill in the first half-wavelength of the tube. Bubbles smaller than the resonant size (see Eqn. 9.1) assemble at the nodes of the standing pressure wave, whilst larger ones collect at the antinodes.

The method does not seem to have been tested in whole blood: this might reveal problems due to haemolysis. It does deserve further investigation, since it could have an important clinical application.

APPENDIXES

A1 ANALOGY BETWEEN MECHANICAL AND ELECTRO-MAGNETIC WAVES

Mechanical waves are discussed in Chapter 1. Analogous electromagnetic waves exist. J. C. Maxwell (1831–1879) predicted that waves can be transmitted in the electromagnetic field, one field supporting and generating the other. The existence of these waves was demonstrated in 1887 by Heinrich Hertz.

The oscillations in the electric and magnetic fields occur in normal planes, designated x and y, perpendicular to the direction of propagation z. The wave equations are:

$$\frac{\partial^2 E_x}{\partial z^2} = \frac{1}{c^2} \frac{\partial^2 E_x}{\partial t^2} \tag{A1.1}$$

and

$$\frac{\partial^2 H_y}{\partial z^2} = \frac{1}{c^2} \frac{\partial^2 H_y}{\partial t^2} \tag{A1.2}$$

where E_x = electric field vector,

$\quad H_y$ = magnetic field vector,

and $\quad c = (1/\epsilon\mu)^{1/2}$

where ϵ = permittivity of propagation medium,

and $\quad \mu$ = permeability of propagation medium.

Equations A1.1 and A1.2 are in the same form as Eqns. 1.16 and 1.20, and c has the meaning of velocity for both forms of wave, whether mechanical or electromagnetic.

Electromagnetic energy is composed of tiny packets, called *quanta* or *photons*. A photon is an elementary particle, in the same sense that an electron is an elementary particle: but it has neither electrical charge nor rest mass. This concept is incompatible with zero velocity. As a wave packet, the photon has a particle mass equivalent m, given by Einstein's relativity equation:

$$E = mc^2 \tag{A1.3}$$

where E is the energy of the photon. In free space, $c = 2.99 \times 10^8$ m s^{-1} for all electromagnetic radiation.

The Heisenberg *uncertainty principle* embodies the concept of wave-particle duality. This is a product of twentieth-century physics, which explained what had for 250 years seemed to be a paradox. Thus, writing about light in 1675, Newton stated "They, that will, may suppose it an aggregate of peripatetic qualities. Others may suppose it multitudes of unimaginable small and swift corpuscles of various sizes . . . let every man here take his fancy; only whatever light be, I suppose it consists of rays differing from one another in contingent circumstances, as bigness, form or vigour." It is now understood that it is impossible simultaneously to know both the exact position and the exact velocity of a particle. The physical meaning of this is that the intensity of a particle wave at any given point is proportional to the probability of finding a particle at that point. Thus, a particle is a highly localized entity, which is situated at a point in space at a particular instant. A wave is a diffuse entity which is spread over a whole region of space. In other respects, waves and particles are the same: they have mass, energy and momentum, and are deflected by gravitational fields.

The energy of the photon is given by the relationship:

$$E = hc/\lambda = hf \qquad (A1.4)$$

where h is Planck's constant (6.63×10^{-34} J s). Hence, from Eqns. A1.3 and A1.4

$$m = h/c\lambda \qquad (A1.5)$$

Thus, the mass of the photon is inversely proportional to the wavelength.

The energy which can be delivered by a single photon spans a range of 10^{16} across the electromagnetic spectrum. This is because the wavelengths of the various kinds of electromagnetic radiation extend from those of γ-rays ($\lambda = 10^{-13}$ m) to the longest radio waves ($\lambda = 10^3$ m). (Light, which is the portion of the spectrum visible to man, is mainly contained within the range 380 nm—violet—to 760 nm—red.)

In considering the biological effects of electromagnetic radiation, the photon energy is a most important factor. The term *"ionizing radiation"* refers to that end of the electromagnetic spectrum where the energies of the photons are sufficient, under ordinary circumstances, to produce ionization in the atoms of the absorbing molecules. An atom which has lost one or more electrons is called an *ion*. The energy needed to remove an electron from inside an atom to a point well outside the atom (strictly to a position at rest an infinite distance from the proton) is called the *ionization energy*. This energy is conveniently measured in electron volts, [eV], defined as the amount of energy released when an electron falls through a potential difference of 1 V; hence 1 $eV = 1.60 \times 10^{-19}$ J. Elements have ionization energies in the range 3–25 eV; some typical values are: hydrogen, 13·6 eV; carbon, 11·2 eV; nitrogen, 14·6 eV; oxygen, 13·7 eV; and sodium, 5·2 eV. If an energy of 3 eV is considered to be the minimum energy required to cause ionization, this corresponds to a wavelength equal to about 400 nm. Radiations with wavelengths of less than 50 nm have energies greater than 25 eV, and are capable of ionizing any element. Where the photons have insufficient energy to cause ionization, the radiation is said to be "*non-ionizing*". Arbitrarily, the lower limit of wavelength for ultraviolet radiation is generally set at 100 nm. Thus, non-ionizing electromagnetic radiation includes some of the ultraviolet, all of the visible spectrum, and the infrared and radio waves.

A2 THE DECIBEL NOTATION

It is often convenient to measure the ratios of pairs of wave amplitudes, or wave intensities, particularly if the *level* of one of these is taken as a reference for comparison with others. In this way, the need for absolute measurement is avoided, and, because ultrasonic waves are generally both generated and detected electrically, relative wave amplitudes can be expressed as ratios of voltages.

Two advantages accrue if such ratios are expressed as *logarithms*. Firstly, this affords a simple method of expressing numbers which extend over many orders of magnitude. Secondly, the arithmetic product of two or more quantities is obtained by addition of their logarithms (and similarly, by subtraction, in the case of division). The logarithmic unit which is most commonly used is the *decibel*, defined as follows:

$$\text{(relative level in decibels)} = 10 \log_{10}(P_2/P_1) = 20 \log_{10}(A_2/A_1) \quad \text{(A2.1)}$$

where P_1 and P_2 are the two powers, and A_1 and A_2 are the corresponding wave amplitudes.

The decibel levels corresponding to a wide range of power and amplitude ratios are listed in Table A2.1.

In the literature, reference is frequently made to the *neper*: this is a logarithmic ratio defined as follows:

$$\text{(relative level in nepers)} = \log_e(A_2/A_1) \quad \text{(A2.2)}$$

Hence, 1 neper = 8·686 dB.

TABLE A2.1

Decibel levels corresponding to various power and amplitude ratios

Negative decibels			Positive decibels	
Amplitude ratio	Power ratio	dB	Amplitude ratio	Power ratio
1·000	1·000	0·0	1·000	1·000
0·989	0·977	0·1	1·012	1·022
0·977	0·955	0·2	1·023	1·047
0·944	0·891	0·5	1·059	1·122
0·891	0·794	1	1·122	1·259
0·794	0·631	2	1·259	1·585
0·708	0·501	3	1·413	1·995
0·631	0·398	4	1·585	2·512
0·562	0·316	5	1·778	3·162
0·501	0·251	6	1·995	3·981
0·447	0·200	7	2·239	5·012
0·398	0·159	8	2·512	6·310
0·355	0·126	9	2·818	7·943
0·316	0·100	10	3·162	10·000
0·282	0·0794	11	3·584	12·59
0·251	0·0631	12	3·981	15·85
0·224	0·0501	13	4·467	19·95
0·200	0·0398	14	5·012	25·12
0·178	0·0316	15	5·623	31·62
0·159	0·0251	16	6·310	39·81
0·141	0·0200	17	7·080	50·12
0·126	0·0159	18	7·943	63·10
0·112	0·0126	19	8·913	79·43
0·100	0·0100	20	10·000	100·00
0·0562	0·003 16	25	17·78	316
0·0316	0·001 00	30	31·62	1000
0·0178	0·000 32	35	56·23	3162
0·0100	0·000 10	40	100·00	10000
0·0056	0·000 03	45	177·80	31620
0·0032	0·000 01	50	316·20	100000
0·001 00	10^{-6}	60	1000	10^6
0·000 32	10^{-7}	70	3162	10^7
0·000 10	10^{-8}	80	10000	10^8
0·000 03	10^{-9}	90	31620	10^9
0·000 01	10^{-10}	100	100000	10^{10}

A3 HISTORICAL REVIEW

This Appendix is a list of some key advances in biomedical ultrasonics, arranged in chronological order of the first significant publications, together with the names of selected pioneer investigators.

1917	Sonar	Langevin
1928	Studies of biological effects	Dunn, Dyer, Dyson, Fry, Harvey, Hill, Hughes, Lele, Nyborg, Taylor, Wood
1937	Ultrasound camera	Sokolov, Jacobs
1939	Measurements of velocity and attenuation in tissue	Carstensen, Dunn, Fry, Goldman, Hueter, Ludwig, Pohlman, Schwan
1946	Pulse–echo in NDT	Firestone, Sproule
1947	Transmission imaging	Dussik, Green
1950	A-scope	Gordon, Leksell, Ludwig, Reid, de Vlieger, White, Wild
1952	Vestibular surgery	Arslan, James, Kossoff, Krejci, Wells
	Two-dimensional B-scope	Baum, Brown, Donald, Greenwood, Holmes, Howry, Kossoff, Reid, Wagai, Wells, Wild
1953	Studies of scattering by biological tissues	Chivers, Hill, Lele, Mountford, Reid
1954	Neurosurgery	Fry, Lele, Lindstrom, Pond, Warwick
	Time position recording	Edler, Hertz
1955	Discovery of lead zirconate titanate	Jaffe
1957	Continuous-wave Doppler	Reid, Satomura, Woodcock
1964	Internal probes for diagnostics	Kimoto, Watanabe
1965	Physiotherapy	Lehmann
1966	Bragg imaging	Korpel
1967	Dental surgery	Balamuth
	Eye surgery	Kelman
	Real-time imaging	Åsberg, Bom, Henry, Roelandt, Somer, Thurstone
	Directional Doppler	Light, McLeod
1968	Direct-view storage tubes	Kossoff
	Acoustical holography	Aldridge, Brendon, Metherell
	Arrays	Bom, Meindl, Somer, Thurstone

1969	Rangefinding Doppler	Baker, Peronneau, Wells
1971	Acoustic microscopes	Kessler, Lemons
1972	Doppler imaging	Fish, Mozersky, Reid, Spencer
	Grey-scale displays	Hill, Kossoff, Taylor
1973	Automatic echoencephalography	Williams
1974	Computerized tomography	Greenleaf
	Time delay spectrometry	Heyser
	Impediography	Jones
1975	Scan converters	Hall
	Correlation methods	Newhouse

REFERENCES

1 Wave fundamentals

Beyer, R. T. (1950). Radiation pressure in a sound wave, *Am. J. Phys.*, **18**, 25–9.
Blitz, J. (1963). "Fundamentals of Ultrasonics", Butterworths, London.
Borgnis, F. E. (1953). Acoustic radiation pressure of plane compressional waves, *Rev. mod. Phys.*, **25**, 653–64.
Gooberman, G. L. (1968). "Ultrasonics, Theory and Application", English Universities Press, London.
Grosso, V. A. del and Mader, C. W. (1972). Speed of sound in pure water, *J. acoust. Soc. Am.*, **52**, 1442–6.
Hueter, T. F. and Bolt, R. H. (1955). "Sonics", Wiley, New York.
Kaye, G. W. C. and Laby, T. H. (1968). "Tables of Physical and Chemical Constants", Longmans, London.
Kinsler, L. E. and Frey, P. (1962). "Fundamentals of Acoustics", Wiley, New York.
Rooney, J. A. (1973). Does radiation pressure depend on B/A? *J. acoust. Soc. Am.*, **54**, 429–30.
Rooney, J. A. and Nyborg, W. L. (1972). Acoustic radiation pressure in a travelling plane wave, *Am. J. Phys.*, **40**, 1825–30.
Wells, P. N. T. (1969). "Physical Principles of Ultrasonic Diagnosis", Academic Press, London.
Wells, P. N. T., Bullen, M. A., Follett, D. H., Freundlich, H. F. and James, J. A. (1963). The dosimetry of small ultrasonic beams, *Ultrasonics*, **1**, 106–10.

2 Radiation

Beaver, W. L. (1974). Sonic nearfields of a pulsed piston radiator, *J. acoust. Soc. Am.*, **56**, 1043–8.
Christie, D. G. (1962). The distribution of pressure in the sound beams from probes used in ultrasonic flaw detection, *Appl. mater. Res.*, **1**, 86–97.
Dehn, J. T. (1960). Interference patterns in the near field of a circular piston, *J. acoust. Soc. Am.*, **32**, 1692–6.
Faran, J. (1951). Sound scattering by solid cylinders and spheres, *J. acoust. Soc. Am.*, **23**, 405–18.
Farn, C. L. S. and Huang, H. (1968). Transient acoustic fields generated by a body of arbitrary shape, *J. acoust. Soc. Am.*, **43**, 252–7.
Filipczyński, L. (1956). Radiation of acoustic waves for pulse ultrasonic flaw detection purposes, *Proc. 2nd Conf. Ultrason.*, *Warsaw*, 29–34.
Filipczyński, L. and Etienne, J. (1973). Theoretical study and experiments on spherical focusing transducers with Gaussian surface velocity distribution, *Acustica*, **28**, 121–8.
Freedman, A. (1970). Sound field of plane or gently curved pulsed radiators, *J. acoust. Soc. Am.*, **48**, 221–7.

Fry, W. J. and Dunn, F. (1962). Ultrasound: analysis and experimental methods in biological research. *In* "Physical Techniques in Biological Research" (ed. W. L. Nastuk), vol. IV, pp. 261–394, Academic Press, New York.

Golis, M. J. (1968). An analysis of the ultrasonic zone lens, *I.E.E.E. Trans. Sonics Ultrason.*, **SU-15**, 105–10.

Haselberg, K. von and Krautkramer, J. (1959). Ein Ultraschall-Strahler fur die Werkstoffprufurg mit verbessertum Nahfeld, *Acustica*, **9**, 359–64.

Kaspar'yants, A. A. (1960). Non-stationary radiation of sound by a piston. *Soviet Phys. Acoust.*, **6**, 52–6.

Kinsler, L. E. and Frey, P. (1962). "Fundamentals of Acoustics", Wiley, New York.

Kossoff, G. (1963). Design of narrow-beamwidth transducers, *J. acoust. Soc. Am.*, **35**, 905–12.

Kossoff, G. (1971). A transducer with uniform intensity distribution, *Ultrasonics*, **9**, 196–200.

Lale, P. G. (1969). Ultrasonic scanning: increased angular resolution by the use of half-wave plate combinations. *Proc. 8th int. Conf. med. biol. Engng*, 10–1.

Lockwood, J. C. and Willette, J. G. (1973a). High-speed method for computing the exact solution for the pressure variations in the nearfield of a baffled piston, *J. acoust. Soc. Am.*, **53**, 735–41.

Lockwood, J. C. and Willette, J. G. (1973b). Erratum: "High-speed method for computing the exact solution for the pressure variations in the nearfield of a baffled piston", *J. acoust. Soc. Am.*, **54**, 1762.

Martin, D. F. and Breazeale, M. A. (1971). A simple way to eliminate diffraction lobes emitted by ultrasonic transducers, *J. acoust. Soc. Am.*, **49**, 1668–9.

Mole, L. A., Hunter, J. L. and Davenport, J. M. (1972). Scattering of sound by air bubbles in water, *J. acoust. Soc. Am.*, **52**, 837–42.

Oberhettinger, F. (1961). On transient solutions of the "baffled piston" problem, *J. Res. natn. Bur. Stand.*, **65B**, 1–6.

Olofsson, F. (1963). An ultrasonic optical mirror system, *Acustica*, **13**, 361–7.

O'Neil, H. T. (1949). Theory of focusing radiators, *J. acoust. Soc. Am.*, **21**, 516–26.

Papadakis, E. P. and Fowler, K. A. (1971). Broad-band transducers: radiation field and selected applications, *J. acoust. Soc. Am.*, **50**, 729–45.

Robinson, D. E., Lees, S. and Bess, L. (1974). Near field transient radiation patterns for circular pistons, *I.E.E.E. Trans. Acoust. Speech Sig. Proc.*, **ASSP-22**, 395–403.

Schoch, A. (1941). Betrachtungen uber das Schallfeld einer Kolbenmembran, *Akust. Z.*, **6**, 318–26.

Sigelmann, R. A. and Reid, J. M. (1973). Analysis and measurement of ultrasound backscattering from an ensemble of scatterers excited by sine-wave bursts, *J. acoust. Soc. Am.*, **53**, 1351–5.

Stenzel, H. (1952). Die akustiche Strahlung der rechteckigen Kolbenmembran, *Acustica*, **2**, 263–81.

Tarnóczy, T. (1965). Sound focussing lenses and waveguides, *Ultrasonics*, **3**, 115–27.

Twersky, V. (1964). Acoustic bulk parameters of random volume distributions of small scatterers, *J. acoust. Soc. Am.*, **36**, 1314–29.

Zemanek, J. (1971). Beam behaviour within the nearfield of a vibrating piston, *J. acoust. Soc. Am.*, **49**, 181–91.

3 Generation and detection

3.1 Transducers

3.1.a Magnetostrictive transducers

Burgt, C. M. van der (1957). Ferroxcube material for piezomagnetic vibrators, *Philips Tech. Rev.*, **18**, 285–316.

Burgt, C. M. van der (1958). Ferroxcube 7A1 and 7A2, new piezomagnetic materials for ultrasonic power transducers, *Matronics*, no. 15, 173–304.

Hueter, T. F. and Bolt, R. H. (1955). "Sonics", Wiley, New York.

3.1.b Piezoelectric transducers

Bechman, R. (1958). Elastic and piezoelectric constants of alpha-quartz, *Phys. Rev.*, (2), **110**, 1060–1.

Cady, W. G. (1946). "Piezoelectricity", McGraw-Hill, New York.

Jaffe, B., Roth, R. S. and Marzullo, S. (1955). Properties of piezoelectric ceramics in solid–solution series lead titanate–lead zirconate–lead oxide: tin oxide and lead titanate–lead hafnate, *J. Res. natn. Bur. Stand.*, **55**, 239–54.

Kawai, H. (1969). The piezoelectricity of poly (vinylidene fluoride), *Jap. J. appl. Phys.*, **8**, 975–6.

Mason, W. P. (1950). "Piezoelectric Crystals and their Application to Ultrasonics", Van Nostrand, Princeton.

3.2 Resonance

3.3 The equivalent electrical circuit

Gooberman, G. L. (1968). "Ultrasonics", pp. 57–65, English Universities Press, London.

3.4 Impedance matching

Kossoff, G. (1966). The effects of backings and matching on the performance of piezo-electric ceramic transducers, *I.E.E.E. Trans. Sonics Ultrason.*, **SU-13**, 20–30.

McSkimmin, H. J. (1955). Transducer design for ultrasonic delay lines, *J. acoust. Soc. Am.*, **27**, 302–9.

3.5 Velocity transformers

James, J. A., Dalton, G. A., Hadley, K. J., Freundlich, H. F., Bullen, M. A., and Wells, P. N. T. (1963). A new 3-megacycle generator for destruction of the vestibular end organ, *Acta oto-lar.*, **36**, 148–53.

Neppiras, E. A. (1953). A high-frequency reciprocating drill, *J. scient. Instrum.* **30**, 72–4.

3.6 Ultrasonic generators

Carome, E. F., Parks, P. E. and Mraz, S. J. (1964). Propagation of acoustic transients in water, *J. acoust. Soc. Am.*, **36**, 946–52.

Coakley, W. T. (1971). Acoustical detectors of single cavitation events in a focused field in water at 1 MHz, *J. acoust. Soc. Am.*, **49**, 792–801.

Connolly, C. C. (1968). An ultrasonic generator giving widely variable ultrasonic parameters, *Biomed. Engng*, **3**, 72–5.

Cook, E. G. (1956). Transient and steady-state response of ultrasonic piezoelectric transducers, *I.R.E. Conv. Rec.*, **4** (9), 61–9.

Fry, W. J. (1958). Intense ultrasound in investigations of the central nervous system, *Adv. biol. med. Phys.*, **6**, 281–348.

Gericke, O. R. (1966). Experimental determination of ultrasonic transducer frequency response, *Mater. Eval.*, **24**, 409–11.

Gordon, G. (1963). Ultrasonic rays in diagnosis and surgery, *Med. Soc. Trans.*, **79**, 173–80.

Higgs, R. W. and Erikson, L. J. (1969). Acoustic decoupling properties of Corprene DC-100, *J. acoust. Soc. Am.*, **46**, 1254–8.

Hughes, D. E. and Cunningham, V. R. (1963). Methods for disrupting cells, *Biochem. Soc. Symp.*, **23**, 8–19.

Jacobsen, E. H. (1960). Sources of sound in piezoelectric crystals, *J. acoust. Soc. Am.*, **32**, 949–53.

James, J. A., Dalton, G. A., Hadley, K. J., Freundlich, H. F., Bullen, M. A. and Wells, P. N. T. (1963). A new 3-megacycle generator for destruction of the vestibular end organ, *Acta oto-lar.*, **56**, 148–53.

Kasai, C., Okuyama, D. and Kikuchi, Y. (1973). Generation and detection of short ultrasonic pulses via piezoelectric transducer with an intermediate layer of quarter wavelength, *Electron. Comm. Jap.*, **56-A**, 43–9.

Kolsky, H. (1956). The propagation of stress pulses in viscoelastic solids, *Phil. Mag.* (8), **1**, 693–710.

Kossoff, G. (1964). Design of the C.A.L. ultrasonic generator for the treatment of Menière's disease, *I.E.E.E. Trans. Sonics Ultrason.*, **SU-11**, 95–101.

Kossoff, G. (1966). The effects of backing and matching on the performance of piezo-electric ceramic transducers, *I.E.E.E. Trans. Sonics Ultrason.*, **SU-13**, 20–30.

Kossoff, G., Robinson, D. E. and Garrett, W. J. (1965). Ultrasonic two dimensional vizualization techniques, *I.E.E.E. Trans. Sonics Ultrason.*, **SU-12**, 31–7.

Kossoff, G., Wadsworth, J. R. and Dudley, P. F. (1967). The round window ultrasonic technique for treatment of Menière's disease, *Archs Otolar.*, **86**, 535–42.

Lele, P. P. (1962). A simple method for production of trackless focal lesions with focused ultrasound: physical factors, *J. Physiol., Lond.*, **160**, 494–512.

Lutsch, A. (1962). Solid mixtures with specified impedances and high attenuation for ultrasonic waves, *J. acoust. Soc. Am.*, **34**, 131–2.

McSkimmin, H. J. (1955). Transducer design for ultrasonic delay lines, *J. acoust. Soc. Am.*, **27**, 302–9.

Neppiras, E. A. (1971). Motional feedback systems for ultrasonic transducers. *In* "Ultrasonics 1971", pp. 56–8, I.P.C. Science and Technology Press, Guildford.

Pellam, J. R. and Galt, J. K. (1946). Ultrasonic propagation in liquids. 1. Application of the pulse technique to velocity and absorption measurements at 15 megacycles, *J. chem. Phys.*, **14**, 608–14.

Petersen, R. G. and Rosen, M. (1967). Use of thick transducers to generate short-duration stress pulses in thin specimens, *J. acoust. Soc. Am.*, **41**, 336–45.

Ponomarev, P. V. (1957). Transients in piezoelectric resonators, *Soviet Phys. Acoust.*, **3**, 260–71.

Redwood, M. (1961). Transient performance of a piezoelectric transducer, *J. acoust. Soc. Am.*, **33**, 527–36.

Redwood, M. (1963). A study of waveforms in the generation and detection of short ultrasonic pulses, *Appl. mater. Res.*, **2**, 76–84.

Redwood, M. (1964). Experiments with the electrical analog of a piezoelectric transducer, *J. acoust. Soc. Am.*, **36**, 1872–81.

Sjöberg, A., Stahle, J., Johnson, S. and Sahl, R. (1963). Treatment of Menière's disease by ultrasonic irradiation, *Acta oto-lar.*, Suppl., 178.

Stuetzer, O. M. (1967). Multiple reflections in a free piezoelectric plate, *J. acoust. Soc. Am.*, **42**, 502–8.

Walker, D. C. B. and Lumb, R. F. (1964). Piezoelectric probes for immersion ultrasonic testing, *Appl. mater. Res.*, **3**, 176–83.

Washington, A. B. G. (1961). The design of piezoelectric ultrasonic probes, *Br. J. non-destr. Test.*, **3**, 56–63.

Wells, P. N. T. (1968). The effect of ultrasonic irradiation on survival of *Daphnia magna*, *Exp. Biol.*, **49**, 61–70.

Wells, P. N. T. (1974). Ultrasonic Doppler probes. *In* "Cardiovascular Applications of Ultrasound" (ed. R. S. Reneman), pp. 125–31, North-Holland, Amsterdam.

Williams, A. R. and Nyborg, W. L. (1970). Microsonation using a transversely oscillating capillary, *Ultrasonics*, **8**, 36–8.

3.7 Ultrasonic detectors

3.7.a Hydrophones

Ackerman, E. and Holak, W. (1954). Ceramic probe microphones, *Rev. scient. Instrum.*, **25**, 857–61.

Aveyard, S. (1962). Radiation patterns from ultrasonic probes, *Br. J. non-destr. Test.*, **4**, 120–4.

Bom, N. (1972). "New Concepts in Echocardiography", pp. 67–8, Stenfert Kroese, Leiden.

Brendel, K. (1972). Hydrophones. *In* "Interaction of Ultrasound and Biological Tissues", (ed. J. M. Reid and M. R. Sikov), pp. 181–2, U.S. Department of Health, Education and Welfare, Publication (FDA) 73–8008.

Christie, D. G. (1962). The distribution of pressure in the sound beams from probes used with ultrasonic flaw detectors, *Appl. Mater. Res.*, **1**, 86–97.

Coakley, W. T. (1971). Acoustical detectors of single cavitation events in a focused field in water at 1 MHz, *J. acoust. Soc. Am.*, **49**, 792–801.

Colbert, J. R., Eggleton, R. C. and Weidner, A. J. (1972). Intensity calibration of pulsed ultrasonic beams. *In* "Interaction of Ultrasound and Biological Tissues", (ed. J. M. Reid and M. R. Sikov), pp. 187–92, U.S. Department of Health, Education and Welfare, Publication (FDA) 73–8008.

Hill, C. R. (1970). Calibration of ultrasonic beams for biomedical applications, *Phys. Med. Biol.*, **15**, 241–8.

Hodgkinson, W. L. (1966). Isosonography, *Ultrasonics*, **4**, 138–42.

Koppelmann, J. (1952). Beitrage zur Ultraschallmesstechnik in Flussigkeiten, *Acustica*, **2**, 92–5.

Okujima, M. (1974). Microphone for measurement of sound pressure radiated from ultrasono-diagnostic equipment, *Abstr. 8th int. Congr. Acoustics*, 353.

Romanenko, P. V. (1957). Miniature piezoelectric ultrasonic receivers, *Soviet Phys. Acoust.*, **3**, 364–70.

Saneyoshi, J., Okujima, M. and Ide, M. (1966). Wide frequency calibrated probe microphones for ultrasound in liquid, *Ultrasonics*, **4**, 64–6.

Schmitt, H. J. (1961). Ceramic capacitors as sound probes in liquids, *Rev. scient. Instrum.*, **32**, 215–7.

Simmons, B. D. and Urick, R. J. (1949). The plane wave reciprocity parameter and its application to the calibration of electroacoustic transducers at close distances, *J. acoust. Soc. Am.*, **21**, 633–5.

3.7.b Electrokinetic probes

Dietrick, H., Yeager, E., Bugosh, J. and Hovorka, F. (1953). Ultrasonic waves and electrochemistry. III. An electrokinetic effect produced by ultrasonic waves, *J. acoust. Soc. Am.*, **25**, 461–5.

3.7.c Electromagnetic transducers

Filipczyński, L. (1967). The absolute method for intensity measurements of liquid-borne ultrasonic pulses with the electrodynamic transducer, *Proc. Vibr. Probl.*, **8**, 21–6.

3.7.d Electrostatic transducers

Curtis, G. (1974). A broadband polymeric foil transducer, *Ultrasonics*, **12**, 148–54.

Filipczyński, L. (1966). Measuring pulse intensity of ultrasonic longitudinal and transverse waves in solids, *Proc. Vibr. Probl.*, **7**, 31–46.

Filipczyński, L. and Lypacewicz, G. (1972). Vibration patterns and properties of piezoelectric ceramic transducers for diagnostic application in medicine. *In* "Ultrasonics in Biology and Medicine", (ed. L. Filipczyński), pp. 81–9, Polish Scientific Publishers, Warsaw.

Gauster, W. B. and Breazeale, M. A. (1966). Detector for measurement of ultrasonic strain amplitudes in solids, *Rev. scient. Instrum.*, **37**, 1544–8.

Kolsky, H. (1956). The propagation of stress pulses in viscoelastic solids, *Phil. Mag.*, (8), **1** 693–710.

Legros, D. and Lewiner, J. (1973). Electrostatic ultrasonic transducers and their utilization with foil electrets, *J. acoust. Soc. Am.*, **53**, 1663–72.

Wintle, H. J. (1973). Introduction to electrets, *J. acoust. Soc. Am.*, **53**, 1578–88.

3.7.e Radiation pressure

Fox, F. E. (1940). Sound pressure on spheres, *J. acoust. Soc. Am.*, **12**, 147–9.

Green, P. S. (1971), A new liquid-surface-relief method of acoustic image conversion. *In* "Acoustical Holography" (ed. A. F. Metherell), vol. 3, pp. 173–87, Plenum Press, New York.

Hasegawa, T. and Yoshioka, K. (1969). Acoustic-radiation force on a solid elastic sphere, *J. acoust. Soc. Am.*, **46**, 1139–43.

Hill, C. R. (1970). Calibration of ultrasonic beams for biomedical applications, *Phys. Med. Biol.* **15**, 241–8.

King, L. V. (1934). On the acoustic radiation pressure on spheres, *Proc. R. Soc. A*, **147**, 212–40.

Kossoff, G. (1962). Calibration of ultrasonic therapeutic equipment, *Acustica*, **12**, 84–90.

Kossoff, G. (1965). Balance technique for the measurement of very low ultrasonic power outputs, *J. acoust. Soc. Am.*, **38**, 880–1.

Newell, J. A. (1963). A radiation pressure balance for the absolute measurement of ultrasonic power, *Phys. Med. Biol.*, **8**, 215–21.

Pohlman, R. (1948). Materialdurchleuchtung Mittels schalloptischer Abbildungen, *Z. angew. Phys.*, **1**, 181–7.

Rooney, J. A. (1973). Determination of acoustic power outputs in the microwatt–milliwatt range, *Ultrasound Med. Biol.*, **1**, 13–6.

Rozenberg, L. D. (1955). Survey of methods used for visualization of ultrasonic fields, *Soviet Phys. Acoust.*, **1**, 105–16.

Sjöberg, A., Stahle, J., Johnson, S. and Sahl, R. (1963). Treatment of Menière's disease by ultrasonic irradiation, *Acta oto-lar.*, Suppl., 178.

Wells, P. N. T., Bullen, M. A., Follett, D. H., Freundlich, H. F. and James, J. A. (1963). The dosimetry of small ultrasonic beams, *Ultrasonics*, **1**, 106–10.

Wells, P. N. T., Bullen, M. A. and Freundlich, H. F. (1964). Milliwatt ultrasonic radiometry, *Ultrasonics*, **2**, 124–8.

Wemlén, A. (1968). A milliwatt ultrasonic servo-controlled balance, *Med. biol. Engng*, **6**, 159–65.

3.7.f Calorimeters

Mikhailov, I. G. and Shutilov, V. A. (1957). Meter for measuring absolute ultrasonic intensity, *Soviet Phys. Acoust.*, **3**, 410–1.

Wells, P. N. T., Bullen, M. A., Follett, D. H., Freundlich, H. F. and James, J. A. (1963). The dosimetry of small ultrasonic beams, *Ultrasonics*, **1**, 106–10.

Zieniuk, J. (1965). On a non-adiabatic non-isothermal calorimeter for measurements of ultrasonic wave power in liquids, *Proc. Vibr. Prob.*, **4**, 367–78.

3.7.g Thermocouple probes

Fry, W. J. and Fry, R. B. (1954a). Determination of absolute sound levels and acoustic absorption coefficients by thermocouple probes—theory, *J. acoust. Soc. Am.*, **26**, 294–310.

Fry, W. J. and Fry, R. B. (1954b). Determination of absolute sound levels and acoustic absorption coefficients by thermocouple probes—experiment, *J. acoust. Soc. Am.*, **26**, 311–17.

Hueter, T. F. (1957). Boundary losses associated with acoustical streaming, *J. acoust. Soc. Am.*, **29**, 735–8.

Yoshioka, K. and Oka, M. (1965). Technical developments of focussed ultrasound and its biological and surgical applications in Japan. *In* "Ultrasonic Energy" (ed. E. Kelly), pp. 190–201, University of Illinois Press, Urbana.

3.7.h Thermistor probes

Szilard, J. (1974). A new device for monitoring ultrasound dosage, *Abstr. 8th int. Congr. Acoustics*, 352.

3.7.i Optical methods

Aldridge, E. E. (1967). A study of the ultrasonic micrometer, *I.E.E.E. Trans. Sonics Ultrason.*, **SU-14**, 89–99.

Deferrari, H. A., Darby, R. A. and Andrews, F. A. (1967). Vibrational displacement and mode-shape measurement by a laser interferometer, *J. acoust. Soc. Am.*, **42**, 982–90.

Erikson, K. R. (1972). Calibration of standard ultrasonic probe transducers using light diffraction. *In* "Interaction of Ultrasound and Biological Tissues" (ed. J. M. Reid and M. R. Sikov), pp. 193–7, U.S. Department of Health, Education and Welfare, Publication (FDA) 73–8008.

Harding, D. C. and Baker, D. W. (1968). Laser schlieren optical system for analyzing ultrasonic fields, *Biomed. Scis Instrum.*, **4**, 223–30.

James, J. A., Dalton, G. A., Bullen, M. A., Freundlich, H. F. and Wells, P. N. T. (1961). The effect of ultrasonics on the temporal bone, *Acta oto-lar.*, **53**, 168–81.

Mezrich, R. S., Etzold, K. F. and Vilkomerson, D. H. R. (1975). System for visualizing and measuring ultrasonic wavefronts. *In* "Acoustical Holography" (ed. N. Booth), vol. 6, pp. 165–91, Plenum Press, New York.

Sjöberg, A., Stahle, J., Johnson, S. and Sahl, R. (1963). Treatment of Menière's disease by ultrasonic irradiation, *Acta oto-lar.*, Suppl., 178.

Willard, G. W. (1947). Ultrasound waves made visible, *Bell Labs. Rec.*, **25**, 194–200.

3.7.j Chemical methods

Chapman, I. V. and Christie, A. D. (1972). Calibration of ultrasonic probes: a rapid method involving lecithin solutions, *Ultrasonics*, **10**, 57–8.

Cook, B. D. and Werchan, R. E. (1971). Mapping ultrasonic fields with cholesteric liquid crystals, *Ultrasonics*, **9**, 101–2.

Ernst, P. J. and Hoffman, C. W. (1952). New methods of ultrasonoscopy and ultrasonography, *J. acoust. Soc. Am.*, **24**, 207–11.

Kossoff, G. (1962). Calibration of ultrasonic therapeutic equipment, *Acustica*, **12**, 84–90.

Lele, P. P. (1962). Irradiation of plastics with focused ultrasound: a simple method for evaluation of dosage factors for neurological applications, *J. acoust. Soc. Am.*, **34**, 412–20.

Trier, H. G., Hagemann, H., Hockwin, O., Reuter, R. and Geissler, G. (1973). The determination of diagnostic ultrasound intensities using ammonium nitrate solutions, *Ophthal. Res.*, **5**, 77–88.

3.7.k Ultrasonic image converters

Brown, P. H., Randall, R. P., Sivyer, R. F. and Wardley, J. (1975). A high resolution, sensitive ultrasonic image converter. *In* "Ultrasonics International 1975", pp. 73–9, I.P.C. Science and Technology Press, Guildford.

Freitag, W., Martin, H. J. and Schellbac, G. (1960). Descriptions and results of investigations of an electronic ultrasonic image converter, *Proc. 2nd int. Conf. med. Electron.*, 373–9.

Goldman, R. G. (1962). Electronic acoustic image converter, *J. acoust. Soc. Am.*, **34**, 514–5.

Jacobs, J. E. (1965). The ultrasound camera, *Science J.*, **1** (4), 60–5.

Jacobs, J. E. (1974). Advances in the Sokoloff tube. *In* "Acoustical Holography" (ed. P. S. Green), vol. 5, pp. 633–45, Plenum Press, New York.

Jacobs, J. E., Berger, H. and Collis, W. J. (1963). An investigation of the limitations to the maximum attainable sensitivity in image converters, *I.E.E.E. Trans. ultrason. Engng*, **UE-10**, 83–8.

Semennikov, I. B. (1958). A study of acoustic image converters, *Soviet Phys. Acoust.*, **4**, 72–83.

Smyth, C. N., Poynton, F. Y. and Sayers, J. F. (1963). The ultrasound image camera, *Proc. I.E.E.*, **110**, 16–28.

3.7.l Pulse–echo methods

Gordon, D. (1964). Comparison of ultrasonic pulse–echo apparatus used in medicine, *Ultrasonics*, **2**, 199–202.

Lypacewicz, G. and Hill, C. R. (1974). Choice of standard target for medical pulse–echo equipment evaluation, *Ultrasound Med. Biol.*, **1**, 287–9.

Panian, F. C. and Valkenburg, H. E. van (1961). Development of ASTM standard reference blocks for ultrasonic inspection, *Non-destruct. Test.*, **19**, 45–57.

Wells, P. N. T. (1966a). Ultrasonics in clinical diagnosis. *In* "Scientific Basis of Medicine—Annual Reviews", pp. 38–53, Athlone Press, London.

Wells, P. N. T. (1966b). Some physical limitations in ultrasonic diagnosis, *Bio-med. Engng*, **1**, 390–4.

3.7.m Reciprocity

Carstensen, E. L. (1947). Self-reciprocity calibration of electro-acoustic transducer, *J. acoust. Soc. Am.*, **19**, 961–5.

MacLean, W. R. (1940). Absolute measurement of sound without a primary standard, *J. acoust. Soc. Am.*, **12**, 140–6.

Reid, J. M. (1974). Self-reciprocity calibration of echo-ranging transducers, *J. acoust. Soc. Am.*, **55**, 862–8.

Simmons, B. D. and Urick, R. J. (1949). The plane wave reciprocity parameter and its application to calibration of electroacoustic transducers at close distances, *J. acoust. Soc. Am.*, **21**, 633–5.

4 Velocity, absorption and attenuation in biological materials

4.1 Propagation velocity

4.2 Methods of velocity measurement

4.2.a Interferometry

Andreae, J. H. and Edmonds, P. D. (1961). Two megacycle interferometer, *J. scient. Instrum.*, **38**, 508.

Goldman, D. E. and Richards, J. R. (1954). Measurement of high frequency sound velocity in mammalian soft tissues, *J. acoust. Soc. Am.*, **26**, 981–3.

Kessler, L. W., Hawley, S. A. and Dunn, F. (1971). Semi-automatic determination of ultrasonic velocity and absorption in liquids, *Acustica*, **24**, 105–7.

4.2.b Pulse transit time measurement

Kossoff, G., Fry, E. K. and Jellins, J. (1973). Average velocity of ultrasound in the human female breast, *J. acoust. Soc. Am.*, **53**, 1730–6.

Papadakis, E. P. (1972). Absolute accuracy of the pulse–echo overlap method and the pulse-superposition method for ultrasonic velocity, *J. acoust. Soc. Am.*, **52**, 843–6.

Pellam, J. R. and Galt, J. K. (1946). Ultrasonic propagation in liquids: I. Application of pulse techniques to velocity and absorption measurements at 15 megacycles, *J. chem. Phys.*, **14**, 608–14.

4.2.c Sing-around technique

Greenspan, M. and Tschiegg, C. E. (1957). Speed of sound in water by a direct method, *J. Res. natn. Bur. Stand.*, **59**, 249–254.

Venrooij, G. E. P. M. van (1971). Measurement of ultrasound velocity in human tissues, *Ultrasonics*, **9**, 240–2.

4.2.d Velocity difference method

Carstensen, E. L. (1954). Measurement of dispersion of velocity of sound in liquids, *J. acoust. Soc. Am.*, **26**, 858–61.

Grosso, V. A. del, and Mader, C. W. (1972). Speed of sound in pure water, *J. acoust. Soc. Am.*, **52**, 1442–6.

4.2.e Reflexion coefficient

Dunn, F. and Fry, W. J. (1961). Ultrasonic absorption and reflection by lung tissue, *Phys. Med. Biol.*, **5**, 401–10.

4.3 Methods of attenuation measurement

4.3.a Pulse techniques

Andreae, J. H., Bass, R., Heasell, E. L. and Lamb, J. (1958). Pulse techniques for measuring ultrasonic absorption in liquids, *Acustica*, **8**, 131–42.

Andreae, J. H. and Joyce, P. L. (1962). 30 to 230 megacycle pulse technique for ultrasonic absorption measurements in liquids, *Br. J. appl. Phys.*, **13**, 462–7.

Chivers, R. C. and Hill, C. R. (1975). Ultrasonic attenuation in human tissues, *Ultrasound Med. Biol.*, **2**, 25–9.

Edmonds, P. D. (1966). Ultrasonic absorption cell for normal liquids, *Rev. scient. Instrum.*, **37**, 367–8.

Edmonds, P. D., Pearce, V. R. and Andreae, J. H. (1962). 1·5 to 28·5 Mc/s pulse apparatus for automatic measurement of sound absorption in liquids and some results for aqueous and other solutions, *Br. J. appl. Phys.*, **13**, 551–60.

Holasek, E., Jennings, W. D., Sokollu, A. and Purnell, E. W. (1973). Recognition of tissue patterns by ultrasonic spectroscopy, *Proc. I.E.E.E. Ultrasonics Symp.*, 73–6.

Hueter, T. F. (1958). "Visco-elastic Losses in Tissues in the Ultrasonic Range", *WADC Tech. Rpt.* 57–706.

Hunter, J. L. and Dardy, H. D. (1964). Ultrahigh-frequency ultrasonic absorption cell, *J. acoust. Soc. Am.*, **36**, 1914–7.

Kessler, L. W., Hawley, S. A. and Dunn, F. (1971). Semi-automatic determination of ultrasonic velocity and absorption in liquids, *Acustica*, **24**, 105–7.

Mountford, R. A. and Wells, P. N. T. (1972). Ultrasonic liver scanning: the A-scan in the normal and cirrhosis, *Phys. Med. Biol.*, **17**, 261–9.

Namery, J. and Lele, P. P. (1972). Ultrasonic detection of myocardial infarction in dog, *Proc. I.E.E.E. Ultrasonics Symp.*, 491–4.

4.3.b Thermocouple probes

Dunn, F. (1962). Temperature and amplitude dependence of acoustic absorption in tissue, *J. acoust. Soc. Am.*, **34**, 1545–7.

Dunn, F. and Fry, W. J. (1961). Ultrasonic absorption and reflection by lung tissue, *Phys. Med. Biol.*, **5**, 401–10.

4.3.c Spherical resonator

Hueter, T. F. (1958). "Visco-elastic Losses in Tissues in the Ultrasonic Range", *WADC Tech. Rpt.* 57–706.

4.4 Data for biological materials

Bakke, T. and Gyfre, T. (1974). Ultrasonic measurement of sound velocity in the pregnant and non-pregnant cervix uteri, *Scand. J. clin. Lab. Invest.*, **33**, 341–6.

Begui, Z. E. (1954). Acoustic properties of the refractive media of the eye, *J. acoust. Soc. Am.*, **26**, 365–8.

Bradley, E. L. and Sacerio, J. (1972). The velocity of ultrasound in human blood under varying physiologic parameters, *J. surg. Res.*, **12**, 290–7.

Buschmann, W., Voss, M. and Kemmerling, S. (1970). Acoustic properties of normal human orbit tissues, *Ophthal. Res.*, **1**, 354–64.

Carstensen, E. L. (1971). Effects of hemolysis on ultrasonic absorption in blood, *Acustica*, **25**, 183.

Carstensen, E. L. and Schwan, H. P. (1959a). Absorption of sound arising from the presence of intact cells in blood, *J. acoust. Soc. Am.*, **31**, 185–9.

Carstensen, E. L. and Schwan, H. P. (1959b). Acoustic properties of hemoglobin solutions, *J. acoust. Soc. Am.*, **31**, 305–11.

Carstensen, E. L., Li, K. and Schwan, H. P. (1953). Determination of the acoustic properties of blood and its components, *J. acoust. Soc. Am.*, **25**, 286–9.

Chivers, R. C. and Hill, C. R. (1975). Ultrasonic attenuation in human tissues, *Ultrasound Med. Biol.*, **2**, 25–9.

Colombati, S. and Petralia, S. (1950). Assorbimento di ultrasuoni in tessuti animali, *Ricerca scient.*, **20**, 71–8.

Craven, J. D., Costantini, M. A., Greenfield, M. A. and Stern, R. (1973). Measurement of the velocity of ultrasound in human cortical bone and its potential clinical importance, *Invest. Radiol.*, **8**, 72–7.

Danckwerts, H.-J. (1974). Discrete relaxation processes as a model of the absorption in liver homogenate, *J. acoust. Soc. Am.*, **55**, 1098–9.

Dunn, F. (1962). Temperature and amplitude dependence of acoustic absorption in tissue, *J. acoust. Soc. Am.*, **34**, 1545–7.

Dunn, F. (1974). Attenuation and speed of ultrasound in lung, *J. acoust. Soc. Am.*, **56**, 1638–9.

Dunn, F. and Fry, W. J. (1961). Ultrasonic absorption and reflection by lung tissue, *Phys. Med. Biol.*, **5**, 401–10.

Dunn, F., Edmonds, P. D. and Fry, W. J. (1969). Absorption and dispersion of ultrasound in biological media. *In* "Biological Engineering" (ed. H. P. Schwan), pp. 205–332, McGraw-Hill, New York.

Edmonds, P. D., Bauld, T. J., Dyro, J. F. and Hussey, M. (1970). Ultrasonic absorption of aqueous hemoglobin solutions, *Biochim. biophys. acta*, **200**, 174–7.

El'piner, I. E., Zaretskii, A. A. and Fursov, K. P. (1970). Absorption of ultrasonic radiation by protein solutions, *Biofizika*, **15**, 585–8.

Esche, R. (1952). Untersuchungen zur Ultraschallabsorption in Tierischen geweben und Kuntstoffen, *Akust. Beih.*, **2**, 71–4.

Floriani, L. P., Devevoise, N. T., and Hyatt, G. W. (1967). Mechanical properties of healing bone by the use of ultrasound, *Surg. Forum.*, **18**, 468–70.

Frucht, A. H. (1953). Die Schallgeschwindigkeit in Menschlichen und Tierischen geweben, *Z. ges. exp. Med.*, **120**, 526–57.

Goldman, D. E. and Hueter, T. F. (1956). Tabular data of the velocity and absorption of high-frequency sound in mammalian tissues, *J. acoust. Soc. Am.*, **28**, 35–7.

Goldman, D. E. and Hueter, T. F. (1957). Errata: tabular data of the velocity and absorption of high-frequency sound in mammalian tissues, *J. acoust. Soc. Am.*, **29**, 655.

Goldman, D. E. and Richards, J. R. (1954). Measurement of high frequency sound velocity in mammalian soft tissues, *J. acoust. Soc. Am.*, **26**, 981–3.

Gramberg, H. (1956). "Absorptionmessungen an biologischen Substanzen bei neidrigen Ultraschall frequenzen", Dissertation, Johann-Wolfgang-Goethe University, Frankfurt am Main.

Grosso, V. A. del and Mader, C. W. (1972). Speed of sound in pure water, *J. acoust. Soc. Am.*, **52**, 1442–6.

Hueter, T. F. (1948). Messung der Ultraschallabsorption in Tierischen geweben und ihre Abhangigkeit von der Frequenz, *Naturwissenschaften*, **35**, 285–6.

Hueter, T. F. (1952). Messung der Ultraschallabsorption in menschlichen Schädel-knocken und ihre Abhangigkeit von der Frequenz, *Naturwissenschaften*, **39**, 21–2.

Hueter, T. F. (1958). "Visco-elastic Losses in Tissues in the Ultrasonic Range", *WADC Tech. Rpt.* 57–706.

Jansson, F. and Sundmark, E. (1961). Determination of the velocity of ultrasound in ocular tissues at different temperatures, *Acta ophthal.*, **39**, 899–910.

Kessler, L. W. (1973). VHF ultrasonic attenuation in mammalian tissue, *J. acoust. Soc. Am.*, **53**, 1759–60.

Kossoff, G., Fry, E. K. and Jellins, J. (1973). Average velocity of ultrasound in the human female breast, *J. acoust. Soc. Am.*, **53**, 1730–6.

Lees, S. (1971). Ultra-sonics in hard tissues, *Int. dent. J.*, **21**, 403–17.

Ludwig, G. D. (1950). The velocity of sound through tissues and the acoustic impedance of tissues, *J. acoust. Soc. Am.*, **22**, 862–6.

Martin, B. and McElhaney, J. H. (1971). The acoustic properties of human skull bone, *J. biomed. mater. Res.*, **5**, 325–32.

Mayer, A. and Vogel, H. (1965). Ultraschallabsorption von Hämoglobinlösungen im MHz-Bereich, *Z. Naturforsch.*, **20b**, 85–92.

Mountford, R. A. and Wells, P. N. T. (1972). Ultrasonic liver scanning: the A-scan in the normal and cirrhosis, *Phys. Med. Biol.*, **17**, 261–9.

Pauly, H. and Schwan, H. P. (1971). Mechanism of absorption of ultrasound in liver tissue, *J. acoust. Soc. Am.*, **50**, 692–9.

Pinkerton, J. M. M. (1949). The absorption of ultrasonic waves in liquids and in relation to molecular constitution, *Proc. phys. Soc. (Lond.)*, **B62**, 129–41.

Pohlman, R. (1939). Uber die Absorption des Ultraschalls in menschlichen Gewebe und ihre Abhangigkeit von der Frequenz, *Phys. Z.*, **40**, 159–61.

Rich, C., Klinik, E., Smith, R. and Graham, B. (1966). Measurement of bone mass from ultrasonic transmission time, *Proc. Soc. exp. Biol. Med.*, **123**, 282–5.

Schneider, F., Muller-Landau, F. and Mayer, A. (1969). Acoustical properties of aqueous solutions of oxygenated and deoxygenated hemoglobin, *Biopolymers*, **8**, 537–44.

Smith, A. and Schwan, H. P. (1971). Acoustic properties of cell nuclei, *J. acoust. Soc. Am.*, **49**, 1329–30.

Theisman, H. and Pfander, F. (1949). Uber die Durchlassigkeit des knochens fur Ultraschall, *Strahlentherapie*, **80**, 607–10.

Venrooij, G. E. P. M. van (1971). Measurement of ultrasound velocity in human tissues, *Ultrasonics*, **9**, 240–2.

Vigoureux, P. (1952). "Ultrasonics", Chapman and Hall, London.

Wells, P. N. T. (1966). Ultrasonics in clinical diagnosis. *In* "Scientific Basis of Medicine—Annual Reviews", pp. 38–53, Athlone Press, London.

White, D. N. and Curry, G. R. (1975). Absorption of ultrasonic energy by the skull. *In* "Ultrasound in Medicine" (ed. D. N. White), vol. 1, p. 289, Plenum Press, New York.

Willocks, J., Donald, I., Duggan, T. C. and Day, N. (1964). Foetal cephalometry by ultrasound, *J. Obstet. Gynaec. Br. Commonw.*, **71**, 11–20.

Wladimiroff, J. W., Craft, I. L. and Talbert, D. G. (1975). *In vitro* measurements of sound velocity in human fetal brain tissue, *Ultrasound Med. Biol.*, **1**, 377–82.

4.5 Relevant theories

4.5.a Classical absorption

Fry, W. J. (1952). Mechanism of acoustic absorption in tissue, *J. acoust. Soc. Am.*, **24**, 412–5.

Hueter, T. F. (1958). "Visco-elastic Losses in Tissues in the Ultrasonic Range", *WADC Tech. Rpt.*, 57–706.

4.5.b Relaxation

Andreae, J. H. and Lamb, J. (1959). Ultrasonic relaxation theory for liquids, *Proc. R. Soc. Lond.*, **B69**, 814–22.

Bhatia, A. B. (1967). "Ultrasonic Absorption", Clarendon Press, Oxford.

Hertzfield, K. F. and Litovitz, T. A. (1959). "Absorption and Dispersion of Ultrasonic Waves", Academic Press, New York.

Litovitz, T. A. (1959). Ultrasonic spectroscopy in liquids, *J. acoust. Soc. Am.*, **31**, 681–91.

Markham, J. J., Beyer, R. T. and Lindsay, R. B. (1951). Absorption of sound in fluids, *Rev. mod. Phys.*, **23**, 353–411.

4.5.c Absorption and dispersion in biological materials

Carstensen, E. L. and Schwan, H. P. (1959). Acoustic properties of hemoglobin solutions, *J. acoust. Soc. Am.*, **31**, 305–11.

Danckwerts, H.-J. (1974). Determination of relaxation processes as a model of the absorption in liver homogenate, *J. acoust. Soc. Am.*, **55**, 1098–9.

Dunn, F., Edmonds, P. D. and Fry, W. J. (1969). Absorption and dispersion of ultrasound in biological media. *In* "Biological Engineering" (ed. H. P. Schwan), pp. 205–332, McGraw-Hill, New York.

Edmonds, P. D. (1962). Ultrasonic absorption of hemoglobin solutions, *Biochim. biophys. acta.*, **63**, 216–9.

Edmonds, P. D., Bauld, T. J., Dyro, J. F. and Hussey, M. (1970). Ultrasonic absorption of aqueous hemoglobin solutions, *Biochim. biophys. acta*, **200**, 174–7.

El'piner, I. E., Zaretskii, A. A. and Fursov, K. P. (1970). Absorption of ultrasonic radiation by protein solutions, *Biofizika*, **15**, 585–8.

Fry, W. J. (1952). Mechanism of acoustic absorption in tissue, *J. acoust. Soc. Am.*, **24**, 412–15.

Fry, W. J. and Dunn, F. (1962). Ultrasound: analysis and experimental methods in biological research. *In* "Physical Techniques in Biological Research" (ed. W. L. Nastuk), vol. IV, pp. 261–394, Academic Press, New York.

Hammes, G. G. and Lewis, T. B. (1966). Ultrasonic absorption in aqueous polyethylene glycol solutions, *J. phys. Chem.*, **70**, 1610–4.

Hueter, T. F. (1958). "Visco-elastic Losses in Tissue in the Ultrasonic Range", *WADC Tech. Rpt.* 57–706.

Kessler, L. W. (1973). VHF ultrasonic attenuation in mammalian tissue, *J. acoust. Soc. Am.*, **53**, 1759–60.

Pauly, H. and Schwan, H. P. (1971). Mechanism of absorption of ultrasound in liver tissue, *J. acoust. Soc. Am.*, **50**, 692–9.

Schneider, F., Muller-Landau, F. and Mayer, A. (1969). Acoustical properties of aqueous solutions of oxygenated and deoxygenated hemoglobin, *Biopolymers*, **8**, 537–44.

4.6 Relaxation processes in biological materials

Applegate, K., Slutsky, L. J. and Parker, R. C. (1968). Kinetics of proton-transfer reactions of amino acids and simple polypeptides, *J. Am. chem. Soc.*, **90**, 6909–13.

Burke, J. J., Hammes, G. G. and Lewis, T. B. (1965). Ultrasonic attenuation measurements in poly-L-glutamic acid solutions, *J. chem. Phys.* **42**, 3520–5.

Hammes, G. G. and Lewis, T. B. (1966). Ultrasonic absorption in aqueous polyethylene glycol solutions, *J. phys. Chem.*, **70**, 1610–4.

Hawley, S. A., Kessler, L. W. and Dunn, F. (1965a). Ultrasonic absorption in aqueous solutions of high-molecular-weight polysaccharides, *J. acoust. Soc. Am.*, **38**, 521–3.

Hawley, S. A., Kessler, L. W. and Dunn, F. (1965b). Errata: ultrasonic absorption in aqueous solutions of high-molecular-weight polysaccharides, *J. acoust. Soc. Am.*, **38**, 1064.

Hueter, T. F. (1952). Messung der Ultraschallabsorption in menschlichen Schädelknocken and ihre Abhangigkeit von der Frequenz, *Naturwissenschaften*, **39**, 21–2.

Hussey, M. and Edmonds, P. D. (1971). Ultrasonic examination of proton-transfer reactions in aqueous solutions of glycine, *J. acoust. Soc. Am.*, **49**, 1309–16.

Kessler, L. W. and Dunn, F. (1969). Ultrasonic investigation of the conformal changes of bovine serum albumin in aqueous solution, *J. phys. Chem.*, **73**, 4256–63.

Kremkau, F. W., Carstensen, E. L. and Aldridge, W. G. (1973). Macromolecular interaction in the absorption of ultrasound in fixed erythrocytes, *J. acoust. Soc. Am.*, **53**, 1448–51.

Michels, B. and Zana, R. (1969). Absorption ultrasonore de solutions aqueuses d'acides polyacrylique et polyméthylacrylique non natralisées, *Koll. Z.*, **234**, 1008–15.

O'Brien, W. D. and Dunn, F. (1972). Ultrasonic absorption mechanisms in aqueous solutions of bovine hemoglobin, *J. phys. Chem.*, **76**, 528–33.

O'Brien, W. D., Christman, C. L. and Dunn, F. (1972). Ultrasonic investigation of aqueous solutions of deoxyribose nucleic acid, *J. acoust. Soc. Am.*, **52**, 1251–5.

Pauly, H. and Schwan, H. P. (1971). Mechanism of absorption of ultrasound in liver tissue, *J. acoust. Soc. Am.*, **50**, 692–9.

Schneider, F., Muller-Landau, F. and Mayer, A. (1969). Acoustical properties of aqueous solutions of oxygenated and deoxygenated hemoglobin, *Biopolymers*, **8**, 537–44.

Sturm, J., Lang, J. and Zana, R. (1971). Ultrasonic absorption of DNA solutions: influence of pH, *Biopolymers*, **10**, 2639–43.

Wada, Y., Sasake, H. and Tomono, M. (1967). Viscoelastic relaxations in solutions of poly (glutamic acid) and gelatin at ultrasonic frequencies, *Biopolymers*, **5**, 887–97.

Zana, R. and Lang, J. (1974). Interaction of ultrasound and amniotic liquid, *Ultrasound Med. Biol.*, **1**, 253–8.

Zana, R., Lang, J., Tondre, C. and Sturm, J. (1972). Interactions of ultrasound with proteins and nucleic acids in solutions. *In* "Interactions of Ultrasound and Biological Tissues" (ed. J. M. Reid and M. R. Sikov), pp. 21–6, U.S. Department of Health, Education and Welfare, Publication (FDA) 73–8008.

Zaretskii, A. A., Zorina, O. M., Fursov, K. P. and El'piner, I. E. (1972). Characteristics of the absorption of ultrasound by protein solutions, *Soviet Phys. Acoust.*, **17**, 397–9.

4.7 Characteristics of other types of tissue
4.7.a Lung

Bauld, T. J. and Schwan, H. P. (1974). Attenuation and reflection of ultrasound in canine lung tissue, *J. acoust. Soc. Am.*, **56**, 1630–7.

Devin, C. (1959). Survey of thermal, radiation, and viscous damping of pulsating air bubbles in water, *J. acoust. Soc. Am.*, **31**, 1654–67.

Dunn, F. (1974). Attenuation and speed of ultrasound in lung, *J. acoust. Soc. Am.*, **56**, 1638–9.

Dunn, F. and Fry, W. J. (1961). Ultrasonic absorption and reflection by lung tissue, *Phys. Med. Biol.*, **5**, 401–10.

4.7.b Bone

Hueter, T. F. (1952). Messung der Ultraschallabsorption in menschlichen Schädelknocken und ihre Abhangigkeit von der Frequenz, *Naturwissenschaften*, **39**, 21–2.

White, D. N. and Curry, G. R. (1975). Absorption of ultrasonic energy by the skull. *In* "Ultrasonics in Medicine" (ed. D. N. White), vol. 1, p. 289, Plenum Press, New York.

4.8 Finite amplitude effects

Dunn, F. (1962). Temperature and amplitude dependence of acoustic absorption in tissue, *J. acoust. Soc. Am.*, **34**, 1545–7.

Fox, F. E. (1950). Dependence of ultrasonic absorption on intensity and the phenomenon of cavitation, *Nuovo cim.*, **7**, ser. ix, Suppl. 2, 198–203.

Fox, F. E. and Wallace, W. A. (1954). Absorption of finite amplitude sound waves, *J. acoust. Soc. Am.*, **26**, 994–1006.

Ryan, R. P., Lutsch, A. G. and Beyer, R. T. (1962). Measurement of the distortion of finite ultrasonic waves in liquids by a pulse method, *J. acoust. Soc. Am.*, **34**, 31–5.

Zarembo, L. K. and Krasil'nikov, V. A. (1959). Some problems in the propagation of ultrasonic waves of finite amplitude in liquids, *Soviet Phys. Usp.*, **2**, 580–99.

4.9 Characteristic impedances of biological materials

Gregg, E. C. and Palagallo, G. L. (1969). Acoustic impedance of tissue, *Invest. Radiol.*, **4**, 357–63.

Wright, H. (1973). Impulse-response function corresponding to reflection from a region of continuous impedance change, *J. acoust. Soc. Am.*, **53**, 1356–9.

5 Scattering by biological materials
5.1 Introduction

Chivers, R. C. (1973). "The Scattering of Ultrasound by Human Tissues", Ph.D. Thesis, University of London.

5.2 The large-obstacle situation

Reid, J. M. (1966). A review of some basic limitations in ultrasonic diagnosis. *In* "Diagnostic Ultrasound" (ed. C. C. Grossman, J. H. Holmes, C. Joyner and E. W. Purnell), pp. 1–12, Plenum Press, New York.

Senapati, N., Lele, P. P. and Woodin, A. (1972). A study of the scattering of sub-millimetre ultrasound from tissues and organs. *Proc. I.E.E.E. Ultrasonics Symp.*, 59–63.

5.3 The small-obstacle situation

Atkinson, P. and Berry, M. V. (1974). Random noise in ultrasonic echoes diffracted by blood, *J. Phys. A*, **7**, 1293–302.

Reid, J. M., Sigelmann, R. A., Nasser, M. G. and Baker, D. W. (1969). The scattering of ultrasound by human blood, *Abstr. 8th int. Congr. med. biol. Engng*, 10–7.

Sigelmann, R. A. and Reid, J. M. (1973). Analysis and measurement of ultrasound backscattering from an ensemble of scatterers excited by sine-wave bursts, *J. acoust. Soc. Am.*, **53**, 1351–5.

Twersky, V. (1964). Acoustic bulk parameters of random volume distributions of small scatters, *J. acoust. Soc. Am.*, **36**, 1314–29.

Waag, R. C. and Lerner, R. M. (1973). Tissue macrostructure determination with swept-frequency ultrasound, *Proc. I.E.E.E. Ultrasonics Symp.*, 63–6.

Wells, P. N. T. (1974). Ultrasonic Doppler probes. *In* "Cardiovascular Applications of Ultrasound" (ed. R. S. Reneman), pp. 125–31, North Holland, Amsterdam.

5.4 Scattering from solid tissues

Chivers, R. C. and Hill, C. R. (1975). A spectral approach to ultrasonic scattering from human tissue: methods, objectives and backscattering measurements, *Phys. Med. Biol.*, **20**, 799–815.

Chivers, R. C., Hill, C. R. and Nicholas, D. (1974). Frequency dependence of ultrasonic back-scattering cross-sections: an indicator of tissue structure characteristics. *In* "Ultrasonics in Medicine" (ed. M. de Vlieger, D. N. White and V. R. McCready), pp. 300–3, Excerpta Medica, Amsterdam.

Gericke, O. R. (1970). Ultrasonic spectroscopy. *In* "Research Techniques in Nondestructive Testing" (ed. R. S. Sharpe), pp. 31–61, Academic Press, London.

Hill, C. R. (1974). Interactions of ultrasound with tissues. *In* "Ultrasonics in Medicine" (ed. M. de Vlieger, D. N. White and V. R. McCready), pp. 14–20, Excerpta Medica, Amsterdam.

Howry, D. H., Stott, D. A. and Bliss, W. R. (1954). The ultrasonic visualization of carcinoma of the breast and other soft tissue structures, *Cancer N.Y.*, **7**, 354–8.

Mountford, R. A. and Wells, P. N. T. (1972a). Ultrasonic liver scanning: the quantitative analysis of the normal A-scan, *Phys. Med. Biol.*, **17**, 14–25.

Mountford, R. A. and Wells, P. N. T. (1972b). Ultrasonic liver scanning: the A-scan in the normal and cirrhosis, *Phys. Med. Biol.*, **17**, 261–9.

Nicholas, D. and Hill, C. R. (1975). Acoustic Bragg diffraction from human tissues, *Nature, Lond.*, **257**, 305–6.

Sigelmann, R. A. and Reid, J. M. (1972). Ultrasound scattering from biological tissues. *In* "Interaction of Ultrasound and Biological Tissues" (ed. J. M. Reid and M. R. Sikov), pp. 245–9, U.S. Department of Health, Education and Welfare, Publication (FDA) 73–80008.

Wild, J. J. and Reid, J. M. (1953). The effects of biological tissues on 15 Mc pulsed ultrasound, *J. acoust. Soc. Am.*, **25**, 270–80.

6 Pulse–echo methods

6.1 Introduction

Boyett, J. D. and Sullivan, J. F. (1970). Zinc and collagen content of cirrhotic liver, *Am. J. dig. Dis.*, **15**, 797–802.

Donald, I., MacVicar, J. and Brown, T. G. (1958). Investigation of abdominal masses by pulsed ultrasound, *Lancet*, **1**, 1188–94.

Fields, S. and Dunn, F. (1973). Correlation of echographic visualizability of tissue with biological composition and physiological state, *J. acoust. Soc. Am.*, **54**, 809–12.

Fry, E. K., Kossoff, G. and Lindeman, H. A. (1972). The potential of ultrasound visualization for detecting the presence of abnormal structures within the female breast, *Proc. I.E.E.E. Ultrasonics Symp.*, 25–30.

Fry, E. K., Okuyama, D. and Fry, F. J. (1971). The influence of biological and instrumentation variables on the characteristics of echosonography. *In* "Ultrasonographica Medica" (ed. J. Böck and K. Ossoinig), vol. I, pp. 387–93, Verlag Wien. Med. Akad., Vienna.

McDicken, W. N., Evans, D. H. and Robertson, D. A. R. (1974). Automatic sensitivity control in diagnostic ultrasonics, *Ultrasonics*, **12**, 173–6.

Mountford, R. A. and Wells, P. N. T. (1972). Ultrasonic liver scanning: the A-scan in the normal and cirrhosis, *Phys. Med. Biol.*, **17**, 241–9.

Robinson, D. E., Kossoff, G. and Garrett, W. J. (1966). Artefacts in ultrasonic echoscopic visualization, *Ultrasonics*, **4**, 186–94.

Wells, P. N. T. (1965). Resonance artifacts, *Ultrasonics*, **3**, 154.

Wells, P. N. T. (1966a). Ultrasonics in clinical diagnosis. *In* "Scientific Basis of Medicine—Annual Reviews", pp. 38–53, Athlone Press, London.

Wells, P. N. T. (1966b). Some physical limitations in ultrasonic diagnosis, *Bio-med. Engng*, **1**, 390–4.

6.2 Timing, switching and gating circuits

Davies, J. G. and Mitchell, M. (1960). Timing of injections for angiocardiography: description of an automatic device, *Clin. Radiol.*, **11**, 214–8.

Hall, A. J. (1970). A positionally incremented timebase display for ultrasonic pictures, *Ultrasonics*, **8**, 211–12.

6.3 Transmitters

Cheney, S. P., Lees, S., Gerhard, F. B. and Kranz, P. R. (1973). Step excitation source for ultrasonic pulse transducers, *Ultrasonics*, **11**, 111–3.

Kossoff, G., Robinson, D. E. and Garrett, W. J. (1965). Ultrasonic two dimensional visualization techniques, *I.E.E.E. Trans. Sonics Ultrason.* **SU-12**, 31–7.

Myers, G. H., Thumin, A., Feldman, S., Santis, G. de and Lupo, F. J. (1972). A miniature pulser-preamplifier for ultrasonic transducers, *Ultrasonics*, **10**, 87–9.

6.4 Radiofrequency amplifiers

Barnes, R. W., Nomeir, A.-M., Pardue, G. T. and Nuss, P. N. (1975). An ultrasound receiver with programmable time gain control, *J. clin. Ultrasound*, **3**, 121–4.

Griffith, J. M. and Henry, W. L. (1975). Switched gain—a technique for simplifying ultrasonic measurement of cardiac thickness, *I.E.E.E. Trans. biomed. Engng*, **BME-22**, 337–40.

Martin, T. B. (1962). Circuit applications of the field-effect transistor: part 2, *Semicond. Prod.*, **5** (3), 30–8.

Morris, A. G. (1965). A constant volume amplifier covering a wide dynamic range, *Electron. Engng*, **37**, 502–7.

Myers, G. H., Thumin, A., Feldman, S., Santis, G. de and Lupo, F. J., (1972). A miniature pulser-preamplifier for ultrasonic transducers, *Ultrasonics*, **10**, 87–9.

Wells, P. N. T., Halliwell, M. and Mountford, R. A. (1974). A method of display dynamic range expansion using system gain wobbulation, *Ultrasound Med. Biol.*, **1**, 179–81.

6.5 Video amplifiers

6.5.a General considerations

Brinker, R. A. (1966). Ultrasonic brain scanning utilizing the contact method. *In* "Diagnostic Ultrasound" (ed. C. C. Grossman, J. H. Holmes, C. Joyner and E. W. Purnell), pp. 186–90, Plenum Press, New York.

Brinker, R. A. and Taveras, J. A. (1966). Ultrasound cross-sectional pictures of the head, *Acta radiol. (D)*, **5**, 745–53.

Railton, R. and Hall, A. J. (1975). A simple approach to grey-scale echography, *Br. J. Radiol.*, **48**, 921–4.

Wells, P. N. T. (1974). The receiver in the pulse–echo system. *In* "Ultrasonics in Medicine" (ed. M. de Vlieger, D. N. White and V. R. McCready), pp. 30–6, Excerpta Medica, Amsterdam.

6.5.b Linear video amplifiers

6.5.c Logarithmic video amplifiers

Lunsford, J. S. (1965). Logarithmic pulse amplifier, *Rev. scient. Instrum.*, **36**, 461–4.

6.5.d Other processing arrangements

Howry, D. H. (1955). Techniques used in ultrasonic visualization of soft tissue structures of the body, *I.R.E. Conv. Rec.*, pt. 9, 75–81.

Hubelbank, M. (1972). Computer enhancement of ultrasound images, *Proc. I.E.E.E. Ultrasonic Symp.*, 22–4.

Ide, M. (1974). Image information processing for pulse echo scanning methods. *In* "Ultrasonic Imaging and Holography" (ed. G. W. Stroke, W. E. Kock, Y. Kikuchi and J. Tsujiuchi), pp. 159–89, Plenum Press, New York.

Kossoff, G. (1972). Improved techniques in cross sectional echography, *Ultrasonics*, **10**, 221–7.

Kossoff, G., Liu, C. N. and Robinson, D. E. (1965). A video logarithmic amplifier with quick recovery, *Electron Engng*, **37**, 306–10.

Kossoff, G., Robinson, D. E. and Garrett, W. J. (1968). Ultrasonic two-dimensional visualization for medical diagnosis, *J. acoust. Soc. Am.*, **44**, 1310–8.

Mars, N. J. I. (1974). Signaalverkerking voor ultrasonore geluidsapparatuser in de medische diagnostick. *Report no. 2. 4.119/1*, Medisch-Fysisch Instituut TNO, Utrecht.

McSherry, D. H. (1974). Digital processing systems for diagnostic ultrasound data. *In* "Ultrasonics in Medicine" (ed. M. de Vlieger, D. N. White and V. R. McCready), pp. 325–31, Excerpta Medica, Amsterdam.

Reid, J. M. (1968). Evaluation of intensity-modulated recording for ultrasonic diagnosis, *J. acoust. Soc. Am.*, **44**, 1319–23.

Wells, P. N. T. (1967). Signal processing in two-dimensional ultrasonography, *Bio-med. Engng*, **2**, 165–7.

6.5.e First echo swept gain trigger circuits

Wells, P. N. T. and Evans, K. T. (1968). An immersion scanner for two-dimensional ultrasonic examination of the human breast, *Ultrasonics*, **6**, 220–8.

6.6 Displays

6.6.a Conventional cathode ray tubes

6.6.b Direct view storage tubes

Anderson, R. H. (1967). A simplified direct-viewing bistable storage tube, *I.E.E.E. Trans. electron. Devices*, **ED-14**, 838–44.

Knoll, M. and Kazan, B. (1956). Viewing storage tubes. *In* "Advances in Electronics and Electron Physics" (ed. L. Martin), vol. 8, pp. 447–501, Academic Press, New York.

6.6.c Scan conversion memory tubes

6.6.d Photographic recording

Land, E. H. (1947). A new one-step photographic process, *J. opt. Soc. Am.*, **37**, 61–77.

6.6.e Grey scale and colour displays

Baum, G. (1970). Aids in ultrasonic diagnosis, *J. acoust. Soc. Am.*, **48**, 1407–12.

Bronson, N. R. and Pickering, N. C. (1975). Real-time color B-scan ultrasonography, *J. clin. Ultrasound*, **3**, 191–7.

Flinn, G. S. (1975). Gray scale color coding of abdominal B-scan ultrasonography, *J. clin. Ultrasound*, **3**, 179–85.

Hall, A. J. and Railton, R. (1975a). The importance of the brilliance control in grey scale echography, *Br. J. Radiol.*, **48**, 320–1.

Hall, A. J. and Railton, R. (1975b). Recording and storage of ultrasonic grey-scale images with a scan converter, *Br. J. Radiol.*, **48**, 1038.

Ide, M. (1974). Image information processing for pulse echo scanning methods. *In* "Ultrasonic Imaging and Holography" (ed. G. W. Stroke, W. E. Kock, Y. Kikuchi and J. Tsujiuchi), pp. 159–89, Plenum Press, New York.

Ito, K., Yokoi, H. and Tatsumi, T. (1974). Quantitative color ultrasonography. Computer aided simultaneous tomogram method. *In* "Ultrasonics in Medicine" (ed. M. de Vlieger, D. N. White and V. R. McCready), pp. 366–72, Excerpta Medica, Amsterdam.

Kobayashi, T., Takatani, O., Hattori, N., and Kimura, K. (1974). Differential diagnosis of breast tumors, *Cancer, N.Y.*, **33**, 940–51.

Kossoff, G. (1974). Display techniques in ultrasound pulse echo investigations: a review, *J. clin. Ultrasound*, **2**, 61–72.

Kossoff, G. and Garrett, W. J. (1972). Ultrasonic film echoscopy for placental localization, *Aust. N.Z. J. Obstet. Gynaec.*, **12**, 117–21.

McCarthy, C. F., Read, A. E. A., Ross, F. G. M. and Wells, P. N. T. (1967). Ultrasonic scanning of the liver, *Q. Jl Med.*, **36**, 517–24.

Milan, J. and Taylor, K. J. W. (1975). The application of the temperature-color scale to ultrasonic imaging, *J. clin. Ultrasound*, **3**, 171–3.

Taylor, K. J. W., Carpenter, D. A. and McCready, V. R. (1973). Grey scale echography in the diagnosis of intrahepatic disease, *J. clin. Ultrasound*, **1**, 184–7.

Wild, J. J. and Reid, J. M. (1952). Further pilot echographic studies on the histologic structure of the living intact human breast, *Am. J. Path.*, **28**, 839–61.

6.6.f Other display methods

Hertz, C. H. and Simonsson, S. I. (1969). Intensity modulation of ink-jet oscillographs, *Med. biol. Engng*, **7**, 337–40.

Hertz, C. H., Månsson, Å. and Simonsson, S.-I. (1967). A method for the intensity modulation of a recording ink jet and its applications, *Acta Univ. Lund.*, **II**, no. 15.

Lee, T. C. (1975). Ultrasound B-scanning with a gray scale video hard copy unit, *J. clin. Ultrasound*, **3**, 129–32.

Lindström, K., Holmer, N.-G., Eriksson, R. and Gudmundsson, B. (1973). The recording of echocardiograms with intensity-modulated ink-jet oscillograph, *I.E.E.E. Trans. biomed. Engng*, **BME-20**, 421–6.

6.7 The A-scope

Schiefer, W., Kazner, E. and Kunze, St (1968). "Clinical Echo-encephalography", John Wright, Bristol.

6.8 The B-scope

6.8.a General considerations

6.8.b The two-dimensional B-scope

Baum, G. and Greenwood, I. (1958). The application of ultrasonic locating techniques to ophthalmology, *A.M.A. Arch. Ophthal.*, **60**, 263–79.

Bom, N. (1972). "New Concepts in Echocardiography", Stenfert Kroese, Leiden.

Brown, T. G. (1960). Direct contact ultrasonic scanning techniques for the visualization of abdominal masses, *Proc. 2nd int. Conf. med. Electron.*, 358–66.

Brown, T. G. and Greening, J. R. (1973). Interactive single-entry-point scanning for medical diagnosis. *In* "Ultrasonics International 1973", pp. 208–13, I.P.C. Science and Technology Press, Guildford.

Eggleton, R. C., Townsend, C., Herrick, J., Templeton, G. and Mitchell, J. H. (1970). Ultrasonic visualization of left ventricular dynamics, *I.E.E.E. Trans. Sonics Ultrason.*, **SU-17**, 143–53.

Evans, G. C., Lehman, J. S., Brady, L. W., Smyth, M. G. and Hart, D. J. (1966). Ultrasonic scanning of abdominal and pelvic organs using B-scan display. *In* "Diagnostic Ultrasound" (ed. C. C. Grossman, J. H. Holmes, C. Joyner and E. W. Purnell), pp. 369–415, Plenum Press, New York.

Filipczyński, L. and Groniowski, J. T. (1967). Visualization of the inside of the abdomen by means of ultrasonics, and two methods for measuring ultrasonic doses, *Dig. 7th int. Conf. med. biol. Engng*, 320.

Filipczyński, L., Etienne, J., Lypacewicz, G. and Salkowski, J. (1967). Visualizing internal structure of the eye by means of ultrasonics, *Proc. Vibr. Probl.*, **4**, 357–680.

Fleming, J. E. E. and Lyons, E. A. (1974). A simple water bath to expand the horizons of the ultrasonic contact scanner, *Med. biol. Engng*, **12**, 864–6.

Fry, W. J., Leichner, G. H., Okuyama, D., Fry, F. J. and Fry, E. K. (1968). Ultrasonic visualization system employing new scanning and presentation methods, *J. acoust. Soc. Am.*, **44**, 1324–38.

Gordon, D. (1962). An improved tomograph for medical diagnosis, *Proc. San Diego Symp. biomed. Engng*, **2**, 20–2.

Greatorex, C. A. and Ireland, H. J. D. (1964). An experimental scanner for use with ultrasound, *Br. J. Radiol.*, **37**, 179–84.

Griffith, J. M. and Henry, W. L. (1974). A sector scanner for real time two-dimensional echocardiography, *Circulation*, **49**, 1147–52.

Hall, A. J. (1970). A positionally-incremented timebase display for ultrasonic pictures, *Ultrasonics*, **8**, 211–2.

Hertz, C. H. and Olofsson, S. (1963). A mirror system for ultrasonic visualization of soft tissues. *In* "Ultrasonic Energy" (ed. E. Kelly), pp. 322–6, University of Illinois Press, Urbana.

Holasek, E. and Sokollu, A. (1972). Direct contact, hand-held, diagnostic B-scanner, *Proc. I.E.E.E. Ultrasonics Symp.*, 38–43.

Holm, H. H. and Northeved, A. (1968). An ultrasonic scanning apparatus for use in medical diagnosis, *Acta chir. scand.*, **134**, 177–81.

Holm, H. H., Kristensen, J. K., Pedersen, J. F., Hancke, S. and Northeved, A. (1975). A new mechanical real time ultrasonic scanner, *Ultrasound Med. Biol.*, **2**, 19–23.

Holmes, J. H., Wright, W., Meyer, E. P., Posakony, G. T. and Howry, D. H. (1965). Ultrasonic contact scanner for diagnostic applications, *Am. J. med. Electron.*, **4**, 147–52.

Howry, D. H. (1957). Techniques used in ultrasonic visualization of soft tissues. *In* "Ultrasound in Biology and Medicine" (ed. E. Kelly), pp. 49–63, A.I.B.S., Washington.

Howry, D. H. (1965). A brief atlas of diagnostic ultrasonic radiologic results, *Radiol. Clin. N. Am.*, **3**, 433–52.

Howry, D. H. and Bliss, W. R. (1952). Ultrasonic visualization of the soft tissue structures of the body, *J. Lab. clin. Med.*, **40**, 579–92.

Jellins, J. and Kossoff, G. (1973). Velocity compensation in water-coupled breast echography, *Ultrasonics*, **11**, 223–6.

Kikuchi, Y., Uchida, R., Tanaka, K. and Wagai, T. (1957). Early cancer diagnosis through ultrasonics, *J. acoust. Soc. Am.*, **29**, 824–33.

Kimoto, S., Omoto, R., Tsunemoto, M., Moroi, T., Atsumi, K. and Uchida, R. (1964). Ultrasonic tomography of the liver and detection of heart atrial septal defect with the aid of ultrasonic intravenous probe, *Ultrasonics*, **2**, 82–6.

Kossoff, G. (1966). The effects of backing and matching on the performance of piezoelectric ceramic transducers, *I.E.E.E. Trans. Sonics Ultrason.*, **SU-13**, 20–30.

Kossoff, G., Garrett, W. J. and Robinson, D. E. (1965). An ultrasonic echoscope for visualizing the pregnant uterus. *In* "Ultrasonic Energy" (ed. E. Kelly), pp. 365–75, University of Illinois Press, Urbana.

Kossoff, G., Robinson, D. E. and Garrett, W. J. (1968). Ultrasonic two-dimensional visualization for medical diagnosis, *J. acoust. Soc. Am.*, **44**, 1310–8.

Krause, W. E. E. and Soldner, R. E. (1967). Ultrasonic imaging technique (B-scan) with high image rate for medical diagnosis—principle and technique of method, *Dig. 7th int. Conf. med. biol. Engng*, 315.

Makow, D. M. and Real, R. R. (1966). Development of a 360° compound immersion head scanner. *In* "Diagnostic Ultrasound" (ed. C. C. Grossman, J. H. Holmes, C. Joyner and E. W. Purnell), pp. 166–85, Plenum Press, New York.

McDicken, W. N. (1970). A fibre optic ultrasonic scanner, *Br. J. Radiol.*, **43**, 356–7.

McDicken, W. N., Bruff, K. and Paton, J. (1974). An ultrasonic instrument for rapid B-scanning of the heart, *Ultrasonics*, **12**, 269–72.

Mountford, R. A., Guibarra, E. J. and Halliwell, M. (1974). Semiautomatic transducer movement for ultrasonic compound B scanning, *Med. biol. Engng*, **12**, 227–32.

Pätzold, J., Krause, W., Kresse, H. and Soldner, R. (1970). Present state of an ultrasonic cross-section procedure with rapid image rate, *I.E.E.E. Trans. biomed. Engng*, **BME-17**, 263–5.

Somer, J. C. (1968). Electronic sector scanning for ultrasonic diagnosis, *Ultrasonics*, **6**, 153–9.

Thurstone, F. L. and Ramm, O. T. von (1974). A new ultrasound imaging technique employing two-dimensional beam steering. *In* "Acoustical Holography" (ed. P. S. Green), vol. 5, pp. 249–59, Plenum Press, New York.

Tomey, G. F. and Reid, J. M. (1969). Rotational compound scan, *Proc. 8th int. Conf. med. biol. Engng*, 22–2.

Vlieger, M. de, Sterke, A. de, Molin, C. E. and Ven, C. van der (1963). Ultrasound for two-dimensional echoencephalography, *Ultrasonics*, **1**, 148–51.

Wells, P. N. T. (1966). Developments in medical ultrasonics, *Wld med. Electron.*, **4**, 272–7.

Wells, P. N. T. and Evans, K. T. (1968). An immersion scanner for two-dimensional ultrasonic examination of the human breast, *Ultrasonics*, **6**, 220–8.

Wild, J. J. and Reid, J. M. (1952a). Application of echo-ranging techniques to the determination of structure of biological tissues, *Science, N.Y.*, **115**, 226–30.

Wild, J. J. and Reid, J. M. (1952b). Further pilot echographic studies of the histologic structure of the living intact human breast, *Am. J. Path.*, **28**, 839–61.

Wild, J. J. and Reid, J. M. (1954). Echographic visualization of lesions of the living intact human breast, *Cancer Res.*, **14**, 277–83.

Wild, J. J. and Reid, J. M. (1957). Progress in the techniques of soft tissue examination by 15 Mc pulsed ultrasound. *In* "Ultrasound in Biology and Medicine" (ed. E. Kelly), pp. 30–45, A.I.B.S., Washington.

6.8.c High speed scanners

Griffith, J. M. and Henry, W. L. (1974). A sector scanner for real time two-dimensional echocardiography, *Circulation*, **49**, 1147–52.

Holm, H. H., Kristensen, J. K., Pedersen, J. F., Hancke, S. and Northeved, A. (1975). A new mechanical real time ultrasonic scanner, *Ultrasound Med. Biol.*, **2**, 19–23.

McDicken, W. N., Bruff, K. and Paton, J. (1974). An ultrasonic instrument for rapid B-scanning of the heart, *Ultrasonics*, **12**, 269–72.

6.8.d Gated displays

Hussey, M., McDicken, W. N. and Robertson, D. A. R. (1973). Ultrasonic B-scanning of the heart with an ECG gated television display, *Ultrasonics*, **11**, 73–6.

6.8.e Considerations in choosing a scanner

Blackwell, R. J., Lachelin, G. C. L., McIntosh, A. S. and Suter, P. E. N. (1973). Technical points influencing the choice of an ultrasonic "B" scanner for obstetric use, *Br. J. Radiol.*, **46**, 259–61.

6.9 Time position recording

Barnes, R. W. and Thurstone, F. L. (1971). An ultrasound moving target indicator system for diagnostic use, *I.E.E.E. Trans. biomed. Engng*, **BME-18**, 4–8.

Hokanson, D. E., Strandness, D. E. and Miller, C. W. (1970). An echo-tracking system for recording arterial wall motion, *I.E.E.E. Trans. Sonics Ultrason.*, **SU-17**, 130–2.

Wells, P. N. T. and Ross, F. G. M. (1969). A time-to-voltage analogue converter for ultrasonic cardiology, *Ultrasonics*, **7**, 171–6.

6.10 Other systems

6.10.a The C-scope

Carson, P. L., Leung, S. S., Hendee, W. R. and Holmes, J. H. (1975). Constant depth ultrasound imaging using computer acquisition, display, and analysis. *In* "Ultrasound in Medicine" (ed. D. N. White), vol. 1, pp. 509–17, Plenum Press, New York.

Hill, C. R. and McCready, V. R. (1975). Ultrasonic scanning apparatus, *Br. Patent* 1 391 903.

Kimoto, S., Omoto, R., Tsunemoto, M., Moroi, T., Atsumi, K. and Uchida, R. (1964). Ultrasonic tomography of the liver and detection of heart atrial septal defect with the aid of ultrasonic intravenous probe, *Ultrasonics*, **2**, 82–6.

McCready, V. R. and Hill, C. R. (1971). A constant depth ultrasonic scanner, *Br. J. Radiol.*, **44**, 747–50.

Northeved, A., Holm, H. H., Kristensen, J. K., Pedersen, J. F. and Rasmussen, S. N. (1974). An automatic ultrasonic spherical section scanner, *Ultrasound Med. Biol.*, **1**, 183–6.

Omoto, R. (1967). Intercardiac scanning of the heart with the aid of ultrasonic intravenous probe, *Jap. Heart J.*, **8**, 569–81.

6.10.b Strongly focused systems

Ardenne, M. von and Millner, R. (1962). The US-focosan method, *I.R.E. Trans. med. Electron.*, **ME-9**, 145–9.

Burckhardt, C. B., Grandchamp, P.-A. and Hoffmann, H. (1974). Methods for increasing the lateral resolution of B-scan. *In* "Acoustical Holography" (ed. P. S. Green), vol. 5, pp. 391–413, Plenum Press, New York.

Burckhardt, C. B., Grandchamp, P.-A. and Hoffmann, H. (1975). Focussing ultrasound over a large depth with an annular transducer, an alternative method, *I.E.E.E. Trans. Sonics Ultrason.*, **SU-22**, 11–15.

Burckhardt, C. B., Hoffmann, H. and Grandchamp, P.-A. (1973). Ultrasound axicon: a device for focussing over a large depth, *J. acoust. Soc. Am.*, **54**, 1628–30.

Fry, F. J. (1968). Intracranial anatomy visualized in vivo by ultrasound, *Invest. Radiol.*, **3**, 243–66.

Kossoff, G. (1972). Improved techniques in ultrasonic cross sectional echography, *Ultrasonics*, **10**, 221–7.

Thurstone, F. L. and McKinney, W. M. (1966a). Resolution enhancement in scanning of tissue, *Ultrasonics*, **4**, 25–7.

Thurstone, F. L. and McKinney, W. M. (1966b). Focused transducer arrays in an ultrasonic scanning system for biologic tissue. *In* "Diagnostic Ultrasound" (ed. C. C. Grossman, J. H. Holmes, C. Joyner and E. W. Purnell), pp. 191–4, Plenum Press, New York.

6.10.c Arrays

Adams, R. N. and McCutcheon, E. P. (1973). Electronically steered ultrasonic beam using a single crystal, *Proc. 26th ann. Conf. Engng Med. Biol.*, 425.

Bom, N. (1972). "New Concepts in Echocardiography," Stenfert Kroese, Leiden.

Bom, N., Lancée, C. T., Honkoop, J. and Hugenholtz, P. G. (1971). Ultrasonic viewer for cross-sectional analysis of moving cardiac structures, *Bio-med. Engng*, **6**, 500–3, 508.

Bom, N., Lancée, C. T., Zwieten, G. van, Kloster, F. E. and Roelandt, J. (1973). Multiscan echocardiography. I. Technical description. *Circulation*, **48**, 1066–74.

Brown, T. G. and Haslett, R. W. G. (1963). Improvements in flaw detection and like systems using pulsed sonic or ultrasonic waves, *Br. Patent* 941 573.

Burckhardt, C. B., Grandchamp, P.-A. and Hoffmann, H. (1974). An experimental 2 MHz synthetic aperture sonar system intended for medical use, *I.E.E.E. Trans. Sonics. Ultrason.*, **SU-21**, 1–6.

Cutrona, L. J. (1970). Synthetic aperture radar. *In* "Radar Handbook" (ed. M. I. Skolnik), pp. 1–25, McGraw-Hill, London.

Doornbos, P. and Somer, J. C. (1972). An electrically variable analogue delay line achieved by fast consecutively commutated capacitors, *Prog. Rpt*, Institute of Medical Physics, Utrecht, 109–13.

Eggleton, R. C., Townsend, C., Herrick, J., Templeton, G. and Mitchell, J. H. (1970). Ultrasonic visualization of left ventricular dynamics, *I.E.E.E. Trans. Sonics Ultrason.*, **SU-17**, 143–53.

Esser, L. J. M. (1974). The peristaltic charge-coupled device for high-speed charge transfer, *Proc. I.E.E.E. int. solid-state Circ. Conf.*, 28–29, 219.

Havlice, J. F., Kino, G. S. and Quate, C. F. (1973). A new acoustic imaging device, *Proc. I.E.E.E. Ultrasonic Symp.*, 13–7.

Hottinger, C. F. and Meindl, J. D. (1973). Ultrasonic transducer array for arterial imaging, *Proc. 26th ann. Conf. Engng Med. Biol.*, 424.

Kossoff, G. (1973). Ultrasonic research in medicine in Australia—a review. *In* "Ultrasonics International 1973", pp. 199–205, I.P.C. Science and Technology Press, Guildford.

Lobdell, D. D. (1968). A non-linearly processed array for enhanced azimuthal resolution, *I.E.E.E. Trans. Sonics Ultrason.*, **SU-15**, 202–8.

Maginness, M. G., Plummer, J. D. and Meindl, J. D. (1974). An acoustic image sensor using a transmit-receive array. *In* "Acoustical Holography" (ed. P. S. Green), vol. 5, pp. 619–31, Plenum Press, New York.

Manoli, S. H. (1974). An intraventricular ultrasound method for measurement of left-ventricular dimensions, *I.E.E.E. Trans. biomed. Engng*, **BME-21**, 333–5.

Martin, R. W., Lindbloom, L. E. and Pollack, G. H. (1974). Ultrasonic catheter tip instrument for measurement of vessel cross-sectional area, *Proc. 27th ann. Conf. Engng Med. Biol.*, 186.

Meindl, J. D., Brody, W. R., Green, P. S., Hileman, R. and Kopel, L. (1974). "Ultrasonic Transducers: Signal Detection and Preprocessing", A.E.M.B., Chevy Chase.

Mountford, R. A., Halliwell, M. and Wells, P. N. T. (1974). Ultrasonic array scanning of the kidney, *Ultrasound Med. Biol.*, 1, 161–77.

Sato, T., Ueda, M. and Tada, H. (1972). Ultrasonic imaging system by using optical pulse compression, *J. opt. Soc. Am.*, 62, 668–71.

Snoeck, B. (1972). Clock pulse generator for driving electrically variable delay circuits, *Prog. Rept*, Institute of Medical Physics, Utrecht, 106–8.

Somer, J. C. (1968). Electronic sector scanning for ultrasonic diagnosis, *Ultrasonics*, 6, 153–9.

Somer, J. C. and Dael, J. W. J. M. van (1972). Application of a non-linear processing technique to ultrasound pulse-echo systems for improving angular resolution. *In* "Ultrasonics in Biology and Medicine" (ed. L. Filipczyński), pp. 201–13, Polish Scientific Publishers, Warsaw.

Suckling, E. E. and Hendrickson, J. R. (1969). Image scanner using diode switches, *J. acoust. Soc. Am.*, 45, 892–4.

Thompsett, M. F. and Zimany, E. J. (1973). Use of charge-coupled devices for delaying analog signals, *I.E.E.E. Trans. solid-state Circ.*, SC-8, 151–7.

Thurstone, F. L. and Ramm, O. T. von (1974). A new ultrasound imaging technique employing two-dimensional electronic beam steering. *In* "Acoustical Holography" (ed. P. S. Green), vol. 5, pp. 149–59, Plenum Press, New York.

Whittingham, T. A. and Evans, J. A. (1975). Ultrasonic visualization of the heart. *In* "Ultrasonics International 1975", pp. 182–9, I.P.C. Science and Technology Press, Guildford.

6.11 Display of three-dimensional data

Baum, G. and Greenwood, I. (1961). Orbital lesion localization by three-dimensional ultrasonography, *N.Y. State J. Med.*, 61, 4149–57.

Brown, T. G. and Greening, J. R. (1973). Interactive single-entry-point scanning for medical diagnosis. *In* "Ultrasonics International 1973", pp. 208–13, I.P.C. Science and Technology Press, Guildford.

Dekker, D. L., Piziali, R. L. and Dong, E. (1974). A system for ultrasonically imaging the human heart in three dimensions, *Comput. biomed. Res.*, 7, 544–53.

Howry, D. H., Posakony, G. J., Cushman, C. R. and Holmes, J. H. (1956). Three-dimensional and stereoscopic observation of body structure by ultrasound, *J. appl. Physiol.*, 9, 304–6.

Leith, E. N., Upatnieks, J., Kozma, A. and Massey, N. (1966). Hologram visual displays, *J. Soc. Motion Pict. Telev. Engrs*, 75, 323–6.

McDicken, W. N., Lindsay, M. and Robertson, D. A. R. (1972). Three-dimensional images using a fibreoptic ultrasonic scanner, *Br. J. Radiol.*, 45, 70–1.

Rasmussen, S. N., Nielsen, S. K., Bartrum, R. J., Stigsby, B. and Holm, H. H. (1974). Three-dimensional imaging of abdominal organs with ultrasound, *Am. J. Roentg.*, 121, 883–8.

Redman, J. D., Walton, W. P., Fleming, J. E. and Hall, A. J. (1969). Holographic display of data from ultrasonic scanning, *Ultrasonics*, 7, 26–9.

Robinson, D. E. (1972). Display of three-dimensional ultrasonic data for medical diagnosis, *J. acoust. Soc. Am.*, 52, 673–87.

Szilard, J. (1974). An improved three-dimensional display system, *Ultrasonics*, **12**, 273–6.

6.12 Analysis of pulse–echo data
6.12.a General considerations

Erikson, J. J. and Brill, A. B. (1970). Digitization of ultrasonic images, *Radiology*, **95**, 589–93.

Fields, S. I., Bowie, J. A., Pai, A. L. and Lichtor, J. L. (1975). Tissue differentiation by semi-automated quantitative analysis of A-scan echography. *In* "Ultrasound in Medicine" (ed. D. N. White), vol. 1, pp. 439–46, Plenum Press, New York.

Goldstein, A., Ophir, J. and Templeton, A. W. (1975). A computerized ultrasound processing, acquisition and display (CUPAD) system: research in ultrasound image generation. *In* "Ultrasound in Medicine" (ed. D. N. White), vol. 1, pp. 475–87, Plenum Press, New York.

Ide, M. and Masuzawa, N. (1975). Electrical recording and reproduction of ultrasono-tomograms using a VTR, *I.E.E.E. Trans. biomed. Engng*, **BME-22**, 340–6.

Kay, M., Shimmins, J., Manson, G. and England, M. E. (1975). A computer interface for digitizing ultrasonic information, *Ultrasonics*, **13**, 18–20.

Kelsey, C., Dunn, F., Edwards, P. D., Nyborg, W. L. and Reid, J. M. (1974). "Interaction of Ultrasonic Energy with Biological Structures", A.E.M.B., Chevy Chase.

Milan, J. (1972). An improved ultrasonic scanning system employing a small digital computer, *Br. J. Radiol.*, **45**, 911–6.

Trier, H. G. and Reuter, R. (1973). Digital computer analysis of time-amplitude ultrasonograms from the human eye. I. Signal acquisition, *J. clin. Ultrasound*, **1**, 150–4.

Vlieger, M. de, Megens, P. and Sluys, J. van der (1974). Recording pulsations in echo-encephalography, *Med. biol. Engng*, **12**, 503–9.

Wells, P. N. T. (1974). The receiver in the pulse-echo system. *In* "Ultrasonics in Medicine" (ed. M. de Vlieger, D. N. White and V. R. McCready), pp. 30–6, Excerpta Medica, Amsterdam.

6.12.b Image enhancement

Hirsch, M., Sanders, W. J., Popp, R. L. and Harrison, D. C. (1973). Computer processing of ultrasonic data from the cardiovascular system, *Comput. biomed. Res.*, **6**, 336–46.

King, J. C. and Wong, A. K. C. (1972). Computer analysis of transcranial echotomographic B-scans, *Comput. biomed. Res.*, **5**, 190–204.

McSherry, D. H. (1974). Digital processing systems for diagnostic ultrasound data. *In* "Ultrasonics in Medicine" (ed. M. de Vlieger, D. N. White and V. R. McCready), pp. 325–31, Excerpta Medica, Amsterdam.

Pai, A. L., Cahill, N. S., Du Broff, R. J. and Brooks, H. L. (1974). Computer analysis of echocardiograms, *Proc. 27th ann. Conf. Engng Med. Biol.*, 265.

6.12.c Amplitude analysis

Chivers, R. C. and Hill, C. R. (1975). A spectral approach to ultrasonic scattering from human tissue: methods, objectives and backscattering measurements, *Phys. Med. Biol.*, **20**, 799–815.

Czarnecki, T. and Kubicki, S. (1970). Observations on the application of ultrasounds in the diagnosis of diffuse liver disease, *Pol. med. J.*, **9**, 79–87.

Decker, D., Epple, E., Leiss, W. and Nagel, M. (1973). Digital computer analysis of time-amplitude ultrasonograms from the human eye. II. Data processing, *J. clin. Ultrasound*, **1**, 156–9.

Fields, S. I., Bowie, J. D., Pai, A. L. and Lichtor, J. L. (1975). Tissue differentiation by semi-automated quantitative analysis of A-scan echography. *In* "Ultrasound in Medicine" (ed. D. N. White), vol. 1, pp. 439–46, Plenum Press, New York.

Grossmann, H. (1971). Automatische Echogrammauswertung bei der Ultraschall-Leberdiagnostik, *Nachrichtentechnik*, **21**, 64–6.

Hill, C. R. (1974). Interactions of ultrasound with tissues. *In* "Ultrasonics in Medicine" (ed. M. de Vlieger, D. N. White and V. R. McCready), pp. 14–20, Excerpta Medica, Amsterdam.

Hounsfield, G. N. (1973). Computerized transverse axial scanning (tomography): Part I. Description of system, *Br. J. Radiol.*, **46**, 1016–22.

Mountford, R. A. and Wells, P. N. T. (1972a). Ultrasonic liver scanning: the quantitative analysis of the normal A-scan, *Phys. Med. Biol.* **17**, 14–25.

Mountford, R. A. and Wells, P. N. T. (1972b). Ultrasonic liver scanning: the A-scan in the normal and cirrhosis, *Phys. Med. Biol.*, **17**, 261–9.

Mountford, R. A., Halliwell, M. and Atkinson, P. (1973). Ultrasonic liver scanning: automated A-scan analysis, *Phys. Med. Biol.*, **18**, 559–69.

Namery, J. and Lele, P. P. (1972). Ultrasonic detection of myocardial infarction in dog, *Proc. I.E.E.E. Ultrasonics Symp.*, 491–4.

Ossoinig, K. C. (1974). Quantitative echography—the basis of tissue differentiation, *J. clin. Ultrasound*, **2**, 33–46.

Rettenmaier, G. (1974). Quantitative criteria of intrahepatic echo patterns correlated with structural alterations. *In* "Ultrasonics in Medicine" (ed. M. de Vlieger, D. N. White and V. R. McCready), pp. 199–206, Excerpta Medica, Amsterdam.

Schentke, K.-U. and Renger, F. (1964). Über die diagnostische Verwertbarkeit des Ultraschallhepatogramms, *Z. ges. inn. Med.*, **21**, 239–40.

Shung, K. P., Sigelmann, R. A. and Schmer, G. (1975). Ultrasonic measurement of blood coagulation time, *I.E.E.E. Trans. biomed. Engng*, **BME-22**, 334–7.

Wells, P. N. T., McCarthy, C. F., Ross, F. G. M. and Read, A. E. A. (1969). Comparison of A-scan and compound B-scan ultrasonography in the diagnosis of liver disease, *Br. J. Radiol.*, **42**, 818–23.

Wild, J. J. and Reid, J. M. (1952). Further pilot echographic studies on the histologic structure of tumors of the living intact human breast, *Am. J. Path.*, **28**, 839–61.

6.12.d Frequency analysis

Chivers, R. C. and Hill, C. R. (1975). A spectral approach to ultrasonic scattering from human tissue: methods, objectives and backscattering measurements, *Phys. Med. Biol.*, **20**, 799–815.

Chivers, R. C., Hill, C. R. and Nicholas, D. (1974). Frequency dependence of ultrasonic backscattering cross-sections: an indicator of tissue structure characteristics. *In* "Ultrasonics in Medicine" (ed. M. de Vlieger, D. N. White and V. R. McCready), pp. 300–3, Excerpta Medica, Amsterdam.

Freese, M. and Hamid, M. A. K. (1974). Lipid content determination in whole fish using ultrasonic pulse backscatter, *Proc. I.E.E.E. Ultrasonics Symp.*, 69–76.

Holasek, E., Gans, L. A., Purnell, E. W. and Sokollu, A. (1975). A method for spectra-color B-scan ultrasonography, *J. clin. Ultrasound*, **3**, 175–8.

Namery, J. and Lele, P. P. (1972). Ultrasonic detection of myocardial infarction in dog, *Proc. I.E.E.E. Ultrasonics Symp.*, 491–4.

Pace, N. G. (1975). Sediment identification using acoustic techniques. *In* "Ultrasonics International 1975", pp. 245–8, I.P.C. Science and Technology Press, Guildford.

6.12.e Signal averaging

Furgason, E. S., Newhouse, V. L., Bilgutay, N. M. and Cooper, G. R. (1975). Application of random signal correlation techniques to ultrasonic flaw detection, *Ultrasonics*, **13**, 11–7.

Lees, S., Gerhard, F. B., Barber, F. E. and Cheney, S. P. (1973). DONAR: a computer processing system to extend ultrasonic pulse-echo testing, *Ultrasonics*, **11**, 165–73.

6.12.f Impediography

Jones, J. P. (1973). Impediography: a new ultrasonic technique for non-destructive testing and medical diagnosis. *In* "Ultrasonics International 1973", pp. 214–18, I.P.C. Science and Technology Press, Guildford.

Jones, J. P. (1975a). Impediography: a new ultrasonic technique for diagnostic medicine. *In* "Ultrasound in Medicine" (ed. D. N. White), vol. 1, pp. 489–97, Plenum Press, New York.

Jones, J. P. (1975b). A preliminary experimental evaluation of ultrasonic impediography. *In* "Ultrasound in Medicine" (ed. D. N. White), vol. 1, pp. 499–508, Plenum Press, New York.

6.12.g Correlation techniques

Furgason, E. S., Newhouse, V. L., Bilgutay, N. M. and Cooper, G. R. (1975). Application of random signal correlation techniques to ultrasonic flaw detection, *Ultrasonics*, **13**, 11–7.

6.13 System performance
6.13.a Introduction

Lypacewicz, G. and Hill, C. R. (1974). Choice of standard target for medical pulse-echo equipment evaluation, *Ultrasound Med. Biol.*, **1**, 287–9.

6.13.b Signal path performance

Blackwell, R. J. (1972). Practical aspects of ultrasonic "B" scanning in medicine, *Bio-med. Engng*, **7**, 356–62.

Buschmann, W. (1965). New equipment and transducers for ophthalmic diagnosis, *Ultrasonics*, **3**, 18–21.

Kossoff, G. (1969). The measurement of peak acoustic intensity generated by pulsed ultrasonic equipment, *Ultrasonics*, **7**, 249–51.

Wells, P. N. T. (1971). The standardisation of electronic systems in ultrasonic pulse-echo diagnosis. *In* "Ultrasonographia Medica" (ed. J. Böck and K. Ossoinig), vol. II, pp. 29–37, Verlag Wien. Med. Akad., Vienna.

6.13.c Registration performance

Blackwell, R. J. (1972). Practical aspects of ultrasonic "B" scanning in medicine, *Bio-med. Engng*, **7**, 356–62.

Fleming, J. E. and Hall, A. J. (1968). Two dimensional compound scanning—effects of maladjustment and calibration, *Ultrasonics*, **6**, 160–6.

Garrett, W. J. and Kossoff, G. (1975). An obstetric test for resolution by ultrasonic echoscopes, *Ultrasonics*, **13**, 217–8.

Hall, A. J. and Fleming, J. E. E. (1975). A method for checking the registration of contact B-scanners, *J. clin. Ultrasound*, **3**, 51–4.

Halliwell, M. and Mountford, R. A. (1973). Physical sources of registration errors in pulse-echo ultrasonic systems. Part I—Velocity and attenuation, *Med. biol. Engng*, **11**, 27–32.

Hudson, A. C. and Bradley, J. L. (1973). Simple simulated human head for checking echoencephalographic equipment, *Med. biol. Engng*, **11**, 359–61.

Mountford, R. A. and Halliwell, M. (1973). Physical sources of registration errors in pulse-echo ultrasonic systems. Part II—Beam deformation, deviation and divergence, *Med. biol. Engng*, **11**, 33–8.

Taylor, K. J. W. and Hill, C. R. (1975). Scanning techniques in grey-scale ultrasonography, *Br. J. Radiol*, **48**, 918–20.

Wells, P. N. T. and Ross, F. G. M. (1969). A time-to-voltage analogue converter for ultrasonic cardiology, *Ultrasonics*, **7**, 171–6.

White, D. N., Clark, J. M., Campbell, J. K., Cheseborough, J. N., Bahuleyan, K. and Curry, G. R. (1969a). Experimental observations on the origin of the M-echo, *Med. biol. Engng*, **7**, 465–79.

White, D. N., Clark, J. M., White, D. A. W., Campbell, J. K., Bahuleyan, K., Kraus, A. S. and Brinker, R. A. (1969b). The deformation of the ultrasonic field in passage across the living and cadaver head, *Med. biol. Engng*, **7**, 607–18.

6.14 Measurement of patient irradiation

Bang, J. (1972). The intensity of ultrasound in the uterus during examination for diagnostic purposes, *Acta path. microbiol. scand.*, **A80**, 341–4.

Hill, C. R. (1971). Acoustic intensity measurements on ultrasonic diagnostic devices. *In* "Ultrasonographia Medica" (ed. J. Böck and K. Ossoinig), vol. II, pp. 21–7, Verlag Wien. Med. Akad., Vienna.

Hutchison, J. M. S. (1974). A dose monitor for medical ultrasonic pulse-echo systems, *Med. biol. Engng*, **12**, 871–2.

Whittingham, T. A. (1973). A method of measuring the worst-case total dose received by a patient in ultrasonic pulse-echo scanning. *In* "Ultrasonics International 1973", pp. 227–32, I.P.C. Science and Technology Press, Guildford.

6.15 Aids for training operators

Hall, A. J., Fleming, J. E. E., Morley, P. and Barnett, E. (1972). Technical pitfalls in ultrasonic B scan examination, *Med. biol. Engng*, **10**, 631–42.

Holm, H. H., Rasmussen, S. N. and Kristensen, J. K. (1971). Identification of ultrasonic scanning pictures of the abdomen, *Ultrasonics*, **9**, 49–53.

Holm, H. H., Rasmussen, S. N. and Kristensen, J. K. (1972). Errors and pitfalls in ultrasonic scanning of the abdomen, *Br. J. Radiol.*, **45**, 835–40.

Holmes, J. H. and Williams, C. L. (1973). Training tank: a method for training technicians in ultrasound scanning, *J. clin. Ultrasound*, **1**, 202–7.

McDicken, W. N. and Evans, D. H. (1975). Labelling planes of scan and calculating location co-ordinates in diagnostic ultrasonics, *Br. J. Radiol.*, **48**, 392–5.

Wells, P. N. T. (1977) (ed.). "Ultrasonics in Clinical Diagnosis", 2nd, edn., Churchill Livingstone, Edinburgh.

6.16 Clinical applications

6.16.a Angiology

Birnholz, J. C. (1973). Alternatives in the diagnosis of abdominal aortic aneurysm: combined use of isotope aortography and ultrasonography, *Am. J. Roentg.*, **118**, 809–13.

Buschmann, W. (1973). Ultrasonic imaging of arterial wall echoes, *Ultrasound Med. Biol.*, **1**, 33–43.

Evans, G. C., Lehman, J. S., Segal, B. L., Likoff, W., Ziskin, M. and Kingsley, B. (1967). Echoaortography, *Am. J. Cardiol.*, **19**, 91–6.

Goldberg, B. B. (1971). Suprasternal ultrasonography, *J. Am. med. Ass.*, **215**, 245–50.

Goldberg, B. B., Ostrum, B. J. and Isard, H. J. (1966). Ultrasonic aortography, *J. Am. med. Ass.*, **198**, 353–8.

Hartley, C. J. and Strandness, D. E. (1969). A potential means for detection of atherosclerosis, *Proc. 8th int. Conf. med. biol. Engng*, 32–7.

Hokanson, D. E., Mozersky, D. J., Sumner, D. S. and Strandness, D. E. (1972). A phase-locked echo tracking system for recording arterial diameter changes in vivo, *J. appl. Physiol.*, **32**, 728–33.

Holm, H. H. (1971). Ultrasonic scanning in the diagnosis of space-occupying lesions of the upper abdomen, *Br. J. Radiol.*, **44**, 24–36.

Holm, H. H., Kristensen, J. K., Mortensen, T. and Gammelgaard, P. A. (1968). Ultrasonic diagnosis of arterial aneurysms, *Scand. J. thor. cardiovasc. Surg.*, **2**, 140–6.

Kristensen, J. K., Eiken, M. and Wowern, F. von (1971). Ultrasonic diagnosis of carotid artery disease, *J. Neurosurg.*, **35**, 40–4.

Kristensen, J. K., Holm, H. H. and Rasmussen, S. N. (1972). Ultrasonic diagnosis of aortic aneurysms, *J. Cardiovasc. Surg.*, **13**, 161–74.

Laustela, E. and Tähti, E. (1968). Echoaortography in abdominal aortic aneutysm, *Annls Chir. Gynaec. Fenn.*, **57**, 506–9.

Lees, S., Barber, F. E. and Aaronson, C. D. (1969). Ultrasonic determination of the cross section of a simulated blood vessel, *Proc. 8th int. Conf. med. biol. Engng*, 10–4.

Leopold, G. R. (1970). Ultrasonic abdominal aortography, *Radiology*, **96**, 9–14.

Leopold, G. R. (1975). Gray scale ultrasonic angiography of the upper abdomen, *J. clin. Ultrasound*, **3**, 665–71.

Mozersky, D. J., Sumner, D. S., Hokanson, D. E. and Strandness, D. E. (1972). Transcutaneous measurement of the elastic properties of the human femoral artery, *Circulation*, **46**, 948–55.

Powell, M. R. (1972). Leg pain and gas bubbles in the rat following decompression from pressure: monitoring by ultrasound, *Aerospace Med.*, **43**, 168–72.

Rubissow, G. J. and MacKay, R. S. (1974). Decompression study and control using ultrasonics, *Aerospace Med.*, **45**, 473–8.

Segal, B. L., Likoff, W., Asperger, F. and Kingsley, B. (1966). Ultrasonic diagnosis of abdominal aortic aneurysm, *Am. J. Cardiol.*, **17**, 101–3.

Skelton, D. K. and Olson, R. M. (1972). A nondestructive technique to measure pulmonary artery diameter and its pulsative variations, *J. appl. Physiol.*, **33**, 542–4.

Taylor, K. J. W. (1975). Ultrasonic investigation of inferior vena-caval obstruction, *Br. J. Radiol.*, **48**, 1024–6.

Tucker, D. G. and Welsby, V. G. (1968). Ultrasonic monitoring of decompression, *Lancet*, **1**, 1253.

Walder, D. N., Evans, A. and Hempleman, H. V. (1968). Ultrasonic monitoring of decompression, *Lancet*, **1**, 1253.

Winsberg, F., Cole-Beuglet, C. and Mulder, D. S. (1974). Continuous ultrasound "B" scanning of abdominal aortic aneurysms, *Am. J. Roentg.*, **121**, 626–33.

6.16.b Cardiology

Åsberg, A. (1967). Ultrasonic cinématography of the living heart, *Ultrasonics*, **5**, 113–7.

Belenkie, I., Carr, M., Schlant, R. C., Nutter, D. O. and Symbas, P. N. (1973). Malfunction of a Cutter–Smeloff mitral ball valve prosthesis: diagnosis by phonocardiography and echocardiography, *Am. Heart. J.*, **86**, 399–403.

Bom, N., Lancée, C. T., Zwieten, G. van, Kloster, F. E. and Roelandt, J. (1973). Multiscan echocardiography. I. Technical description. *Circulation*, **48**, 1066–74.

Bom, N., Hugenholtz, P. G., Kloster, F. E., Roelandt, J., Popp, R. L., Pirdie, R. B. and Sahn, D. J. (1974). Evaluation of structure recognition with the multiscan echocardiograph, *Ultrasound Med. Biol.*, **1**, 243–52.

Carson, P. and Kanter, L. (1971). Left ventricular wall movement in heart failure, *Br. med. J.*, **4**, 77–9.

Chesler, E., Joffe, H. S., Beck, W. and Schrire, V. (1971). Echocardiography in the diagnosis of congenital heart disease, *Pediat. Clin. N. Am.*, **18**, 1163–90.

Chung, K. J., Manning, J. A. and Gramiak, R. (1974). Echocardiography in coexisting hypertrophic subaortic stenosis and fixed left ventricular outflow obstruction, *Circulation*, **49**, 673–7.

Corya, B. C., Feigenbaum, H., Rasmussen, S. and Black, M. J. (1974). Anterior left ventricular wall echoes in coronary artery disease, *Am. J. Cardiol.*, **34**, 652–7.

Diamond, M. A., Dillon, J. C., Haine, C. L., Chang, S. and Feigenbaum, H. (1971). Echographic features of atrial septal defect, *Circulation*, **43**, 129–35.

Dillon, J. C., Haine, C. L., Chang, S. and Feigenbaum, H. (1970). Use of echocardiography in patients with prolapsed mitral valve, *Circulation*, **43**, 503–7.

Duchak, J. M., Chang, S. and Feigenbaum, H. (1972). Echocardiographic features of torn chordae tendineae, *Am. J. Cardiol.*, **29**, 260.

Edler, I. (1961). Ultrasoundcardiography, *Acta med. scand.*, **170**, Suppl. 370.

Edler, I. (1964). Ultrasoundcardiography. *In* "Ultrasound as a Diagnostic and Surgical Tool" (ed. D. Gordon), pp. 124–44, E. & S. Livingstone, Edinburgh.

Edler, I. (1965). The diagnostic use of ultrasound in heart disease. *In* "Ultrasonic Energy" (ed. E. Kelly), pp. 303–21, University of Illinois Press, Urbana.

Edler, I. (1966). Mitral valve function studied by the ultrasound echo method. *In* "Diagnostic Ultrasound" (ed. C. C. Grossman, J. H. Holmes, C. Joyner and E. W. Purnell), pp. 198–228, Plenum Press, New York.

Edler, I. and Hertz, C. H. (1954). The use of the ultrasonic reflectoscope for the continuous recording of the movements of heart walls, *K. fysiogr. Sällsk. Lund Förh.*, **24**, 40–58.

Effert, S., Bleifeld, W., Deupmann, F. J. and Karitsiotis, J. (1964). Diagnostic value of ultrasonic cardiography, *Br. J. Radiol.*, **37**, 920–7.

Feigenbaum, H. (1972). "Echocardiography", Lea and Febiger, Philadelphia.

Feigenbaum, H., Wolfe, S. B., Popp, R. L., Haine, C. L. and Dodge, H. T. (1969). Correlation of ultrasound with angiocardiography in measuring left ventricular diastolic volume, *Am. J. Cardiol.*, **23**, 111.

Feigenbaum, H., Zaky, A. and Nasser, W. K. (1967a). Use of ultrasound to measure left ventricular stroke volume, *Circulation*, **35**, 1092–9.

Feigenbaum, H., Zaky, A. and Waldhausen, J. A. (1967b). Use of reflected ultrasound in detecting pericardial effusion, *Am. J. Cardiol.*, **19**, 84–90.

Feizi, Ö. and Emanuel, R. (1975). Echocardiographic spectrum of hypertropic cardiomyopathy, *Br. Heart. J.*, **37**, 1286–302.

Feizi, Ö., Symons, C. and Yacoub, M. (1974). Echocardiography of the aortic valve. 1: studies of the normal aortic valve, aortic stenosis, aortic regurgitation and mixed aortic valve disease, *Br. Heart J.*, **36**, 341–51.

Fortuin, N. J. and Craige, E. (1972). On the mechanism of the Austin Flint murmur, *Circulation*, **45**, 558–70.

Fortuin, N. J., Hood, W. P., Sherman, M. E. and Craige, E. (1971). Determination of left ventricular volumes by ultrasound, *Circulation*, **44**, 575–84.

Gibson, D. G. (1973). Estimation of left ventricular size by echocardiography, *Br. Heart J.*, **35**, 128–34.

Gibson, D. G. and Brown, D. J. (1974). Relation between diastolic left ventricular wall stress and strain in man, *Br. Heart J.*, **36**, 1066–77.

Gimenez, J. L., Winters, W. L., Davita, J. C., Connell, J. and Klein, K. S. (1965). Dynamics of the Starr–Edwards ball valve prosthesis—a cinéfluorographic and ultrasonic study in humans, *Am. J. med. Sci.*, **250**, 652–7.

Goldberg, B. B. and Pollack, H. M. (1973). Ultrasonically guided pericardiocentesis, *Am. J. Cardiol.*, **31**, 490–3.

Goldberg, B. B. and Ziskin, M. C. (1973). Echo patterns with an aspiration ultrasonic transducer, *Invest. Radiol.*, **8**, 78–83.

Gordon, D. (1974). A new ultrasonic technique for lung diagnosis. *In* "Ultrasonics in Medicine" (ed. M. de Vlieger, D. N. White and V. R. McCready), pp. 207–11, Excerpta Medica, Amsterdam.

Gramiak, R. and Shah, P. M. (1970). Echocardiography of the normal and diseased aortic valve, *Radiology*, **96**, 1–8.

Gramiak, R. and Shah, P. M. (1971). Cardiac ultrasonography. A review of current applications. *Radiol. Clin. N. Am.*, **9**, 469–90.

Gramiak, R., Shah, P. M. and Kramer, D. H. (1969). Ultrasound cardiography: contrast studies in anatomy and function, *Radiology*, **92**, 939–48.

Gramiak, R., Nanda, N. C. and Shah, P. M. (1972). Echographic detection of the pulmonary valve, *Radiology*, **102**, 153–7.

Gramiak, R., Waag, R. C. and Simon, W. (1973). Ciné ultrasound cardiography, *Radiology*, **107**, 175–80.

Griffith, J. M. and Henry, W. L. (1974). A sector scanner for real time two-dimensional echocardiography, *Circulation*, **49**, 1147–52.

Henry, W. L., Clark, C. E., Roberts, W. C., Morrow, A. G. and Epstein, S. E. (1974). Differences in distribution of myocardial abnormalities in patients with obstructive and non-obstructive asymmetric septal hypertrophy (ASH), *Circulation*, **50**, 447–55.

Hileman, R. E., Dick, D. E. and Cooper, D. (1975). Economical dynamic cardiac imaging. *In* "Ultrasound in Medicine" (ed. D. N. White), vol. 1, pp. 519–26, Plenum Press, New York.

Hussey, M., McDicken, W. N. and Robertson, D. A. R. (1973). Ultrasonic B-scanning of the heart with an ECG gated television display, *Ultrasonics*, **11**, 73–6.

Joyner, C. R., Herman, R. J. and Reid, J. M. (1967a). Reflected ultrasound in the detection and localization of pleural effusion, *J. Am. med. Ass.*, **200**, 399–402.

Joyner, C. R., Hey, E. B., Johnson, J. and Reid, J. M. (1967b). Reflected ultrasound in the diagnosis of tricuspid stenosis, *Am. J. Cardiol.*, **19**, 66–73.

Kerber, R. E. and Abboud, F. M. (1973). Echocardiographic detection of regional myocardial infarction, *Circulation*, **48**, 997–1005.

Kerber, R. E., Kioschos, J. M. and Laner, R. M. (1974). Use of an ultrasonic contrast method in the diagnosis of valvular regurgitation and intracardiac shunts, *Am. J. Cardiol.*, **34**, 722–7.

Kimoto, S., Omoto, R., Tsunemoto, M., Moroi, T., Atsumi, K. and Uchida, R. (1964). Ultrasonic tomography of the liver and detection of heart atrial septal defect with the aid of ultrasonic intravenous probes, *Ultrasonics*, **2**, 82–6.

King, D. L. (1973). Cardiac ultrasonography, *Circulation*, **47**, 843–7.

King, D. L., Steeg, C. N. and Ellis, K. (1971). Demonstration of transposition of the great arteries by cardiac ultrasonography, *Radiology*, **107**, 181–6.

Kingsley, B. and Segal, B. (1969). Ultrasound diagnosis of idiopathic hypertrophic subaortic stenosis, *Proc. 8th int. Conf. med. biol. Engng*, 32–12.

Kisslo, J., Wolfson, S., Ross, A., Pasternak, R., Hammond, G. and Cohen, L. S. (1973). Ultrasound assessment of left ventricular function following aortocoronary saphenous vein bypass grafting, *Circulation*, **48**, Suppl. 3, 156–61.

Kisslo, J., Ramm, O. T. von and Thurstone, F. L. (1975). Thaumascan: clinical cardiac imaging. *In* "Ultrasound in Medicine" (ed. D. N. White), vol. 1, pp. 379–83, Plenum Press, New York.

Kratochwil, A., Jantsch, C., Mösslachev, H., Slany, J. and Wenger, R. (1974). Ultrasonic tomography of the heart, *Ultrasound Med. Biol.*, **1**, 275–81.

Kremkau, F. W., Gramiak, R., Carstensen, E. L., Shah, P. M. and Kramer, D. H. (1970). Ultrasonic detection of cavitation at catheter tips, *Am. J. Roentg.*, **110**, 177–83.

Ludbrook, P., Karliner, N. S., London, A., Peterson, K. L., Leopold, G. R. and O'Rourke, R. A. (1974). Posterior wall velocity: an unreliable index of total left ventricular performance in patients with coronary artery disease, *Am. J. Cardiol.*, **33**, 475–82.

Mary, D. A. S., Pakrashi, B. C., Catchpole, R. W. and Ionescu, M. I. (1974). Echocardiographic studies of stented fascia lata grafts in the mitral position, *Circulation*, **49**, 237–45.

Matsumoto, M., Nimura, Y., Matsuo, H., Nagata, S., Mochizuki, S., Sakakibara, H. and Abe, H. (1975). Interatrial septum in B-mode and conventional echograms—a clue for the diagnosis of congenital heart diseases, *J. clin. Ultrasound*, **3**, 29–37.

McLaurin, L. P., Gibson, T. C., Waider, W., Grossman, W. and Craige, E. (1973). An appraisal of mitral valve echograms mimicking mitral stenosis in conditions with right ventricular pressure overload, *Circulation*, **48**, 801–9.

Miller, H. C., Stephens, J. and Gibson, D. (1973). Echocardiographic features of mitral Starr–Edwards prosthetic regurgitation, *Br. Heart J.*, **35**, 560.

Miller, L. D., Joyner, C. R., Dudrick, S. J. and Eskin, D. J. (1967). Clinical use of ultrasound in the early diagnosis of pulmonary embolism, *Ann. Surg.*, **166**, 381–92.

Murray, J. A., Johnston, W. and Reid, J. M. (1972). Echocardiographic determination of left ventricular dimensions, volumes and performance, *Am. J. Cardiol.* **30**, 252–7.

Murphy, K. F., Kotler, N. M., Reichek, N. and Perloff, J. K. (1975). Ultrasound in the diagnosis of congenital heart disease, *Am. Heart J.*, **89**, 638–56.

Nanda, N. C., Gramiak, R., Robinson, T. I. and Shah, P. M. (1974). Echocardiographic evaluation of pulmonary hypertension, *Circulation*, **50**, 575–81.

Omoto, R. (1967). Intracardiac scanning of the heart with the aid of ultrasonic intravenous probe, *Jap. Heart J.*, **8**, 569–81.

Paraskos, J. A., Grossman, W., Saltz, S., Dalen, J. E. and Dexter, L. (1971). A noninvasive technique for the determination of velocity of circumferential fiber shortening in man, *Circulation Res.*, **29**, 610–15.

Paulev, P.-E. and Pedersen, J. F. (1973). Myocardial contraction velocity and acceleration in man measured by ultrasound echography differentiation, *Cardiovasc. Res.*, **7**, 266–76.

Paulev, P.-E., Pedersen, J. F. and Neumann, F. (1973). Myocardial contraction velocity measured by ultrasound echocardiography—differentiation and evaluated by left ventricular pressures in pigs, *Cardiovasc. Res.*, **7**, 277–81.

Pell, R. L. (1964). Ultrasound for routine clinical investigations, *Ultrasonics*, **2**, 87–9.

Pridie, R. B. and Turnbull, T. A. (1968). Diagnosis of pericardial effusion by ultrasound, *Br. med. J.*, **3**, 356–7.

Pridie, R. B., Benham, R. and Oakley, C. M. (1971). Echocardiography of the mitral valve in aortic valve disease, *Br. Heart J.*, **33**, 296–340.

Pombo, J. F., Russell, R. O., Rackley, C. E. and Foster, G. L. (1971). Comparison of stroke volume and cardiac output determination by ultrasound and dye dilution in acute myocardial infarction, *Am. J. Cardiol.*, **27**, 630–5.

Popp, R. L. and Harrison, D. C. (1969). Ultrasound in the diagnosis and evaluation of idiopathic hypertrophic subaortic stenosis, *Circulation*, **40**, 905–14.

Quinones, M. A., Gaasch, W. H., Waisser, E. and Alexander, J. K. (1974). Reduction in the rate of diastolic descent of the mitral valve echogram in patients with altered left ventricular diastolic pressure–volume relations, *Circulation*, **49**, 246–54.

Ramm, O. T. von, Thurstone, F. L. and Kisslo, J. (1975). Cardiovascular diagnosis with real time ultrasound imaging. *In* "Acoustical Holography" (ed. N. Booth), vol. 6, pp. 91–102, Plenum Press, New York.

Ratshin, R. A., Rackley, C. E. and Russell, R. O. (1974). Determination of left ventricular preload and afterload by quantitative echography in man, *Circulation Res.*, **34**, 711–8.

Redwood, D. R., Henry, W. L. and Epstein, S. E. (1974). Evaluation of the ability of echocardiography to measure acute alterations in left ventricular volume, *Circulation*, **50**, 901–4.

Reid, J. M. and Bor, I. (1969). Ultrasound cardiogram of artificial mitral valves (Starr–Edwards prosthesis), *Z. Kreislaufforsch.*, **58**, 979–83.

Roelandt, J., Kloster, K. E., Cate, F. J. ten, Dorp, W. G. van, Honkoop, J., Bom, N. and Hugenholtz, P. G. (1974). Multidimensional echocardiography, *Br. Heart J.*, **36**, 29–43.

Ross, A. M., Genton, E. and Holmes, J. H. (1968). Ultrasonic examination of the lung, *J. lab. clin. Med.*, **72**, 556–64.

Ross, F. G. M. (1972). Ultrasonic investigation of the heart. *In* "Ultrasonics in Clinical Diagnosis" (ed. P. N. T. Wells), pp. 120–42, Churchill Livingstone, Edinburgh

Sahn, D. J., Deely, W. J., Hagan, A. D. and Friedman, W. F. (1974). Echocardiographic assessment of left ventricular performance in normal newborns, *Circulation*, **49**, 232–6.

Sahn, D. J., Terry, R., O'Rourke, R., Leopold, G. and Friedman, W. F. (1974). Multiple crystal cross-sectional echography in the diagnosis of cyanotic congenital heart disease, *Circulation*, **50**, 230–8.

Segal, B. L., Likoff, W. and Kingsley, B. (1967a). Echocardiography. Clinical application in combined mitral stenosis and mitral regurgitation, *Am. J. Cardiol.*, **19**, 42–9.

Segal, B. L., Likoff, W. and Kingsley, B. (1967b). Echocardiography. Clinical application in mitral regurgitation, *Am. J. Cardiol.*, **19**, 50–8.

Shah, P. M., Gramiak, R. and Kramer, D. H. (1969). Ultrasound localization of left ventricular outflow obstruction in hypertrophic obstructive cardiomyopathy, *Circulation*, **40**, 3–11.

Siggers, D. C., Srivongse, S. A. and Deuchar, D. (1971). Analysis of dynamics of mitral Starr–Edwards valve prosthesis using reflected ultrasound, *Br. Heart J.*, **33**, 401–8.

Sjögren, A.-L. (1974). Left ventricular wall thickness measured ultrasonically in patients with recent myocardial infarction, *Ann. clin. Res.*, **6**, 177–86.

Tanaka, M., Neyazaki, T., Kosaka, S., Sugi, H., Oka, S., Ebina, T., Terasawa, Y., Unno, K. and Nitta, K. (1971). Ultrasonic evaluation of anatomical abnormalities of heart in congenital and acquired heart diseases, *Br. Heart J.*, **33**, 686–98.

Taylor, K. J. W. (1974). Use of ultrasound in opaque hemithorax, *Br. J. Radiol.*, **47**, 199–200.

Ultan, L. B., Segal, B. L. and Likoff, W. (1967). Echocardiography in congenital heart disease, *Am. J. Cardiol.*, **19**, 74–83.

Waag, R. C. and Gramiak, R. (1974). Computer-controlled two-dimensional cardiac motion imaging, *Proc. I.E.E.E. Ultrasonics Symp.*, 12–5.

Weissler, A. M. (1974). Non-invasive methods of assessing left ventricular performance in man, *Am. J. Cardiol.*, **34**, 111–4.

Weyman, A. E., Dillon, J. C., Feigenbaum, H. and Chang, S. (1974a). Echocardiographic patterns of pulmonic valve motion with pulmonary hypertension, *Circulation*, **50**, 905–10.

Weyman, A. E., Dillon, J. C., Feigenbaum, H. and Chang, S. (1974b). Echocardiographic patterns of pulmonary valve motion in valvular pulmonary stenosis, *Am. J. Cardiol.*, **34**, 644–51.

Wharton, C. F. P., Smithen, C. S. and Sowton, E. (1971). Changes in left ventricular wall movement after acute myocardial infarction measured by reflected ultrasound, *Br. med. J.*, **4**, 75–7.

White, D. N. (ed.) (1975). "Ultrasound in Medicine", vol. 1, Plenum Press, New York.

Winters, W. L., Gimenez, J. and Soloff, L. A. (1967). Clinical application of ultrasound in the analysis of prosthetic ball function, *Am. J. Cardiol.*, **19**, 97–107.

Wolfe, S. B., Popp, R. L. and Feigenbaum, H. (1969). Diagnosis of atrial tumors by ultrasound, *Circulation*, **39**, 615–22.

Yuste, P., Aza, V., Minguez, I., Cerezo, L. and Martinez-Bordia, C. (1974). Dissecting aortic aneurysm diagnosed by echocardiography, *Br. Heart J.*, **36**, 111–2.

Ziskin, M. C., Bonakdarpour, A., Weinstein, D. P. and Lynch, P. R. (1972). Contrast agents for diagnostic ultrasound, *Invest. Radiol.*, **7**, 500–5.

6.16.c Endocrinology

Bearman, S., Sanders, R. C. and Oh Kook Sang (1973). B-scan ultrasound in the evaluation of pediatric abdominal masses, *Radiology*, **108**, 111–7.

Birnholz, J. C. (1973). Ultrasound imaging of adrenal mass lesions, *Radiology*, **109**, 163–6.

Blum, M., Weiss, B. and Hemberg, J. (1971). Evaluation of thyroid nodules by A-mode echography, *Radiology*, **101**, 651–6.

Damascelli, M. D., Lattuada, A., Musumeci, R. and Severini, A. (1968). Two-dimensional ultrasonic investigation of the urinary tract, *Br. J. Radiol.*, **41**, 837–43.

Davidson, J. K., Morley, P., Hurley, G. D. and Holford, N. G. H. (1975). Adrenal venography and ultrasound in the investigation of the adrenal gland: an analysis of 58 cases, *Br. J. Radiol.*, **48**, 435–50.

Goldberg, B. B., Capitanio, N. A. and Kirkpatrick, J. A. (1972). Ultrasound evaluation of masses in pediatric patients, *Am. J. Roentg.*, **116**, 667–84.

Holm, H. H. (1971). Ultrasonic scanning in the diagnosis of space-occupying lesions of the upper abdomen, *Br. J. Radiol.*, **44**, 24–36.

Hunig, R. (1971). Ultraschall Tomographie am Kindlichen, *Helv. Paed. Acta Suppl.*, **24**, 3–22.

Jellins, J., Kossoff, G., Wiseman, J., Reeve, T. and Hales, I. (1975). Ultrasonic grey scale visualization of the thyroid gland, *Ultrasound Med. Biol.*, **1**, 405–10.

Lyons, E. A., Murphy, A. V. and Arneil, G. C. (1972). Sonar and its uses in kidney disease in children, *Archs Dis. Child.*, **47**, 777–84.

Miskin, M., Rosen, I. B. and Wallfish, P. C. (1973). B-mode ultrasonography in assessment of thyroid gland lesions, *Ann. intern. Med.*, **79**, 505–10.

Ramsay, I. and Meire, H. (1975). Ultrasonics in the diagnosis of thyroid disease, *Clin. Radiol.*, **26**, 191–7.

Rasmussen, S. N., Christiansen, N. J. B., Jorgensen, J. S. and Holm, H. H. (1971). Differentiation between cystic and solid thyroid nodules by ultrasonic examination, *Acta. chir. scand.*, **137**, 331–3.

Tanaka, K., Wagai, I., Kikuchi, Y., Uchida, R. and Uematsu, S. (1966). Ultrasonic diagnosis in Japan. *In* "Diagnostic Ultrasound" (ed. C. C. Grossman, J. H. Holmes, C. Joyner and E. W. Purnell), pp. 27–45, Plenum Press, New York.

Taylor, K. J. W., Carpenter, D. A. and McCready, V. R. (1975). Grey scale ultrasonography and radioisotope scanning as complementary investigations of thyroid swellings. *In* "Ultrasound in Medicine" (ed. D. N. White), vol. 1, pp. 305–8, Plenum Press, New York.

Thijs, L. G., Roos, P. and Wiener, J. D. (1972). Use of ultrasound and digital scintiphoto analysis in the evaluation of solitary thyroid lesions, *J. nucl. Med.*, **13**, 504–9.

6.16.d Gastroenterology

Asher, W. M., Nebel, O. and Huber, K. (1975). Demonstration of the normal pancreas with gray scale ultrasound. *In* "Ultrasound in Medicine" (ed. D. N. White), vol. 1, p. 194, Plenum Press, New York.

Burcharth, F. and Rasmussen, S. N. (1974). Localization of the porta hepatis by ultrasonic scanning prior to percutaneous transhepatic portography, *Br. J. Radiol.*, **47**, 598–602.

Daly, C. H. and Wheeler, J. B. (1971). The use of ultra-sonic thickness measurement in the clinical evaluation of the oral soft tissues, *Int. dent. J.*, **21**, 418–29.

Doust, B. D. and Maklad, N. F. (1974). Ultrasonic B-mode examination of the gall bladder, *Radiology*, **110**, 643–7.

Engelhart, G. and Blauenstein, U. W. (1970). Ultrasound in the diagnosis of malignant pancreatic tumours, *Gut*, **11**, 443–9.

Filly, F. A. and Freimanis, A. K. (1970). Echographic diagnosis of pancreatic lesions, *Radiology*, **96**, 575–82.

Gilby, E. D. and Taylor, K. J. W. (1975). Ultrasound monitoring of hepatic metatases during chemotherapy, *Br. med. J.*, **1**, 371–3.

Goldberg, B. B., Goodman, G. A. and Clearfield, H. R. (1970). Evaluation of ascites by ultrasound, *Radiology*, **96**, 15–22.

Goldberg, B. B., Harris, K. and Brooker, W. (1974). Ultrasonic and radiographic cholecystography, *Radiology*, **111**, 405–9.

Hancke, S., Holm, H. H. and Koch, F. (1975). Ultrasonically guided percutaneous fine needle biopsy of the pancreas, *Surg. Gynec. Obstet.*, **140**, 361–4.

Hayashi, S., Wagai, T., Miyazawa, R., Ito, K., Ishikawa, S., Uematsu, K., Kikuchi, Y. and Uchida, R. (1962). Ultrasonic diagnosis of breast tumor and cholelithiasis, *West. J. Surg. Obstet. Gynec.*, **70**, 34–40.

Hill, M. J. and McColl, I. (1961). Ultrasonic detection of choledocholithiasis, *Nature, Lond.*, **190**, 627.

Holm, H. H. (1971). Ultrasonic scanning in the diagnosis of space-occupying lesions of the upper abdomen, *Br. J. Radiol.*, **44**, 24–36.

Howry, D. H. and Bliss, W. R. (1952). Ultrasonic visualization of soft tissue structures of the body, *J. lab. clin. Med.*, **40**, 579–92.

Hublitz, U. F., Kahn, P. C. and Sell, L. A. (1972). Cholecystosonography: an approach to the non-visualized gall-bladder, *Radiology*, **103**, 645–9.

Hünig, R. and Kinser, J. (1973). The diagnosis of ascites by ultrasonic tomography (B-scan), *Br. J. Radiol.*, **46**, 325–8.

Kardel, T., Holm, H. H., Rasmussen, S. N. and Mortensen, T. (1971). Ultrasonic determination of liver and spleen volumes, *Scand. J. clin. Lab. Invest.*, **27**, 123–8.

Knight, P. R. and Newell, J. A. (1963). Operative use of ultrasonics in cholelithiasis, *Lancet.*, **1**, 1023–5.

Kossoff, G. and Sharpe, C. J. (1966). Examination of the contents of the pulp cavity in teeth, *Ultrasonics*, **4**, 77–83.

Kratochwil, A., Rosenmayr, F. and Howanietz, L. (1973). Diagnosis of a traumatic pancreas cyst by means of ultrasound, *Ultrasound Med. Biol.*, **1**, 49–52.

Lees, S. (1972). Some capabilities of ultrasonics in dental diagnostics and dental research. *In* "Interaction of Ultrasound and Biological Tissues" (ed. J. M. Reid and M. R. Sikov), pp. 281–5, U.S. Department of Health, Education and Welfare, Publication (FDA) 73–8008.

Lees, S. and Barber, F. E. (1971). Looking into the teeth and its surfaces with ultrasonics, *Ultrasonics*, **9**, 95–100.

Lees, S., Gerhard, F. B. and Oppenheim, F. G. (1973). Ultrasonic measurement of dental demineralization, *Ultrasonics*, **11**, 269–73.

Lehman, J. S., Evans, G. C. and Brody, L. W. (1966). Ultrasound exploration of the spleen. *In* "Diagnostic Ultrasound" (ed. C. C. Grossman, J. H. Holmes, C. Joyner and E. W. Purnell), pp. 264–95, Plenum Press, New York.

Leyton, B., Halpern, S., Leopold, G. and Hagen, S. (1973). Correlation of ultrasound and colloid scintiscan studies of the normal and diseased liver, *J. nucl. Med.*, **14**, 27–33.

Ludwig, G. D. and Struthers, F. W. (1950). Detecting gall-stones with ultrasonics, *Electronics*, **23** (2), 172–8.

Lutz, H. (1975). Sonographic pancreas diagnosis, *Electromedica*, **43**, 74–7.

Lutz, H. and Rettenmaier, G. (1973). Sonographic pattern of tumors of the stomach and the intestine, *Excerpta Medica International Congress Series*, **277**, 31.

Macridis, C. A., Kouloulas, A., Koatsimbelas, B. and Yannoulis, G. (1975). Diagnosis of the tumours of the salivary glands by ultrasonography, *Electromedica*, **43**, 130–4.

Matthews, A. W., Gough, K. R., Davies, E. R., Ross, F. G. M. and Hinchliffe, A. (1973). The use of combined ultrasonic and isotope scanning in the diagnosis of amoebic liver disease, *Gut*, **14**, 50–3.

McCarthy, C. F. (1972). Ultrasonic investigation of the liver. *In* "Ultrasonics in Clinical Diagnosis" (ed. P. N. T. Wells), pp. 105–19, Churchill Livingstone, Edinburgh

McCarthy, C. F., Read, A. E. A., Ross, F. G. M. and Wells, P. N. T. (1967). Ultrasonic scanning of the liver, *Q. Jl Med.*, **36**, 517–24.

McCarthy, C. F., Wells, P. N. T., Ross, F. G. M. and Read, A. E. A. (1969). The use of ultrasound in the diagnosis of cystic lesions of the liver and upper abdomen and in the detection of ascites, *Gut*, **10**, 904–12.

McCarthy, C. F., Davies, E. R., Wells, P. N. T., Ross, F. G. M., Follett, D. H., Muir, K. M. and Read, A. E. (1970). A comparison of ultrasonic and isotope scanning in the diagnosis of liver disease, *Br. J. Radiol.*, **43**, 100–9.

Mittelstaedt, C. (1975). Ultrasonic diagnosis of omental cysts, *J. clin. Ultrasound*, **3**, 673–6.

Monroe, L. S., Leopold, G. R., Brown, J. W. and Smith, J. L. (1971). The ultrasonic scan in the management of amebic hepatic abscess, *Am. J. dig. Dis.*, **16**, 523–8.

Palo, P. and Tähti, E. (1971). Ultrasonic measurement of the spleen. *In* "Ultrasonographia Medica" (ed. J. Böck and K. Ossoinig), vol. III, pp. 43–5, Verlag Wien. med. Akad., Vienna.

Rasmussen, S. N. (1972). Liver volume determination by ultrasonic scanning, *Br. J. Radiol.*, **45**, 579–85.

Rasmussen, S. N., Holm, H. H., Kristensen, J. K. and Barlebo, H. (1972). Ultrasonically-guided liver biopsy, *Br. med. J.*, **2**, 500–2.

Rasmussen, S. N., Holm, H. H., Kristensen, J. K., Pedersen, J. F. and Hancke, S. (1973). Ultrasound in the diagnosis of liver disease, *J. clin. Ultrasound*, **1**, 220–6.

Rasmussen, S. N., Kardel, T. and Jurgensen, B. J. (1975). Liver volume estimated by ultrasonic scanning before and after portal decompression surgery, *Scand. J. Gastroent.*, **10**, 25–8.

Rettenmaier, G. (1974). Quantitative criteria of intrahepatic echo patterns correlated with structural alterations. *In* "Ultrasonics in Medicine" (ed. M. de Vlieger, D. N. White and V. R. McCready), pp. 199–206, Excerpta Medica, Amsterdam.

Rettenmaier, G. and Gail, K. (1972). Echographie pancréatique, *J. Radiol. Electrol. Med. nucl.*, **53**, 745–7.

Smirnow, R. (1966). Diagnostic ultrasonics in dentistry. *In* "Diagnostic Ultrasound" (ed. C. C. Grossman, J. H. Holmes, C. Joyner and E. W. Purnell), pp. 300–5, Plenum Press, New York.

Smith, E. H. and Bartrum, R. J. (1975). Percutaneous aspiration of abscesses with ultrasound. *In* "Ultrasound in Medicine" (ed. D. N. White), vol. 1, pp. 177–81, Plenum Press, New York.

Smith, E. H., Bartrum R. J., Cheng, Y. C., D'Orsi, C. J., Lokich, J., Abbruzzese, A. and Dontano, J. (1975). Percutaneous aspiration biopsy of the pancreas under ultrasonic guidance, *New Engl. J. Med.*, **292**, 825–8.

Stigsby, B. and Rasmussen, S. N. (1971). A semi-automatic method for liver volume determination based on ultrasonic scanning, *Comput. Prog. Biomed.*, **2**, 66–70.

Stuber, J. L., Templeton, A. W. and Bishop, K. (1972). Sonographic diagnosis of pancreatic lesions, *Am. J. Roentg.*, **116**, 406–12.

Tabrisky, J., Lindstrom, R. R., Herman, M. W., Castagna, J. and Sarti, D. (1975). Value of gallbladder B-scan ultrasonography, *Gastroentrology*, **68**, 1246–52.

Tala, P., Lieto, J., Kerminen, T. and Laustala, E. (1966). Ultrasonic diagnosis of cholelithiasis, *Annls Chir. Gynaec. Fenn.*, **55**, 124–8.

Taylor, K. J. W. (1974). Ultrasonic patterns of tumors of the liver, *J. clin. Ultrasound.*, **2**, 74–8.

Taylor, K. J. W. and Carpenter, D. A. (1974). Grey-scale ultrasonography in the investigation of obstructive jaundice, *Lancet*, **2**, 586–7.

Taylor, K. J. W. and Carpenter, D. A. (1975a). Comparison of radioisotope and ultrasound examination in the investigation of hepatobiliary disease. *In* "Ultrasound in Medicine" (ed. D. N. White), vol. 1, pp. 159–67, Plenum Press, New York.

Taylor, K. J. W. and Carpenter, D. A. (1975b). The anatomy and pathology of the porta hepatis demonstrated by gray scale ultrasonography, *J. clin. Ultrasound*, **3**, 117–19.

Taylor, K. J. W., Carpenter, D. A. and McCready, V. R. (1973). Grey scale echography in the diagnosis of intrahepatic disease, *J. clin. Ultrasound*, **1**, 284–7.

Wagai, T., Miyazawa, R., Ito, K. and Kikuchi, Y. (1965). Ultrasonic diagnosis of intracranial disease, breast tumors and abdominal diseases. *In* "Ultrasonic Energy" (ed. E. Kelly), pp. 346–60, University of Illinois Press, Urbana.

Wells, P. N. T. (1971). Physical factors controlling the diagnostic value of two-dimensional ultrasonic liver scans. *In* "Ultrasonographia Medica" (ed. J. Böck and K. Ossoinig), vol. I, pp. 169–76, Verlag Wien. med. Akad., Vienna.

6.16.e Neurology

Avant, W. S. (1966). Pulsatile echoencephalography, *Neurology*, **16**, 1033–40.

Braak, J. W. G. ter and Vlieger, M. de (1965). Cerebral pulsations in echoencephalography, *Acta neurochir.*, **12**, 678–94.

Brinker, R. A. and Taveras, J. M. (1966). Ultrasound cross-sectional pictures of the head, *Acta radiol. (D)*, **5**, 745–53.

Brinker, R. A., King, D. L. and Taveras, J. M. (1965). Echoencephalography, *Am. J. Roentg.*, **93**, 781–90.

Curry, G. R., Stevenson, R. J. and White, D. N. (1973). The orbit and superior orbital fissure as an acoustic window, *Med. biol. Engng*, **11**, 293–309.

Freund, H.-J. (1974). Electronic sector scanning in cerebral diagnostics. III. Visualization of intracranial structures and brain arteries. *In* "Ultrasonics in Medicine" (ed. M. de Vlieger, D. N. White and V. R. McCready), pp. 314–7, Excerpta Medica, Amsterdam.

Fry, F. J. (1968). Intracranial anatomy visualized *in vivo* by ultrasound, *Invest. Radiol..*, **3**, 243–66.

Fry, F. J. (1970). Ultrasonic visualization of human brain structure, *Invest. Radiol.*, **5**, 117–21.

Fry, F. J., Eggleton, R. C. and Heimburger, R. F. (1974). Transkull visualization of brain using ultrasound: an experimental model study. *In* "Ultrasonics in Medicine" (ed. M. de Vlieger, D. N. White and V. R. McCready), pp. 97–103, Excerpta Medica, Amsterdam.

Galicich, J. H. and Williams, J. B. (1971). A computerized echoencepholograph, *J. Neurosurg.*, **35**, 453–60.

Garrett, W. J., Kossoff, G. and Jones, R. F. C. (1975). Ultrasonic cross-sectional visualization of hydrocephalus in infants, *Neuroradiology*, **8**, 279–88.

Gordon, D. (1959). Echoencephalography: ultrasonic rays in diagnostic radiology, *Br. med. J.*, **1**, 1500–4.

Heimburger, R. F., Fry, F. J. and Eggleton, R. C. (1973). Ultrasound visualization in human brain: the internal capsule, a preliminary report, *Surg. Neurol.*, **1**, 56–8.

Jenkins, C. O., Campbell, J. K., White, D. N. and Clark, J. M. (1971). Ultrasonic echo pulsations in range. A study of rise times and delay times, *Acta neurochir.*, **24**, 1–10.

Jeppsson, S. (1964). Echoencephalography. V. A method for recording the intra-cranial pressure with the aid of the echoencephalographic technique, *Acta chir. scand.*, **128**, 218–24.

Kamphuisen, H. A. C. (1974). Electronic sector scanning in cerebral diagnostics. II. Space occupying processes and hydrocephalus. *In* "Ultrasonics in Medicine" (ed. M. de Vlieger, D. N. White and V. R. McCready), pp. 309–13, Excerpta Medica, Amsterdam.

Kazner, E. and Hopman, H. (1973). Possibilities and reliability of echoventriculography, *Ultrasound Med. Biol.*, **1**, 17–32.

Kienast, H. W., Hussman, L. H. and Selner, R. L. (1971). The phenomenon of the vanishing midline echo in dying patients. *In* "Ultrasonographia Medica" (ed. J. Böck and K. Ossoinig), vol. I, 289–93, Verlag Wien. med. Akad., Vienna.

Kossoff, G., Garrett, W. J. and Radavanovich, G. (1974). Ultrasonic atlas of normal brain of infant, *Ultrasound Med. Biol.*, **1**, 259–66.

Leksell, L. (1956). Echo-encephalography. 1. Detection of intracranial complications following brain injury. *Acta chir. scand.*, **110**, 301–15.

Lithander, B. (1960). A control method for echo-encephalography, *Acta psychiat. neurol. scand.*, **35**, 235–40.

Makow, D. M. and Real, R. R. (1965). Immersion ultrasonic brain examination—360° degree compound scan, *Ultrasonics*, **3**, 75–80.

Müller, H. R. (1972). Transdural and transorbital ultrasonic exploration of the brain. *In* "Ultrasonics in Biology and Medicine" (ed. L. Filipczyński), pp. 163–70, Polish Scientific Publishers, Warsaw.

Oka, M., Nishii, T., Marusasa, Y. and Moriwaki, H. (1974). Intracranial echo pulsation in brain death, brain tumor and intracranial hypertension. *In* "Ultrasonics in Medicine" (ed. M. de Vlieger, D. N. White and V. R. McCready), pp. 112–9, Excerpta Medica, Amsterdam.

Quaknine, G., Kosary, I. Z., Braham, J., Czerniak, P. and Nathan, H. (1973). Laboratory criteria of brain death, *J. Neurosurg.*, **39**, 429–33.

Richardson, A., Eversden, I. D. and Sternbergh, W. C. A. (1972). Detecting intracranial pressure waves with ultrasound, *Lancet*, **1**, 355–7.

Robinson, D. E. and Kossoff, G. (1966). An ultrasonic echo-encephaloscope for the examination of the human brain, *Proc. I.R.E.*, **27**, 39–44.

Schiefer, W., Kazner, E. and Kunze, St (1968). "Clinical Echo-encephalography", John Wright, Bristol.

Somer, J. C. (1968). Electronic sector scanning for ultrasonic diagnosis, *Ultrasonics*, **6**, 153–9.

Vlieger, M. de (1967). Evolution of echo-encephalography in neurology—a review, *Ultrasonics*, **6**, 91–7.

Vlieger, M. de, Sterke, A. de, Molin, C. E. and Ven, C. van der (1963). Ultrasound for two-dimensional echo-encephalography, *Ultrasonics*, **1**, 148–51.

Wagai, T., Miyazawa, R., Ito, K. and Kikuchi, Y. (1965). Ultrasonic diagnosis of intracranial disease, breast tumors and abdominal diseases. *In* "Ultrasonic Energy" (ed. E. Kelly), pp. 346–60, University of Illinois Press, Urbana.

Wealthall, S. R. and Todd, J. H. (1972). A soft-ended probe for echo-encephalography, *Br. J. Radiol.*, **45**, 867.

Wealthall, S. R. and Todd, J. H. (1973). B-scope echoencephalography in the infant, *Dev. Med. Child Neurol.*, **15**, 338–47.

White, D. N. (1966). Studies in ultrasonic echoencephalography. IV. A critical analysis of the amplitude-averaging, A-scan technique. *Neurology*, **16**, 358–66.

White, D. N. (1967). The limitations of echo-encephalography, *Ultrasonics*, **5**, 88–90.

White, D. N. (1972). Ultrasonic investigation of the brain. *In* "Ultrasonics in Clinical Diagnosis" (ed. P. N. T. Wells), pp. 41–73, Churchill Livingstone, Edinburgh.

White, D. N. (1974). Computerised axial tomography and its implications for ultrasonic encephalography. *In* "Ultrasonics in Medicine" (ed. M. de Vlieger. D. N. White and V. R. McCready), pp. 69–81, Excerpta Medica, Amsterdam,

White, D. N. and Blanchard, J. B. (1966). Studies in echo-encephalography. An objective technique for the A-scan presentation of the cerebral mid-line structures. *Acta radiol. (D)*, **5**, 936–52.

White, D. N. and Curry, G. R. (1974). Registration errors in midline echoencephalography, *Med. biol. Engng*, **12**, 712–9.

White, D. N. and Hanna, L. F. (1974). Automatic midline echoencephalography, *Neurology*, **24**, 80–93.

White, D. N. and Stevenson, R. J. (1975). The causes of transient variations in the magnitude of systolic pulsations in amplitude of echoes recorded from cerebral interfaces: the absence of any relationship with variations in regional blood flow. *In* "Ultrasound in Medicine" (ed. D. N. White), vol. 1, pp. 251–63, Plenum Press, New York.

White, D. N., Clark, J. M., White, D. A. W., Kraus, A. S., Campbell, J. K., Bahuleyan, K. and Brinker, R. A. (1969). The deformation of the ultrasonic field in passage across the living and cadaver head, *Med. biol. Engng*, **7**, 607–18.

White, D. N., Kraus, A. S., Clark, J. M. and Campbell, J. K. (1969). Interpreter error in echoencephalography, *Neurology*, **19**, 775–85.

Williams, J. B. (1973). Automatic encephalography, *Proc. I.E.E.E. Ultrasonics Symp.*, 49–51.

6.16.f Obstetrics and gynaecology

Aanta, K. (1971). Location of the placenta—a comparison between radiography, ultrasound, thermography, isotopes, *Acta radiol. (D).*, Suppl. 303.

Abramowski, P. K., Kopecky, P. and Auterman, R. (1971). The "Rapid" ultrasonic section image as a valuable aid during intrauterine—intraperitoneal transfusion, *Electromedica*, **39**, 155–6.

Bang, J. and Northeved, A. (1972). A new ultrasonic method for transabdominal amniocentesis, *Am. J. Obstet. Gynec.*, **114**, 599–601.

Birnholz, J. C. and Barnes, A. B. (1973). Early diagnosis of hydatidiform by ultrasound imaging, *J. Am. med. Ass.*, **225**, 1359–60.

Boddy, K. and Dawes, G. S. (1975). Foetal breathing, *Br. med. Bull.*, **31**, 3–7.

Boddy, K. and Mantell, C. D. (1972). Observations of fetal breathing movements transmitted through maternal abdominal wall, *Lancet*, **2**, 1219–20.

Boddy, K. and Robinson, J. S. (1971). External method for detection of fetal breathing *in utero*, *Lancet*, **2**, 1231–3.

Bowley, A. R., Christie, A. D. and Nicol, C. (1972). A new fetal cephalometer, *Ultrasonics*, **10**, 37–9.

Bowley, A. R., Christie, A. D. and Nicol, C. (1973). A digital electronic caliper, *Ultrasonics*, **11**, 227–9.

Brown, A. A. and Young, G. B. (1972). A study of four methods of placental localisation, *Am. J. Obstet. Gynec.*, **114**, 24–8.

Campbell, S. (1968). An improved method of fetal cephalometry by ultrasound, *J. Obstet. Gynaec. Br. Commonw.*, **75**, 568–76.

Campbell, S. (1969). The prediction of fetal maturity by ultrasonic measurement of the biparietal diameter, *J. Obstet. Gynaec. Br. Commonw.*, **76**, 603–9.

Campbell, S. (1973). The antenatel detection of fetal abnormality by ultrasonic diagnosis. *In* "Birth Defects" (ed. A. G. Motulsky and W. Leng), pp. 240–7, Excerpta Medica, Amsterdam.

Campbell, S. and Dewhurst, C. J. (1970). Quintuplet pregnancy diagnosed and assessed by ultrasonic compound scanning, *Lancet*, **1**, 101–3.

Campbell, S. and Kohorn, E. I. (1968). Placental localization by ultrasonic compound scanning, *J. Obstet. Gynaec. Br. Commonw.*, **75**, 1007–13.

Campbell, S. and Kurjak, A. (1972). Comparison between urinary oestrogen assay and serial ultrasonic cephalometry in assessment of fetal growth retardation, *Br. med. J.*, **4**, 336–40.

Campbell, S., Johnstone, F. D., Holt, E. M. and May, P. (1972). Anencephaly: early ultrasonic diagnosis and active management, *Lancet*, **2**, 1226–7.

Campbell, S., Wladimiroff, J. W. and Dewhurst, C. J. (1973). The antenatal measurement of fetal urine production, *J. Obstet. Gynaec. Br. Commonw.*, **80**, 680–6.

Campbell, S., Pryse-Davies, J., Coltart, T. M., Seller, M. and Singer, J. D. (1975a). Ultrasound in the diagnosis of spina bifida, *Lancet*, **2**, 1065.

Campbell, S., Pryce-Davies, J., Coltart, T. M., Seller, M. and Singer, J. D. (1975b). Ultrasound in the diagnosis of spina bifida, *Lancet*, **2**, 1336.

Christie, A. D. (1974). Diagnostic procedures in obstetrics. A review of commonly accepted scanning techniques with associated limitations and errors. *In* "Ultrasonics in Medicine" (ed. M. de Vlieger, D. N. White and V. R. McCready), pp. 171–6, Excerpta Medica, Amsterdam.

Cohen, W. N., Chaudhun, T. K., Christie, J. H., and Goplerud, C. P. (1972). Correlation of ultrasound and radioisotope placentography, *Am. J. Roentg.*, **116**, 643–6.

Davison, J. M., Lind, T., Farr, V. R. and Whittingham, T. A. (1973). The limitations of ultrasonic fetal cephalometry, *J. Obstet. Gynaec. Br. Commonw.*, **80**, 769–75.

Dawes, G. S. (1973). Revolutions and cyclical rhythms in prenatal life: fetal respiratory movements rediscovered, *Pediatrics*, **51**, 965–71.

Dawes, G. S. (1974). Breathing before birth in animals and man. An essay in developmental medicine, *New Engl. J. Med.*, **290**, 557–9.

Dawes, G. S., Fox, H. E., Leduc, B. M., Liggins, G. C. and Richards, R. T. (1972). Respiratory movements and rapid eye movement sleep in the fetal lamb, *J. Physiol., Lond.*, **220**, 119–43.

Donald, I. (1963). The use of ultrasonics in the diagnosis of abdominal swellings. *Br. med. J.*, **2**, 1154–5.

Donald, I. (1972). Ultrasonic investigations in obstetrics and gynaecology. *In* "Ultrasonics in Clinical Diagnosis" (ed. P. N. T. Wells), pp. 74–93, Churchill Livingstone, Edinburgh.

Donald, I. (1974). New problems in sonar diagnosis in obstetrics and gynecology, *Am. J. Obstet. Gynec.*, **118**, 299–309.

Donald, I. and Abdulla, U. (1968). Placentography by sonar, *J. Obstet. Gynaec. Br. Commonw.*, **75**, 993–1006.

Donald, I. and Brown, T. G. (1961). Demonstration of tissue interfaces within the body by ultrasonic echo sounding, *Br. J. Radiol.*, **34**, 539–46.

Donald, I., Morley, P. and Barnett, E. (1972). The diagnosis of blighted ovum by sonar, *J. Obstet. Gynaec. Br. Commonw.*, **79**, 304–10.

Durkan, J. P. and Russo, G. L. (1966). Ultrasonic fetal cephalometry: accuracy, limitations and applications, *Obstet. Gynec., N.Y.*, **27**, 399–403.

Farman, D. J. and Thomas, G. (1975). The use of ultrasound for monitoring foetal breathing movements, *Bio-med. Engng*, **10**, 172–4.

Farman, D. J., Thomas, G. and Blackwell, R. J. (1975). Errors and artifacts encountered in the monitoring of fetal respiratory movements using ultrasound, *Ultrasound Med. Biol.*, **2**, 31–6.

Fisher, C. C., Garrett, W. J. and Kossoff, G. (1975). Anencephaly in one of twins diagnosed by ultrasonic echography, *Aust. N.Z. J. Obstet. Gynaec.*, **15**, 108–10.

Flamme, P. (1972). Ultrasonic fetal cephalometry: percentiles curve, *Br. med. J.*, **3**, 384–5.

Fleming, J. E. E. (1974). The design of a new system for ultrasonic foetal cephalometry, *Bio-med. Engng*, **9**, 290–5.

Garrett, W. J., Grunwald, G. and Robinson, D. E. (1970). Prenatal diagnosis of fetal polycystic kidney by ultrasound, *Aust. N.Z. J. Obstet. Gynaec.*, **10**, 7–9.

Garrett, W. J., Kossoff, G. and Lawrence, R. (1975a). Gray scale echography in the diagnosis of hydrops due to fetal lung tumor, *J. clin. Ultrasound*, **3**, 45–50.

Garrett, W. J., Kossoff, G. and Osborn, R. A. (1975b). The diagnosis of fetal hydronephrosis, megaureter and urethral obstruction by ultrasonic echography, *Br. J. Obstet. Gynaec.*, **82**, 115–20.

Goldie, D. J. and Monk, A. M. (1975). Ultrasound in the diagnosis of spina bifida, *Lancet*, **2**, 1336.

Gottesfeld, K. R., Thompson, H. E., Holmes, J. H. and Taylor, E. S. (1966). Ultrasonic placentography—a new method for placental localization, *Am. J. Obstet. Gynec.*, **96**, 538–47.

Gray, F. (1975). Ultrasound in the diagnosis of spina bifida, *Lancet*, **2**, 1336.

Hall, A. J., Fleming, J. E. E. and Abdulla, U. (1970). Ultrasonic fetal cephalometry —some improvements and future developments, *Ultrasonics*, **8**, 34–5.

Hansmann, M. and Voigt, U. (1973). Ultrasonic fetal thoracometry: an additional parameter for determining fetal growth, *Excerpta Medica International Congress Series*, **277**, 22.

Hellman, L. M., Kobayashi, M., Tolles, W. E. and Cromb, E. (1970). Ultrasonic studies on the volumetric growth of the human placenta, *Am. J. Obstet. Gynec.*, **108**, 740–50.

Hohler, C. W. and Fox, H. E. (1975). Real-time gray-scale B-scan ultrasound recording of human fetal breathing movements *in utero*, *Abst. 20th ann. Conf. Am. Inst. Ultrasound Med.*, 70–1.

Ianniruberto, A. and Gibbons, J. M. (1971). Predicting fetal weight by ultrasonic B-scan cephalometry, *Obstet. Gynec., N.Y.*, **37**, 689–94.

Janssens, D., Vrijens, M., Thiery, M. and Kets, H. van (1973). Ultrasonic detection, localization and typing of intrauterine contraceptive devices (IUDs), *Excerpta Medica International Congress Series*, **277**, 23.

Jonatha, W. (1974). Amniocentesis in early pregnancy under ultrasonic visual control, *Electromedica*, **42**, 94–6.

Kitau, M. J., Leighton, P., Gordon, Y. B. and Chard, T. (1975). Ultrasound in the diagnosis of spina bifida, *Lancet*, **2**, 1336.

Kukard, R. F. P. and Freeman, M. E. (1973). The clinical application of ultrasonic placentography, *J. Obstet. Gynaec. Br. Commonw.*, **80**, 433–7.

Kossoff, G. and Garrett, W. J. (1972a). Ultrasonic film echoscopy for placental localisation, *Aust. N.Z. J. Obstet. Gynaec.*, **12**, 117–21.

Kossoff, G. and Garrett, W. J. (1972b). Intracranial detail in fetal echograms, *Invest. Radiol.*, **7**, 159–63.

Kossoff, G., Garrett, W. J. and Radavanovich, G. (1974). Gray scale echography in obstetrics and gynaecology, *Aust. Radiol.*, **18**, 62–111.

Loveday, B. J., Barr, J. A. and Aitken, J. (1975). The intra-uterine demonstration of duodenal atresia by ultrasound, *Br. J. Radiol.*, **48**, 1031–2.

Lunt, R. M. and Chard, T. (1974). Reproducibility of measurement of fetal biparietal diameter by ultrasonic cephalometry, *J. Obstet. Gynaec. Br. Commonw.*, **81**, 682–5.

MacKay, D. H. and Mowat, J. (1974). Translocation of intrauterine contraceptive devices, *Lancet*, **1**, 652–3.

MacVicar, J. and Donald, I. (1963). Sonar in the diagnosis of early pregnancy and its complications, *J. Obstet. Gynaec. Br. Commonw.*, **70**, 387–95.

Meire, H. B., Fish, P. J. and Wheeler, T. (1975). Ultrasound recording of fetal breathing, *Br. J. Radiol.*, **48**, 477–80.

Miskin, M., Doran, T. A., Malone, R. M., Gardner, H. A., Rudd, N. and Benzie, R. (1975). Ultrasound in prenatal genetic diagnosis. *In* "Ultrasound in Medicine" (ed. D. N. White), vol. 1, pp. 201–11, Plenum Press, New York.

Morrison, J., Lachelin, G. C. and Blackwell, R. J. (1972). The accuracy of diagnosing placenta praevia with compound ultrasonic scanning, *Aust. N.Z. J. Obstet. Gynaec.*, **12**, 220–4.

Murata, Y., Takemura, H. and Kurachi, K. (1971). Observation of fetal cardiac motion by M-mode ultrasonic cardiography, *Am. J. Obstet. Gynec.*, **111**, 287–94.

Robinson, H. P. (1972). Detection of fetal heart movement in the first trimester of pregnancy using pulsed ultrasound. *Br. med. J.*, **4**, 466–8.

Robinson, H. P. (1973). Sonar measurement of fetal crown-rump length as a means of assessing maturity in the first trimester of pregnancy, *Br. med. J.*, **4**, 28–31.

Robinson, H. P. (1975). The diagnosis of early pregnancy failure by sonar, *Br. J. Obstet. Gynaec.*, **82**, 849–57.

Robinson, H. P. and Shaw-Dunn, J. (1973). Fetal heart rates as determined by sonar in early pregnancy, *J. Obstet. Gynaec. Br. Commonw.*, **80**, 805–9.

Robinson, H. P., Chatfield, W. R., Logan, R. W., Tweedie, A. K. and Barnard, W. P. (1973). A scoring system for the assessment of multiple methods of monitoring fetal growth, *J. Obstet. Gynaec. Br. Commonw.*, **80**, 230–5.

Sundén, B. (1964). On the diagnostic value of ultrasound in obstetrics and gynaecology, *Acta obstet. gynec. scand.*, **43**, suppl. 6.

Thompson, H. E. (1973). Ultrasonic diagnostic procedures in obstetrics and gynecology, *J. clin. Ultrasound*, **1**, 160–71.

Thompson, H. E., Holmes, J. H., Gottesfeld, K. R. and Taylor, E. S. (1965). Fetal development as determined by ultrasonic pulse-echo techniques, *Am. J. Obstet. Gynec.*, **92**, 44–50.

Varma, T. R. (1974). Prediction of fetal weight by ultrasound cephalometry, *Aust. N.Z. J. Obstet. Gynec.*, **14**, 83–7.

Vrijens, M., Thiery, M. and Defoort, P. (1974). Translocation of intrauterine contraceptive devices, *Lancet*, **1**, 1165.

Watmough, D. J., Crippin, D. and Haddad, D. (1974a). A modified method of ultrasonic fetal cephalometry, *Br. J. Radiol.*, **47**, 352–5.

Watmough, D., Crippin, D. and Mallard, J. R. (1974b). A critical assessment of ultrasonic fetal cephalometry, *Br. J. Radiol.*, **47**, 24–33.

Whittingham, T. A. (1971). The ultrasonic biparietal diameter, expressed in time units, *Br. J. Radiol.*, **44**, 481–2.

Whittingham, T. A. (1973). An ultrasonic fetal cephalometer with a facility for automatic instantaneous measurement, *Ultrasonics*, **11**, 230–3.

Willocks, J., Donald, I., Duggan, T. C. and Day, N. (1964). Foetal cephalometry by ultrasound, *J. Obstet. Gynaec. Br. Commonw.*, **71**, 11–20.

Wladimiroff, J. W. and Campbell, S. (1974). Fetal urine-production rates in normal and complicated pregnancy, *Lancet*, **1**, 151–4.

Wladimiroff, J. W., Craft, I. L. and Talbert, D. G. (1975). *In vitro* measurements of sound velocity in human fetal brain tissue, *Ultrasound Med. Biol.*, **1**, 377–82.

Ylöstalo, P. (1974). Measurement of fetal body dimensions by the ultrasound B-scan method, *Annls Chir. Gynaec. Fenn.*, **63**, 20–3.

Zelnick, E., Saary, Z. and Gershowitz, M. (1975). Ultrasonic localization of "Missing I.U.C.D.'s". *In* "Ultrasound in Medicine" (ed. D. N. White), vol. 1, pp. 233–9, Plenum Press, New York.

6.16.g Oncology

Asher, W. M. and Freimanis, A. K. (1969). Echographic diagnosis of retroperitoneal lymph node enlargement, *Am. J. Roentg.*, **105**, 438–45.

Brascho, D. J. (1972). Clinical applications of diagnostic ultrasound in abdominal malignancy, *S. med. J.*, **65**, 1331–9.

Brascho, D. J. (1974). Computerized radiation treatment planning with ultrasound, *Am. J. Roentg.*, **120**, 213–23.

Cole-Bueglet, C. and Beique, R. A. (1975). Continuous ultrasound B-scanning of palpable breast masses, *Radiology*, **117**, 123–8.

Damascelli, B., Bonadonna, G., Musumeci, R. and Uslenghi, C. (1969). Two-dimensional pulsed echo detection of para-aortic lymph nodes, *Surg. Gynec. Obstet.*, **128**, 772–6.

Damascelli, B., Fossati, F., Livraghi, T. and Severini, A. (1969). B-scan ultrasound exploration of neoplastic disease, *Am. J. Roentg.*, **105**, 428–37.

Damascelli, B., Musumeci, R. and Orefice, S. (1970). Sonar information about breast tumors, *Radiology*, **96**, 583–6.

Deland, F. H. (1969). A modified technique of ultrasonography for the detection and differential diagnosis of breast lesions, *Am. J. Roentg.*, **105**, 446–52.

Eule, J., Bockenstedt, F. and Salzman, E. (1973). Diagnostic ultrasonic scanning: a valuable aid in radiation therapy planning, *Am. J. Roentg.*, **117**, 139–45.

Evans, G. C., Lehman, J. S., Brody, L. W., Smyth, M. G. and Hart, D. J. (1966). Ultrasonic scanning of abdominal and pelvic organs using B-scan display. *In* "Diagnostic Ultrasound" (ed. C. C. Grossman, J. H. Holmes, C. Joyner and E. W. Purnell), pp. 369–415, Plenum Press, New York.

Fry, E. K., Kossoff, G. and Hindman, H. A. (1972). The potential of ultrasound vizualization for detecting the presence of abnormal structures within the female breast, *Proc. I.E.E.E. Ultrasonics Symp.*, 25–30.

Goldberg, B. B., Sklaroff, D. M. and Isard, H. J. (1968). Echoencephalography in the management of patients receiving radiation therapy, *Radiology*, **91**, 363–6.

Hayashi, S., Wagai, T., Miyazawa, R., Ito, K., Ishikawa, S., Uematsu, K., Kikuchi, Y. and Uchida, R. (1962). Ultrasonic diagnosis of breast tumor and chol-elithisis, *West. J. Surg. Obstet. Gynec.*, **70**, 34–40.

Heimburger, R. F., Eggleton, R. C. and Fry, F. J. (1973). Ultrasonic visualization in determination of tumor growth rate, *J. Am. med. Ass.*, **224**, 497–501.

Herring, D. F. and Compton, D. M. J. (1971). Degree of precision required in radiation dose delivered in cancer radiotherapy, *Br. J. Radiol.*, Special Report Series No. 5, 51–8.

Holm, H. H. (1971). Ultrasonic scanning in the diagnosis of space-occupying lesions of the upper abdomen, *Br. J. Radiol.*, **44**, 24–36.

Howry, D. H., Stott, D. A. and Bliss, W. R. (1954). The ultrasonic visualization of carcinoma of the breast and other soft-tissue structures, *Cancer, N.Y.* **7**, 354–8.

Jackson, S. M., Naylor, G. P. and Kerby, I. J. (1970). Ultrasonic measurement of post-mastectomy chest wall thickness, *Br. J. Radiol.*, **43**, 458–61.

Jellins, J. and Kossoff, G. (1973). Velocity compensation in water-coupled breast echography, *Ultrasonics*, **11**, 223–6.

Jellins, J., Kossoff, G., Buddee, F. W. and Reeve, T. S. (1971). Ultrasonic visualization of the breast, *Med. J. Aust.*, **1**, 305–7.

Jellins, J., Kossoff, G. and Reeve, T. S. (1975a). The ultrasonic appearance of pathology in the male breast, *Ultrasound Med. Biol.*, **2**, 43–4.

Jellins, J., Kossoff, G., Reeve, T. S. and Barraclough, B. H. (1975b). Ultrasonic gray scale visualization of breast disease, *Ultrasound Med. Biol.*, **1**, 393–404.

Jentzsch, K., Kärcher, K. H. and Böhm, B. (1974). Ultraschall in der Strahlen-therapie: bei der Bestrahlungsplanung und Überwachung des Therapieerfolges, *Ultrasound Med. Biol.*, **1**, 149–59.

Kobayashi, T. (1975). Ultrasonic diagnosis of breast cancer, *Ultrasound Med. Biol.*, **1**, 383–91.

Kobayashi, T., Takatani, O., Hattori, N. and Kimura, K. (1972a). Clinical investigation of ultrasonographic patterns of malignant abdominal tumor in special reference to changes of its pattern after irradiation or chemotherapy (preliminary report), *Med. Ultrasonics*, **10**, 18–22.

Kobayashi, T., Takatani, O., Hattori, N. and Kimura, K. (1972b). Clinical investigation of ultrasonotomographic patterns of malignant abdominal tumor in special reference to changes of its pattern after irradiation or chemotherapy (II), *Med. Ultrasonics*, **10**, 132–5.

Kobayashi, T., Takatani, O., Hattori, N. and Kimura, K. (1972c). Study of sensitivity graded ultrasonotomography (Preliminary report)—Evaluation upon 64 cases with breast tumor and representation of "malignant echo-like pattern" seen in two cases with fat necrosis in breast, *Med. Ultrasonics*, **10**, 38–40.

Kobayashi, T., Takatani, O., Kimura, K., Watanabe, H. and Abe, O. (1972d). Clinical investigation for the differential diagnosis of breast tumor by means of the graded sensitivity method of ultrasonotomography (2nd report)— Proposal of new differential diagnostic criteria: tadpole-tail sign with lateral shadow (benign) and acoustic middle shadow sign (malignant) and its clinical significance and evaluation, *Med. Ultrasonics*, **10**, 81–6.

Kobayashi, T., Takatani, O., Hattori, N., and Kimura, K. (1974). Echographic evaluation of abdominal tumor regression during antineoplastic treatment, *J. clin. Ultrasound*, **2**, 131–41.

Laustela, E., Kerminen, T., Lieto, J. and Tala, P. (1966). Studies of ultrasonic diagnosis of breast tumours, *Annls Chir. Gynaec. Fenn.*, **55**, 173–5.

Mayer, E. G., Galindo, J., Connor, W. G., Hicks, J. A. and Aristizibal, S. A. (1975). Evaluation of B-mode ultrasound as a means of improving radium dosimetry in the treatment of gynecologic cancer, *Radiology*, **117**, 141–7.

Sanders, R. C., Hughes, B. and Hazra, T. A. (1974). Ultrasound localization of kidneys for radiation therapy, *Br. J. Radiol.*, **47**, 196–7.

Slater, J. M., Neilsen, I. R., Chu, W. T., Carlsen, E. N. and Chrispens, J. E. (1974). Radiotherapy treatment planning using ultrasound—sonic graph pen-computer system, *Cancer, N.Y.*, **34**, 96–9.

Tolbert, D. D., Zagzebski, J. A., Banjavic, R. A. and Wiley, A. L. (1974). Quantitation of tumour volumes and response to therapy with ultrasound B-scans, *Radiology*, **113**, 705–8.

Wagai, T., Miyazawa, R., Ito, K. and Kikuchi, Y. (1965). Ultrasonic diagnosis of intracranial disease, breast tumors and abdominal diseases. *In* "Ultrasonic Energy" (ed. E. Kelly), pp. 346–60, University of Illinois Press, Urbana.

Wagai, T., Takahashi, S., Ohashi, H. and Ichikawa, H. (1967). A trial for quantitative diagnosis of breast tumor by ultrasono-tomography, *Med. Ultrasonics*, **5**, 39–40.

Weiss, L. (1974). Some pathobiological considerations of detection of breast cancer by ultrasonic holography. *In* "Ultrasonic Imaging and Holography" (ed. G. W. Stroke, W. E. Koch, Y. Kikuchi and J. Tsujiuchi), pp. 567–85, Plenum Press, New York.

Wells, P. N. T. and Evans, K. T. (1968). An immersion scanner for two-dimensional ultrasonic examination of the human breast, *Ultrasonics*, **6**, 220–8.

Whittingham, P. D. G. V. (1962). Measurement of tissue thickness by ultrasound, *Aerospace Med.*, **33**, 1121–8.

Wild, J. J. and Reid, J. M. (1952). Further pilot echographic studies on the histologic structure of the living intact human breast, *Am. J. Path.*, **28**, 839–61.

6.16.h Ophthalmology

Aldridge, E. E., Clare, A. B. and Shepherd, D. A. (1974). Scanned ultrasonic holography for ophthalmic diagnosis, *Ultrasonics*, **12**, 155–60.

Baum, G. and Greenwood, I. (1958). The application of ultrasonic locating techniques to ophthalmology, *Archs ophthal.*, **60**, 263–79.

Bronson, N. R. (1965). Techniques of ultrasonic localisation and extraction of intra- and extra-ocular foreign bodies, *Am. J. Ophthal.*, **60**, 596–603.

Bronson, N. R. (1972). Development of a simple B-scan ultrasonoscope, *Trans. Am. ophthal. Soc.*, **70**, 365–408.

Bronson, N. R. (1974). Contact B-scan ultrasonography, *Am. J. Ophthal.*, **77**, 181–91.

Buschmann, W. (1965). New equipment and transducers for ophthalmic diagnosis, *Ultrasonics*, **3**, 18–21.

Coleman, D. J. (1972a). Reliability of ocular and orbital diagnosis with B-scan ultrasound. 1. Ocular diagnosis. *Am. J. Ophthal.*, **73**, 501–16.

Coleman, D. J. (1972b). Reliability of ocular and orbital diagnosis with B-scan ultrasound. 2. Orbital diagnosis. *Am. J. Ophthal.*, **74**, 704–18.

Coleman, D. J. and Carlin, B. (1967). Transducer alignment and electronic measurement of visual axis dimensions in the human eye using time-amplitude ultrasound. *In* "Ultrasonics in Ophthalmology, Symp. Münster", pp. 207–14, Karger, Basle.

Coleman, D. J. and Jack, R. L. (1973). B-scan ultrasonography in diagnosis and management of retinal detachments, *Archs ophthal.*, **90**, 29–34.

Coleman, D. J., Konig, W. F. and Katz, L. (1969). A hand-operated ultrasound scan system for ophthalmic evaluation, *Am. J. Ophthal.*, **68**, 256–63.

Dadd, M. J., Hughes, H. L. and Kossoff, G. (1975). Ultrasonic characteristics of choroidal melanoma, *Bibl. ophthal.*, **83**, 155–62.

Dadd, M., Kossoff, G. and Hughes, H. (1974). Ultrasonic display of the orbital contents, *Med. J. Aust.*, **1**, 580–4.

Giglio, E. J. and Meyers, R. R. (1969). An automatic probe transport to the eye for ultrasound, *Am. J. Optom.*, **46**, 275–82.

Giglio, E. J., Ludlam, W. M. and Wittenberg, S. (1968). Improvement in the measurement of intraocular distances using ultrasound, *J. acoust. Soc. Am.*, **44**, 1359–64.

Jansson, F. (1963). Determination of axis length of the eye roentgenologically and by ultrasound, *Acta ophthal.*, **41**, 236–46.

Leary, G. A. (1967). Basic techniques for applying ultrasonics to ophthalmic measurements and diagnosis, *Ultrasonics*, **6**, 84–7.

Mundt, G. H. and Hughes, W. F. (1956). Ultrasonics in ocular diagnosis, *Am. J. Ophthal.*, **41**, 488–98.

Oksala, A. (1968). A-scan echography in the diagnosis of intraocular diseases, *Proc. int. Symp., diag. Ultrasound Ophth.*, pp. 5–30, Documenti Italseber, Turin.

Ossoinig, K. C. (1974). Quantitative echography—an important aid for the acoustic differentiation of tissues. *In* "Ultrasonics in Medicine" (ed. M. de Vlieger, D. N. White and V. R. McCready), pp. 49–54, Excerpta Medica, Amsterdam.

Sorsby, A., Leary, G. A., Richards, M. J. and Chaston, J. (1963). Ultrasonic measurement of the components of ocular refraction in life, *Vision Res.*, **2**, 499–505.

Sutherland, G. R. and Forrester, J. V. (1974). B-scan ultrasonography in ophthalmology, *Br. J. Radiol.*, **47**, 383–6.

Sutherland, G. R. and Forrester, J. V. (1975). Demonstration of abnormalities of the lens by echography, *Br. J. Radiol.*, **48**, 1019–22.

Sutherland, G. R., Forrester, J. V. and Railton, R. (1975). Echography in the diagnosis and management of retinal detachment, *Br. J. Radiol.*, **48**, 796–800.

6.16.i Orthopaedics and rheumatology

Abendschein, W. and Hyatt, G. W. (1972). Ultrasonics and the physical properties of healing bone, *J. Trauma*, **12**, 297–301.

Booth, K. A., Goddard, B. A. and Paton, A. (1966). Measurement of fat thickness in man: a comparison of fat thickness, Harpenden calipers and electrical conductivity, *Br. J. Nutr.*, **20**, 719–25.

Bullen, B. A., Quaade, F., Olesen, E. and Lund, S. A. (1965). Ultrasonic reflection used for measuring subcutaneous fat in humans, *Hum. Biol.*, **37**, 375–84.

Davies, G. T. and Wells, P. N. T. (1971). Ulnar resonant frequency determination and its relevance to the assessment of osteoporosis, *Phys. Med. Biol.*, **16**, 148.

Holmes, J. H. and Howry, D. H. (1958). Ultrasonic visualization of edema, *Trans. Am. clin. climat. Ass.*, **70**, 225–35.

Horn, C. A. and Robinson, D. (1965). Assessment of fracture healing by ultrasonics, *J. Coll. Radiol. Aust.*, **9**, 165–7.

Howry, D. H. (1965). A brief atlas of diagnostic ultrasonic radiologic results, *Radiol. Clin. N. Am.*, **3**, 433–52.

Jackson, S. M., Naylor, G. P. and Kerby, I. J. (1970). Ultrasonic measurement of post-mastectomy chest wall thickness, *Br. J. Radiol.*, **43**, 458–61.

Jurist, J. M. (1970a). *In vivo* determination of the elastic response of bone. I. Method of ulnar resonant frequency determination, *Phys. Med. Biol.*, **15**, 417–26.

Jurist, J. M. (1970b). *In vivo* determination of the elastic response of bone. II. Ulnar resonant frequency in osteoporotic, diabetic and normal subjects. *Phys. Med. Biol.*, **15**, 427–34.

Jurist, J. M. and Kianian, K. (1973). Three models of the vibrating ulna, *J. Biomechanics*, **6**, 331–42.

McDonald, D. G. and Leopold, G. R. (1972). Ultrasound B-scanning in the differentiation of Baker's cyst and thrombophlebitis, *Br. J. Radiol.*, **45**, 729–32.

Meire, H. B., Lindsay, D. J., Swinson, D. R. and Hamilton, E. B. D. (1974). Comparison of ultrasound and positive contrast arthography in the diagnosis of popliteal and calf swellings, *Ann. rheum. Dis.*, **33**, 221–4.

Ramsden, D., Peabody, C. O. and Speight, R. G. (1967). The use of ultrasonics to investigate soft tissue thickness on the human chest, "U.K.A.E.A. Reactor Group Report", A.E.E.W.-R493, H.M.S.O., London.

Rich, C., Klinik, E., Smith, R. and Graham, B. (1966). Measurement of bone mass from ultrasonic transmission time, *Proc. Soc. exp. Biol. Med.*, **123**, 282–5.

Sloan, A. W. (1967). Estimation of body fat in young men, *J. appl. Physiol.*, **23**, 311–5.

Whittingham, P. D. V. G. (1962). Measurement of tissue thickness by ultrasound, *Aerospace Med.*, **33**, 1121–8.

6.16.j Otorhinolaryngology

Brezińska, H. (1972). Application of the ultrasonic echo method for laryngological diagnostics in children. *In* "Ultrasonics in Biology and Medicine" (ed. L. Filipczyński), pp. 29–33, Polish Scientific Publishers, Warsaw.

Hamlet, S. L. (1972). Vocal fold articulatory activity during whispered sibilants, *Archs Otolar.*, **95**, 211–3.

Hertz, C. H., Lindström, K. and Sonesson, B. (1970). Ultrasonic recording of the vibrating vocal folds, *Acta oto-lar.*, **69**, 223–30.

Johnson, S., Sjöberg, A. and Stahle, J. (1966). Studies of the otic capsule. 1. Reduced dead time ultrasonic probe for the measurement of bone thickness. *Acta oto-lar.*, **62**, 532–64.

Kelsey, C. A., Crummy, A. B. and Schulman, E. Y. (1969a). Comparison of ultrasonic and cineradiographic measurements of lateral pharyngeal wall motion, *Invest. Radiol.*, **4**, 241–5.

Kelsey, C. A., Hixon, T. J. and Minifie, F. D. (1969b). Ultrasonic measurement of lateral pharyngeal wall displacement, *I.E.E.E. Trans. biomed. Engng*, **BME-16**, 143–7.

6.16.k Urology

Alftan, O. and Mattson, T. (1969). Ultrasonic method of measuring residual urine, *Annls Chir. Gynaec. Fenn.*, **58**, 300–3.

Asher, W. M. and Leopold, G. R. (1972). A streamlined approach to renal mass lesions with renal echogram, *J. Urol.*, **108**, 205–7.

Barnett, E. and Morley, P. (1971). Ultrasound in the investigation of space-occupying lesions of the urinary tract, *Br. J. Radiol.*, **44**, 733–42.

Barnett, E. and Morley, P. (1972). Diagnostic ultrasound in renal disease, *Br. med. Bull.*, **28**, 196–9.

Berlyne, G. M. (1961). Ultrasonics in renal biopsy. An aid to the determination of kidney position, *Lancet*, **2**, 750–1.

Damascelli, B., Fossati, F., Livraghi, T. and Severini, A. (1968). B-scan ultrasound exploration of neoplastic disease, *Am. J. Roentg.*, **105**, 428–37.

Goldberg, B. B. and Pollack, H. M. (1971). Differentiation of renal masses using A-mode ultrasound, *J. Urol.*, **105**, 765–71.

Goldberg, B. B. and Pollack, H. M. (1973). Ultrasonically guided renal cyst aspiration, *J. Urol.*, **109**, 5–7.

Goldberg, B. B., Ostrum, B. J. and Isard, H. J. (1968). Nephrosonography: ultrasound differentiation of renal masses, *Radiology*, **90**, 1113–8.

Heap, G. (1968). Localization of urinary calculi by ultrasound, *Br. J. Urol.*, **40**, 485.

Holmes, J. H. (1966a). Ultrasonic studies of the bladder and kidney. *In* "Diagnostic Ultrasound" (ed. C. C. Grossman, J. H. Holmes, C. Joyner and E. W. Purnell), pp. 465–80, Plenum Press, New York.

Holmes, J. H. (1966b). Ultrasonic studies of the bladder, *J. Urol.*, **97**, 654–63.

Hünig, R. and Kinser, J. (1973). Ultrasonic diagnosis of Wilms' tumors, *Am. J. Roentg.*, **117**, 119–27.

King, W. W., Wilkiemeyer, R. M., Boyce, W. H. and McKinney, W. M. (1973). Current status of prostatic echography, *J. Am. med. Ass.*, **226**, 444–7.

Kristensen, J. K., Gammelgaard, P. A., Holm, H. H. and Rasmussen, S. N. (1972). Ultrasound in the demonstration of renal masses, *Br. J. Urol.*, **44**, 517–27.

Lyons, E. A., Murphy, A. V. and Arneil, G. C. (1972). Sonar and its use in kidney disease in children, *Archs Dis. Child.*, **47**, 777–86.

Micsky, L. von, Radkowski, M. A., Hecker, J. and Finby, N. (1974). Optimal diagnosis of renal masses in children by combining and correlating diagnostic features of sonography and radiography, *Am. J. Roentg.*, **120**, 438–47.

Miskin, M. and Bain, J. (1974). B-mode ultrasonic examination of the testes, *J. clin. Ultrasound*, **2**, 307–11.

Miller, S. S., Garvie, W. H. H. and Christie, A. D. (1973). The evaluation of prostate size by ultrasonic scanning: a preliminary report, *Br. J. Urol.*, **45**, 187–91.

Morley, P., Barnett, E., Bell, P. R. F., Briggs, J. K., Calman, K. C., Hamilton, D. N. H. and Paton, A. M. (1975). Ultrasound in the diagnosis of fluid collections following renal transplantation, *Clin. Radiol.*, **26**, 199–207.

Mountford, R. A., Ross, F. G. M., Burwood, R. J. and Knapp, M. S. (1971). The use of ultrasound in the diagnosis of renal disease, *Br. J. Radiol.*, **44**, 860–9.

Schlegal, J. U., Diggdon, P. and Cuellar, J. (1961). The use of ultrasound for localizing renal calculi, *J. Urol.*, **86**, 367–9.

Takahashi, H. and Ouchi, T. (1963). Ultrasonic diagnosis in the field of urology: first report, *Jap. med. Ultrason.*, **1**, 7–10.

Watanabe, H., Kaiho, H., Tanaka, M. and Terasawa, Y. (1971). Diagnostic application of ultrasonotomography to the prostate, *Invest. Urol.*, **8**, 548–59.

Whittingham, T. A. and Bishop, R. (1973). Ultrasonic estimation of the volume of the enlarged prostate, *Br. J. Radiol.*, **46**, 68–70.

7 Doppler methods

7.1 Transmission methods

Baldes, E. J., Farral, W. R., Haugen, M. C. and Herrick, J. F. (1957). A forum on an ultrasonic method for measuring the velocity of blood. *In* "Ultrasound in Biology and Medicine" (ed. E. Kelly), pp. 165–76, A.I.B.S., Washington.

Blumenfeld, W., Wilson, P. D. and Turney, S. (1974). A mathematical model for the ultrasonic measurement of respiratory flow, *Med. biol. Engng*, **12**, 621–5.

Borgnis, F. (1974). A novel design for intravascular measurement of blood velocity in arteries and veins based on the transit-time principle. *In* "Cardiovascular Applications of Ultrasound" (ed. R. S. Reneman), pp. 173–82, North-Holland, Amsterdam.

Farral, W. R. (1959). Design considerations for ultrasonic flowmeters, *I.R.E. Trans. med. Electron.*, **ME-6**, 198–201.

Franklin, D. L., Baker, D. W., Ellis, R. M. and Rushmer, R. F. (1959). A pulsed ultrasonic flowmeter, *I.R.E. Trans. med. Electron.*, **ME-6**, 204–6.

Franklin, D. and Kemper, W. S. (1974). Frequency modulated ultrasonic transit-time flowmeter. *In* "Cardiovascular Applications of Ultrasound" (ed. R. S. Reneman), pp. 145–9, North-Holland, Amsterdam.

Fricke, G., Studer, V. and Schen, H. D. (1970). Pulsatile velocity of blood in the pulmonary artery of dogs: measurement by an ultrasound gauge, *Cardiovasc. Res.*, **4**, 371–9.

Kalmus, H. P. (1954). Electronic flowmeter system, *Rev. scient. Instrum.*, **25**, 201–6.

7.2 Reflexion methods

7.2.a Basic principles

Michie, D. D. and Cain, C. P. (1971). Effect of hematocrit upon the shift in Doppler frequency, *Proc. Soc. exp. Biol. Med.*, **138**, 768–72.

Reid, J. M. and Baker, D. W. (1971). Physics and electronics of the ultrasonic Doppler method. *In* "Ultrasonographia Medica" (ed. J. Böck and K. Ossoinig), vol. I, pp. 109–20, Verlag Wien. med. Akad., Vienna.

7.2.b Transducer arrangements and beam directivities

Baker, D. W. (1970). Pulsed ultrasonic Doppler blood-flow sensing, *I.E.E.E. Trans. Sonics Ultrason.*, **SU-17**, 170–85.

Baker, D. W. and Yates, W. G. (1973). Technique for studying the sample volume of ultrasonic Doppler devices, *Med. biol. Engng*, **11**, 766–70.

Benchimol. A., Stagall, H. F., Maroko, P. R., Gartlan, J. L. and Brener, L. (1969). Aortic flow velocity in man during cardiac arrhythmias measured with Doppler catheter-flowmeter system, *Am. Heart J.*, **78**, 649–59.

Duck, F. A. and Hodson, C. J. (1973). A practical method of eliminating the angular dependence of Doppler flow measurements, *Excerpta Medica International Congress Series*, **277**, 15–6.

Duck, F. A., Hodson, C. J. and McMannamon, P. J. (1972). An intravenous Doppler probe for arterial flow monitoring, *Proc. 3rd int. Conf. med. Phys.*, **35**, 10.

Fahrbach, K. (1970). Ein Beitrag zur Blutgeschwindigkeitsmessung unter Anwendung des Doppler effektes, *Electromed.*, **15**, 26–31.

Higgs, R. W. and Erikson, L. J. (1969). Acoustic decoupling properties of Corprene DC-100, *J. acoust. Soc. Am.*, **46**, 1254–8.

Jethwa, C. P., Kaveh, M., Cooper, G. R. and Saggio, F. (1975). Blood flow measurements using ultrasonic pulsed random signal Doppler system, *I.E.E.E. Trans. Sonics Ultrason.*, **SU-22**, 1–11.

Lubé, V. M., Safonov, Y. D. and Yakiemenkov, L. I. (1967). Ultrasonic detection of the motions of cardiac valves and muscle, *Soviet Phys. Acoust.*, **13**, 59–65.

Peronneau, P., Xhaard, M., Nowicki, A., Pellet, M., Delouche, P. and Hinglais, J. (1972). Pulsed Doppler ultrasonic flow pattern analysis. *In* "Blood Flow Measurement" (ed. C. Roberts), pp. 24–8, Sector, London.

Reid, J. M., Davis, D. L., Ricketts, H. J. and Spencer, M. P. (1974). A new Doppler flowmeter system and its operation with catheter mounted transducers. *In* "Cardiovascular Applications of Ultrasound" (ed. R. S. Reneman), pp. 183–92, North-Holland, Amsterdam.

Satomura, S. (1957). Ultrasonic Doppler method for the inspection of cardiac functions, *J. acoust. Soc. Am.*, **29**, 1181–5.

Side, C. D. and Gosling, R. G. (1971). Non-surgical assessment of cardiac function, *Nature, Lond.*, **232**, 335–6.

Wells, P. N. T. (1970). The directivities of some ultrasonic Doppler probes, *Med. biol. Engng*, **8**, 241–56.

Wells, P. N. T. (1974). Ultrasonic Doppler probes. *In* "Cardiovascular Applications of Ultrasound" (ed. R. S. Reneman), pp. 125–31, North-Holland, Amsterdam.

Woodcock, J. P. (1975). Development of the ultrasonic flowmeter, *Ultrasound Med. Biol.*, **2**, 11–8.

7.2.c Analysis of backscattered Doppler signals

Arts, M. G. J. and Roevros, J. M. J. G. (1972). On the instantaneous measurement of bloodflow by ultrasonic means, *Med. biol. Engng*, **10**, 23–34.

Coghlan, B. A., Taylor, M. G. and King, D. H. (1974). On-line display of Doppler-shift spectra by a new time compression analyser. *In* "Cardiovascular Applications of Ultrasound" (ed. R. S. Reneman), pp. 55–65, North-Holland, Amsterdam.

Flax, S. W., Webster, J. G. and Updike, S. J. (1971). Statistical evaluation of the Doppler ultrasonic blood flowmeter, *Instrum. Soc. Am. Trans.*, **10**, 1–20.

Koenig, W., Dunn, H. K. and Lacy, L. Y. (1946). The sound spectrograph, *J. acoust. Soc. Am.*, **18**, 19–49.

Light, L. H. (1970). A recording spectrograph for analysing Doppler blood velocity signals (particularly from aortic flow) in real time, *J. Physiol., Lond.*, **207**, 42P–44P.

Lunt, M. J. (1975). Accuracy and limitations of the ultrasonic Doppler blood velocimeter and zero crossing detector, *Ultrasound Med. Biol.*, **2**, 1–10.

Reneman, R. S. and Spencer, M. P. (1974). Difficulties in processing of an analogue Doppler flow signal; with special reference to zero-crossing meters and quantification. *In* "Cardiovascular Applications of Ultrasound" (ed. R. S. Reneman), pp. 32–42, North-Holland, Amsterdam.

Reneman, R. S., Clarke, H. F., Simmons, N. and Spencer, M. P. (1973). *In vivo* comparison of electromagnetic and Doppler flowmeters: with special attention to the processing of the analogue Doppler flow signal, *Cardiovasc. Res.*, **7**, 557–66.

Rice, S. O. (1944). Mathematical analysis of random noise, *Bell Syst. tech. J.*, **23**, 282–332.

Rice, S. O. (1945). Mathematical analysis of random noise, *Bell Syst. tech. J.*, **24**, 1–162.

7.2.d Directional detectors

Arts, M. G. J. and Roevros, J. M. J. G. (1972). On the instantaneous measurement of blood flow by ultrasonic means, *Med. biol. Engng*, **10**, 23–34.

Cross, G. and Light, L. H. (1971). Direction resolving Doppler instrument with improved rejection of tissue artefacts, *J. Physiol., Lond.*, **217**, 5.

Haase, W. C., Foletta, W. S. and Meindl, J. D. (1973). A directional ratiometric ultrasonic blood flowmeter, *Proc. I.E.E.E. Ultrasonics Symp.*, 81–5.

Jong, D. A. de, Megens, P. H. A., Vlieger, M. de, Thön, H. and Holland, W. P. J. (1975). A directional quantifying Doppler system for measurement of transport velocity of blood, *Ultrasonics*, **13**, 138–41.

McLeod, F. D. (1967). A directional Doppler flowmeter, *Dig. 7th int. Conf. med. biol. Engng*, 213.

Nippa, J. H. (1975). Ultrasonic Doppler velocity meter for quantitating forward and reverse blood flow velocities. *In* "Ultrasound in Medicine" (ed. D. N. White), vol. 1, pp. 459–62, Plenum Press, New York.

Nippa, J. H., Hokanson, D. E., Lee, D. R., Sumner, D. S. and Strandness, D. E. (1975). Phase rotation for separating forward and reverse blood velocity signals, *I.E.E.E. Trans. Sonics Ultrason.*, **SU-22**, 340–6.

7.2.e Phase detectors

Baker, D. W., Reid, J. M. and Simmons, V. E. (1967). Transcutaneous detection of arterial wall motion using phase lock Doppler, *Dig. 7th int. Conf. med. biol. Engng*, 325.

Reid, J. M., Baker, D. W. and Simmons, V. E. (1967). Phase detection of Doppler signals for measurement of biological displacements, *Dig. 7th int. Conf. med. biol. Engng*, 214.

7.2.f Rangefinding Doppler methods

Atkinson, P. (1974). "On the Measurement of Bloodflow by Ultrasound", Ph.D. Dissertation, University of Bristol.

Baker, D. W. (1970). Pulsed ultrasonic Doppler blood-flow sensing, *I.E.E.E. Trans. Sonics Ultrason.*, **SU-17**, 170–85.

Baker, D. W. and Watkins, D. (1967). A phase coherent pulse Doppler system for cardiovascular measurement, *Proc. 20th ann. Conf. Engng Med. Biol.*, **27**, 2.

Bendick, P. J. and Newhouse, V. L. (1974). Ultrasonic random-signal flow measurement system, *J. acoust. Soc. Am.*, **56**, 860–5.

Brown, J. and Glazier, E. V. D. (1964). "Telecommunications", Chapman and Hall, London.

Flaherty, J. J. and Strauts, E. J. (1969). Ultrasonic pulse Doppler instrumentation, *Proc. 8th int. Conf. med. biol. Engng*, 10–10.

Gill, R. W. and Meindl, J. D. (1973). Optimal system design of the pulsed Doppler ultrasonic blood flowmeter, *Proc. I.E.E.E. Ultrasonics Symp.*, 88–93.

Haase, W. C., Foletta, W. S. and Meindl, J. D. (1973). A directional ratiometric ultrasonic blood flowmeter, *Proc. I.E.E.E. Ultrasonics Symp.*, 81–5.

Jethwa, C. P., Kaveh, M., Cooper, G. R. and Saggio, F. (1975). Blood flow measurements using ultrasonic pulsed random signal Doppler system, *I.E.E.E. Trans. Sonics Ultrason.*, **SU-22**, 1–11.

Jorgensen, J. E., Campau, D. N. and Baker, D. W. (1973). Physical characteristics and mathematical modelling of the pulsed ultrasonic flowmeter, *Med. biol. Engng*, **11**, 404–21.

McCarty, K. and Woodcock, J. P. (1975). Frequency modulated ultrasonic Doppler flowmeter, *Med. biol. Engng*, **13**, 59–64.

Peronneau, P. A. and Leger, F. (1969). Doppler ultrasonic pulsed blood flowmeter, *Proc. 8th int. Conf. med. biol. Engng*, 10–11.

Peronneau, P. A., Hinglais, J. R., Pellet, H. M. and Leger, F. (1970). Vélocimètre sanguin par effet Doppler à émission ultra-sonore pulsée, *Onde élect.*, **50**, 369–84.

Waag, R. C., Myklebust, J. B., Rhoads, W. L. and Gramiak, R. (1972). Instrumentation for noninvasive cardiac chamber flow rate measurement, *Proc. I.E.E.E. Ultrasonics Symp.*, 74–7.

Wells, P. N. T. (1969). A range-gated ultrasonic Doppler system, *Med. biol. Engng*, **7**, 641–52.

7.2.g Two-dimensional Doppler imaging

Barber, F. E., Baker, D. W., Nation, A. W. C., Strandness, D. E. and Reid, J. M. (1974). Ultrasonic duplex echo-Doppler scanner, *I.E.E.E. Trans. biomed. Engng*, **BME-21**, 109–13.

Evans, T. C., Green, P. S. and Greenleaf, J. F., (1974). Development of high resolution ultrasonic imaging techniques for detection and clinical assessment of cardiovascular disease, *Report no. NO1-HT-4-2904-1*, N.T.I.S., Springfield.

Fish, P. (1972). Visualising blood vessels by ultrasound. *In* "Blood Flow Measurement" (ed. C. Roberts), pp. 29–32, Sector, London.

Hottinger, C. F. and Meindl, J. D. (1975). Real-time Doppler imaging for unambiguous measurement of blood volume flow. *In* "Acoustical Holography" (ed. N. Booth), vol. 6, pp. 247–58, Plenum Press, New York.

Mozersky, D. J., Hokanson, D. E., Baker, D. W., Sumner, D. S. and Strandness, D. E. (1971). Ultrasonic arteriography, *Archs Surg.*, **103**, 663–7.

Reid, J. M. and Spencer, M. P. (1972). Ultrasonic Doppler technique for imaging blood vessels, *Science, N.Y.*, **176**, 1235–6.

Spencer, M. P., Reid, J. M., Davis, D. L. and Paulson, P. S. (1974). Cervical carotid imaging with a continuous-wave Doppler flowmeter, *Stroke*, **5**, 145–54.

7.2.h Activity monitors

Haines, J. (1974). An ultrasonic system for measuring activity, *Med. biol. Engng*, **12**, 378–81.

7.3 Clinical applications

7.3.a Angiology

Allan, J. S. and Terry, H. J. (1969). The evaluation of an ultrasonic flow detector for the assessment of peripheral vascular disease, *Cardiovasc. Res.*, **3**, 503–9.

Barber, F. E., Baker, D. W., Nation, A. W. C., Strandness, D. E. and Reid, J. M. (1974). Ultrasonic duplex echo-Doppler scanner, *I.E.E.E. Trans. biomed. Engng*, **BME-21**, 109–13.

Bracey, D. W. (1973). Hazard of ultrasonic detection of deep vein thrombosis, *Br. med. J.*, **1**, 420.

Edmonds-Seal, J. and Maroon, J. C. (1969). Air embolism diagnosed with ultrasound, *Anaesthesia*, **24**, 438–40.

Evans, A. and Walder, D. N. (1970). Detection of circulating bubbles in the intact mammal, *Ultrasonics*, **8**, 216–7.

Evans, D. S. (1971). The early diagnosis of thrombo-embolism by ultrasound, *Ann. R. Coll. Surg. Enghl.*, **49**, 225–49.

Fish, P. J. (1972). Visualising blood vessels by ultrasound. *In* "Blood Flow Measurement" (ed. C. Roberts), pp. 29–32, Sector, London.

Fish, P. J., Kakkar, V. V., Corrigan, T. and Nicolaides, A. N. (1972). Arteriography using ultrasound, *Lancet*, **1**, 1269–70.

Fitzgerald, D. E. and Carr, J. (1975). Doppler ultrasound diagnosis and classification as an alternative to arteriography, *Angiology*, **26**, 283–8.

Fitzgerald, D. E., Gosling, R. G. and Woodcock, J. P. (1971). Grading dynamic capability of arterial collateral circulation, *Lancet*, **1**, 66–7.

Gillis, M. F., Peterson, P. L. and Karagianes, M. T. (1968). *In-vivo* detection of circulating gas emboli associated with decompression sickness using the Doppler flowmeter, *Nature, Lond.*, **217**, 965–7.

Gosling, R. G. and King, D. H. (1974). Continuous wave ultrasound as an alternative and complement to X-rays in vascular examination. *In* "Cardiovascular Applications of Ultrasound" (ed. R. S. Reneman), pp. 266–82, North-Holland, Amsterdam.

Hills, B. A. and Grulke, D. C. (1975). Evaluation of ultrasonic bubble detectors in vitro using calibrated microbubbles at selected velocities, *Ultrasonics*, **13**, 181–4.

Histand, B. and Miller, C. W. (1972). A comparison of velocity profiles measured in unexposed and exposed arteries, *Biomed. Scis. Instrum.*, **9**, 121–4.

Histand, M. B., Miller, C. W. and McLeod, F. D. (1973). Transcutaneous measurement of blood velocity profiles and flow, *Cardiovasc. Res.*, **7**, 703–12.

Hodson, C. J. and Duck, F. A. (1973). Blood-flow monitoring in deeply-situated arteries, *Invest. Radiol.*, **8**, 160–6.

James, P. B. and Galloway, R. W. (1971). The ultrasonic blood velocity detector as an aid to arteriography, *Br. J. Radiol.*, **44**, 743–6.

Johnston, K. W. and Kakkar, V. V. (1974). Non-invasive measurement of systolic pressure slope, *Archs Surg.*, **108**, 52–6.

Keitzer, W. F., Lichti, E. L., Brossart, F. A. and Wesse, M. S. de (1972). Use of the Doppler ultrasonic flowmeter during arterial vascular surgery, *Archs Surg.*, **105**, 308–12.

Kelly, G. L., Dodi, G. and Eiseman, B. (1972). Ultrasound detection of fat emboli, *Surg. Forum*, **23**, 459–61.

Lewis, J. D., Papathanaiou, C., Yao, S. T. and Eastcott, H. H. G. (1972). Simultaneous flow and pressure measurements in intermittent claudication, *Br. J. Surg.*, **59**, 418–22.

Lewis, J. D., Parsons, D. C. S., Needham, T. N., Douglas, J. N., Lawson, J., Hobbs, J. T. and Nicolaides, A. N. (1973). The use of various pressure measurements and directional Doppler recordings in distinguishing between superficial and deep valvular incompetence in patients with deep venous insufficiency, *Br. J. Surg.*, **60**, 312.

Manley, D. M. J. P. (1969). Ultrasonic detection of gas bubbles in blood, *Ultrasonics*, **7**, 102–5.

Maroon, J. C., Goodman, J. M., Horner, T. G. and Campbell, R. L. (1968). Detection of minute venous air emboli with ultrasound, *Surg. Gynec. Obstet.*, **127**, 1236–8.

Maroon, J. C., Edmonds-Seal, J. and Campbell, R. L. (1969). An ultrasonic method for detecting air bubbles, *J. Neurosurg.*, **31**, 196–201.

McIrroy, R. F. (1972). The routine use of ultrasound for the diagnosis of post-operative deep-vein thrombosis in a district general hospital, *Br. J. Surg.*, **59**, 133–5.

Miller, S. S. and Foote, A. V. (1974). The ultrasonic detection of incompetent perforating veins, *Br. J. Surg.*, **61**, 653–6.

Mol, J. M. F. and Rijcken, W. J. (1974). Doppler haematotachographic investigation in cerebral circulation disturbances. *In* "Cardiovascular Applications of Ultrasound" (ed. R. S. Reneman), pp. 305–14, North-Holland, Amsterdam.

Moore, R. D., Pryce, W. I. J. and Todd, J. H. (1973). The use of the ultrasonic Doppler test in the detection of deep vein thrombosis, *Phys. Med. Biol.*, **18**, 142–3.

Morris, S. J., Woodcock, J. P. and Wells, P. N. T. (1975). Impulse response of a segment of artery derived from transcutaneous blood-velocity measurements, *Med. biol. Engng*, **13**, 803–12.

Mozersky, D. J., Hokanson, D. E., Baker, D. W., Sumner, D. S. and Strandness, D. E. (1971). Ultrasonic arteriography, *Archs Surg.*, **103**, 663–7.

Mozersky, D. J., Hokanson, D. E., Sumner, D. S. and Strandness, D. E. (1972). Ultrasonic visualization of the arterial lumen, *Surgery, St. Louis*, **72**, 253–9.

Müller, H. R. and Gonzalez, R. R. (1974). Evaluation of cranial blood flow with ultrasonic Doppler techniques. *In* "Ultrasonics in Medicine" (ed. M. de Vlieger, D. N. White and V. R. McCready), pp. 89–96, Excerpta Medica, Amsterdam.

Negus, D. (1972). The diagnosis of deep-vein thrombosis, *Br. J. Surg.*, **59**, 830–4.

Olson, R. M. (1974). Human carotid artery wall thickness, diameter, and blood flow by a noninvasive technique, *J. appl. Physiol.*, **37**, 955–60.

Planiol, T. and Pourcelot, L. (1974). Doppler effect study of carotid circulation. *In* "Ultrasonics in Medicine" (ed. M. de Vlieger, D. N. White and V. R. McCready), pp. 104–11, Excerpta Medica, Amsterdam.

Ramsey, S. D., Taenzer, J. C., Holzemer, J. F., Suarez, J. R. and Green, P. S. (1975). A real-time ultrasonic B-scan/Doppler artery-imaging system, *Proc. I.E.E.E. Ultrasonics Symp.*, 10–2.

Rittenhouse, E. A. and Brockenbrough, E. C. (1969). A method for assessing the circulation distal to a femoral artery obstruction, *Surg. Gynec. Obstet.*, **129**, 538–44.

Sigel, B., Popky, G. L., Wagner, D. K., Boland, J. P., Mapp, E. McD. and Feigl, P. (1968). Comparison of clinical and Doppler ultrasound evaluation of confirmed lower extremity venous disease, *Surgery, St. Louis*, **64**, 332–8.

Somerville, J. J. F., Byrne, P. J. and Fegan, W. G. (1974). Analysis of flow patterns in venous insufficiency, *Br. J. Surg.*, **61**, 40–4.

Spencer, M. P., Reid, J. M., Davis, D. L. and Paulson, P. S. (1974). Cervical carotid imaging with a continuous-wave Doppler flowmeter, *Stroke*, **5**, 145–54.

Strandness, D. E., Schultz, R. D., Sumner, D. S. and Rushmer, R. F. (1967). Ultrasonic flow detection. A useful technic in the evaluation of peripheral vascular disease. *Am. J. Surg.*, **113**, 311–20.

Thomas, G. I., Spencer, M. P., Jones, T. W., Edmark, K. W. and Stavney, L. S. (1974). Noninvasive carotid bifurcation mapping, *Am. J. Surg.*, **128**, 168–74.

Walder, D. N., Evans, A. and Hempleman, H. V. (1968). Ultrasonic monitoring of decompression, *Lancet*, **1**, 897–8.

Wells, M. K., Bhagat, P. K. and Gross, D. R. (1973). Coronary artery blood velocity waveforms using a pulsed Doppler velocity meter, *Proc. 26th ann. Conf. Engng Med. Biol.*, 86.

Woodcock, J. P. (1970). The significance of changes in the velocity/time waveform in occlusive arterial disease of the leg. *In* "Ultrasonics in Biology and Medicine" (ed. L. Filipczyński), pp. 243–50, Polish Scientific Publishers, Warsaw.

Woodcock, J. P., Alexander, S. and Durkin, M. (1974). Differential diagnosis of ischaemic ulceration of the leg using ultrasound, *Br. J. Dermat.*, **91**, 77–80.

Woodcock, J. P., Morris, S. J. and Wells, P. N. T. (1975). Significance of the velocity impulse response and cross-correlation of the femoral and popliteal blood-velocity/time waveforms in disease of the superficial femoral artery, *Med. biol. Engng*, **13**, 813–8.

Wyatt, A. P., Ratnavel, K. and Loxton, G. E. (1973). The technique and possible application of supra-orbital artery blood-pressure estimation, *Br. J. Surg.*, **60**, 741–3.

Yao, S. T., Needham, T. N. and Ashton, J. P. (1970). Transcutaneous measurement of blood flow by ultrasound, *Bio-med. Engng*, **5**, 230–5.

Ziskin, M. D., Bonakdarpour, A., Weinstein, D. P. and Lynch, P. R. (1972). Contrast agents for diagnostic ultrasound, *Invest. Radiol.*, **7**, 500–5.

7.3.b Cardiology

Bellet, S. and Kostis, J. (1968). Study of the cardiac arrhythmias by the ultrasonic Doppler method, *Circulation*, **38**, 721–36.

Benchimol, A. (1967). Arterial flow in normal and diseased states, *Proc. 20th ann. Conf. Engng Med. Biol.*, 27.6.

Benchimol, A., Desser, K. B. and Gartlan, J. L. (1973). Left ventricular blood flow velocity in man studied with the ultrasonic flowmeter, *Am. Heart J.*, **85**, 294–301.

Benchimol, A., Harris, C. L. and Desser, K. B. (1973). Non-invasive diagnosis of tricuspid insufficiency utilizing the external Doppler flowmeter probe, *Am. J. Cardiol.*, **32**, 868–73.

Blumenfeld, W., Turney, S. Z. and Denman, R. J. (1975). A coaxial ultrasonic pneumotachometer, *Med. biol. Engng*, **13**, 855–60.

Duck, F. A., Hodson, C. J. and Tomlin, P. J. (1974). An esophageal Doppler probe for aortic flow monitoring, *Ultrasound Med. Biol.*, **1**, 233–41.

Dweck, H. S., Reynolds, D. W. and Cassady, G. (1974). Indirect blood pressure measurement in newborns, *Am. J. Dis. Child.*, **127**, 492–4.

Elseed, A. M., Shinebourne, E. A. and Joseph, M. C. (1973). Assessment of techniques for measurement of blood pressure in infants and children, *Archs Dis. Child.*, **48**, 932–6.

Fixler, D. E., Stage, L., Rudolph, A. M., Buckberg, G. D. and Archie, J. P. (1973). Evaluation of a Doppler catheter probe to measure cardiac output, *J. surg. Res.*, **15**, 243–50.

Forlini, F. J. (1974). Indirect measurement of systolic blood pressure during + Gz acceleration, *J. appl. Physiol.*, **37**, 584–6.

Harken, A. H. and Smith, R. M. (1973). Aortic pressure versus Doppler-measured peripheral arterial pressure, *Anesthesiology*, **38**, 184–6.

Hochberg, H. M., George, M. E. D., Schmalzbach, E. L. and Caceres, C. A. (1973). Automatic ECG and blood pressure measurements in multitesting: correlation of blood pressure and ECG abnormalities, *Am. Heart J.*, **86**, 764–70.

Huntsman, L. L., Gams, E., Johnson, C. C. and Fairbanks, E. (1975). Transcutaneous determination of aortic blood-flow velocities in man, *Am. Heart J.*, **89**, 605–12.

Johnson, S. L., Baker, D. W., Lute, R. A. and Dodge, H. T. (1973). Doppler echocardiography. The localization of cardiac mumurs, *Circulation*, **48**, 810–22.

Kalmanson, D., Veyrat, C., Chiche, P. and Witchitz, S. (1974). Non-invasive diagnosis of right heart diseases and of left-to-right shunts using directional Doppler ultrasound. *In* "Cardiovascular Applications of Ultrasound" (ed. R. S. Reneman), pp. 361–70, North-Holland, Amsterdam.

Kardon, M. B., Stegall, H. F., Stone, H. L., Bishop, V. S., Ware, R. W. and Kemmerer, W. L. (1967). Indirect measurement of blood pressure using Doppler-shifted ultrasound, *Dig. 7th int. Conf. med. biol. Engng*, 324.

Kirby, R. R., Kemmerer, W. T. and Morgan, J. L. (1969). Transcutaneous Doppler measurement of blood pressure, *Anesthesiology*, **31**, 86–9.

Knutti, J. W., Meindl, J. D., Angell, W. W., Rossiter, S. J. and Gibbons, J. A. (1974). Postoperative monitoring of human blood flow using the pulsed Doppler ultrasonic blood flowmeter, *Proc. 27th ann. Conf. Engng Med. Biol.*, 342.

Kopczynski, H. D. (1974). Airborne blood pressure measurement using ultrasonics, *Aerospace Med.*, **45**, 1307–9.

Kostis, J. B., Mavrogeorgis, E., Slater, A. and Bellet, S. (1972). Use of a range-gated, pulsed ultrasonic Doppler technique for continuous measurement of velocity of the posterior heart wall, *Chest*, **62**, 597–604.

Labarthe, D. R., Hawkins, C. M. and Remington, R. D. (1973). Evaluation of performance of selected devices for measuring blood pressure, *Am. J. Cardiol.*, **32**, 546–53.

Light, L. H. (1969). Non-injurious ultrasonic technique for observing flow in the human aorta, *Nature, Lond.*, **224**, 1119–21.

Light, L. H. (1974). Initial evaluation of transcutaneous aortovelography—a new non-invasive technique for haemodynamic measurements in the major thoracic vessels. *In* "Cardiovascular Applications of Ultrasound" (ed. R. S. Reneman), pp. 325–60, North-Holland, Amsterdam.

Light, H. and Cross, G. (1972). Cardiovascular data by transcutaneous aorto-velography. *In* "Blood Flow Measurement" (ed. C. Roberts), pp. 60–3, Sector, London.

Light, L. H., Cross, G. and Hansen, P. L. (1974). Non-invasive measurement of blood velocity in the major thoracic vessels, *Proc. R. Soc. Med.*, **67**, 142–4.

Lubé, V. M., Safonov, Y. D. and Yakiemenkov, L. I. (1967). Ultrasonic detection of the motions of cardiac valves and muscle, *Soviet Phys. Acoust.*, **13**, 59–65.

Mackay, R. S. and Hechtman, H. B. (1975). Continuous cardiac output measurement: aspects of Doppler frequency analysis, *I.E.E.E. Trans. biomed. Engng*, **BME-22**, 346–50.

Olson, R. M. and Cooke, J. P. (1974). A nondestructive ultrasonic technique to measure diameter and blood flow in arteries, *I.E.E.E. Trans. biomed. Engng*, **BME-21**, 168–71.

Peronneau, P., Xhaard, M., Nowicki, A., Pellet, M., Delouche, P. and Hinglais, J. (1972). Pulsed Doppler ultrasonic flowmeter and flow pattern analysis. *In* "Blood Flow Measurement" (ed. C. Roberts), pp. 24–8, Sector, London.

Poppers, P. J. (1973). Controlled evaluation of ultrasonic measurement of systolic and diastolic blood pressures in pediatric patients, *Anesthesiology*, **38**, 187–91.

Stegall, H. F. (1967). Remote respirometry by phase-shifted ultrasound, *Dig. 7th int. Conf. med. biol. Engng*, 438.

Stegall, H. F., Flanagan, W. J., Richardson, B. D. and Rosenbaum, R. H. (1973). An ultrasonic apnea monitor, *Proc. 26th ann. Conf. Engng Med. Biol.*, 426.

Thompson, P. D. and Mennel, R. G. (1969). Transcutaneous Doppler flowmeter detection of aortic insufficiency, *Proc. 8th int. Conf. med. biol. Engng*, 32–9.

Wells, P. N. T. (1969). A range-gated ultrasonic Doppler system, *Med. biol. Engng*, **7**, 641–52.

Yoshida, T., Mori, M., Nimura, Y., Hikita, G., Takagishi, S., Nakanishi, K. and Satomura, S. (1961). Analysis of heart motion with ultrasonic Doppler method, and its clinical application, *Jap. Heart J.*, **61**, 61–75.

7.3.c Gastroenterology

Atkinson, P. (1974). "On the Measurement of Bloodflow by Ultrasound", Ph.D. Dissertation, University of Bristol.

Loisance, D. Y., Peronneau, P. A., Pellet, M. M. and Lenriot, J. P. (1973). Hepatic circulation after side-to-side portacaval shunt in dogs: velocity pattern and flow rate changes studied by an ultrasonic velocimeter, *Surgery, St. Louis*, **73**, 43–52.

7.3.d Obstetrics

Baskett, T. F. and Ko, K. S. (1974). Sinusoidal fetal heart pattern. A sign of fetal hypoxia. *Obstet. Gynec., N.Y.*, **44**, 379–82.

Beard, R. W., Filshie, G. M., Knight, C. A. and Roberts, G. M. (1971). The significance of the changes in the continuous fetal heart rate in the first stage of labour, *J. Obstet. Gynaec Br. Commonw.*, **78**, 865–81.

Bishop, E. H. (1966). Obstetric uses of the ultrasonic motion sensor, *Am. J. Obstet. Gynec.*, **96**, 863–7.

Callagan, D. A., Rowland, T. C. and Goldman, D. E. (1964). Ultrasonic Doppler observation of the fetal heart, *Obstet. Gynec., N.Y.*, **23**, 637.

Cooper, J. A., John, A. H., Ross, F. G. M. and Davies, E. R. (1969). Placental localization using an ultrasonic fetal pulse detector, *J. reprod. Med.*, **3**, 271–7.

Cousin, A. J., Smith, K. C., Rowe, I. H. and Organ, L. W. (1974). A cardiac pre-ejection period monitor for foetal assessment during labour, *Med. biol. Engng*, **12**, 479–81.

Hon, E. H. (1962). Electronic evaluation of the fetal heart rate, *Am. J. Obstet. Gynec.*, **83**, 333–53.

Hunt, K. M. (1969). Placental localization using the Doptone fetal pulse detector, *J. Obstet. Gynaec. Br. Commonw.*, **76**, 144–7.

Johnson, W. L., Stegall, H. F., Lein, J. N. and Rushmer, R. F. (1965). Detection of fetal life in early pregnancy with an ultrasonic Doppler flowmeter, *Obstet. Gynec., N.Y.*, **26**, 305–7.

Liu, D. T. Y., Thomas, G. and Blackwell, R. J. (1975). Progression in response patterns of fetal heart rate throughout labour, *Br. J. Obstet. Gynaec.*, **82**, 943–51.

Murata, Y. and Martin, C. B. (1974). Systolic time intervals of the fetal cardiac cycle, *Obstet. Gynec., N.Y.*, **44**, 224–32.

Nelson, C. R. and Parkes, J. R. (1974). Placental localisation using the Doppler portable ultrasonic apparatus, *S. Afr. med. J.*, **48**, 2393–5.

Organ, L. W., Bernstein, A., Rowe, I. H. and Smith, K. C. (1973a). The preejection period of the fetal heart: detection during labor with Doppler ultrasound, *Am. J. Obstet. Gynec.*, **115**, 369–76.

Organ, L. W., Milligan, J. E., Goodwin, J. W. and Bain, M. J. C. (1973b). The preejection period of the fetal heart: response to stress in the term fetal lamb, *Am. J. Obstet. Gynec.*, **115**, 377–86.

Thomas, D. L., Torbet, T., Hansen, S. and Hay, D. M. (1973). A comprehensive system for monitoring the foetal heartrate and uterine contractions, *Med. biol. Engng.*, **11**, 703–9.

Thomas, G. and Blackwell, R. J. (1975). The analysis of continuous fetal heart rate traces in the first and second stages of labour, *Br. J. Obstet. Gynaec.*, **82**, 634–42.

Tushuizen, P. B. T., Stoot, J. E. G. M. and Ubachs, J. M. H. (1974). Fetal heart rate monitoring of the dying fetus, *Am. J. Obstet. Gynec.*, **120**, 922–41.

7.3.e Otorhinolaryngology

Minifie, F. D., Kelsey, C. A. and Hixon, T. J. (1968). Measurement of vocal fold motion using an ultrasonic Doppler velocity monitor, *J. acoust. Soc. Am.*, **43**, 1165–9.

7.3.f Psychiatry

Haines, J. (1974). An ultrasonic system for measuring activity, *Med. biol. Engng*, **12**, 378–81.

Johnson, C. F. (1972). Limits on the measurement of activity level in children using ultrasound and photoelectric cells, *Am. J. ment. Defic.*, **77**, 301–10.

Peacock, L. J. and Williams, M. (1962). An ultrasonic device for recording activity, *Am. J. Psychol.*, **75**, 648–52.

7.3.g Urology

Albright, R. J. and Harris, J. H. (1975). Diagnosis of urethral flow parameters by ultrasonic backscatter, *I.E.E.E. Trans. biomed. Engng*, **BME-22**, 1–11.

Albright, R. J., Harris, J. H. and Zinner, N. R. (1969). Ultrasonic diagnosis of micturition, *Proc. 8th int. Conf. med. biol. Engng*, 32–1.

Marchioro, T. L., Strandness, D. E. and Krugmire, W. J. (1969). The ultrasonic velocity detector for determining vascular patency in renal homografts, *Transplantation*, **8**, 296–8.

Pedersen, J. F., Holm, H. H. and Hald, T. (1975). Torsion of the testis diagnosed by ultrasound. *In* "Ultrasound in Medicine" (ed. D. N. White), vol. 1, p. 193, Plenum Press, New York.

Sampson, D. (1969). Ultrasonic method for detecting rejection of human renal allotransplants, *Lancet*, **2**, 976–8.

Sampson, D., Abramczyk, J. and Murphy, G. P. (1972). Ultrasonic measurement of blood flow changes in canine renal allografts, *J. surg. Res.*, **12**, 388–93.

8 Other diagnostic methods

8.1 Transmission methods

8.1.a Attenuation measurements

Ballantine, H. T., Bolt, R. H., Hueter, T. F. and Ludwig, G. D. (1950). On the detection of intracranial pathology by ultrasound, *Science, N.Y.*, **112**, 525–8.

Ballantine, H. T., Hueter, T. F. and Bolt, R. H. (1954). On the use of ultrasound for tumor detection, *J. acoust. Soc. Am.*, **26**, 581.

Bracewell, R. N., and Roberts, J. A. (1954). Aerial smoothing in radioastronomy, *Aust. J. Phys.*, **74**, 615–40.

Brooks, R. A. and DiChiro, G. (1975). Theory of image reconstruction in computed tomography, *Radiology*, **117**, 561–72.

Clark, R. E., Dietz, D. R. and Miller, J. G. (1974). Quantification of microemboli in extracorporeal circulation systems, *Surg. Forum*, **25**, 139–41.

Crawford, H. D., Wild, J. J., Wolf, P. I. and Fink, J. S. (1959). Transmission of ultrasound through living human thorax, *I.R.E. Trans. med. Electron.*, **ME-6**, 141–6.

Dietz, D., Heyman, J. S., Miller, J. G. and Clark, R. E. (1974). Continuous wave ultrasonic microemboli monitor for use in extracorporeal perfusion, *Proc. 27th ann. Conf. Engng Med. Biol.*, 188.

Dussik, K. T., Dussik, F. and Wyt, L. (1947). Auf dem Wege zur Hyperphonographie des Gehirnes, *Wien. med. Wschr.*, **97**, 425–9.

Fry, F. J. and Jethwa, C. P. (1975). Ultrasonic transmission imaging using continuous Gaussian noise source. *In* "Ultrasound in Medicine" (ed. D. N. White), vol. 1, pp. 551–8, Plenum Press, New York.

Green, P. S., Schaefer, L. F., Jones, E. D. and Suarez, J. R. (1974). A new high-performance ultrasonic camera. *In* "Acoustical Holography" (ed. P. S. Green), vol. 5, pp. 493–503, Plenum Press, New York.

Greenleaf, J. F., Johnson, S. A., Lee, S. L., Herman, G. T. and Wood, E. H. (1974). Algebraic reconstruction of spatial distributions of acoustic absorption within tissue from their two-dimensional acoustic projections. *In* "Acoustical Holography" (ed. P. S. Green), vol. 5, pp. 591–603, Plenum Press, New York.

Greenleaf, J. F., Johnson, S. A., Samaoya, W. F. and Duck, F. A. (1975). Algebraic reconstruction of spatial distributions of acoustic velocities in tissue from their time-of-flight profiles. *In* "Acoustical Holography" (ed. N. Booth), vol. 6, pp. 71–90, Plenum Press, New York.

Güttner, W., Fielder, G. and Pätzold, J. (1952). Über ultraschallabbildungen am Menschlichen Schädel, *Acustica*, **2**, 148–56.

Hamlet, S. L., and Reid, J. M. (1972). Transmission of ultrasound through the larynx as a means of determining vocal-fold activity, *I.E.E.E. Trans. biomed. Engng*, **BME-19**, 34–7.

Harrold, S. O. (1969). Solid state ultrasonic camera, *Ultrasonics*, **7**, 95–101.

Herman, G. T. and Rowland, S. (1971). Resolution in ART: an experimental investigation of the resolving power of an algebraic picture reconstruction technique, *J. theor. Biol.*, **33**, 213–23.

Heyser, R. C. and Croissette, D. H. le (1974). A new ultrasonic imaging system using time delay spectrometry, *Ultrasound Med. Biol.*, **1**, 119–31.

Holasek, E., Jennings, W. D., Sokollu, A. and Purnell, E. W. (1973). Recognition of tissue patterns by ultrasonic spectroscopy, *Proc. I.E.E.E. Ultrasonics Symp.*, 73–6.

Horn, C. A. and Robinson, D. (1965). Assessment of fracture healing by ultrasonics, *J. Coll. Radiol. Aust.*, **9**, 165–7.

Hounsfield, G. N. (1973). Computerized transverse axial scanning (tomography): Part 1. Description of system. *Br. J. Radiol.*, **46**, 1016–22.

Hueter, T. F. and Bolt, R. H. (1951). An ultrasonic method for outlining the cerebral ventricles, *J. acoust. Soc. Am.*, **23**, 160–7.

Jacobs, J. E. (1965). The ultrasound camera, *Science, J.* **1** (4), 60–5.

Jacobs, J. E. (1967). Performance of the ultrasound microscope, *Mater. Eval.*, **25** (3), 41–5.

Kossoff, G. (1975). An historical review of ultrasonic investigations at the National Acoustic Laboratories, *J. clin. Ultrasound*, **3**, 39–43.

Kossoff, G. and Sharpe, C. J. (1966). Examination of the contents of the pulp cavity in teeth, *Ultrasonics*, **4**, 77–83.

Marich, K. W., Zatz, L. M., Green, P. S., Suarez, J. R. and Macovski, A. (1975). Real-time imaging with a new ultrasonic camera: Part I, In vitro experimental studies on transmission imaging of biological structures, *J. clin. Ultrasound*, **3**, 5–16.

Smyth, C. N., Poynton, F. Y. and Sayers, J. F. (1963). The ultrasound image camera, *Proc. I.E.E.*, **110**, 16–28.

Suarez, J. R., Marich, K. W., Holzemer, J. F., Taenzer, J. and Green, P. S. (1975). Biomedical imaging with the SRI ultrasonic camera. *In* "Acoustical Holography" (ed. N. Booth), vol. 6, pp. 1–13, Plenum Press, New York.

Zatz, L. M. (1975). Initial clinical evaluation of a new ultrasonic camera, *Radiology*, **117**, 399–404.

Zatz, L. M., Marich, K. W., Green, P. S., Lipton, M. J., Suarez, J. R. and Macovski, A. (1975). Real-time imaging with a new ultrasonic camera: Part II, Preliminary studies in normal adults, *J. clin. Ultrasound*, **3**, 17–22.

8.1.b Transit time measurements

Greenleaf, J. F., Johnson, S. A., Samoaya, W. F., and Duck, F. A. (1975). Algebraic reconstruction of spatial distributions of acoustic velocities in tissue from their time-of-flight profiles. *In* "Acoustical Holography" (ed. N. Booth), vol. 6, pp. 71–90, Plenum Press, New York.

Guntheroth, W. G. (1974). Changes in left ventricular wall thickness during the cardiac cycle, *J. appl. Physiol.*, **36**, 308–12.

Häusler, E. and Klauck, J. (1970). Measurement of the volume of a cat's heart by means of ultrasound, *I.E.E.E. Trans. Sonics Ultrason.*, **SU-17**, 140–2.

Heyser, R. C. and Croissette, D. H. le (1974). A new ultrasonic imaging system using time delay spectrometry, *Ultrasound Med. Biol.*, **1**, 119–31.

Horwitz, L. D., Bishop, V. S., Stone, H. L. and Stegall, H. F. (1968). Continuous measurement of internal left ventricular diameter, *J. appl. Physiol.*, **24**, 738–40.

Kardon, M. B., O'Rourke, R. A. and Bishop, V. S. (1971). Measurement of left ventricular internal diameter by catheterization, *J. appl. Physiol.*, **31**, 613–5.

McGough, G. A., Beazeale, D., Mullins, G. L., and Guntheroth, W. G. (1973). An ultrasonic displacement instrument with greater beam dispersal, *Cardiovasc. Res.*, **7**, 713–8.

Mullins, G. L. and Guntheroth, W. G. (1966). Continuous recording of changes in mesenteric blood volume, *Ultrasonics*, **4**, 24–5.

Rich, C., Klinik, E., Smith, R. and Graham, B. (1966). Measurement of bone mass from ultrasonic transmission time, *Proc. Soc. exp. Biol. Med.*, **123**, 282–5.

Rushmer, R. F., Franklin, D. L. and Ellis, R. M. (1956). Left ventricular dimensions recorded by sonocardiometry, *Circulation Res.*, **4**, 684–8.

Stegall, H. F. (1974). Ultrasonic measurement of organ dimensions. *In* "Cardiovascular Applications of Ultrasound" (ed. R. S. Reneman), pp. 150–61, North-Holland, Amsterdam.

Stinson, E. B., Rahmoeller, G. and Tecklenberg, P. L. (1974). Measurement of internal left ventricular diameter by tracking sonomicrometer, *Cardiovasc. Res.*, **8**, 283–9.

Suga, H. and Sagawa, K. (1974). Assessment of absolute volume from diameter of the intact canine left ventricular cavity, *J. appl. Physiol.*, **36**, 496–9.

Wolfson, R. N. and Neuman, M. R. (1973). Measurement of fetal descent during labor by ultrasonic time-of-flight, *Proc. 26th ann. Conf. Engng Med. Biol.*, 9.

Zador, I., Wolfson, R. N. and Neuman, M. R. (1974). Ultrasonic measurement of cervical dilatation during labor, *Proc. 27th ann. Conf. Engng Med. Biol.*, 187.

8.1.c Microscopy

Devey, G. B. (1953). Ultrasonic microscope, *Radio-electron. Engng* (2), 8–9. (Translation of Sokolov, S.Y. (1949). *Akad. Nauk S.S.S.R. Doklady*, **64**, 333–45.)

Dunn, F. and Fry, W. J. (1959). Ultrasonic absorption microscope, *J. acoust. Soc. Am.*, **31**, 632–3.

Jacobs, J. E. (1967). Performance of the ultrasound microscope, *Mater. Eval.*, **25** (3), 41–5.

Kessler, L. W. (1974). Review of progress and applications in acoustic microscopy, *J. acoust. Soc. Am.*, **55**, 909–18.

Kessler, L. W., Korpel, A. and Palermo, P. R. (1972). Simultaneous acoustic and optical microscopy of biological specimens, *Nature, Lond.*, **239**, 111–2.

Kompfner, R. (1975). Recent advances in acoustical microscopy, *Br. J. Radiol.*, **48**, 615–27.

Korpel, A., Kessler, L. W. and Palermo, P. R. (1971). Acoustic microscope operating at 100 MHz, *Nature, Lond.*, **232**, 110–1.

Lemons, R. A. and Quate, C. F. (1974). Integrated circuits as viewed with an acoustic microscope, *Appl. Phys. Lett.*, **25**, 251–3.

Lemons, R. A. and Quate, C. F. (1975a). Acoustical microscopy: biomedical applications, *Science, N.Y.*, **188**, 905–11.

Lemons, R. A. and Quate, C. F. (1975b). Acoustic microscopy—a tool for medical and biological research. *In* "Acoustical Holography" (ed. N. Booth), vol. 6, pp. 305–17, Plenum Press, New York.

8.1.d Thermo-acoustic sensing technique

Sachs, T. D. (1973). Potential of TAST for measurements of perfusion, ultrasonic absorption and intensity at a point, *Proc. I.E.E.E. Ultrasonics Symp.*, 52–9.

Sachs, T. D., Welt, A. J. and Slayton, P. W. (1972). Thermo-acoustic sensing technique—TAST, *Proc. I.E.E.E. Ultrasonics Symp.*, 54–8.

8.2 Holography

Aldridge, E. E., Clare, A. B., Lloyd, G. A. S., Shepherd, D. A. and Wright, J. E. (1971). A preliminary investigation of the use of ultrasonic holography in ophthalmology, *Br. J. Radiol.*, **44**, 126–30.

Aldridge, E. E., Clare, A. B. and Shepherd, D. A. (1974). Scanned ultrasonic holography for ophthalmic diagnosis, *Ultrasonics*, **12**, 155–60.

Anderson, R. E. and Curtin, H. R. (1973). Ultrasonic holography. A promising medical imaging tool. *Radiology*, **109**, 417–21.

Brendon, B. B. (1974). Ultrasonic holography—a practical system. *In* "Ultrasonic Imaging and Holography" (ed. G. W. Stroke, W. E. Kock, Y. Kikuchi and J. Tsujiuchi), pp. 87–103, Plenum Press, New York.

Chivers, R. C. (1974). B-scanning and holography in ophthalmic diagnosis, *Ultrasonics*, **12**, 209–13.

Erikson, K. R., O'Loughlin, B. J., Flynn, J. J., Pisa, E. J., Wreede, J. E., Greer, R. E., Stauffer, B. and Metherell, A. F. (1975a). Acoustical holography medical imaging—a report on work in progress. *In* "Ultrasound in Medicine" (ed. D. N. White), vol. 1, pp. 463–73, Plenum Press, New York.

Erikson, K. R., O'Loughlin, B. J., Flynn, J. J., Pisa, E. J., Wreede, J. E., Greer, R. E., Stauffer, B. and Metherell, A. F. (1975b). Through-transmission acoustical holography for medical imaging—a status report. *In* "Acoustical Holography" (ed. N. Booth), vol. 6, pp. 15–55, Plenum Press, New York.

Gabor, D. (1974). A project of ultrasonic tomography ("Sonoradiography"). *In* "Ultrasonic Imaging and Holography" (ed. G. W. Stroke, W. E. Kock, Y. Kikuchi and J. Tsujiuchi), pp. 151–8, Plenum Press, New York.

Halstead, J. (1968). Ultrasound holography, *Ultrasonics*, **6**, 79–87.

Holbrooke, D. R., McCurry, E. E., Richards, V. and Shibata, H. (1973). Acoustical holography for surgical diagnosis, *Ann. Surg.*, **178**, 547–58.

Holbrooke, D. R., McCurry, E. E. and Richards, V. (1974). Medical uses of acoustical holography. *In* "Acoustical Holography" (ed. P. S. Green), vol. 5, pp. 415–51, Plenum Press, New York.

Korpel, A. and Desmares, P. (1969). Rapid sampling of acoustic holograms by laser-scanning techniques, *J. acoust. Soc. Am.*, **45**, 881–4.

Lafferty, A. J. and Stephens, R. W. B. (1971). The Pohlman cell as a means of producing acoustic holograms, *Optics Laser Technol.*, **3**, 232–3.

Metherell, A. F. (1968). Holography with sound, *Science J.*, **4** (11), 57–62.

Metherell, A. F. (1974). Linearized subfringe interferometric holography. *In* "Acoustical Holography" (ed. P. S. Green), vol. 5, pp. 41–58, Plenum Press, New York.

Metherell, A. F., Erikson, K. R., Wreede, J. E., Norton, R. E. and Watts, R. M. (1974). A medical imaging acoustical holography system using linearized subfringe holographic interferometry. *In* "Acoustical Holography" (ed. P. S. Green), vol. 5, pp. 453–70, Plenum Press, New York.

Weiss, L. and Holyoke, E. D. (1969). Detection of tumors in soft tissues by ultrasonic holography, *Surg. Gynec. Obstet.*, **128**, 953–62.

8.3 Bragg imaging

Keyani, H., Landry, J. and Wade, G. (1974). Bragg-diffraction imaging: a potential technique for medical diagnosis and material inspection, Part II. *In* "Acoustical Holography" (ed. P. S. Green), vol. 5, pp. 25–39, Plenum Press, New York.

Korpel, A. (1966). Visualization of the cross section of a sound beam by Bragg diffraction of light, *Appl. Phys. Lett.*, **9**, 425–6.

Landry, J., Powers, J. and Wade, G. (1969). Ultrasonic imaging of internal structure by Bragg diffraction, *Appl. Phys. Lett.*, **15**, 186–8.

8.4 Fluctuation measurements

Atkinson, P. (1975). An ultrasonic fluctuation velocimeter, *Ultrasonics*, **13**, 275–8.

9 Biological effects

9.1 Early investigations

Harvey, E. N. (1930). Biological aspects of ultrasonic waves; a general survey, *Biol. Bull. mar. biol. Lab., Woods Hole*, **59**, 306–25.

Harvey, E. N. and Loomis, A. L. (1928). High frequency sound waves of small intensity and their biological effects, *Nature, Lond.*, **12**, 622–4.

Harvey, E. N. and Loomis, A. L. (1931). High speed photomicrography of living cells subjected to supersonic vibrations, *J. gen. Physiol.*, **15**, 147–53.

Johnson, C. H. (1929). The lethal effects of ultrasonic irradiation, *J. Physiol., Lond.*, **67**, 356–9.

Schmitt, F. O. (1929). Ultrasonic micromanipulation, *Protoplasma*, **7**, 332–40.

Schmitt, F. O., Olson, A. R. and Johnson, C. H. (1928). Effects of high-frequency sound waves on protoplasm, *Proc. Soc. exp. Biol. Med.*, **25**, 718–20.

Wood, R. W. and Loomis, A. L. (1927). The physical and biological effects of high-frequency sound waves of great intensity, *Phil. Mag.*, (7), **4**, 417–36.

9.2 Thermal effects

Arslan, M. and Sala, O. (1965). Action of ultrasound on the internal ear. *In* "Ultrasonic Energy" (ed. E. Kelly), pp. 160–76, University of Illinois Press, Urbana.

Barnett, S. B., Kossoff, G. and Clark, G. M. (1973). Histological changes in the inner ear of sheep following a round window ultrasonic irradiation, *J. oto-lar. Soc. Aust.*, **3**, 508–12.

Basauri, L. and Lele, P. P. (1962). A simple method for production of trackless focal lesions with focussed ultrasound: statistical evaluation of the effects of irradiation on the central nervous system of the cat, *J. Physiol., Lond.*, **160**, 513–34.

Baum, G. (1956). The effect of ultrasonic radiation upon the eye and ocular adnexa, *Am. J. Ophthal.*, **42**, 696–706.

Brain, P. J., Coleman, B. H., Lumsden, R. B. and Ogilvie, R. F. (1960). The effects of ultrasound on the internal ear: a histological investigation, *J. Lar. Otol.*, **74**, 628–58.

Carney, S. A., Lawrence, J. C. and Ricketts, C. R. (1972). Some effects of ultrasound on guinea-pig ear skin, *Br. J. industr. Med.*, **29**, 214–20.

Chapman, I. V. (1974). The effect of ultrasound on the potassium content of rat thymocytes *in vitro*, *Br. J. Radiol.*, **47**, 411–5.

Crysdale, W. S. and Stahle, J. (1972). Ultrasonic irradiation of the guinea-pig cochlea, *Ann. Otol.*, **81**, 87–98.

Drettner, B., Johnson, S., Sjöberg, A. and Stahle, J. (1967). Thermal effects of ultrasound in the inner ear, *Acta oto-lar.*, **64**, 464–76.

Fry, W. J., Brennan, J. F., and Barnard, J. W. (1957). Histological study of changes produced by ultrasound in gray and white matter of the central nervous system. *In* "Ultrasound in Biology and Medicine" (ed. E. Kelly), pp. 110–30, A.I.B.S., Washington.

Herrick, J. F. (1953). Temperatures produced in tissues by ultrasound: experimental study using various technics, *J. acoust. Soc. Am.*, **25**, 12–6.

Hodgkin, A. L. and Katz, B. (1949). The effect of temperature on the electrical activity of the giant axon of the squid, *J. Physiol., Lond.*, **109**, 240–9.

Hughes, D. E. (1965). Biological implications of the action of weak ultrasound. *In* "Ultrasonic Energy" (ed. E. Kelly), pp. 9–18, University of Illinois Press, Urbana.

Hughes, D. E., Chou, J. T. Y., Warwick, R. and Pond, J. (1963). The effect of focussed ultrasound on the permeability of frog muscle, *Biochim. biophys. Acta*, **75**, 137–9.

James, J. A. (1963). New developments in the ultrasonic therapy of Menière's disease, *Ann. R. Coll. Surg. Engl.*, **33**, 226–44.

James, J. A., Dalton, G. A., Freundlich, H. F., Bullen, M. A., Wells, P. N. T., Hughes, D. E. and Chou, J. T. Y. (1964). Histological, thermal and biochemical effects of ultrasound on the labyrinth and temporal tone, *Acta oto-lar.*, **57**, 306–11.

Lehmann, J. F. (1953). The biophysical mode of action of biologic and therapeutic ultrasonic reactions, *J. acoust. Soc. Am.*, **25**, 17–25.

Lele, P. P. (1963). Effects of focussed ultrasonic radiation on peripheral nerve, with observations on local heating, *Expl. Neurol.*, **8**, 47–83.

Lele, P. P. and Pierce, A. D. (1972). The thermal hypothesis of the mechanism of ultrasonic focal destruction in organized tissues. *In* "Interaction of Ultrasound and Biological Tissue" (ed. J. M. Reid and M. R. Sikov), pp. 121–8, U.S. Department of Health, Education and Welfare, Publication (FDA) 73-8008.

Lindstrom, P. A. (1954). Prefrontal ultrasonic irradiation—a substitute for lobotomy, *Archs Neurol. Psychiat.*, Chicago, **72**, 399–425.

Lundquist, P.-G., Igarashi, M., Wersäll, J., Guilford, F. R. and Wright, W. K. (1971). The acute effect of ultrasonic irradiation upon ampullar sensory epithelia of the guinea-pig, *Acta oto-lar.*, **72**, 68–79.

Madsden, P. W. and Gersten, J. W. (1961). The effect of ultrasound on conduction velocity of peripheral nerve, *Archs phys. Med. Rehabil.*, **42**, 645–9.

McLay, K., Flinn, M. and Ormerod, F. C. (1961). Histological changes in the inner ear resulting from the application of ultrasonic energy, *J. Lar. Otol.*, **75**, 345–57.

Shealy, C. N. and Henneman, E. (1962). Reversible effects of ultrasound on spinal reflexes, *Archs Neurol.*, Chicago, **6**, 374–86.

Sjöberg, A., Stahle, J., Johnson, S. and Sahl, R. (1963). The treatment of Menière's disease by ultrasonic irradiation, *Acta oto-lar.*, Suppl. 178.

Smith, A. N., Fisher, G. W., Macleod, I. B., Preshaw, R. M., Stavney, L. S. and Gordon, D. (1966). The effect of ultrasound on the gastric mucosa and its secretion of acid, *Br. J. Surg.*, **53**, 720–5.

Torchia, R. T., Purnell, E. W. and Sokollu, A. (1967). Cataract production by ultrasound, *Am. J. Ophth.*, **64**, 305–9.

Warwick, R. and Pond, J. (1968). Trackless lesions in nervous tissues produced by high intensity focused ultrasound (high-frequency mechanical waves), *J. Anat.*, **102**, 387–405.

Wells, P. N. T. (1966a). Ultrasonics in clinical diagnosis. *In* "Scientific Basis of Medicine—Annual Reviews", pp. 38–53, Athlone Press, London.

Wells, P. N. T. (1966b). "Some Biological Effects of Ultrasound", Ph.D. Dissertation, University of Bristol.

Young, R. R. and Henneman, E. (1961). Reversible block of nerve conduction by ultrasound, *Archs Neurol.*, Chicago, **4**, 83–9.

9.3 Evidence of non-thermal effects

Bell, E. (1957). The action of ultrasound on the mouse liver, *J. cell. comp. Physiol.*, **50**, 83–103.

Curtis, J. C. (1965). Action of intense ultrasound on the intact mouse liver. *In* "Ultrasonic Energy" (ed. E. Kelly), pp. 85–109, University of Illinois Press, Urbana.

Freundlich, H. and Gillings, D. W. (1938). The influence of ultrasonic waves on the viscosity of colloidal solutions, *Trans. Faraday Soc.*, **34**, 649–60.

Fry, W. J., Wulff, V. J., Tucker, D. and Fry, F. J. (1950). Physical factors involved in ultrasonically induced changes in living systems: I. Identification of non-temperature effects, *J. acoust. Soc. Am.*, **22**, 867–76.

Fry, W. J., Tucker, D., Fry, F. J. and Wulff, V. J. (1951). Physical factors involved in ultrasonically induced changes in living systems: II. Amplitude duration relations and the effect of hydrostatic pressure for nerve tissue. *J. acoust. Soc. Am.*, **23**, 364–8.

Johnsson, A. and Lindvall, A. (1969). Effects of low-intensity ultrasound on viscous properties of Helodea cells, *Naturwissenschaften*, **56**, 40.

Ravitz, M. J. and Schnitzler, R. M. (1970). Morphological changes induced in the frog semitendinosus muscle fiber by localized ultrasound, *Expl. Cell. Res.*, **60**, 78–85.

Takagi, S. F., Higashiro, S., Shibuya, T. and Osawa, N. (1960). The actions of ultrasound on the myelinated nerve, the spinal chord, and the brain, *Jap. J. Physiol.*, **10**, 183–93.

Talbert, D. G. (1975). Spontaneous smooth muscle activity as a means of detecting biological effects of ultrasound. *In* "Ultrasonics International 1975", pp. 279–84, I.P.C. Science and Technology Press, Guildford.

Wells, P. N. T. (1968). The effect of ultrasonic irradiation on the survival of *Daphnia magna*, *J. exp. Biol.*, **49**, 61–70.

9.4 Cavitation: physical considerations

Flynn, H. G. (1964). Physics of acoustic cavitation in liquids. *In* "Physical Acoustics" (ed. W. P. Mason), vol. IB, pp. 57–172, Academic Press, New York.

9.4.a Transient cavitation

Blake, F. G. (1949). "The Onset of Cavitation in Liquids. I. Cavitation Threshold Sound Pressures in Water as a Function of Temperature and Hydrostatic Pressure", Tech. Mem. 12, Acoustics Research Laboratory, Department of Engineering Sciences and Applied Physics, Harvard University, Cambridge.

Él'piner, I. E. (1964). "Ultrasound—Physical, Chemical and Biological Effects", Consultants' Bureau, New York.

Esche, R. (1952). Untersuchungen zur Ultraschallabsorption in tierischen Geweben und Kuntstoffen, *Akust. Beih.*, **2**, 71–4.

Gaertner, W. (1954). Frequency dependence of ultrasonic cavitation, *J. acoust. Soc. Am.*, **26**, 977–80.

Griffing, V. (1950). Theoretical explanation of the chemical effects of ultrasonics, *J. chem. Phys.*, **18**, 997–8.

Griffing, V. (1952). The chemical effects of ultrasonics, *J. chem. Phys.*, **20**, 939.

Harvey, E. N., Whiteley, A. H., McElroy, W. D., Pease, D. C. and Barnes, D. K. (1944). Bubble formation in animals. II. Gas nuclei and their distribution in blood and tissues. *J. cell. comp. Physiol.*, **24**, 23–34.

Harvey, E. N., McElroy, W. D. and Whiteley, A. H. (1947). On cavity formation in water, *J. appl. Phys.*, **18**, 162–72.

Noltingk, B. E. and Neppiras, E. A. (1950). Cavitation produced by ultrasonics, *Proc. phys. Soc. B*, **63**, 674–85.

Sette, D. and Wanderlingh, F. (1962). Nucleation by cosmic rays in ultrasonic cavitation, *Phys. Rev.*, **125**, 409–17.
Sirotyuk, M. G. (1963). Ultrasonic cavitation, *Soviet Phys. Acoust.*, **8**, 201–13.

9.4.b Stable cavitation

Minnaert, M. (1933). On musical air-bubbles and the sounds of running water, *Phil. Mag.*, (7), **16**, 235–48.

9.4.c Cavitation thresholds

Apfel, R. E. (1970). The role of impurities in cavitation-threshold determination, *J. acoust. Soc. Am.*, **48**, 1179–86.
Blake, F. G. (1949). "The Onset of Cavitation in Liquids. I. Cavitation Threshold Sound Pressures in Water as a Function of Temperature and Hydrostatic Pressure," Tech. Mem. 12, Acoustics Research Laboratory, Department of Engineering Sciences and Applied Physics, Harvard University, Cambridge.
Briggs, H. B., Johnson, J. B. and Mason, W. P. (1947). Properties of liquids at high sound pressure, *J. acoust. Soc. Am.*, **19**, 664–77.
Coakley, W. T. (1971). Acoustical detection of single cavitation events in a focused field in water at 1 MHz, *J. acoust. Soc. Am.*, **49**, 792–801.
Eller, A. I. (1972). Bubble growth by diffusion in an 11-kHz sound field, *J. acoust. Soc. Am.*, **52**, 1447–9.
Eller, A. and Flynn, H. G. (1969). Generation of subharmonics of order one-half by bubbles in a sound field, *J. acoust. Soc. Am.*, **46**, 722–7.
Esche, R. (1952). Untersuchungen zur Ultraschallabsorption in tierischen Geweben und Kuntstoffen, *Akust. Beih.*, **2**, 71–4.
Evans, A. and Walder, D. N. (1969). Significance of gas micronuclei in the aetiology of decompression sickness, *Nature, Lond.*, **222**, 251–2.
Flynn, H. G. (1964). Physics of acoustic cavitation in liquids. *In* "Physical Acoustics" (ed. W. P. Mason), vol. IB, pp. 57–172, Academic Press, New York.
Harvey, E. N., Barnes, D. K., McElroy, W. D., Whiteley, A. H. and Pease, D. C. (1945). Removal of gas nuclei from liquids and surfaces, *J. Am. chem. Soc.*, **67**, 156–7.
Hill, C. R. (1972). Ultrasonic exposure thresholds for changes in cells and tissues, *J. acoust. Soc. Am.*, **52**, 667–72.
Hill, C. R., Clarke, P. R., Crowe, M. R. and Hammick, J. W. (1969). Biophysical effects of cavitation in a 1 MHz ultrasonic beam. *In* "Ultrasonics for Industry", pp. 26–30, Iliffe, Guildford.
Iernetti, G. (1971). Cavitation threshold dependence on volume, *Acustica*, **24**, 191–6.
Lauterborn, W. (1969). Zu einer Theorie der Kavitationsschwellen, *Acustica*, **22**, 48–54.
Lele, P. P., Senapati, N. and Hsu, W. (1974). Mechanisms of tissue-ultrasound interaction. *In* "Ultrasonics in Medicine" (ed. M. de Vlieger, D. N. White and V. R. McCready), pp. 345–52, Excerpta Medica, Amsterdam.
Neppiras, E. A. (1969). Subharmonic and other low-frequency emission from bubbles in sound-irradiated liquids, *J. acoust. Soc. Am.*, **46**, 587–601.
Santis, P. de, Sette, D. and Wanderlingh, F. (1967). Cavitation detection: the use of subharmonics, *J. acoust. Soc. Am.*, **42**, 514–6.
Storm, D. L. (1974). Interfacial distortions of a pulsating gas bubble. *In* "Finite-amplitude Wave Effects in Fluids" (ed. L. Bjørnø), pp. 234–9, I.P.C. Science and Technology Press, Guildford.

Walder, D. N. and Evans, A. (1974). *In vivo* nuclear fission in the aetiology of decompression sickness, *Nature, Lond.*, **252**, 696–7.

Weissler, A., Cooper, H. W. and Snyder, S. (1950). Chemical effects of ultrasonic waves: oxidation of potassium iodide solution by carbon tetrachloride, *J. Am. chem. Soc.*, **72**, 1769–75.

9.5 Acoustic streaming: physical considerations

Elder, S. A. (1959). Cavitation microstreaming, *J. acoust. Soc. Am.*, **31**, 54–64.

Nyborg, W. L. (1958). Acoustic streaming near a boundary, *J. acoust. Soc. Am.*, **30**, 329–39.

Nyborg, W. L. (1965). Acoustic streaming. *In* "Physical Acoustics" (ed. W. P. Mason), vol. IIB, pp. 265–331, Academic Press, New York.

Nyborg, W. L. (1968). Mechanisms for nonthermal effects of sound, *J. acoust. Soc. Am.*, **44**, 1302–9.

Nyborg, W. L. and Rooney, J. A. (1969). Radiation pressure on a vibrating hemispherical meniscus, *J. acoust. Soc. Am.*, **45**, 384–5.

Sanders, M. F. and Coakley, W. T. (1972). Factors affecting disruption of biological material by an ultrasonically vibrating wire, *Expl. Cell. Res.*, **73**, 410–14.

Williams, A. R. (1972). Disorganization and disruption of mammalian and amoeboid cells by acoustic microstreaming, *J. acoust. Soc. Am.*, **52**, 688–93.

Williams, A. R., Hughes, D. E. and Nyborg, W. L. (1970). Hemolysis near a transversely oscillating wire, *Science, N.Y.*, **169**, 871–3.

9.6 Biological effects of transient cavitation

Ackerman, E. (1952). Cellular fragilities and resonances observed by means of sonic vibrations, *J. cell. comp. Physiol.*, **39**, 167–90.

Ackerman, E. (1954). Mechanical resonances of *Amphiuma* erythrocytes, *J. acoust. Soc. Am.*, **26**, 257–8.

Ackerman, E. (1960). Surface modes of resonance of biological cells in ultrasonic fields, *Proc. 3rd int. Conf. med. Electron.*, 437–44.

Bronskaya, L. M., Vigderman, V. S., Sokol'skaya, A. V. and Él'piner, I. E. (1968). Influence of static pressure on ultrasonic chemical and biological effects, *Soviet Phys. Acoust.*, **13**, 374–5.

Coakley, W. T. and Dunn, F. (1971). Degradation of DNA in high-intensity focused ultrasonic fields at 1 MHz, *J. acoust. Soc. Am.*, **50**, 1539–45.

Coakley, W. T., Hampton, D. and Dunn, F. (1971). Quantitative relationships between ultrasonic cavitation and effects upon amoebae at 1 MHz, *J. acoust. Soc. Am.*, **50**, 1546–53.

Doty, P., McGill, B. B. and Rice, S. A. (1958). The properties of sonic fragments of deoxyribose nucleic acid, *Proc. natn. Acad. Sci. U.S.A.*, **44**, 432–8.

Freifelder, D. and Davison, P. F. (1962). Studies on the sonic degradation of deoxyribonucleic acid, *Biophys. J.*, **2**, 235–47.

Goldman, D. E. and Lepeschkin, W. W. (1952). Injury to living cells in standing sound waves, *J. cell. comp. Physiol.*, **40**, 255–68.

Hamrick, P. E. and Cleary, S. F. (1969). Breakage of tobacco mosaic virus by acoustic transients: a hydrodynamic model, *J. acoust. Soc. Am.*, **45**, 1–6.

Howkins, S. D. and Weinstock, A. (1970). The effect of focused ultrasound on human blood, *Ultrasonics*, **8**, 174–6.

Hughes, D. E. and Cunningham, V. R. (1963). Methods for disrupting cells, *Biochem. Soc. Symp.*, **23**, 8–19.

Neppiras, E. A. and Hughes, D. E. (1964). Some experiments on the disintegration of yeast by high intensity ultrasound, *Biotechnol. Bioengng*, **6**, 247–70.

Neppiras, E. A. and Noltingk, B. E. (1951). Cavitation produced by ultrasonics: theoretical conditions for the onset of cavitation, *Proc. phys. Soc. B*, **64**, 1032–8.

Pritchard, N. J., Hughes, D. E. and Peacocke, A. R. (1966). The ultrasonic degradation of biological macromolecules under conditions of stable cavitation. I. Theory, methods and application to deoxyribonucleic acid. *Biopolymers*, **4**, 259–73.

Thacker, J. (1973). An approach to the mechanisms of killing of cells in suspension by ultrasound, *Biochem. biophys. Acta*, **304**, 240–8.

Tomlinson, J. A., Walkey, D. G. A., Hughes, D. E. and Watson, D. H. (1965). Multiple transverse breakage of the filamentous particles of turnip mosaic virus by ultrasonic vibration, *Nature, London.*, **207**, 495–7.

9.7 Biological effects of acoustic streaming

Child, S. Z., Carstensen, E. L. and Miller, M. W. (1975). Growth of pea roots exposed to pulsed ultrasound, *J. acoust. Soc. Am.*, **58**, 1109–10.

Dunn, F. and MacLeod, R. M. (1968). Effects of intense noncavitating ultrasound on selected enzymes, *J. acoust. Soc. Am.*, **44**, 932–40.

Freifelder, D. and Davison, P. F. (1962). Studies on the sonic degradation of deoxyribonucleic acid, *Biophys. J.*, **2**, 235–47.

Gershoy, A. and Nyborg, W. L. (1973). Perturbation of plant-cell contents by ultrasonic micro-irradiation, *J. acoust. Soc. Am.*, **54**, 1356–67.

Harrington, R. E. and Zimm, B. H. (1965). Degradation of polymers by controlled hydrodynamic shear, *J. phys. Chem., Ithaca*, **69**, 161–75.

Hawley, S. A., MacLeod, R. M. and Dunn, F. (1963). Degradation of DNA by intense, noncavitating ultrasound, *J. acoust. Soc. Am.*, **35**, 1285–7.

Hill, C. R., Clarke, P. R., Crowe, M. R. and Hammick, J. W. (1969). Biophysical effects of cavitation in a 1 MHz ultrasonic beam. *In* "Ultrasonics for Industry", pp. 26–30, Iliffe, Guildford.

Howkins, S. D. (1965). Measurements of the resonant frequency of a bubble near a rigid boundary, *J. acoust. Soc. Am.*, **37**, 504–8.

Hughes, D. E. and Nyborg, W. L. (1962). Cell disruption by ultrasound, *Science, N.Y.*, **138**, 108–14.

Jackson, F. J. and Nyborg, W. L. (1958). Small scale acoustic streaming near a locally excited membrane, *J. acoust. Soc. Am.*, **30**, 614–9.

Levinthal, C. and Davison, P. F. (1961). Degradation of deoxyribonucleic acid under hydrodynamic shearing forces, *J. molec. Biol.*, **3**, 674–83.

Nyborg, W. L. (1965). Physical principles involved in the action of weak ultrasound. *In* "Ultrasonic Energy" (ed. E. Kelly), pp. 1–5, University of Illinois Press, Urbana.

Nyborg, W. L. (1974). Cavitation in biological systems. *In* "Finite-amplitude Wave Effects in Fluids" (ed. L. Bjørnø), pp. 245–51, I.P.C. Science and Technology Press, Guildford.

Nyborg, W. L. and Dyer, H. J. (1960). Ultrasonically induced motions in single plant cells, *Proc. 2nd int. Conf. med. Electron.*, 391–6.

Peacocke, A. R. and Pritchard, N. J. (1968). The ultrasonic degradation of biological macromolecules under conditions of stable cavitation. II. Degradation of deoxyribonucleic acid. *Biopolymers*, **6**, 605–23.

Pritchard, N. J., Hughes, D. E. and Peacocke, A. R. (1966). The ultrasonic degradation of biological macromolecules under conditions of stable cavitation. I. Theory, methods and application to deoxyribonucleic acid. *Biopolymers*, **4**, 259–73.

Robinson, H. P., Sharp, F., Donald, I., Young, H. and Hall, A. J. (1972). The effect of pulsed and continuous wave ultrasound on the enzyme histochemistry of placental tissue *in vitro*, *J. Obstet. Gynaec. Br. Commonw.*, **79**, 821–7.

Rooney, J. A. (1972). Shear as a mechanism for sonically induced biological effects, *J. acoust. Soc. Am.*, **52**, 1718–24.

Selman, G. G. and Jurand, A. (1964). An electron microscope study of the endoplasmic reticulum in newt notochord cells after disturbance with ultrasonic treatment and subsequent regeneration, *J. cell. Biol.*, **20**, 175–83.

Williams, A. R. and Slade, J. S. (1971). Ultrasonic dispersal of aggregates of Sarcina lutea, *Ultrasonics*, **9**, 85–7.

Williams, A. R., Hughes, D. E. and Nyborg, W. L. (1970a). Hemolysis near a transversely oscillating wire, *Science, N.Y.*, **169**, 871–3.

Williams, A. R., Stafford, D. A., Callely, A. G. and Hughes, D. E. (1970b). Ultrasonic dispersal of activated sludge flocs, *J. appl. Bact.*, **33**, 656–63.

Wilson, W. L., Wiercinski, F. J., Nyborg, W. L., Schnitzler, R. M. and Sichel, F. J. (1966). Deformation and motion produced in isolated living cells by localised ultrasonic vibration, *J. acoust. Soc. Am.*, **40**, 1363–70.

Woodcock, J. P. and Connolly, C. C. (1969). The effect of non-cavitating ultrasound on the hydrolysis of sucrose solutions, *Acustica*, **21**, 45–50.

9.8 Dosimetry

Wells, P. N. T. (1973). Letter to the editor, *Ultrasound Med. Biol.*, **1**, 53.

9.9 Frequency dependence of biological effects

Fry, F. J., Kossoff, G., Eggleton, R. C. and Dunn, F. (1970). Threshold ultrasonic dosages for structural changes in mammalian brain, *J. acoust. Soc. Am.*, **48**, 1413–7.

Hill, C. R. (1972). Ultrasonic exposure thresholds for changes in cells and tissues, *J. acoust. Soc. Am.*, **52**, 667–72.

Joshi, G. P., Hill, C. R. and Forrester, J. A. (1973). Mode of action of ultrasound on the surface charge of mammalian cells *in vitro*, *Ultrasound Med. Biol.*, **1**, 45–8.

Taylor, K. J. W. and Newman, D. L. (1972). Electrophoretic mobility of Ehrlich cell suspensions exposed to ultrasound of varying parameters, *Phys. Med. Biol.*, **17**, 270–6.

Taylor, K. J. W. and Pond, J. B. (1972). A study of the production of haemorrhagic injury and paraplegia in rat spinal cord by pulsed ultrasound of low megahertz frequencies in the context of the safety for clinical usage, *Br. J. Radiol.*, **45**, 343–53.

9.10 Cumulative effects

Clarke, P. R. and Hill, C. R. (1970). Physical and chemical aspects of ultrasonic disruption of cells, *J. acoust. Soc. Am.*, **47**, 649–53.

Fry, W. J., Wulff, V. J., Tucker, D. and Fry, F. J. (1950). Physical factors involved in ultrasonically induced changes in living systems: I. Identification of non-temperature effects. *J. acoust. Soc. Am.*, **22**, 867–76.

Joshi, G. P., Hill, C. R. and Forrester, J. A. (1973). Mode of action of ultrasound on the surface charge of mammalian cells *in vitro*, *Ultrasound Med. Biol.*, **1**, 45–8.

Taylor, K. J. W. (1970). Ultrasonic damage to spinal cord and the synergistic effect of hypoxia, *J. Path.*, **102**, 41–7.

Taylor, K. J. W. and Connolly, C. C. (1969). Differing hepatic lesions caused by the same dose of ultrasound, *J. Path.*, **98**, 291–3.

Taylor, K. J. W. and Newman, D. L. (1972). Electrophoretic mobility of Ehrlich cell suspensions exposed to ultrasound of varying parameters, *Phys. Med. Biol.*, **17**, 270–6.

9.11 Other investigations of biological effects

9.11.a Production of focal lesions in brain

Dunn, F., Lohnes, J. E. and Fry, F. J. (1975). Frequency dependence of ultrasonic dosage for irreversible structural changes in mammalian brain, *J. acoust. Soc. Am.*, **58**, 512–14.

Fallon, J. T., Stehbens, W. E. and Eggleton, R. C. (1972). Effect of ultrasound on arteries, *Archs Path.*, **94**, 380–8.

Fry, F. J., Kossoff, G., Eggleton, R. C. and Dunn, F. (1970). Threshold ultrasonic dosages for structural changes in mammalian brain, *J. acoust. Soc. Am.*, **48**, 1413–17.

Fry, W. J. (1958). Intense ultrasound in investigations of the central nervous system. *Adv. biol. med. Phys.*, **6**, 281–348.

Lele, P. P., Senapati, N. and Hsu, W. (1974). Mechanisms of tissue-ultrasound interaction. *In* "Ultrasonics in Medicine" (ed. M. de Vlieger, D. N. White and V. R. McCready), pp. 345–52, Excerpta Medica, Amsterdam.

Lerner, R. M., Carstensen, E. L. and Dunn, F. (1973). Frequency dependence of thresholds for ultrasonic production of thermal lesions in tissue, *J. acoust. Soc. Am.*, **54**, 504–6.

Pierce, A. D. (1973). Temperature rise in biological tissue during focused ultrasonic irradiation: some theoretical subtleties, *J. acoust. Soc. Am.*, **53**, 381.

Pond, J. B. (1970). The role of heat in the production of ultrasonic focal lesions, *J. acoust. Soc. Am.*, **47**, 1607–11.

Robinson, T. C. and Lele, P. P. (1972). An analysis of lesion development in the brain and in plastics by high-intensity focused ultrasound at low-megahertz frequencies, *J. acoust. Soc. Am.*, **51**, 1333–51.

9.11.b Synergistic effect with hypoxia

Taylor, K. J. W. (1970). Ultrasonic damage to spinal cord and the synergistic effect of hypoxia, *J. Path.*, **102**, 41–7.

Taylor, K. J. W. and Pond, J. B. (1972). A study of the production of haemorrhagic injury and paraplegia in rat spinal cord by pulsed ultrasound of low megahertz frequencies in the context of the safety for clinical usage, *Br. J. Radiol.*, **45**, 343–53.

9.11.c Synergistic effect with sterilizing chemicals

Last, A. J. and Boucher, R. M. G. (1973). Sono-synergistic sterilization of surgical and dental instruments. *In* "Ultrasonics International 1973", pp. 233–7, I.P.C. Science and Technology Press, Guildford.

9.11.d Effect on blood flow

Baker, N. V. (1972). Segregation and sedimentation of red blood cells in ultrasonic standing waves, *Nature, Lond.*, **239**, 398–9.

Dyson, M. and Pond, J. B. (1973). The effects of ultrasound on circulation, *Physiotherapy*, **59**, 284–7.

Dyson, M., Woodward, B. and Pond, J. B. (1971). Flow of red blood cells stopped by ultrasound, *Nature, Lond.*, **232**, 572–3.

Dyson, M., Pond, J. B., Woodward, B. and Broadbent, J. (1974). The production of blood cell stasis and endothelial damage in the blood vessels of chick embryos treated with ultrasound in a stationary wave, *Ultrasound Med. Biol.*, **1**, 133–48.

Gould, R. K. and Coakley, W. T. (1974). The effects of acoustic forces on small particles in suspension. *In* "Finite-amplitude Wave Effects in Fluids" (ed. L. Bjørnø), pp. 252–7, I.P.C. Science and Technology Press, Guildford.

Nyborg, W. L. and Gershoy, A. (1974). Micro-sonation of cells under near-threshold conditions. *In* "Ultrasonics in Medicine" (ed. M. de Vlieger, D. N. White and V. R. McCready), pp. 360–5, Excerpta Medica, Amsterdam.

Pond, J. B., Woodward, B. and Dyson, M. (1971). A microscope viewing ultrasonic irradiation chamber, *Phys. Med. Biol.*, **16**, 521–4.

Taylor, K. J. W. and Dyson, M. (1972). Possible hazards of diagnostic ultrasound, *Br. J. hosp. Med.*, **8**, 571–7.

Wladimiroff, J. W. and Talbert, D. G. (1973). The changing fine structure of erythrocyte formations when trapped in ultrasonic standing waves, *Phys. Med. Biol.*, **18**, 888–9.

9.11.e Effects on malignant tumours

Cerino, L. E., Ackerman, E. and Janes, J. M. (1966). Effects of heat and ultrasound on Vx-2 carcinoma in bones of rabbits: a preliminary report, *J. acoust. Soc. Am.*, **40**, 916–8.

Clarke, P. R., Hill, C. R. and Adams, K. (1970). Synergism between ultrasound and X-rays in tumour therapy, *Br. J. Radiol.*, **43**, 97–9.

Gavrilov, L. R., Kalendo, G. S., Ryabukhin, V. V., Shaginyan, K. A. and Yarmonenko, S. P. (1975). Ultrasonic enhancement of the gamma radiation of malignant tumors, *Soviet Phys. Acoust.*, **21**, 119–21.

Heimburger, R. F., Fry, F. J., Franklin, T. D. and Eggleton, R. C. (1975). Ultrasound potentiation of chemotherapy for brain malignancy. *In* "Ultrasound in Medicine" (ed. D. N. White), vol. 1, pp. 273–81, Plenum Press, New York.

Lehmann, J. F. and Krusen, F. H. (1955). Biophysical effects of ultrasonic energy on carcinoma and their possible significance, *Archs phys. Med. Rehabit.*, **36**, 452–9.

Muckle, D. S. (1974). The selective effect of heat in cancer, *Ann. R. Coll. Surg.*, **54**, 72–7.

Pospíšilová, J. (1968). Viscosity changes of synovia after application of water treated with ultrasound, *Experientia*, **24**, 139.

Southam, C. M., Beyer, H. and Allen, A. C. (1953). The effects of ultrasonic irradiation upon normal and neoplastic tissues in the intact mouse, *Cancer, N.Y.*, **6**, 390–6.

Woeber, K. (1965). The effect of ultrasound in the treatment of cancer. *In* "Ultrasonic Energy" (ed. E. Kelly), pp. 137–47, University of Illinois Press, Urbana.

9.11.f Effect on tissue regeneration

Dyson, M., Pond, J. B., Joseph, J. and Warwick, R. (1968). The stimulation of tissue regeneration by means of ultrasound, *Clin. Sci.*, **35**, 273–85.

Pond, J. and Dyson, M. (1967). A device for the study of the effects of ultrasound in tissue grown in rabbits' ears, *J. sci. Instrum.*, **44**, 165–6.

9.11.g Effect on cell surface charge

Joshi, G. P., Hill, C. R. and Forrester, J. A. (1973). Mode of action of ultrasound on the surface charge of mammalian cells *in vitro*, *Ultrasound Med. Biol.*, **1**, 45–8.

Repacholi, M. H., Woodcock, J. P., Newman, D. L. and Taylor, K. J. W. (1971). Interaction of low intensity ultrasound and ionizing radiation with tumour cell surface, *Phys. Med. Biol.*, **16**, 221–7.

Taylor, K. J. W. and Newman, D. L. (1972). Electrophoretic mobility of Ehrlich cell suspensions exposed to ultrasound of varying parameters, *Phys. Med. Biol.*, **17**, 270–6.

9.11.h Effect on recalcification time of platelet rich plasma

Williams, A. R. (1974). Release of serotonin from human platelets by acoustic microstreaming, *J. acoust. Soc. Am.*, **56**, 1640–3.

Williams, A. R. (1975). An ultrasonic technique to generate intravascular microstreaming. *In* "Ultrasonics International 1975", pp. 266–8, I.P.C. Science and Technology Press, Guildford.

9.11.i Evidence of genetic effects

Abdulla, U., Campbell, S., Dewhurst, C. J., Talbert, D., Lucas, M. and Mullarkey, M. (1971). Effect of diagnostic ultrasound on maternal and fetal chromosomes, *Lancet*, **2**, 829–31.

Andrew, D. S. (1964). Ultrasonography in pregnancy—an enquiry into its safety, *Br. J. Radiol.*, **37**, 185–6.

Baethman, A., Oeckler, R. and Kazner, E. (1974). Experimental studies on brain tissue response to ultrasonic radiation (USR) during enchoencephalography: preliminary results. *In* "Ultrasonics in Medicine" (ed. M. de Vlieger, D. N. White and V. R. McCready), pp. 82–5, Excerpta Medica, Amsterdam.

Bang, J. (1971). The effect of continuous ultrasound on pregnant mice and measurement of intra-uterine energy levels. *In* "Ultrasonographia Medica" vol. I (ed. J. Böck and K. Ossoinig), pp. 495–501, Verlag Wien. Med. Akad., Vienna.

Bernstine, R. L. (1969). Safety studies with ultrasonic Doppler technic, *Obstet. Gynec., N.Y.*, **34**, 707–9.

Bleaney, B. I. and Oliver, R. (1972). The effect of irradiation of *vicia faba* roots with 1·5 MHz ultrasound, *Br. J. Radiol.*, **45**, 358–61.

Bleaney, B. I., Blackbourn, P. and Kirkley, J. (1972). Resistance of CHLF hamster cells to ultrasonic radiation of 1·5 MHz frequency, *Br. J. Radiol.*, **45**, 354–7.

Bobrow, M., Blackwell, N., Unrau, A. E. and Bleaney, B. (1971). Absence of any observed effect of ultrasonic irradiation on human chromosomes, *J. Obstet. Gynaec. Br. Commonw.*, **78**, 730–6.

Boyd, E., Abdulla, U., Donald, I., Fleming, J. E. E., Hall, A. J. and Ferguson-Smith, M. A. (1971). Chromosome breakage and ultrasound, *Br. med. J.*, **2**, 501–2.

Braeman, J., Coakley, W. T. and Gould, R. K. (1974). Human lymphocyte chromosomes and ultrasonic cavitation, *Br. J. Radiol.*, **47**, 158–61.

Brock, R. D., Peacock, W. J., Geard, C. R., Kossoff, G. and Robinson, D. E. (1973). Ultrasound and chromosome aberrations, *Med. J. Aust.*, **2**, 533–6.

Brown, R. C. and Coakley, W. T. (1975). Unchanged growth patterns of *Acanthamoeba* exposed to intermediate intensity ultrasound, *Ultrasound Med. Biol.*, **2**, 37–41.

Buckton, K. E. and Baker, N. V. (1972). An investigation into possible chromosome damaging effects of ultrasound on human blood cells, *Br. J. Radiol.*, **45**, 340–2.

Bugnon, C., Cottin, Y., Kraehenbuhl, J. and Weill, F. (1972). Aberrations chromosomiques provoquées par des ultra-sons diagnostiqués sur des lymphocytes humains en culture, *J. Radiol. Electrol. Med. nucl.*, **53**, 750–5.

Clarke, P. R. and Hill, C. R. (1969). Biological action of ultrasound in relation to the cell cycle, *Expl. Cell. Res.*, **58**, 443–4.

Coakley, W. T., Hughes, D. E., Slade, J. S. and Laurence, K. M. (1971). Chromosome aberrations after exposure to ultrasound, *Br. med. J.*, **1**, 109–10.

Coakley, W. T., Slade, J. S., Braeman, J. M. and Moore, J. L. (1972). Examination of lymphocytes for chromosome aberrations after ultrasonic irradiation, *Br. J. Radiol.*, **45**, 328–32.

Combes, R. D. (1975). Absence of mutation following ultrasonic treatment of *Bacillus subtilis* cells and transforming deoxyribonucleic acid, *Br. J. Radiol.*, **48**, 306–11.

Donald, I., MacVicar, J. and Brown, T. G. (1958). Investigation of abdominal masses by means of ultrasound, *Lancet*, **1**, 1188–94.

Eames, F. A., Carstensen, E. L., Miller, M. W. and Li, M. (1975). Ultrasonic heating of *Vicia faba* roots, *J. acoust. Soc. Am.*, **57**, 1192–4.

Fischer, P., Golob, E., Kratochwil, A. and Kunze-Mühl, E. (1967). Chromosomenuntersuchung nach Ultraschalleinwirkung, *Wien klin. Wschr.*, **79**, 436–7.

Fischman, H. (1973). Ultrasound and marrow-cell chromosomes, *Lancet*, **2**, 920–1.

Ford, R. M. (1974). Clinical–pathological studies on brain tissue response to ultrasonic radiation: preliminary results. *In* "Ultrasonics in Medicine" (ed. M. de Vlieger, D. N. White and V. R. McCready), pp. 85–8, Excerpta Medica, Amsterdam.

French, L. A., Wild, J. J. and Neal, D. (1951). Attempts to determine harmful effects of pulsed ultrasonic vibration, *Cancer, N.Y.*, **4**, 342–4.

Fritz-Niggli, H. and Böni, A. (1950). Biological experiments on *Drosophila melanogaster* with supersonic vibrations, *Science, N.Y.*, **112**, 120–2.

Galperin-Lemaitre, H., Gustot, P. and Levi, S. (1973). Ultrasound and marrow-cell chromosomes, *Lancet*, **2**, 505–6.

Garg, A. G. and Taylor, A. R. (1967). An investigation into the effect of pulsed ultrasound on the brain, *Ultrasonics*, **5**, 208–12.

Garrison, B. M., Bo, W. J., Krueger, W. A., Kremkau, F. W. and McKinney, W. M. (1973). The influence of ovarian sonication on fetal development in the rat, *J. clin. Ultrasound*, **1**, 316–9.

Gregory, W. D., Miller, M. W., Carstensen, E. L., Cataldo, F. L. and Reddy, M. M. (1974). Non-thermal effects of 2 MHz ultrasound on the growth and cytology of *Vicia faba* roots, *Br. J. Radiol.*, **44**, 122–9.

Hall, E. J. (1963). Dose response relationship for reproductive integrity of *Vicia faba* deduced from protracted irradiation experiments, *Radiat. Res.*, **20**, 195–202.

Hellman, L. M., Duffus, G. M., Donald, I. and Sundén, B. (1970). Safety of diagnostic ultrasound in obstetrics, *Lancet*, **1**, 1133–5.

Hering, E. R. and Shepstone, B. J. (1972). The effect of irradiation of "Vicia faba" roots with 1·5 MHz ultrasound, *Br. J. Radiol.*, **45**, 786–7.

Hering, E. R., Shepstone, B. J. and Davey, D. A. (1974). Lack of effect of the ultrasonic radiation from the diasonograph on the roots of *Zea mays*, *S. Afr. med. J.*, **48**, 2126.

Hill, C. R., Joshi, G. P. and Revell, S. H. (1972). A search for chromosome damage following exposure of Chinese hamster cells to high intensity, pulsed ultrasound, *Br. J. Radiol.*, **45**, 333–4.

Ikeuchi, T., Sasaki, M., Oshimura, M., Azumi, J. and Tsuji, K. (1973). Ultrasound and embryonic chromosomes, *Br. med., J.* **1**, 112.

Kato, M. (1966). Visible mutation induced in *Drosophila* by ultrasonic vibration, *Bull. Osaka med. Sch.*, **12**, 114–8.

Kirsten, E. B., Zinssler, H. H. and Reid, J. M. (1963). Effect of 1 Mc ultrasound on the genetics of mouse, *I.E.E.E. Trans. Ultrason. Engng*, **UE-10**, 112–6.

Kohorn, E. I., Pritchard, J. W. and Hobbins, J. C. (1967). The safety of clinical ultrasonic examination, *Obstet. Gynec., N.Y.*, **29**, 272–4.

Kremkau, F. W. and Witcofski, R. L. (1974). Mitotic reduction in rat liver exposed to ultrasound, *J. clin. Ultrasound*, **2**, 123–6.

Kunze-Mühl, E. and Golob, E. (1972). Chromosomenanalysen nach Ultraschalleinwirkung, *Humangenetik*, **14**, 237–46.

Leeman, S., Khokhar, M. T. and Oliver, R. (1975). Ultrasonic irradiation of bean roots and the influence of exposure parameters, *Br. J. Radiol.*, **48**, 954.

Loch, E. G., Fischer, A. B. and Kuwert, E. (1971). Effect of diagnostic and therapeutic intensities of ultrasonics on normal and malignant human cells in vitro, *Am. J. Obstet. Gynec.*, **110**, 457–60.

Lyon, M. F. and Simpson, G. M. (1974). An investigation into the possible genetic hazards of ultrasound, *Br. J. Radiol.*, **47**, 712–22.

Macintosh, I. J. C. and Davey, D. A. (1970). Chromosome aberrations induced by an ultrasonic fetal pulse detector, *Br. med. J.*, **4**, 92–3.

Macintosh, I. J. C. and Davey, D. A. (1972). Relationship between intensity of ultrasound and induction of chromosome aberrations, *Br. J. Radiol.*, **45**, 320–7.

Macintosh, I. J. C., Brown, R. C. and Coakley, W. T. (1975). Ultrasound and "in vitro" chromosome aberrations, *Br. J. Radiol.*, **48**, 230–2.

Mahoney, M. J. and Hobbins, J. C. (1973). Ultrasound and growth of amniotic fluid cells, *Lancet*, **2**, 454–5.

Mannor, S. M., Serr, D. M., Tamari, I., Meshorev, A. and Frei, E. H. (1972). The safety of ultrasound in fetal monitoring, *Am. J. Obstet. Gynec.*, **113**, 653–61.

Mermut, S., Katayama, K. P., Castillo, R. del and Jones, H. W. (1973). The effect of ultrasound on human chromosomes in vitro, *Obstet. Gynec., N.Y.*, **41**, 4–6.

McClain, R. M., Hoar, R. M. and Saltzman, M. B. (1972). Teratologic study of rats exposed to ultrasound, *Am. J. Obstet. Gynec.*, **114**, 39–42.

Robinson, A. (1973). Intrauterine diagnosis and ultrasound, *Lancet*, **2**, 1504.

Rott, H.-D., Huber, H. J., Soldner, R. and Schwanitz, G. (1972). Examinations of chromosomes after in-vitro exposure of human lymphocytes to ultrasound, *Electromedica*, **40**, 14–6.

Selman, G. G. and Counce, S. J. (1953). Abnormal embryonic development in *Drosophila* induced by ultrasonic treatment, *Nature, Lond.*, **172**, 503–4.

Serr, D. M., Padeh, B., Zakut, H., Shaki, R., Mannor, S. M. and Kalner, B. (1971). Studies on the effects of ultrasonic waves on the fetus. *In* "Proc. 2nd Europ. Congr. perinatal Medicine" (ed. P. J. Huntingford), pp. 302–7, Karger, Basel.

Shoji, R., Momma, E., Shimizu, T. and Matsuda, S. (1971). An experimental study on the effect of low-intensity ultrasound on developing mouse embryos, *J. Fac. Sci., Hokkaido Univ.* (VI), *Zool.*, **18**, 51–6.

Shoji, R., Momma, E., Shimizu, T. and Matsuda, S. (1972). Experimental studies on the effect of ultrasound on mouse embryos, *Teratology*, **6**, 119.

Šlotova, J., Karpfel, Z. and Hrazdiva, I. (1967). Chromosome aberrations caused by the effect of ultrasound in the meristematic cells of *Vicia faba, Biol. Plant. (Praha)*, **9**, 49–55.

Smyth, M. G. (1966). Animal toxicity studies with ultrasound at diagnostic power levels. *In* "Diagnostic Ultrasound" (ed. C. C. Grossman, J. H. Holmes, C. Joyner and E. W. Purnell), pp. 296–9, Plenum Press, New York.

Taylor, K. J. W. and Dyson, M. (1974). Toxicity studies on the interaction of ultrasound on embryonic and adult tissues. *In* "Ultrasonics in Medicine" (ed. M. de Vlieger, D. N. White and V. R. McCready), pp. 353–9, Excerpta Medica, Amsterdam.

Thacker, J. (1973). The possibility of genetic hazard from ultrasonic radiation, *Curr. Top. radiat. Res. Q.*, **8**, 235–58.

Thacker, J. (1974). An assessment of ultrasonic radiation hazard using yeast genetic systems, *Br. J. Radiol.*, **47**, 130–8.

Wallace, R. H., Bushnell, R. J. and Newcomer, E. H. (1948). The induction of cytogenic variations by ultrasonic waves, *Science, N.Y.*, **107**, 577–8.

Warwick, R., Pond, J. B., Woodward, B. and Connolly, C. C. (1970). Hazards of diagnostic ultrasonography—a study with mice, *I.E.E.E. Trans. Sonics Ultrason.*, **SU-17**, 158–64.

Watts, P. L. and Stewart, C. R. (1972). The effect of fetal heart monitoring by ultrasound on maternal and fetal chromosomes, *J. Obstet. Gynaec. Br. Commonw.*, **79**, 715–6.

Watts, P. L., Hall, A. J. and Fleming, J. E. E. (1972). Ultrasound and chromosome damage, *Br. J. Radiol.*, **45**, 335–9.

Wolff, S. (1968). Chromosome aberrations and the cell cycle, *Radiat. Res.*, **33**, 609–19.

9.11.j Effects on plants

Gordon, A. G. (1971). Beneficial effects of ultrasound on plants—a review, *Ultrasonics*, **9**, 88–94.

9.12 Possibily of hazard in diagnostics

David, H., Weaver, J. B. and Pearson, J. F. (1975). Doppler ultrasound and fetal activity, *Br. med. J.*, **2**, 62–4.

Edmonds, P. D. (1972). Interactions of ultrasound with biological structures—a survey of data. *In* "Interaction of Ultrasound and Biological Tissue" (ed. J. M. Reid and M. R. Sikov), pp. 299–317, U.S. Department of Health, Education and Welfare, Publication (FDA), 73–8008.

Grimwade, J. C., Walker, D. W., Bartlett, M., Gordon, S. and Wood, C. (1971). Human fetal heart rate change and movement in response to sound and vibration, *Am. J. Obstet. Gynec.*, **109**, 86–90.

Ulrich, W. D. (1971). Ultrasound dosage for experimental use in human beings, *Report no. 2, Project M 4306.01–1010 BXX9*, Naval Medical Research Institute, Bethesda.

Ulrich, W. D. (1974). Ultrasound dosage for nontherapeutic use on human beings—extrapolations from a literature survey, *I.E.E.E. Trans. biomed. Engng*, **BME-21**, 48–51.

Wells, P. N. T. (1974). The possibility of harmful biological effects in ultrasonic diagnosis. *In* "Cardiovascular Applications of Ultrasound" (ed. R. S. Reneman), pp. 1–17, North-Holland, Amsterdam.

9.13 Effects of airborne sound and ultrasound on mammals

Acton, W. I. (1968). A criterion for the prediction of auditory and subjective effects due to airborne noise from ultrasonic sources, *Ann. occ. Hyg.*, **11**, 227–34.

Acton, W. I. (1974). The effects of industrial airborne ultrasound on humans, *Ultrasonics*, **12**, 124–8.

Hill, V. H. (1970). Why 92 dB A? *Am. ind. Hyg. Ass. J.*, **31**, 189–97.

Knight, J. J. (1967). Effects of airborne ultrasound on man. *In* "Ultrasonics for Industry", pp. 39–42, Iliffe, Guildford.

9.14 Biological effects of low-frequency vibrations

10 Functional modification: clinical applications

10.1 Physiotherapy

Abramson, D. I., Burnett, C., Bell, Y., Tuck, S., Rejal, H. and Fleischer, C. J. (1960). Changes in blood flow, oxygen uptake and tissue temperature produced by therapeutic physical agents. I. Effect of ultrasound. *Am. J. phys. Med.*, **39**, 51–62.

Bickford, R. H. and Duff, R. S. (1953). Influence of ultrasonic irradiation on temperature and blood flow in human skeletal muscle, *Circulation Res.*, **1**, 534–8.

Buchan, J. F. (1970). The use of ultrasonics in physical medicine, *Practitioner*, **205**, 319–26.

Chan, A. K., Sigelmann, R. A., Guy, A. W. and Lehmann, J. F. (1973). Calculation by the method of finite differences of the temperature distribution in layered tissues, *I.E.E.E. Trans. biomed. Engng.*, **BME-20**, 86–90.

Chan, A. K., Sigelmann, R. A. and Guy, A. W. (1974). Calculations of therapeutic heat generated by ultrasound in fat-muscle-bone layers, *I.E.E.E. Trans. biomed. Engng.*, **BME-21**, 280–4.

Dyson, M. and Pond, J. B. (1973). The effects of ultrasound on circulation, *Physiotherapy*, **59**, 284–7.

Howkins, S. D. (1969). Diffusion rates and the effect of ultrasound, *Ultrasonics*, **7**, 129–30.

Lanfear, R. T. and Clarke, W. B. (1972). The treatment of tenosynovitis in industry, *J. chart. Soc. Physio.*, **58**, 128–9.

Lehmann, J. F. (1965). Ultrasound therapy. *In* "Therapeutic Heat and Cold" (ed. S. Licht), pp. 321–86, Waverly Press, Baltimore.

Lehmann, J. F. and Guy, A. W. (1972). Ultrasound therapy. *In* "Interaction of Ultrasound and Biological Tissue" (ed. J. M. Reid and M. R. Sikov), pp. 141–52, U.S. Department of Health, Education and Welfare, Publication (FDA) 73-8008.

Lehmann, J. F. and Krusen, F. H. (1958). Therapeutic application of ultrasound in physical medicine, *Am. J. phys. Med.*, **37**, 173–83.

Paaske, W. P., Hovind, H. and Sejrsen, P. (1973). Influence of therapeutic ultrasonic irradiation on blood flow in human cutaneous, subcutaneous, and muscular tissues, *Scand. J. clin. Lab. Invest.*, **31**, 389–94.

Patrick, M. K. (1971). Experience with ultrasonic therapy in clinic practice. *In* "Ultrasonics 1971", pp. 71–2, I.P.C. Science and Technology Press, Guildford.

Patrick, M. K. (1973). Ultrasonic therapy—has it a place in the 70s? *Physiotherapy*, **59**, 282–3.

Pätzold, J., Güttner, W. and Bastir, R. (1951). Beitrag zum Dosiproblem in der Uttaschall-therapie, *Strahlentherapie*, **86**, 298–305.

Roman, M. P. (1960). A clinical evaluation of ultrasound by use of a placebo technic, *Physical Ther. Rev.*, **40**, 649–52.

Sokollu, A. (1972). Future uses of ultrasound in diagnosis and surgery. *In* "Interaction of Ultrasound and Biological Tissue" (ed. J. M. Reid and M. R. Sikov), pp. 287–91, U.S. Department of Health, Education and Welfare, Publication (FDA) 73-8008.

Stewart, H. F., Harris, G. R., Herman, B. A., Robinson, R. A., Haran, M. E., McCall, G. R., Carless, G. and Rees, D. (1973). "Survey of Use and Performance of Ultrasonic Therapy Equipment in Pinellas County, Florida", U.S. Department of Health, Education and Welfare, Report, no. FDA 73-8039.

Summer, W. and Patrick, M. K. (1964). "Ultrasonic Therapy", Elsevier, Amsterdam.

Wells, P. N. T. (1966). "Some Biological Effects of Ultrasound", Ph.D. Dissertation, University of Bristol.

10.2 Neurosurgery

Fry, W. J., Mosberg, W. H., Barnard, J. W. and Fry, F. J. (1954). Production of focal destructive lesions in the central nervous system with ultrasound, *J. Neurosurg.*, **11**, 471–8.

Lindstrom, P. A. (1954). Prefrontal ultrasonic irradiation—a substitute for lobotomy, *Archs Neurol. Psychiat.*, *Chicago*, **72**, 399–425.

Lindstrom, P. A. and Beck, E. C. (1963). Suppression of epileptic movements in the presence of grand mal seizure discharges, *J. Neurosurg.*, **20**, 97–104.

Lynn, J. G. and Putnam, T. J. (1944). Histology of cerebral lesions produced by focussed ultrasound, *Am. J. Path.*, **20**, 637–47.

Meyers, R., Fry, F. J., Fry, W. J., Eggleton, R. C. and Schultz, D. F. (1960). Determination of topologic human brain representations and modifications of signs and symptoms of some neurologic disorders by the use of high level ultrasound, *Neurology*, **10**, 271–7.

Warwick, R. and Pond, J. (1968). Trackless lesions in nervous tissues produced by high intensity focused ultrasound (high-frequency mechanical waves), *J. Anat.*, **102**, 387–405.

10.2.a Treatment of Parkinson's disease

Cotzias, G. C., Woert, M. H. van, and Schiffer, L. M. (1967). Aromatic amino acids and modification of parkinsonism, *New Engl. J. Med.*, **276**, 374–9.

Meyers, R., Fry, W. J., Fry, F. J., Dreyer, L. L., Schultz, D. F. and Noyes, R. F. (1959). Early experiences with ultrasonic irradiation of the pallidofugal and nigral complexes in hyperkinetic and hypertonic disorders, *J. Neurosurg.*, **16**, 32–54.

10.2.b Hypophysectomy

Arslan, M. (1964). Ultrasonic hypophysectomy, *J. Lar. Otol.*, **20**, 73–85.

Arslan, M. (1967). Ultrasonic selective hypophysectomy, *Ultrasonics*, **5**, 98–101.

Arslan, M., Crepaldi, G., Grandesso, R., Molinari, G. A., Muggeo, M. and Ricci, V. (1973). "Direct Ultrasonic Irradiation of the Hypophysis", Piccin Medical Books, Padua.

Giancarlo, H. R. and Mattucci, K. F. (1971). Effect of ultrasonic hypophysectomy on diabetic retinopathy, *Laryngoscope*, **81**, 452–64.

Hickey, R. C., Fry, W. J., Meyers, R., Fry, F. J. and Bradbury, J. T. (1961). Human pituitary irradiation with focused ultrasound, *Archs Surg.*, **83**, 620–33.

Hickey, R. C., Fry, W. J., Meyers, R., Fry, F. J., Bradbury, J. T. and Eggleton, R. C. (1963). Ultrasound irradiation of the hypophysis in disseminated breast cancer, *Am. J. Roentg.*, **89**, 71–7.

James, J. A. (1969). Transphenoidal hypophysectomy. *In* "Disorders of the Skull Base Region" (ed. C.-A. Hamberger and J. Wersäll), pp. 163–9, Wiley, New York.

Krumins, R., Kelly, E., Fry, F. J. and Fry, W. J. (1965). The use of high-intensity ultrasound to alter the structure of the anterior pituitary. *In* "Ultrasonic Energy" (ed. E. Kelly), pp. 77–83, University of Illinois Press, Urbana.

Lawrence, J. H., Tobias, C. A., Born, J. L., Gottschalk, A., Linfoot, J. A. and Kling, R. P. (1963). Alpha particle and proton beams in therapy, *J. Am. med. Ass.*, **186**, 236–45.

Rand, R. W., Heuser, G., Dashe, A., Adams, D. and Roth, N. (1969). Stereotaxic transsphenoidal biopsy and cryosurgery of pituitary tumors, *Am. J. Roentg.*, **105**, 273–86.

Rand, R. W., Dashe, A. M., Paglia, D. E., Conway, L. W. and Solomon, D. H. (1964). Stereotactic cryohypophysectomy, *J. Am. med. Ass.*, **189**, 255–9.

Rand, R. W., Dashe, A. M., Solomon, D. H., Westover, J. L., Crandall, P. H., Brown, J. and Tranquada, R. (1962). Stereotaxic yttrium-90 hypophysectomy for metastic mammary carcinoma, *Ann. Surg.*, **156**, 986–93.

Yoshioka, K. and Oka, M. (1965). Technical developments of focused ultrasound and its biological and surgical applications in Japan. *In* "Ultrasonic Energy" (ed. E. Kelly), pp. 190–200, University of Illinois Press, Urbana.

10.2.c Ultrasonic focal lesions in neuro-anatomical studies

Basauri, L. and Lele, P. P. (1962). A simple method for production of trackless focal lesions with focused ultrasound: statistical evaluation of the effects of irradiation on the central nervous system of the cat, *J. Physiol., Lond.*, **160**, 513–34.

Fry, F. J. (1972). The role of ultrasonically generated lesions in the determination of quantitative organizational aspects of brain stem nuclei. *In* "Interaction of Ultrasound and Biological Tissue" (ed. J. M. Reid and M. R. Sikov), p. 297, U.S. Department of Health, Education and Welfare, Publication (FDA) 73-8008.

Lele, P. P. (1962). A simple method for production of trackless focal lesions with focused ultrasound: physical factors, *J. Physiol., Lond.*, **140**, 494–512.

Manlapaz, J. S., Åstrom, K. E., Ballantine, H. T. and Lele, P. P. (1964). Effects of ultrasonic radiation in experimental focal epilepsy in the cat, *Expl Neurol.*, **10**, 345–56.

Young, G. F. and Lele, P. P. (1964). Focal lesions in the brain of growing rabbits produced by focused ultrasound, *Expl Neurol.*, **9**, 502–11.

10.2.d Commissurotomy

Collins, W. F., Nulsen, F. E. and Randt, C. T. (1960). Relation of peripheral nerve fiber size and sensation in man, *Archs Neurol., Chicago*, **3**, 381–5.

Griffith, H. B., Brownell, B., Bowes, J. B., Halliwell, M. and Wells, P. N. (1973). Arterial damage by trackless lesions in the spinal cord made by focused ultrasound, *Br. J. Surg.*, **60**, 899.

Richards, D. E., Typer, C. F. and Shealy, C. N. (1966). Focused ultrasonic spinal commissurotomy: experimental evaluation, *J. Neurosurg.*, **24**, 701–7.

Shaffron, M. and Collins, W. F. (1964). Ascending spinal pathways of centre median nucleus in cat, *J. Neurosurg.*, **21**, 874–9.

10.2.e Reversible ultrasonic lesions

Lele, P. P. (1966). Concurrent detection of the production of ultrasonic lesions, *Med. biol. Engng*, **4**, 451–6.

Lele, P. P. (1967). Production of deep focal lesions by focused ultrasound—current status, *Ultrasonics*, **5**, 105–12.

Matison, G. G. and Lele, P. P. (1974). Scattering of ultrasonic plane waves by ultrasonic focal lesions in tissues, *Proc. I.E.E.E. Ultrasonics Symp.*, 446–52.

10.3 Non-invasive stimulation of neural elements

Fry, W. J. (1968). Electrical stimulation of brain localized without probes—theoretical analysis of a proposed method, *J. acoust. Soc. Am.*, **44**, 919–31.

10.4 Vestibular surgery

Arslan, M. (1955). Quoted by: James, J. A., Dalton, G. A., Bullen, M. A., Freundlich, H. F. and Hopkins, J. C. (1960). The ultrasonic treatment of Menière's disease, *J. Lar. Otol.*, **74**, 730–57.

Arslan, M. (1958). Ultrasonic surgery of the labyrinth in patients with Menière's syndrome, *Sci. med. Ital.*, **7**, 301–26.

Arslan, M. (1968). Ultrasonic selective irradiation of the ear windows, as a new treatment of vertigo and tinnitus, *Acta oto-lar.*, **65**, 224–35.

Cutt, R. A., Wolfson, R. J., Ishiyama, E., Rothwarf, F. and Myers, D. (1965). Preliminary results with experimental cryosurgery of the labyrinth, *Archs Otolar.*, **82**, 147–58.

Gordon, D. (1962). An improved ultrasonic transducer for the surgery of the labyrinth, *Proc. San Diego Symp. biomed. Engng*, 23–4.

House, W. F. (1966). Cryosurgical treatment of Menière's disease, *Archs Otolar.* **84**, 616–28.

James, J. A. (1963). New developments in the ultrasonic therapy of Menière's disease, *Ann. R. Coll. Surg. Engl.*, **33**, 226–44.

James, J. A. and Halliwell, M. (1970). Thermal effects of ultrasound on the temporal bone, *Med. biol. Engng*, **8**, 477–81.

James, J. A., Dalton, G. A., Bullen, M. A., Freundlich, H. F. and Hopkins, J. C. (1960). The ultrasonic treatment of Menière's disease, *J. Lar. Otol.*, **74**, 730–57.

James, J. A., Dalton, G. A., Hadley, K. J., Freundlich, H. F., Bullen, M. A. and Wells, P. N. T. (1963). A new 3-megacycle generator for destruction of the vestibular end organ, *Acta oto-lar.*, **56**, 148–53.

Johnson, S. J. (1967). An ultrasonic unit for the treatment of Menière's disease, *Ultrasonics*, **5**, 173–6.

Kossoff, G. (1964). Design of the C.A.L. ultrasonic generator for the treatment of Menière's disease, *I.E.E.E. Trans. Sonics Ultrason.*, **SU-11**, 95–101.

Kossoff, G. (1972a). Safety factors of the ultrasonic round window irradiation technique, *Archs Otolar.*, **96**, 113–6.

Kossoff, G. (1972b). Current status of ultrasonic treatment of Menière's disease. *In* "Interaction of Ultrasound and Biological Tissue" (ed. J. M. Reid and M. R. Sikov), pp. 293–4, U.S. Department of Health, Education and Welfare, Publication (FDA) 73-8008.

Kossoff, G. and Khan, A. E. (1966). Treatment of vertigo using the ultrasonic generator, *Archs Otolar.*, **84**, 181–8.

Kossoff, G., Wadsworth, J. R. and Dudley, P. F. (1967). The round window ultrasonic technique for treatment of Menière's disease, *Archs Otolar.*, **86**, 535–42.

Krejci, F. (1952). Experimentelle Grundlagen einer extralabyrinthären chirurgischen Behandlungsmethode der Ménièreschen Erkankung. *Practica otorhino-lar.*, **14**, 18–37.

Wells, P. N. T. (1962). "The Production of Controlled Ultrasound, with particular reference to the Surgical Therapy of Menière's Disease", M.Sc. Dissertation, University of Bristol.

10.5 Other applications of high-frequency ultrasound

10.5.a Treatment of warts

Braatz, J. H., McAlistair, B. R. and Broaddus, M. D. (1974). Ultrasound and plantar warts. A double blind study. *Milit. Med.*, **139**, 199–201.

Cherup, N., Urben, J. and Bender, L. F. (1963). The treatment of plantar warts with ultrasound, *Archs phys. Med. Rehabil.*, **44**, 602–4.

Kent, H. (1969). Warts and ultrasound, *Archs Dermat.*, **100**, 79–81.

Rowe, R. J. and Gray, J. M. (1960). Ultrasound therapy of plantar warts, *Archs Dermat.*, **82**, 1008–9.

Rowe, R. J. and Gray, J. M. (1965). Ultrasound treatment of plantar warts, *Archs phys. Med. Rehabil.*, **46**, 273–4.

10.5.b Treatment of laryngeal papillomatosis

Birk, H. G. and Manhart, H. E. (1963). Ultrasound for juvenile laryngeal papillomatosis, *Archs Otolar.*, **77**, 603–8.

Fairman, H. D. (1972). Papillomatosis of the larynx, *Proc. R. Soc. Med.*, **65**, 619–24.

Jenkins, J. C. (1967). Preliminary report on the treatment of multiple juvenile laryngeal papillomata by ultrasound, *J. Lar. Otol.*, **81**, 385–90.

White, A., Halliwell, M. and Fairman, H. D. (1974). Ultrasonic treatment of laryngeal papillomata, *J. Lar. Otol.*, **88**, 249–60.

10.5.c Termination of pregnancy

Sikov, M. R. (1973). Ultrasound: its potential use for the termination of pregnancy, *Contraception*, **8**, 429–38.

10.6 Surgical procedures dependent upon the direct mechanical effects of ultrasonic vibrations

Ensminger, D., (1973). "Ultrasonics", Dekker, New York.

10.6.a Dental applications

Balamuth, L. (1967). The application of ultrasonic energy in the dental field. *In* "Ultrasonic Techniques in Biology and Medicine" (ed. B. Brown and D. Gordon), pp. 194–205, Iliffe, London.

Lees, S. (1972). Some capabilities of ultrasonics in dental diagnostics and dental research. *In* "Interaction of Ultrasound and Biological Tissue" (ed. J. M. Reid and M. R. Sikov), pp. 281–5, U.S. Department of Health, Education and Welfare, Publication (FDA) 73–8008.

10.6.b Disintegration of calculi

Davies, H., Schwartz, R., Pfister, R. and Barnes, F. (1974). Transmitted ultrasound for relief of obstruction in ureters and arteries: current status, *J. clin. Ultrasound*, **2**, 217–20.

Goodfriend, R. (1973). Effects of ultrasound on the dog ureter and a clinical trial, *Proc. West. pharm. Soc.*, **16**, 280–1.

Howard, S. S., Merrill, E., Harris, S. and Cohen, J. (1972). Effect of ultrasonic irradiation on urinary calculi and urothelium, *Surg. Forum*, **23**, 542–44.

Lamport, H. and Newman, H. F. (1956). Ultrasonic lithotresis in the ureter, *J. Urol.*, **76**, 520–9.

Velea, S., Achimescu, V. and Popescu, A. (1972). Ultrasound effects to therapeutical intensities and frequencies on biliari and renali calculi, *Proc. 3rd int. Conf. mod. Phys.*, 30.2.

10.6.c Emulsification and aspiration of cataracts

Arnott, E. (1973). The ultrasonic technique for cataract removal, *Trans. ophthal. Soc. U.K.*, **93**, 33–8.

Kelman, C. D. (1967). Phaco-emulsification and aspiration, *Am. J. Ophthal.*, **64**, 23–35.

Kelman, C. D. (1969). Phaco-emulsification and aspiration, *Am. J. Ophthal.*, **67**, 464–77.

Phillips, C. I. and Williams, A. R. (1972). Cataracts: ultrasonic disintegration with Mason horn, *Ultrasonics*, **10**, 212.

10.6.d Other applications in eye surgery

Sokollu, A. (1972). Destructive effect of ultrasound on ocular tissues. *In* "Interaction of Ultrasound and Biological Tissue" (ed. J. M. Reid and M. R. Sikov), pp. 129–34, U.S. Department of Health, Education and Welfare, Publication (FDA) 73-8008.

Youdin, M. (1969). Applications of the therapeutic ultrasonic radiation in retinal detachment surgery, *Proc. 8th int. Congr. med. biol. Engng*, 32–6.

10.6.e Cleaning and decalcifying blood vessels and cardiac valves

Brown, A. H. and Davies, P. G. H. (1972). Ultrasonic decalcification of calcified cardiac valves and annuli, *Br. med. J.*, **3**, 274–7.

Davies, H., Schwartz, R., Pfister, R. and Barnes, F. (1974). Transmitted ultrasound for relief of obstruction in ureters and arteries: current status, *J. clin. Ultrasound*, **2**, 217–20.

Stumpff, U., Pohlman, R. and Trübestein, G. (1975). A new method to cure thrombi by ultrasonic cavitation. *In* "Ultrasonics International 1975", pp. 273–5, I.P.C. Science and Technology Press, Guildford.

Yeas, J. and Barnes, F. S. (1970). An ultrasonic drill for cleaning blood vessels, *Biomed. scis. Instrum.*, **7**, 165–7.

10.6.f Cutting and welding procedures

Goliamina, I. P. (1974). Ultrasonic surgery, *Proc. 8th int. Congr. Acoust.*, 63–9.

Nikolaev, G. A. (1973). Welding and cutting biological tissues with ultrasound, *Russ. Ultrason.*, **3**, 13–20 (translation of *Svarochnoe Proizvodstro*, 1972, 12).

Volkov, M. V. and Shepeleva, I. S. (1974). The use of ultrasonic instrumentation for the transection and uniting of bone tissue in orthopaedic surgery, *Reconstr. Surg. Traumatol.*, **14**, 147–52.

10.6.g Stapes surgery

Anon. (1967). Ultrasound in a new attempt at safe stapedectomy, *World Med.*, **2**, (11), 20.

10.7 Cell disintegration as a manufacturing process

Brown, R. C., Coakley, W. T. and James, C. J. (1974). The biological integrity of proteins exposed to cavitating ultrasound, *Proc. 8th int. Cong. Acoust.*, 364.

Coakley, W. T. and James, C. J. (1971). Activity of enzymes released from yeast by sonication. *In* "Ultrasonics 1971", pp. 33–6, I.P.C. Science and Technology Press, Guildford.

Hughes, D. E. (1961). The disintegration of bacteria and other micro-organisms by the M. S. E.-Mullard ultrasonic disintegrator, *J. biochem. microbiol. Technol. Engng*, **3**, 405–33.

10.8 Preparation of tissue specimens for histological examination

Gagnon, J. and Katyk, N. (1960). Les ultrasons en technique histologique, *Archs d'Anat. Path.*, **8**, 203–8.

Poston, F. (1967). Bone decalcification expedited by ultrasonic sound, *Am. J. med. Technol.*, **33**, 263–8.

Thorpe, E. J., Bellomy, B. B. and Sellers, R. F. (1963). Ultrasonic decalcification of bone. An experimental and clinical study. *J. Bone Jt. Surg.*, **45-A**, 1257–9.

10.9 Aerosol therapy

Boucher, R. M. G. and Kreuter, J. (1968). The fundamentals of the ultrasonic atomization of medicated solutions, *Ann. Allerg.*, **26**, 591–600.

Cheney, F. W. and Butler, J. (1968). The effects of ultrasonically-produced aerosols on airway resistance in man, *Anesthesiology*, **29**, 1099–1106.

Goddard, R. F., Mercer, T. T., O'Neil, P. X. F., Flores, R. L. and Sanchez, R. (1968). Output characteristics and clinical efficacy of ultrasonic nebulizers, *J. Asthma Res.*, **5**, 355–68.

Long, R. J. (1962). Ultrasonic atomization of liquids, *J. acoust. Soc. Am.*, **34**, 6–8.

Miller, W. F., Johnston, F. F. and Tarkoff, M. P. (1968). Use of ultrasonic aerosols with ventilatory assistors, *J. Asthma Res.*, **5**, 335–54.

Ringrose, R. E., McKown, B., Felton, F. G., Barclay, B. O., Muchmore, H. G. and Rhoades, E. R. (1968). A hospital outbreak of *Serratia marcescens* associated with ultrasonic nebulizers, *Ann. intern. Med.*, **69**, 719–29.

10.10 Elimination of oxygen bubbles from the circulation

Macedo, I. C. and Young, W.-J. (1973). Acoustic effects on gas bubbles in the flows of viscous fluids and whole blood, *J. acoust. Soc. Am.*, **53**, 1327–35.

A1 Analogy between mechanical and electromagnetic waves

A2 The decibel notation

A3 Historical review

AUTHOR INDEX

Numbers in italics are those pages on which references are listed.

23

SUBJECT INDEX